Recent Progress in Veterinary Medicine

Recent Progress in Veterinary Medicine

Edited by Mel Roth

SYRAWOOD
PUBLISHING HOUSE

New York

Published by Syrawood Publishing House,
750 Third Avenue, 9th Floor,
New York, NY 10017, USA
www.syrawoodpublishinghouse.com

Recent Progress in Veterinary Medicine
Edited by Mel Roth

© 2017 Syrawood Publishing House

International Standard Book Number: 978-1-68286-440-1 (Hardback)

Cataloging-in-publication Data

Recent progress in veterinary medicine / edited by Mel Roth.
    p. cm.
Includes bibliographical references and index.
ISBN 978-1-68286-440-1
1. Veterinary medicine. 2. Veterinary medicine--Methodology. 3. Animals--Diseases. I. Roth, Mel.
SF745 .R43 2017
636.089--dc23

Printed in the United States of America.

TABLE OF CONTENTS

PREFACE

Veterinary medicine is defined as the branch of medicine that deals with the causes, diagnosis and treatment of diseases and injuries of animals. This book traces the progress of this field from its early stages to its modern research advancements. The topics included in this book on veterinary medicine are of utmost significance and bound to provide incredible insights to readers. From theories to research to practical applications, case studies related to all contemporary topics of relevance to this field have been included in this book. It is a complete source of knowledge on the present status of this important field. Researchers and students associated with veterinary medicine will be assisted by this text.

The world is advancing at a fast pace like never before. Therefore, the need is to keep up with the latest developments. This book was an idea that came to fruition when the specialists in the area realized the need to coordinate together and document essential themes in the subject. That's when I was requested to be the editor. Editing this book has been an honour as it brings together diverse authors researching on different streams of the field. The book collates essential materials contributed by veterans in the area which can be utilized by students and researchers alike.

Each chapter is a sole-standing publication that reflects each author's interpretation. Thus, the book displays a multi-facetted picture of our current understanding of applications and diverse aspects of the field. I would like to thank the contributors of this book and my family for their endless support.

Editor

1

Effectiveness of Action in India to Reduce Exposure of *Gyps* Vultures to the Toxic Veterinary Drug Diclofenac

Richard Cuthbert[1], Mark A. Taggart[2,3], Vibhu Prakash[4], Mohini Saini[5], Devendra Swarup[5], Suchitra Upreti[5], Rafael Mateo[2], Soumya Sunder Chakraborty[4], Parag Deori[4], Rhys E. Green[1,6]*

1 Royal Society for the Protection of Birds, Sandy, United Kingdom, 2 Instituto de Investigación en Recursos Cinegéticos, IREC (CSIC-UCLM-JCCM), Ciudad Real, Spain, 3 Department of Plant and Soil Science, School of Biological Sciences, University of Aberdeen, Aberdeen, United Kingdom, 4 Bombay Natural History Society, Mumbai, India, 5 Centre for Wildlife Conservation, Management and Disease Surveillance, Indian Veterinary Research Institute, Izatnagar, Uttar Pradesh, India, 6 Conservation Science Group, Department of Zoology, University of Cambridge, Cambridge, United Kingdom

Abstract

Contamination of their carrion food supply with the non-steroidal anti-inflammatory drug diclofenac has caused rapid population declines across the Indian subcontinent of three species of *Gyps* vultures endemic to South Asia. The governments of India, Pakistan and Nepal took action in 2006 to prevent the veterinary use of diclofenac on domesticated livestock, the route by which contamination occurs. We analyse data from three surveys of the prevalence and concentration of diclofenac residues in carcasses of domesticated ungulates in India, carried out before and after the implementation of a ban on veterinary use. There was little change in the prevalence and concentration of diclofenac between a survey before the ban and one conducted soon after its implementation, with the percentage of carcasses containing diclofenac in these surveys estimated at 10.8 and 10.7%, respectively. However, both the prevalence and concentration of diclofenac had fallen markedly 7–31 months after the implementation of the ban, with the true prevalence in this third survey estimated at 6.5%. Modelling of the impact of this reduction in diclofenac on the expected rate of decline of the oriental white-backed vulture (*Gyps bengalensis*) in India indicates that the decline rate has decreased to 40% of the rate before the ban, but is still likely to be rapid (about 18% year^{-1}). Hence, further efforts to remove diclofenac from vulture food are still needed if the future recovery or successful reintroduction of vultures is to be feasible.

Editor: Stephen G. Willis, University of Durham, United Kingdom

Funding: This project was funded by the Darwin Initiative of the United Kingdom government http://darwin.defra.gov.uk/ and the Royal Society for the Protection of Birds (RSPB) http://www.rspb.org.uk. RC and REG are authors of the paper and members of the research staff of the Conservation Science Department of RSPB. Beyond this, the funders had no role in study design, data collection and analysis, decision to publish or preparation of the manuscript.

Competing Interests: The authors have declared that no competing interests exist.

* E-mail: reg29@cam.ac.uk

Introduction

Three species of vultures endemic to South Asia, oriental white-backed vulture (*Gyps bengalensis*), long-billed vulture (*G. indicus*) and slender-billed vulture (*G. tenuirostris*), are listed as being threatened with extinction after rapid population declines in the Indian subcontinent, which began in the 1990s [1,2,3]. The oriental white-backed vulture population in India in 2007 was estimated at one-thousandth of its level in the early 1990s [3]. Veterinary use of the non-steroidal anti-inflammatory drug (NSAID) diclofenac is the major cause of these declines [4,5,6,7]. Diclofenac has been used to treat symptoms of disease and injury in domesticated ungulates in many parts of the subcontinent since the 1990s [8]. The effects of diclofenac on captive oriental white-backed vulture, African white-backed vulture (*G. africanus*), Cape griffon vulture (*G. coprotheres*) and Eurasian griffon vulture (*G. fulvus*) have been studied experimentally. In all species, death occurred within a few days and extensive visceral gout and kidney damage were observed post mortem [4,9,10]. Vultures that died in these experiments showed similar pathology to that found in the majority of vulture carcasses collected from the wild since declines began [4,5,6,9,11]. A large-scale survey of the amount of diclofenac in liver tissue from carcasses of domesticated ungulates available to vultures as food in India in 2004–2005 showed that the prevalence and concentration of the drug was sufficient to cause the observed rapid population declines [7,12]. Approximately 10% of carcasses were found to have detectable levels of diclofenac [12].

After research had indicated the adverse effects of diclofenac on vultures, the governments of India, Pakistan and Nepal commenced actions to prevent the contamination of vulture food supplies with the drug [13]. India's National Board for Wildlife recommended a ban on veterinary use on 17 March 2005. In May 2006, a directive from the Drug Controller General of India was circulated to relevant officials, requiring the withdrawal of manufacturing licences for veterinary formulations of diclofenac. This directive was further strengthened in 2008, when it was made an imprisonable offence to manufacture, retail or use diclofenac for veterinary purposes.

In this paper, we analyse data from three surveys of diclofenac concentrations in liver samples from carcasses of domesticated ungulates in India before and after the ban [12,14] in order to estimate the change in the expected rate of mortality caused by diclofenac in oriental white-backed vultures and the expected trend in their population. Our analysis is restricted to oriental white-backed vulture because this is the only species for which the relationship between dose and mortality has been measured [4,9].

However, we expect that our conclusions concerning this species will also be relevant to the conservation of the two other threatened *Gyps* species in South Asia.

Methods

Field sampling

Liver samples were collected from carcasses of domesticated ungulates during three survey periods: T1 = May 2004–July 2005, T2 = April–December 2006, T3 = January 2007–December 2008. Samples were collected from carcasses deposited at carcass dumps managed by local government corporations, co-operatives, private companies and individuals, and cattle welfare charities. Sampling locations were typical of sites formerly used by large numbers of foraging *Gyps* vultures. Samples were also collected from slaughterhouses during T1 (15% of samples), but not during subsequent surveys. Protocols for sample collection and storage have been reported previously [12,14].

GPS co-ordinates of sample collection sites were recorded. Each site in the T2 and T3 surveys was assigned to one of 21 site clusters previously identified during an analysis of the T1 survey data [7]. Site-cluster assignment was based upon the site being nearer to the geodesic centroid of a particular cluster than to that of any other cluster. Sample sites were always within 186 km of the geodesic centroid of their cluster. Samples were gathered opportunistically when and where it was possible to obtain access and permission to collect. For logistical reasons the geographical distribution of sampling effort differed among the three surveys. Site clusters covered in T2 and T3 were a subset of those covered during T1. The number of samples taken in each cluster differed among surveys.

Sample extraction and quantification of diclofenac concentration

Weighed sub-samples of ungulate liver were homogenized in acetonitrile. Diclofenac concentrations in the extracts were determined by liquid chromatography-electrospray ionisation mass spectrometry. The limit of quantification (LOQ) for this technique, back-calculated to the concentration in wet tissue, was 0.01 ppm (0.01 mg kg^{-1}). Detailed protocols for sample extraction and diclofenac quantification have been reported previously [12,14].

Statistical analysis

The objectives of our analyses were to estimate (1) changes in the level of exposure of vultures to diclofenac over time, (2) consequent changes in the average proportion of oriental white-backed vultures expected to be killed by diclofenac per meal of carrion consumed, and (3) the expected annual rate of decline of a model population of oriental white-backed vultures that would have been stable in the absence of diclofenac. The analysis followed Steps 1–8 of the procedure described in a previous analysis of the T1 survey data [7], except that Step 2 of the procedure was omitted. This was because the previous analysis showed that variation in the measured diclofenac concentration among sub-samples taken from the liver of the same ungulate had a negligible effect on the outcome of the analysis. This source of variation could therefore be ignored. The procedure fits a statistical model to the frequency distribution of the concentrations of diclofenac measured in samples of liver taken from carcasses of domesticated ungulates. It then estimates from the data for liver the distribution of diclofenac concentrations averaged over all edible tissues of the ungulate carcasses and, from that, the distribution of doses of diclofenac per unit vulture body mass

ingested by vultures feeding on a mixture of tissues. The expected average proportion of vultures killed per meal is then obtained and this result is used in a simulation model of the vulture population to estimate its expected rate of decline.

Step 1 of the procedure required a more elaborate treatment than that used in the previous analysis because the present study compares data from three surveys rather than reporting just one. This step determines the cumulative distribution function (cdf) $V(d_{liver})$ of the concentrations d_{liver} of diclofenac in ungulate livers. For the purpose of the present analysis, it is necessary to determine $V(d_{liver})$ for each survey period (T1, T2 and T3), whilst avoiding, as far as possible, the potential bias introduced by differences among surveys in the geographical distribution of sampling sites. In previous analysis of the T1 data [7], $V(d_{liver})$ was assumed to be $1 + f(U(d_{liver}) - 1)$, where f is the true prevalence of diclofenac, i.e., the proportion of livers that contained residues of the drug, and $U(d_{liver})$ is the cdf of diclofenac concentrations in samples that contained the drug. A proportion of the livers sampled $(1 - f)$ have no trace of the drug. In previous analysis [7], a third order complementary log-log distribution was used for $U(d_{liver})$ because this distribution gave a good fit to the data. However, this distribution requires the estimation of four parameters, in addition to f. To reduce the number of fitted parameters required to describe the diclofenac distributions for the three survey periods, we instead assumed that $U(d_{liver})$ was a Weibull distribution, which is determined by just two parameters; a scale parameter a and a shape parameter b. Using this formulation, $U(d_{liver}) = 1 - \exp(-a\ d_{liver}{}^b)$ and $V(d_{liver}) = 1 - f\exp(-a\ d_{liver}{}^b)$. To check whether simplifying the model in this way resulted in an appreciably poorer fit, we compared the Weibull and third order complementary log-log distributions when fitted to the data for samples with detectable diclofenac levels from each of the three surveys. We fitted truncated distributions using a maximum-likelihood method [15], left-censored at the LOQ. We assessed the fit of each distribution using a Kolmogorov-Smirnov one sample test [16]. As expected, because of its larger number of fitted parameters, the third order complementary log-log (CL-L3) distribution gave a better fit than the Weibull for all three surveys. Kolmogorov-Smirnov's D values for CL-L3 vs Weibull for T1, T2 and T3 were 0.042 vs 0.049, 0.030 vs 0.035, 0.043 vs 0.048 respectively, but these differences are small and the fit of all models was good. The significance of the Kolmogorov-Smirnov test was $P>0.40$ in all cases. Hence, we concluded that the Weibull gave an adequate fit, thus allowing a reduction in the number of fitted parameters required and a simplification of subsequent analysis.

If the number and thus the proportion of samples taken within each site cluster had remained the same for all three surveys, it would have been acceptable to estimate f, a and b separately for each survey and then make a direct comparison of these estimates. However, given that some of the site clusters sampled in T1 were not sampled in T2 or T3 or both, and that different numbers of samples were taken within clusters that were sampled in more than one survey, we considered it necessary to model the prevalence and concentration of diclofenac as varying with site cluster (S) and time period (T) (see Table 1 and Figure 1 for the distribution of samples in surveys T1 to T3). Site cluster and survey period were treated as factors in the Weibull models. This allowed us to simulate the prevalence and concentration of diclofenac that would be expected if the geographical distribution of sampling had actually been the same in all three surveys. Since models with site-cluster effects were only used to estimate changes over time, we reduced the number of fitted parameters required by combining data for the seven site clusters that were only sampled in the T1

Table 1. Numbers of ungulate liver samples collected in each of 21 site clusters in three survey periods: T1 = May 2004–July 2005, T2 = April–December 2006, T3 = January 2007–December 2008.

	Number of liver samples		
Cluster	T1	T2	T3
1	28	164	85
2	163	200	0
3	38	58	74
4	159	152	151
5	26	41	262
6	150	187	152
7	90	169	0
8	63	171	0
9	83	110	0
10	92	106	236
11	59	0	0
12	134	0	127
13	150	0	0
14	161	0	143
15	42	0	0
16	25	20	21
17	64	0	0
18	52	0	0
19	54	0	0
20	121	0	0
21	94	110	0
Total samples	1848	1488	1251
Samples with diclofenac	186	165	70
Percentage with diclofenac	10.1	11.1	5.6
Mean concentration (ppm)	0.994	0.874	0.569

	Percentage of samples		
Species	T1	T2	T3
Camel	0.1	0.0	0.2
Cattle	48.3	63.8	60.1
Water buffalo	46.6	29.7	34.9
Sheep	2.6	2.6	2.4
Goat	0.2	3.6	2.2
Horse	2.3	0.3	0.2
Unidentified	0.0	0.1	0.0

Also shown are the total numbers of samples taken, the number and proportion of them in which diclofenac was detected, the arithmetic mean concentration of diclofenac (ppm wet weight) in the samples in which the compound was detected and the species composition of the ungulates from which liver tissue was sampled.

survey and treating these as if they came from just one cluster in all analyses. We used different approaches to represent site-cluster and survey-period variation in the parameters for the prevalence and concentration components of the model. For true prevalence f, which is a proportion, we assumed that the odds of a sample

containing diclofenac were the product of two constants; a site-cluster effect g and a survey-period effect h. Hence, for the ith site cluster and the jth survey period, $f_{ij}/(1 - f_{ij})$, the logit transformation of f_{ij} was assumed to be given by the product $g_i h_j$. The scale and shape parameters a and b of the Weibull model were assumed to be products of site-cluster (m and q) and survey-period (n and r) effects so that $a_{ij} = m_i n_j$ and $b_{ij} = q_i r_j$. The g, m and q factors had a number of levels equal to the number of site clusters, except that the site clusters only sampled in T1 were pooled (as explained above). The h, n and r factors each had three levels, one for each survey period, but the parameter values for the first period, h_1, n_1 and r_1 were fixed at 1, so there were two parameters to be estimated for each factor. We call these the S+T formulations of the model for true prevalence, scale parameter and shape parameter.

Our eventual goal was to fit a single statistical model to the data from all three surveys with appropriate S+T formulations for the parameters that determined prevalence and concentration. However, we first conducted preliminary analyses separately for (1) the prevalence and (2) the concentration components of the model to compare the effects on model fit of the S+T formulations of the different model parameters and other plausible model formulations. In the analyses of prevalence, this was done by fitting logistic regression models to the data on apparent prevalence. Apparent prevalence was the proportion of samples with diclofenac concentrations above the LOQ, not including the undetected contaminated samples with levels of diclofenac below the LOQ. A logistic regression model with the presence/absence of detectable diclofenac as the binary dependent variable and the additive main effects of site cluster and survey period included as factors is equivalent to the S+T formulation of the model of true prevalence described above. In separate analyses of diclofenac concentrations, we fitted a truncated Weibull distribution of concentrations, left-censored at the LOQ, using a maximum-likelihood method [15]. This analysis only used data for samples with detectable diclofenac. For both the logistic regression analyses of apparent prevalence and the truncated Weibull models of concentration, plausible alternative models of apparent prevalence and concentration with various formulations were fitted and compared by calculating their Akaike Information Criterion (AIC) values.

After completing the preliminary analyses of apparent prevalence and concentration, a combined Weibull model including both components, with the selected S+T formulation, was fitted to the full dataset using a maximum-likelihood method [15]. Confidence limits for the parameters of the model were obtained by taking 10,000 bootstrap samples of the data, with bootstrapping being performed by site cluster. The model was then fitted to each bootstrap sample and the central 9,500 estimates of each parameter were taken to be the 95% confidence limits.

We estimated the impact of the observed level of diclofenac contamination on the proportion of oriental white-backed vultures killed by diclofenac per meal using Steps 3 – 7 of the procedure developed previously [7]. Estimates of the parameters required for the calculations were taken from this earlier analysis. The procedure requires the following assumptions. (a) Vultures eat a meals of ungulate tissue of uniform size at intervals F of either two or three days, such that that their energetic requirements are met. (b) The concentration of diclofenac in each meal is that found in all edible tissues of the ungulate combined, which is proportional to the diclofenac concentration in the animal's liver, as determined previously [7]. (c) The distribution of diclofenac concentrations in meals is given by the product of the ratio of concentration in the

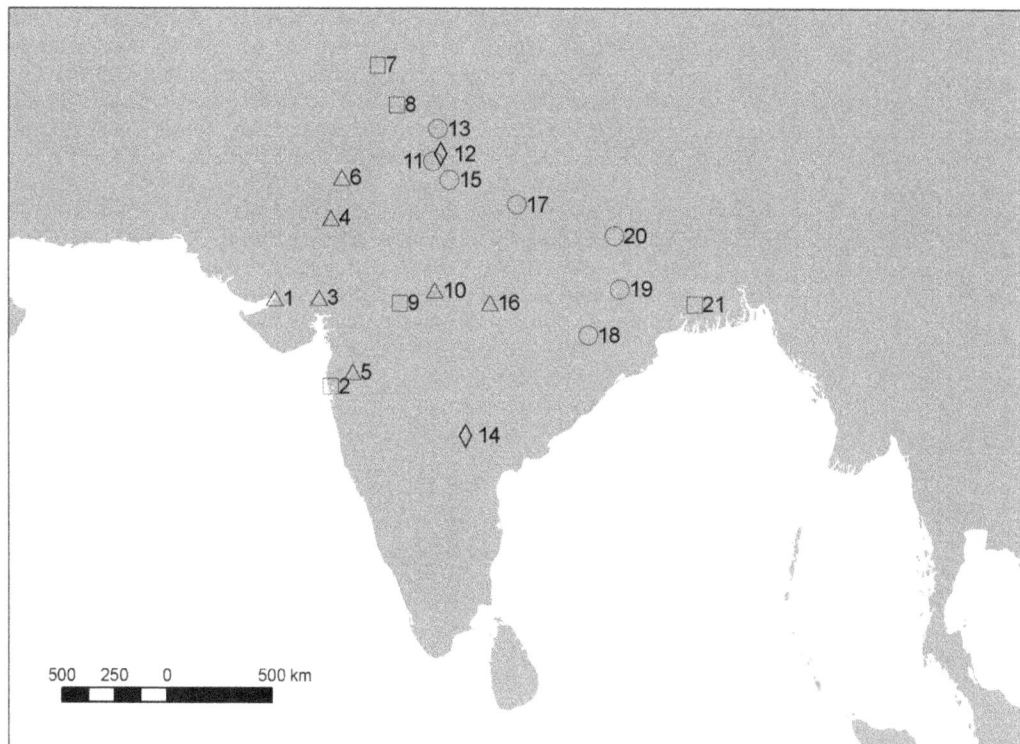

Figure 1. Locations of sampling site clusters in India. The map shows centroids of 21 site clusters at which liver samples were obtained from carcasses of domesticated ungulates. Numbers next to the symbols identify site clusters listed in Table 1. Triangles show clusters sampled in all three surveys (T1, T2, T3), squares show clusters sampled in T1 and T2, diamonds, T1 and T3, and circles T1 only.

whole carcase to that in the liver and the distribution of liver concentrations fitted to the results of the survey of ungulate carcasses described above. (d) The proportion of vultures killed by a given dose of diclofenac is specified by a relationship fitted to data from a dosing experiment conducted previously on captive oriental white-backed vultures [4,9]. We used a version of this dose-response curve that was fitted after excluding an outlier (Vulture 11) [4,9], since inclusion of this datum leads to unrealistically high estimates of the rate of population decline [7]. The average proportion of vultures killed per meal, averaged across all meals taken by the vulture population, was then obtained from the probability density function of the dose of diclofenac per unit vulture body weight per meal and the dose-response relationship between diclofenac dose and the proportion of vultures killed. Integration under the curve given by the product of these two functions gives the average proportion of vultures killed per meal [7].

The final step in the procedure (Step 8) [7] used the death rate per meal, as calculated above, in a simple model of the vulture population [5] to estimate the population's expected rate of decline. The model assumes that the population would have demographic rates such that it is stable in the absence of diclofenac, and that the annual adult survival rate S_0 is either 0.90 or 0.97. These survival values were considered to span the plausible range in a previous modelling study [5]. The interval between meals F is assumed to be either 2 or 3 days. Other details of the model have been described previously [5]. Confidence limits for death rate per meal and population decline rate were obtained using sets of 10,000 bootstrap and Monte Carlo parameter estimates as described previously [7].

Results

Differences among surveys in diclofenac prevalence and concentration

Liver samples were taken from a large number of sites distributed across the northern half of India (Table 1, Figure 1), and came predominantly from carcasses of cattle (*Bos indicus, B. taurus* and hybrids) and water buffalo (*Bubalus bubalis*). The proportion of samples with detectable diclofenac (apparent prevalence), the cumulative distribution of diclofenac concentrations and the arithmetic mean concentration in those samples with detectable levels were broadly similar between the two surveys conducted before and just after the implementation of the ban on diclofenac use for veterinary purposes (T2 cf. T1, Table 1). However, apparent prevalence and mean concentration were both substantially lower in the third survey than in the previous two (T3 cf. T2 and T1, Table 1, Figure 2).

The geographical distribution of samples differed among the three surveys (Table 1, Figure 1). Only seven of the 21 site clusters were sampled in all three surveys. Five site clusters were sampled in T1 and T2, but not in T3, two site clusters were sampled in T1 and T3, but not in T2, and seven site clusters were only sampled in T1 (Table 1). A higher proportion of the site clusters located in western India were sampled in more than one survey than was the case for clusters in the east (Figure 1).

Differences in the distribution of sampling sites among surveys might lead to spurious differences in prevalence or the distribution of concentrations of diclofenac if (a) these varied consistently with location, and (b) site clusters covered in surveys T2 and T3 differed in prevalence or concentration distribution

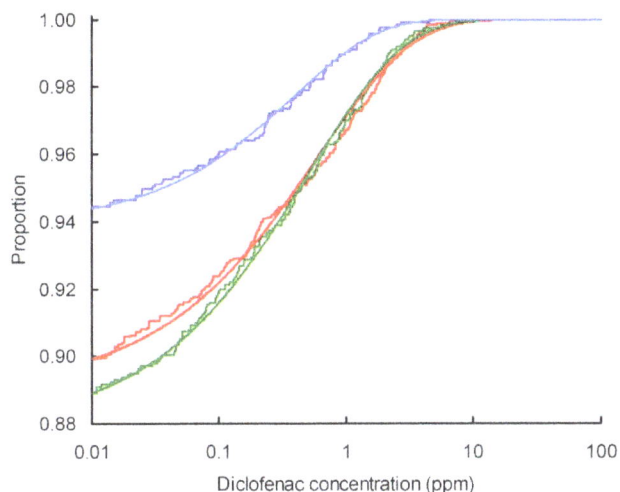

Figure 2. Comparison of the distributions of diclofenac concentrations before and after the ban on the veterinary use of diclofenac. Cumulative distributions of diclofenac concentration (ppm wet weight) in ungulate liver samples from three surveys: red = T1, pre-ban, green = T2, soon after the ban, blue = T3, 7–31 months after the ban are shown by the stepped lines. The curves show cumulative Weibull distributions fitted separately to the data for each survey. Fitted values of prevalence f, the scale a and shape b parameters respectively were T1, 0.110, 1.336 and 0.592; T2, 0.122, 1.458 and 0.597; T3, 0.061, 1.844 and 0.673.

from the site clusters not covered in the later surveys, or covered to a lesser extent. A previous analysis of data from T1 has already revealed significant geographical variation in apparent prevalence [12]. Comparison of apparent prevalence between pairs of survey periods indicated that significant positive correlations also existed across site clusters. Clusters with higher than average apparent prevalence in one survey also tended to have high prevalence in other surveys (Spearman correlation coefficients [16]: T1 vs T2, $r_S = 0.504$, one-tailed $P = 0.05$; T1 vs T3, $r_S = 0.483$, one-tailed $P = 0.10$; T2 vs T3, $r_S = 0.714$, one-tailed $P = 0.05$). Hence, apparent prevalence not only varied geographically, but the pattern of variation among site clusters tended to be consistent through time. However, the equivalent correlation analyses for mean diclofenac concentration in those samples with detectable levels gave no indication that mean concentrations varied consistently among site clusters in different time periods (Spearman correlation coefficients: T1 vs T2, $r_S = -0.067$; T1 vs T3, $r_S = 0.321$, one-tailed $P = 0.25$; T2 vs T3, $r_S = 0.143$, one-tailed $P > 0.25$).

Although differences among surveys in the geographical distribution of sampling sites were present and might cause spurious differences in estimates of diclofenac prevalence and concentration distribution, simple non-parametric analyses indicated that differences between surveys remained even after site-cluster differences had been allowed for. A Wilcoxon signed ranks test [16] on differences between pairs of apparent prevalence values for the same cluster during different time periods indicated that apparent prevalence was significantly lower in T3 than in T1 ($T^+ = 39$, $N = 9$, one-tailed $P = 0.021$). However, there was no significant difference for comparisons among the other survey pairs (T2 vs T1, $T^+ = 43$, $N = 12$, one-tailed $P = 0.396$; T3 vs T2, $T^+ = 19$, $N = 7$, one-tailed $P = 0.234$). The equivalent analyses for mean diclofenac concentrations in those samples with detectable levels indicated that concentrations were also lower in T3 than in

T1 ($T^+ = 27$, $N = 7$, one-tailed $P = 0.016$), and had a marginally significant tendency to be lower in T3 than T2 ($T^+ = 18$, $N = 6$, one-tailed $P = 0.078$). There was no significant difference between mean concentrations in T2 and T1 ($T^+ = 35$, $N = 10$, one-tailed $P = 0.246$).

These analyses suggest that both the apparent prevalence of diclofenac and its concentration were lower in T3 than in the previous two surveys. However, they also indicate that there was a consistent geographical variation in prevalence, so quantification of the changes requires more elaborate modelling to adjust for differences among surveys in the geographical distribution of sampling.

Site-cluster and time-period effects on apparent prevalence and diclofenac concentration

Adjustments for possible biases caused by differences among surveys in the geographical distribution of sampling required models of the prevalence and concentration of diclofenac that had independent main effects of site cluster (S) and time period (T). We call these S+T models and described the way we used them in the Methods section. We performed two preliminary analyses, separately for data for apparent prevalence and concentration, to see how the fit of the S+T models compared with that of other plausible model formulations.

Comparisons of AIC values among logistic regression models of apparent prevalence in relation to site cluster and time period indicated that those models with the effects of S and T included on their own fitted the data substantially better than did the null model (Table 2; Models B and C cf. Model A). The effect upon AIC of site cluster was considerably larger than that of time period. However, a model in which the odds of a sample having detectable diclofenac were given by the product of a site-cluster effect and a survey-period effect (S+T) had a considerably lower AIC than either of the single factor models (Table 2; Model D cf. Models B and C). A full model, with proportions specific to each site-time combination (S.T), gave an even lower AIC value, but the AIC difference between this and the S+T model was modest, indicating that the S+T model (Model D) provides an adequate description of the data on apparent prevalence.

Comparisons of AIC values were made among truncated Weibull distribution models of the distributions of diclofenac concentrations in those samples with detectable levels (Table 3). In this case, it was possible to formulate the model so that the scale parameter a and the shape parameter b were separately or both affected by S and T. A model in which the scale parameter varied with time period but not site cluster, and in which the shape parameter did not vary with S or T, gave the lowest AIC value of all models considered (Table 3; Model 2). However, there was only a small difference in AIC between this model and one with an S+T formulation of the scale parameter and a constant shape parameter (Table 3; Model 10). Other models which had the shape parameter as well as the scale parameter dependent on S and/or T did not give a substantial reduction in AIC compared with Model 10. Given that an S+T formulation is necessary to allow adjustment for possible bias caused by differences among surveys in the geographical distribution of sampling, we concluded that the S+T model (Model 10) of concentration fits sufficiently well to be used for this purpose. Hence, we decided that the combined model of prevalence and concentration should have the same formulation as that in Model D of apparent prevalence and that in Model 10 of diclofenac concentration.

Table 2. Comparisons between the residual deviance and Akaike Information Criterion (AIC) of various logistic regression models of the variation among site clusters (S) and survey time periods (T) in the apparent prevalence of diclofenac (the proportion of liver samples with detectable levels of the drug).

Model	Model specification	Residual deviance	Number of parameters	AIC	ΔAIC
A	C	184.39	1	186.39	114.39
B	T	154.45	3	160.45	88.45
C	S	53.84	15	83.84	11.84
D	S+T	40.81	17	74.81	2.81
E	S.T	0.00	36	72.00	0.00

A null model in which the proportion was assumed to be constant (C) across site clusters and time periods was compared with models in which the odds of a sample having detectable diclofenac varied either among site clusters or time periods or was given by the product of a site-cluster effect and a time-period effect (denoted S+T). A full model with proportions specific to each site-time combination is denoted S.T.

Combined Weibull model of diclofenac prevalence and concentration

We fitted a combined model in which both the true prevalence of diclofenac f and the scale parameter a of the Weibull distribution of diclofenac concentrations had an S+T formulation, whilst the shape parameter b of the Weibull distribution was assumed not to vary with S or T. We then used a maximum-likelihood method [15] to estimate the values of the true prevalence f_1 and the scale parameter a_1 across all clusters using the data for the first survey period (T1) alone. This was done by estimating the values of f_1 and a_1 whilst ignoring the effects of site cluster, and with the shape parameter b fixed at the value obtained from the combined model of the data from all three surveys with an S+T formulation for both prevalence and the scale parameter.

The values of the time-period effects on prevalence and on the scale parameter were then taken from the combined analysis (the h and n effects: see Methods) and used to calculate f_2 and f_3 and a_2 and a_3 values for surveys T2 and T3 respectively. The time-period effects h on the prevalence parameter were multiplied by $f_1/(1 - f_1)$ and then back-transformed to give f_2 and f_3. The time-period effects n on the scale parameter were multiplied by a_1 to give a_2 and a_3. This procedure simulated the results expected if the geographical distribution of samples in T2 and T3 had been the same as that in T1. These time-period specific estimates of f and a, together with the estimate of the shape parameter b (assumed to be common to all three time periods) are shown in Table 4. The arithmetic mean diclofenac concentration, calculated across all samples that contained residues of the drug, including those with

Table 3. Comparisons between the residual deviance and Akaike Information Criterion (AIC) of various Weibull models of the variation among site clusters (S) and survey time periods (T) in the concentration of diclofenac in liver samples with detectable levels.

Model	Model specification a	Model specification b	Residual deviance	Number of parameters	AIC	ΔAIC
1	C	C	6391.58	2	6395.58	1.42
2	T	C	6386.16	4	6394.16	0.00
3	C	T	6390.24	4	6398.24	4.08
4	T	T	6385.46	6	6397.46	3.30
5	S	C	6366.60	16	6398.60	4.44
6	C	S	6375.62	16	6407.62	13.45
7	S	S	6336.39	30	6396.39	2.23
8	S	T	6365.56	18	6401.56	7.40
9	T	S	6370.11	18	6406.11	11.95
10	S+T	C	6359.26	18	6395.26	1.10
11	C	S+T	6375.01	18	6411.01	16.84
12	S+T	T	6358.27	20	6398.27	4.10
13	T	S+T	6369.89	20	6409.89	15.73
14	S+T	S+T	6331.04	34	6399.04	4.88
15	S.T	T	6347.35	36	6419.35	25.18
16	S.T	S.T	6283.50	66	6415.50	21.34

A null model in which the scale and shape parameters a and b of the Weibull distribution of concentrations of diclofenac were assumed to be constant (C) across sites and time periods is compared with models in which the scale parameter a and/or the shape parameter b varied with site cluster or time period or were given by the product of S and T effects (denoted by S+T). The full model with parameters specific to each site cluster and time combination is denoted by S.T.

Table 4. Estimates of the parameters of a model which describes the true prevalence *f* of diclofenac in liver samples taken during three surveys of ungulate carcasses (T1, T2, T3) and the scale *a* and shape *b* parameters of the Weibull distribution of diclofenac concentrations (ppm wet weight).

Parameter	T1				T2				T3			
	Estimate	95% C.L.			Estimate	95% C.L.			Estimate	95% C.L.		
f	0.108	0.086	-	0.130	0.107	0.085	-	0.129	0.065	0.021	-	0.101
a	1.305	0.700	-	1.951	1.444	0.763	-	2.115	2.071	1.020	-	3.150
b	0.630	0.578	-	0.697	0.630	0.578	-	0.697	0.630	0.578	-	0.697
Mean concentration	0.927	0.229	-	1.565	0.789	0.214	-	1.363	0.446	0.082	-	0.800

The value *b* is assumed to be common to all three surveys. Also shown is the arithmetic mean concentration of diclofenac (ppm wet weight) for those samples which contained the compound, calculated from *a* and *b*. Parameter estimates and their bootstrap 95% confidence limits are shown for each of three surveys.

concentrations less than the LOQ, was obtained using the *a* and *b* values for each survey period. The adjusted estimates from the combined model showed that the true prevalence of diclofenac was similar in T1 and T2, but that true prevalence in T3 was lower than in T1 and in T2 (Table 4). The ratio of values in T3 to those from the earlier surveys indicated a reduction in the true prevalence of diclofenac in T3 to about 60% of its value in T1 and T2 (Table 5).

A similar pattern was seen for the mean concentration of diclofenac in those samples in which the drug was estimated to be present, which was also lower in T3 than in T1 or T2 (Table 4). Calculation of the ratio of values in T3 to those from the earlier surveys indicated a reduction in mean concentration in T3 to 48% and 57% of the values in T1 and T2 respectively (Table 5). Probability density functions (pdfs) calculated from the combined model illustrate this pattern, with the density being lower across all diclofenac concentrations for T3 than for T1 and T2, showing lower prevalence in T3, and the peak of the probability density function occurred at a lower concentration in T3 than in T1 and T2 (Figure 3).

Proportion of vultures expected to be killed per meal

We estimated the impact of the observed levels of diclofenac contamination on the proportion of oriental white-backed vultures that would be killed per meal using Steps 3 – 7 of the procedure developed earlier for the analysis of the T1 data [7]. The calculation is illustrated in Figure 4, which shows the curve that is obtained by multiplying together the probability density function of the dose of diclofenac per unit vulture body weight per meal and the dose-response relationship between the proportion of vultures killed and the dose of diclofenac ingested. The example shown is for the interval between meals $F = 3$. The integral under this curve gives the proportion of birds killed per meal. For both of the feeding intervals, $F = 2$ and $F = 3$, the death rate per meal was slightly lower in T2 than in T1, but, markedly lower in T3 than in both T2 and T1 (Table 6). The death rate per meal in T3 was 21 – 24% of that in T1 and 26 – 30% of that in T2 (Table 5).

Expected rate of decline of the oriental white-backed vulture population in India

The decline rate of the Indian oriental white-backed vulture population, expected from the exposure to diclofenac indicated by survey T1, was 78 – 79% per year with $F = 2$, and 80 – 81% per year with $F = 3$. For both feeding intervals the rate of expected population decline was slightly lower in T2 than in T1, but markedly lower in T3 than in T2 and T1 (Table 6). The decline rate in T3 was 35–41% of that in T1 and 39 - 45% of that in T2 (Table 5). Hence, there was little change in the expected rate of population decline in period T2, immediately after the implementation of the ban on veterinary manufacture of diclofenac in 2006,

Table 5. Estimates of changes between three surveys of ungulate carcasses (T1, T2, T3) in the true prevalence *f* of diclofenac, the arithmetic mean concentration of diclofenac in livers of animals in which it was present (ppm wet weight), the estimated mean percentage of vultures killed by a meal of mixed tissues, and the annual percentage rate of decline of the vulture population.

Parameter	*F*	S_0	T2:T1				T3:T1				T3:T2			
			Ratio	95% C.L.			Ratio	95% C.L.			Ratio	95% C.L.		
f	-	-	0.987	0.971	-	1.007	0.598	0.253	-	0.859	0.605	0.252	-	0.874
Mean conc.	-	-	0.851	0.699	-	1.003	0.480	0.360	-	0.601	0.565	0.430	-	0.699
Death rate	2	-	0.803	0.608	-	1.054	0.211	0.050	-	0.407	0.262	0.065	-	0.483
Death rate	3	-	0.828	0.655	-	1.044	0.244	0.073	-	0.443	0.295	0.094	-	0.513
Decline rate	2	0.90	0.906	0.655	-	1.019	0.357	0.057	-	0.884	0.394	0.074	-	0.886
Decline rate	2	0.97	0.903	0.654	-	1.020	0.351	0.057	-	0.879	0.388	0.073	-	0.881
Decline rate	3	0.90	0.924	0.721	-	1.017	0.413	0.089	-	0.869	0.447	0.114	-	0.872
Decline rate	3	0.97	0.921	0.719	-	1.017	0.406	0.087	-	0.863	0.440	0.113	-	0.866

The interval between meals *F* was assumed to be two or three days and annual adult survival in the absence of diclofenac S_0 was assumed to be either 0.90 or 0.97. Ratios of parameter estimates and their bootstrap 95% confidence limits are shown for each pairwise comparison of surveys.

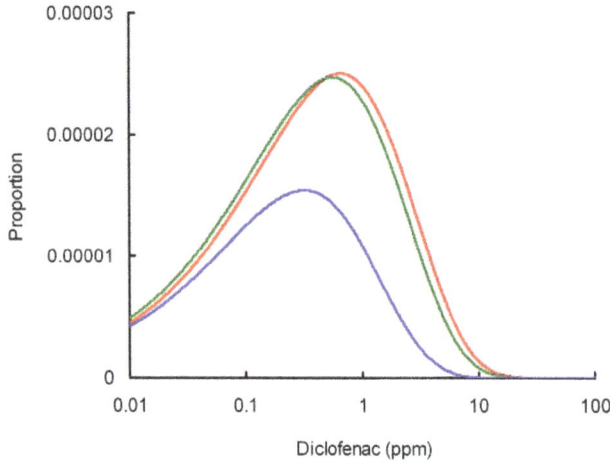

Figure 3. Comparison of probability density functions of diclofenac concentrations in ungulate liver before and after the ban on the veterinary use of diclofenac. Fitted probability density functions are shown of diclofenac concentration (ppm wet weight) in ungulate liver samples from three surveys: red = T1, pre-ban, dark green = T2, soon after the ban, dark blue = T3, 7–31 months after the ban. The curves are derived from a Weibull model in which both the true prevalence of diclofenac f (including those with concentrations < LOQ) and the scale parameter a of the Weibull distribution of concentrations of diclofenac in those samples are determined by a site-cluster effect and a survey period effect. The shape parameter b of the Weibull distribution is assumed not to vary with site-cluster or survey period. Values of f and a in all three surveys were adjusted so that the results simulate those expected if the 21 site-clusters covered by the T1 (pre-ban) survey had been covered at the same sampling intensity in the second T2 and third T3 surveys.

but by 2007 – 2008 (T3) the expected rate of decline had slowed appreciably (Figure 5).

Discussion

Our study shows that both the prevalence and concentration of diclofenac in carcasses of domesticated ungulates available as food for vultures in India has fallen markedly since a ban on the veterinary use of diclofenac was implemented. Between the period prior to the ban and the period 7–31 months after the first implementation by the Government of India of measures to prevent the use of diclofenac for veterinary purposes (period T3) decreased by about about half. The estimates of true prevalence, adjusted for samples with low-level contamination below the limit of quantification and for site-cluster effects, were 6.5% in T3, compared with 10.8% and 10.7% in surveys T1 and T2 respectively. Hence, our conclusion about the change in prevalence between surveys holds with or without the statistical adjustments. Similarly, the unadjusted estimates of mean concentration in Table 1 and the adjusted values for mean concentration in Table 4 both show the same pattern of little difference between T1 and T2 but a substantial decline by period T3. We consider that these declines in prevalence and concentration are likely to be representative of the situation in north-western India because of the wide distribution of sampling sites and scale of sampling undertaken (>4,500 carcass samples analysed in T1 – T3). The magnitude of the decline in diclofenac prevalence was probably slightly underestimated because some T1 samples, but no T2 or T3 samples, were taken from slaughterhouses, where diclofenac prevalence was lower than at carcass dumps [12]. However, because only seven of the samples taken at slaughterhouses in the T1 survey were from a site cluster which was sampled in later surveys, this effect is extremely small.

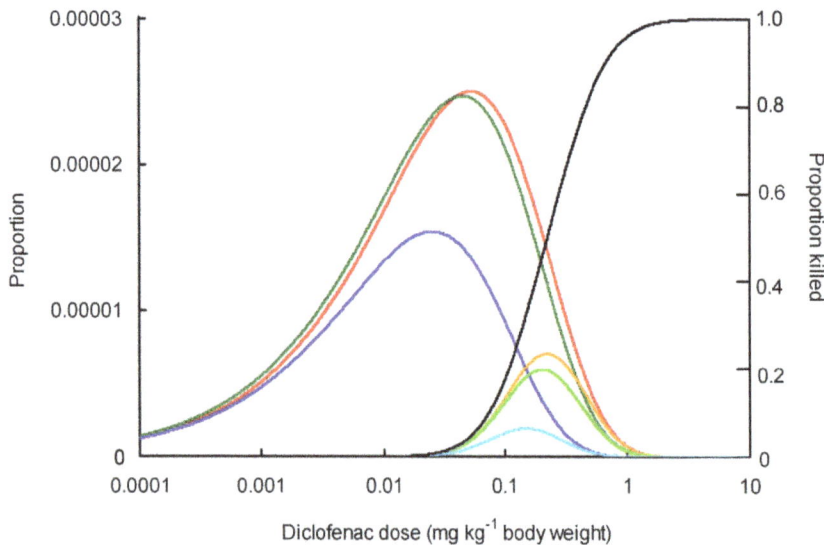

Figure 4. Comparison of probability density functions of diclofenac dose per unit vulture body weight from ungulate tissue before and after the ban on the veterinary use of diclofenac. Probability density functions are shown of estimated diclofenac dose (mg kg^{-1} wet weight) per meal for birds eating a mixture of all edible ungulate tissues and feeding at intervals of three days. Results are shown for three surveys: red = T1, pre-ban, dark green = T2, soon after the ban, dark blue = T3, 7–31 months after the ban. The proportion of vultures expected to be killed by a given dose of diclofenac is shown by the dose-response curve (black, with right-hand y axis). The products of the dose probability density functions and the dose-response curve are shown by the orange, light green and light blue curves for surveys T1, T2 and T3 respectively. The areas under these curves give the estimated proportion of vultures killed per meal.

Table 6. Estimates of the mean percentage of vultures killed by a meal of mixed tissues assuming that the interval between meals F was two or three days, and the annual percentage rate of decline of the vulture population, assuming the two values of F and annual adult survival in the absence of diclofenac S_0 of either 0.90 or 0.97.

Parameter	F	S_0	T1 Estimate	T1 95% C.L.			T2 Estimate	T2 95% C.L.			T3 Estimate	T3 95% C.L.		
Death rate	2	-	0.821	0.076	-	3.451	0.660	0.049	-	3.072	0.173	0.004	-	1.231
Death rate	3	-	1.303	0.202	-	4.367	1.080	0.146	-	3.946	0.318	0.016	-	1.649
Decline rate	2	0.90	79.2	14.5	-	99.9	71.8	9.8	-	99.7	28.3	0.9	-	88.4
Decline rate	2	0.97	78.3	14.0	-	99.9	70.7	9.5	-	99.7	27.5	0.9	-	87.9
Decline rate	3	0.90	81.1	23.3	-	99.7	74.9	17.9	-	99.4	33.5	2.1	-	86.2
Decline rate	3	0.97	80.2	22.5	-	99.6	73.8	17.3	-	99.4	32.5	2.0	-	85.7

Parameter estimates and their bootstrap 95% confidence limits are shown for each of three surveys of ungulate carcasses (T1, T2, T3).

Our estimates of the expected vulture death rate per meal and the expected decline rate of the oriental white-backed vulture population based upon the T1 carcass survey carried out before the ban on diclofenac use was introduced were very similar to those made previously using the same data but with a different method for modelling the distribution of concentrations [7]. This indicates that the changes made in the present analysis to the methods, principally the replacement of the complementary log-log distribution by the Weibull distribution, had a negligible effect on the results.

Based on the data on prevalence and concentration of diclofenac residues presented here and the results of modelling the impact of these residues on the vulture population, the expected rate of decline of the Indian oriental white-backed vulture population has been cut by more than half compared with what it was before the ban. We showed previously that the expected rate of vulture population decline estimated by our method from surveys of diclofenac in ungulate carcasses was higher, though not significantly so, than that observed using repeated counts of vultures during the same period [7]. There are

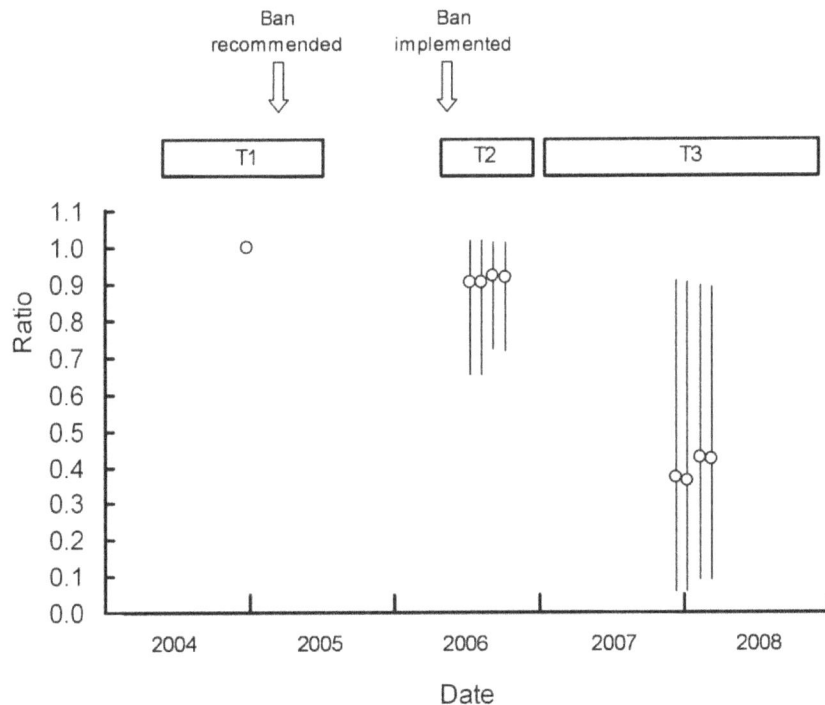

Figure 5. Changes in the expected rate of decline of the oriental white-backed vulture population in India. Circles show the estimated rate of population decline, as a ratio relative to that determined from the T1 survey results in 2004 – 2005. Values are plotted at the mean sampling time for each of the surveys. Horizontal rectangles show the duration of the period covered by the sample collection for each survey. Vertical lines show 95% confidence limits for the ratios. Each of the four adjacent points in a set represents the result for a combination of assumptions (from left to right: $F = 2$, $S_0 = 0.90$; $F = 2$, $S_0 = 0.97$; $F = 3$, $S_0 = 0.90$; $F = 3$, $S_0 = 0.97$). Arrows show the timing of the recommendation by the National Board for Wildlife for a ban on the veterinary use of diclofenac and the withdrawal by the Drug Controller General of manufacturing licences for veterinary formulations of the drug.

several possible reasons for this difference, if it is real. For example, the restriction of the remaining vultures to areas with lower than average diclofenac prevalence and potential selection for vultures with a higher resistance to the toxic effects of diclofenac [7]. However, despite the possibility of a discrepancy in its absolute level, it seems probable that our conclusion about the decrease in the expected rate of population decline is reliable, because the same assumptions and modelling procedure were used for all three survey periods.

Although the observed reduction in the level of diclofenac contamination of the vulture food supply in India is an encouraging sign of a potential future solution to this urgent conservation problem, it is clear from the continued presence of diclofenac in many carcasses that the problem has not yet been overcome. The most recent estimate of the rate of decline in the oriental white-backed vulture population in India from repeated road transect counts is an annual decline of 44% year^{-1} between 2000 and 2007 [3]. Our ungulate carcase survey results from survey period T3 suggest a recent reduction of the expected rate of decline to less than half of the rate before the ban on diclofenac use. Hence, by scaling down the rate of decline from road transect surveys in 2000–2007 by the ratio of expected decline rates before and after the ban reported in this paper, we estimate an annual decline rate in 2007–2008 at 18% year^{-1}. This remains a rapid rate of population decline compared with rates for most other threatened bird populations [17] and one that is unlikely to be fully counteracted by compensatory *in situ* conservation measures such as nest protection and supplementary feeding. Only a very low proportion (< 1%) of ungulate carcasses is required to contain a lethal levels of diclofenac in order to account for the rapid pre-ban population declines of *Gyps* vultures [5], so it may be necessary to remove nearly all diclofenac from the vulture food supply if populations are to recover or be re-introduced successfully from captive-bred stock. There is also a possibility that an Allee effect may occur, caused by reduced social facilitation of foraging at low vulture population densities [18]. This also suggests that almost complete elimination of diclofenac from vulture food may be needed.

Our results indicate that a substantial decrease has occurred in the level of diclofenac contamination in India, but the continued presence of levels of diclofenac lethal to vultures in ungulate carcasses remains a source of major concern. It is now illegal to import, manufacture, retail or use diclofenac for veterinary purposes in India and the continued presence of residues of the

drug in ungulate carcasses in 2007–2008 must therefore be caused by illegal veterinary use. Surveys of pharmacy shops in India confirm that, while diclofenac packaged and labelled for veterinary use was rarely offered for sale for use on livestock after the 2006 ban, human formulations of drug were being sold widely for veterinary use in place of veterinary formulations. A similar situation probably exists in Nepal and Pakistan. Pharmacies in India often dispense both human and veterinary medicines, in which case their holding stocks of human diclofenac is not an offence. Dispensing human formulations of diclofenac for use on livestock, together with informal and illegal dispensing of human diclofenac for veterinary purposes by unregistered people, probably accounts for the continued contamination of ungulate carcasses we have observed. Restrictions on the size of vials of injectable human diclofenac to make it less easy to use human formulations on livestock may help to eliminate these illegal practices. A similar situation may also exist in the Punjab province of Pakistan, where diclofenac-caused mortality of oriental white-backed vultures continued after government action to prevent its veterinary use [19]. If the recovery of wild vulture populations is to be achieved, additional efforts are needed to complete the removal of diclofenac from their food supply and to prevent its replacement by other lethal NSAIDs such as ketoprofen [14,20]. Further effort is also needed to promote the use of the alternative veterinary NSAIDs known not to pose a risk to vultures. At present, the only veterinary NSAID used in India that is known to have low toxicity to vultures is meloxicam [21,22].

Acknowledgments

We thank the Director and Joint Director (Research) at the Indian Veterinary Research Institute for providing the necessary facilities for carrying out the work. For assistance in the field and laboratory we thank Anant Kot, Kamal Kumar Kashyap, Kalu Ram Senacha and Suchitra Upreti. We are grateful to the Wildlife Institute of India and the University of Aberdeen for their roles in the first two surveys. We thank Asad Rahmani for advice and support and Ian Newton and Juliet Vickery for comments on a draft.

Author Contributions

Conceived and designed the experiments: RC MAT VP MS DS RM REG. Performed the experiments: RC MAT MS SSC RM PD SU. Analyzed the data: RC MAT REG SU. Contributed reagents/materials/ analysis tools: MAT MS. Wrote the paper: RC MAT MS REG.

References

1. IUCN (2010) IUCN Red List of Threatened Species. Version 2010.3. www.iucnredlist.org via the Internet. Downloaded on 20 September 2010.
2. Gilbert M, Watson RT, Virani MZ, Oaks JL, Ahmed S, et al. (2006) Rapid population declines and mortality clusters in three Oriental white-backed vulture Gyps bengalensis colonies in Pakistan due to diclofenac poisoning. Oryx 40: 388–399.
3. Prakash V, Green RE, Pain DJ, Ranade SP, Saravanan S, et al. (2007) Recent changes in populations of resident Gyps vultures in India. Journal of the Bombay Natural History Society 104: 129–135.
4. Oaks JL, Gilbert M, Virani MZ, Watson RT, Meteyer CU, et al. (2004) Diclofenac residues as the cause of vulture population declines in Pakistan. Nature 427: 630–633.
5. Green RE, Newton I, Shultz S, Cunningham AA, Gilbert M, et al. (2004) Diclofenac poisoning as a cause of vulture population declines across the Indian subcontinent. Journal of Applied Ecology 41: 793–800.
6. Shultz S, Baral HS, Charman S, Cunningham AA, Das D, et al. (2004) Diclofenac poisoning is widespread in declining vulture populations across the Indian subcontinent. Proc Royal Soc Lond B (Suppl) 271: S458–S460.
7. Green RE, Taggart MA, Senacha KR, Raghavan B, Pain DJ, et al. (2007) Rate of Decline of the Oriental White-Backed Vulture Population in India Estimated from a Survey of Diclofenac Residues in Carcasses of Ungulates. PloS ONE 2: e686.
8. Risebrough RW (2006) Diclofenac: A New Environmental Poison In South Asia. Journal of the Bombay Natural History Society 103: 239–250.
9. Swan GE, Cuthbert R, Quevedo M, Green RE, Pain DJ, et al. (2006) Toxicity of diclofenac to Gyps vultures. Biology Letters 2: 279–282.
10. Naidoo V, Wolter K, Cuthbert R, Duncan N (2009) Veterinary diclofenac threatens Africa's endangered vulture species. Regulatory Toxicology and Pharmacology 53: 205–208.
11. Meteyer CU, Rideout BA, Gilbert M, Shivaprasad HL, Oaks JL (2005) Pathology and pathophysiology of diclofenac poisoning in free-living and esperimentally exposed oriental white-backed vultures (Gyps bengalensis). J Wildl Dis 414: 707–716.
12. Taggart MA, Senacha KR, Green RE, Jhala YV, Raghavan B, et al. (2007) Diclofenac residues in carcasses of domestic ungulates available to vultures in India. Environment International 33: 759–765.
13. Pain DJ, Bowden CGR, Cunningham AA, Cuthbert R, Das D, et al. (2008) The race to prevent the extinction of South Asian vultures. Bird Conservation International 18: S30–S48.
14. Taggart MA, Senacha KR, Green RE, Cuthbert R, Jhala YV, et al. (2009) Analysis of Nine NSAIDs in Ungulate Tissues Available to Critically Endangered Vultures in India. Environmental Science & Technology 43: 4561–4566.
15. Kalbfleisch JG (1985) Probability and Statistical Inference. Vol. II. New York: Springer-Verlag.
16. Seigel S, Castellan NJ (1988) Nonparametric Statistics for the Behavioral Sciences. New York: McGraw-Hill.

17. Green RE, Hirons GJM (1991) The relevance of population studies to the conservation of threatened birds. In: Perrins CM, Lebreton J-D, Hirons GJM, eds. Bird population studies: their relevance to conservation and management. Oxford: Oxford University Press. pp 594–636.
18. Jackson AL, Ruxton GD, Houston DC (2008) The effect of social facilitation on foraging success in vultures: a modelling study. Biology Letters 4: 311–313.
19. Arshad M, Chaudhary NJI, Wink M (2009) High mortality and sex ratio imbalance in a critically declining Oriental White-backed Vulture population (*Gyps bengalensis*) in Pakistan. J Ornithol 150: 495–503.
20. Naidoo V, Wolter K, Cromarty D, Diekmann M, Duncan N, et al. (2010) Toxicity of non-steroidal anti-inflammatory drugs to *Gyps* vultures: a new threat from ketoprofen. Biology Letters 6: 339–341.
21. Swan G, Naidoo V, Cuthbert R, Green RE, Pain DJ, et al. (2006) Removing the Threat of Diclofenac to Critically Endangered Asian Vultures. PLoS Biology 4: 396–402.
22. Swarup D, Patra RC Prakash V, Cuthbert R, Das D, et al. (2007) Safety of meloxicam to critically endangered Gyps vultures and other scavenging birds. Animal Conservation 10: 192–198.

2

A Molecular Diagnostic Tool to Replace Larval Culture in Conventional Faecal Egg Count Reduction Testing in Sheep

Florian Roeber[1]*, John W. A. Larsen[2], Norman Anderson[2], Angus J. D. Campbell[1,2], Garry A. Anderson[1], Robin B. Gasser[1]*, Aaron R. Jex[1]

1 Faculty of Veterinary Science, The University of Melbourne, Parkville, Victoria, Australia, **2** Mackinnon Project, The University of Melbourne, Werribee, Victoria, Australia

Abstract

The accurate diagnosis of parasitic nematode infections in livestock (including sheep and goats) is central to their effective control and the detection of the anthelmintic resistance. Traditionally, the faecal egg count reduction test (FECRT), combined with the technique of larval culture (LC), has been used widely to assess drug-susceptibility/resistance in strongylid nematodes. However, this approach suffers from a lack of specificity, sensitivity and reliability, and is time-consuming and costly to conduct. Here, we critically assessed a specific PCR assay to support FECRT, in a well-controlled experiment on sheep with naturally acquired strongylid infections known to be resistant to benzimidazoles. We showed that the PCR results were in close agreement with those of total worm count (TWC), but not of LC. Importantly, albendazole resistance detected by PCR-coupled FECRT was unequivocally linked to *Teladorsagia circumcincta* and, to lesser extent, *Trichostrongylus colubriformis*, a result that was not achievable by LC. The key findings from this study demonstrate that our PCR-coupled FECRT approach has major merit for supporting anthelmintic resistance in nematode populations. The findings also show clearly that our PCR assay can be used as an alternative to LC, and is more time-efficient and less laborious, which has important practical implications for the effective management and control strongylid nematodes of sheep.

Editor: David Joseph Diemert, The George Washington University Medical Center, United States of America

Funding: This research was supported by the Australian Research Council (RBG). The funders had no role in study design, data collection and analysis, decision to publish, or preparation of the manuscript.

Competing Interests: The authors have declared that no competing interests exist.

* E-mail: robinbg@unimelb.edu.au (RBG); f.roeber@pgrad.unimelb.edu.au (FR)

Introduction

Strongylid nematodes of ruminants are responsible for sub-stantial economic losses due to the diseases that they cause and the costs associated with their treatment and control [1]. These parasites impose a major financial burden on livestock industries globally. Small ruminants, such as sheep, can become infected with multiple strongylid nematodes, including species of *Teladorsagia*, *Trichostrongylus*, *Haemonchus*, *Nematodirus*, *Cooperia*, *Chabertia* and/or *Oesophagostomum* [2], which differ in their geographical distribution, pathogenicity and susceptibility to various anthelmintics [3].

The accurate diagnosis of nematode infections is central to their effective control, supports investigations into their epidemiology and ecology, and, importantly, can assist substantially in the monitoring of anthelmintic resistance in strongylid populations. Such resistance has emerged as a major economic and bionomic problem [4], predominantly as the result of an excessive and uncontrolled use of broad-spectrum anthelmintics (representing three main classes: benzimidazoles, imidazothiazoles and macro-cyclic lactones). Although there has been a recent breakthrough in the development of a new drug, monepantel, representing an alternative compound class (amino-acetonitrile derivatives, AADs) [5], success in the discovery of new anthelmintics has been scarce over the last two decades [6]. Therefore, although there is hope for

new, effective anthelmintics, there is also a major need to preserve compounds that we currently have at our disposal. Hence, monitoring the drug-susceptibility and -resistance status of strongylid nematode populations in livestock needs to be a high priority, and should underpin integrated management strategies.

Various *in vitro* methods, such as egg hatch- and larval development assays, have been used for estimating levels of drug-susceptibility/resistance in strongylid nematodes of small ruminants, cattle and horses. However, these assays can suffer from a lack of reliability, reproducibility and sensitivity [7]. The method most widely used to assess the efficacy of different anthelminthics in live sheep is the faecal egg count reduction test (FECRT) [8]. The diagnostic component of this test involves the enumeration of strongylid eggs in faecal samples before and after treatment of the animals with an anthelmintic compound. From the results, the percentage of reduction in the number of strongylid eggs per gram (EPG) following treatment provides an estimate of the susceptibility/resistance of nematode populations to a particular compound, and a population of worms is considered resistant if the reduction is <95% [9]. However, strongylid populations usually comprise multiple species, and it is, thus, not possible to assess the effect of a drug on different species in the populations, because eggs in faeces cannot be delineated to genus or species based on morphology (with the exception of *Nematodirus*). Therefore, the technique of larval culture (LC) is required to allow eggs to develop through to third-stage larvae (L3s), which can then be differentiated morphologically. However, LC has intrinsic limitations, which relate predominantly to the different requirements for hatching and larval development of individual nematode species [10], methodological differences among diagnostic laboratories, and the inability to unequivocally identify and differentiate particular genera and/or species [11].

There have been significant advances in establishing molecular methods for the genus- or species-specific diagnosis of strongylid infections in livestock [12]. Recently, we evaluated the performance of a PCR method for the diagnosis of naturally acquired strongylid nematode infections in sheep [13]. We established the diagnostic sensitivity (98%) and specificity (100%) of this assay by comparison with a conventional faecal flotation method, and also applied a system to rank the contribution of particular strongylid nematodes to EPGs in individual sheep with mixed-species infections. The ability to rapidly identify and rank nematodes according to their numerical contribution to observed faecal egg count results represents a major advantage over routine coprological methods, and shows clear potential to replace the conventional technique of LC. Therefore, we proposed that this PCR tool [13] can be used as a practical adjunct to conventional FECRT to enable the rapid inference of which species or genera of strongylid nematodes are susceptible or resistant to particular anthelmintic drugs. Here, we assess this tool for this purpose in a controlled experiment on sheep with naturally acquired infections of strongylids known to be resistant to benzimidazoles. We directly compared the results from the PCR evaluation with those obtained from routine LC and worm counts.

Materials and Methods

Experimental Design

The present study was conducted on a farm in Rokewood with owners permission [37°53′S/143°43′E], Victoria, Australia, with a known resistance problem in strongylid nematodes against one or more benzimidazoles; Relevant permission was granted from the owner of this farm to undertake this observational field study, which involved routine anthelmintic treatment of sheep and collection of faecal samples from sheep on this farm in Rokewood. This study was approved by the Animal Ethics Committee (AEC no. 0810850.1) of the University of Melbourne. Merino sheep (n = 80; 15 months of age; 36–59 kg; with ear tag identification) were available for FECRT and were shown previously to have average faecal egg counts of ≥150 EPG. Sheep were divided randomly into four groups (of 20 each), designated AB (albendazole-treated), ABC (albendazole-untreated control), MP (monepantel-treated) and MPC (monepantel-untreated control), respectively. For one sheep in group AB, no faecal sample was obtained after repeated sampling attempts, such that 19 samples could be collected. Groups AB and ABC were kept on the same pasture as were MP and MPC. Albendazole (Valbazen®, Coopers Animal Health) and monepantel (Zolvix®, Novartis) were administered orally by a qualified veterinarian using a syringe at a dose of 4.75 mg/kg (albendazole) and 2.5 mg/kg (monepantel), according to the bodyweight of the heaviest sheep in groups AB and MP, respectively. The experiment was conducted over a period of 13 days. Faecal samples were collected from sheep on days 0 and 10. Groups AB and MP were treated on day 0. A total number of 30 sheep (see subsection 2.3) were necropsied on day 13.

Procurement of Faecal Samples and Conventional Coprological Testing

Fresh faecal samples (6.5–20 g) were collected directly from the rectum of individual sheep into plastic bags, chilled for transport and then stored at 4°C for a maximum of 1 week [14]. The numbers of small- to medium-sized (i.e. <100 μm in length and <50 μm in width), thin-walled 'strongylid eggs' per gram (EPG) of faeces were counted using a standard flotation method [15] with a theoretical detection limit of 10 EPG.

For each of the four experimental groups, an equal amount of faeces (2.5 g) from each individual sample was used to set up a 50 g composite LC in a plastic beaker. The cultures were incubated at 25°C for 10 days. L3s were then recovered by filling each beaker with water (25°C) and inverting it on to a Petridish [16]. The sheath extension lengths [17] of 100 L3s from each of the four cultures were measured to differentiate among *Teladorsagia/Trichostrongylus*, *Haemonchus* and *Chabertia/Oesophagostomum* L3s. Total lengths of L3s were measured to differentiate *Teladorsagia* from *Trichostrongylus*, according to the criteria of three different authors [18–20]. To further refine the delineation *Te. circumcincta* and *Trichostrongylus*, 50 L3s from each culture were exsheathed in aqueous hypochlorite (5%), and their caudal morphology examined for the presence/absence and number of tubercles [20].

Total Worm Counts (TWC)

Three days following the second collection of faecal samples (on day 13), nine, nine, nine and three sheep were selected randomly from groups AB, ABC, MP and MPC, respectively, and then necropsied (approval granted through AEC no. 0810850.1). The entire gastrointestinal tract was removed from each of these sheep. Ligations were positioned anterior and posterior to the abomasum. TWC was performed as described by Anderson [21]. In brief, the entire contents of the abomasum and the proximal six meters of the small intestine were collected separately and each diluted in one litre of water. An aliquot (250 ml) thereof was fixed in formaldehyde (final concentration: 5%). The large intestine was opened longitudinally, distal to the spiral colon, and the worms recovered were fixed in 70% ethanol. Individual adult worms were identified morphologically to species according to Gibbons [22].

PCR Testing

Genomic DNA from strongylid eggs, isolated from individual faecal samples, were column-purified and diluted (1/50) as described previously [23]. PCR-based testing was carried out as reported recently [13], employing primer pairs HAE-NC2, TEL-NC2, TRI-NC2, CHO-NC2 and OEV-NC2, in separate reactions, for the specific amplification from the second internal transcribed spacer (ITS-2) of nuclear ribosomal DNA from *Haemonchus contortus*, *Teladorsagia circumcincta*, *Trichostrongylus* spp., *Chabertia ovina* and *Oesophagostomum venulosum*, respectively. In addition, primer pair NC1–NC2 [24] was used, as a control, to assess inhibition in, and amplification efficiency for individual genomic DNA samples. Individual samples were identified as test-positive on the basis of the detection of an amplicon and also of a single, specific melt-peak that was consistent with that of an homologous control (for each PCR run). The specificity of the PCR, the cycling conditions and the products were verified by selective sequencing of amplicons using an established approach [25] and the subsequent comparison of individual sequence tags against known reference sequences for *Te. circumcincta*, *T. axei*, *T. colubriformis*, *T. vitrinus* and *C. ovina* (GenBank accession nos. AY439025.1, AY439026.1, AB503252.1, AY439027.1 and AY439021.1, respectively).

Any suspected inhibition in the PCR assay, potentially linked to faecal constituents (e.g., humic acids, phenolic compounds and/or polysaccharides), was assessed for all samples for which there was a discrepancy in results between faecal egg count and PCR. In brief, aliquots (2 μl) from samples that were test-negative by PCR, but were shown to contain strongylid eggs by coproscopic examination, were spiked with a limited amount (1 pg) of genomic DNA from *H. contortus* and then subjected to PCR. The amplification results from these aliquots were compared directly (in the same experiment) with that from 1 pg of *H. contortus* DNA alone and a sample without DNA (no-template control).

Statistical Analysis

Samples were tested in conventional methods and PCR in a blinded manner. The reduction in EPG was calculated using the program RESO FECRT v4.0 (http://www.vetsci.usyd.edu.au/sheepwormcontrol/index.html). A population of stronglid nematodes was defined as resistant to an anthelmintic if the reduction in EPG was <95% and the lower confidence limit of the percentage of reduction was <90% [9]. The proportion of sheep that remained test-positive from day 0 to day 10 by PCR was compared between groups using Fisher's exact test in the program Stata v.12.0 (StataCorp, USA). The performance (i.e., sensitivity, specificity and Kappa value) of individual PCR assays was calculated using an established approach [26]. The sensitivity and specificity as well as Kappa statistics of PCR were assessed in relation to results of TWC for 30 sheep, employing the program WinEpiscope 2.0 (http://www.clive.ed.ac.uk./winepiscope/); 95% confidence intervals (CI) for sensitivity and specificity values were calculated using the exact binomial method in Stata. The sensitivity of the specific PCRs for the detection of patent strongylid nematode infections was calculated by comparing the presence of adult female worms of individual species and the corresponding PCR results (because the PCR is based on the specific amplification of genomic DNA from thin-shelled strongylid eggs; [23]). The performance of the PCR assay using primer pair TRI-NC2 was calculated for all infected sheep as well as for those with a minimum TWC of ≥100 adult female *Trichostrongylus*.

Results

Results from FECRT Coupled to Conventional Coproscopic Testing and PCR

The coprological testing of 158 individual faecal samples collected from 79 sheep showed that 136 (86%) of these samples contained strongylid eggs. The arithmetic mean EPG in group AB decreased from 142 (day 0) to 41 (day 10), whereas there was no decrease in their corresponding (untreated) control group. The mean number of EPG in the group MP decreased from 177 (day 0) to 5 (day 10), whereas the numbers increased slightly in group-MPC (see Table 1) during the 10-day period. Based on this reduction in EPG numbers in groups AB and MP, calculated efficacies (with reference to their untreated control) were 64% (95% CI, 31–82%) and 97% (95% CI, 93–99%), respectively. For ten of the 136 samples with an EPG of 10–250, no PCR amplification was detected for any species. With the exception of one sample, these ten samples were from sheep that had received anthelmintic treatment (i.e., three, six and one sample from groups AB, MP and MPC, respectively) and all had an EPG of <50. Microscopic examination of the strongylid eggs in these samples indicated that they were damaged/degraded, with the exception of the sample from group MPC. Molecular screening by PCR showed that 135 (85%) faecal samples were test-positive for one or more of the target nematode species (which included *Te.*

circumcincta, Trichostrongylus and *C. ovina*). Of these samples, there were nine, for which no strongylid eggs were detected by faecal flotation. The molecular analysis of 79 individual faecal samples collected on day 0 revealed that the largest percentage of test-positive faecal samples related to *Te. circumcincta* (84%), *Trichostrongylus* (92%) and, to a lesser extent, *C. ovina* (56%), which was a consistent pattern for all four groups on day 0 (Table 1). No sample was test-positive by PCR for *H. contortus* or *O. venulosum*.

Using the PCR assay, 19 sheep in group AB were test-positive on day 0 and 15 sheep were test-positive on day 10. In contrast, all 20 sheep in group ABC were test-positive by PCR on days 0 and 10 (*P* = 0.047). On day 10, all of the 15 test-positive samples in group AB related to *Te. circumcincta*, and three to *Trichostrongylus*, whereas *C. ovina* was not detected (see Table 1). In group MP, of the 20 samples that were test-positive by PCR on day 0, three were test-positive for *Te. circumcincta* only on day 10. In contrast, all 19 samples from group MPC were test-positive by PCR on day 0 and also on day 10 (*P*<0.001). The melting-curve analysis of all 301 amplicons produced in this study (irrespective of experimental group) as well as selective sequencing and comparison of resultant sequence tags (*n* = 26) with reference sequences demonstrated unequivocally the specificity of both the amplicons and the PCR conditions employed.

Comparison of Results Achieved by Routine Larval Culture (LC) and Total Worm Counts (TWC) with those from Molecular Testing

On day 10, a pooled faecal sample representing all animals in each experimental group was tested by LC (Table 2). L3s of *Te. circumcincta* and *Trichostongylus* were identified in cultures representing three of the four experimental groups, and no larvae were detected for group MP. L3s of *Chabertia/Oesophagostomum* were identified in cultures representing both control groups (ABC and MPC) but not in the others. Morphometric comparisons of these L3s, according to Gordon [19] and McMurtry [20], consistently inferred *Te. circumcincta* as the most abundant parasite for each group, followed by *Trichostrongylus* spp., whereas *Chabertia/Oesophagostomum* were least abundant. This relationship was most pronounced in group AB, wherein >90% of the L3s were identified as *Te. circumcincta*. Measurements of total body length of L3s with a sheath extension of 30–40 μm inferred *Te. circumcincta* and *Trichostrongylus* spp. in groups ABC and MPC, and mainly *Te. circumcincta* in group AB (Fig. 1). These findings were similar to the results achieved by PCR testing of individual faecal samples from each of the four groups of sheep, although LC appeared to under-estimate the contribution of *Chabertia/Oesophagostomum* relative to the PCR, which can be explained by the 'sensitivity' of the molecular method. Notably, morphometric boundaries, as defined by Dikmans and Andrews [18], yielded results that were markedly different from those achieved using the criteria of Gordon [19] and McMurtry [20], with L3s of *Trichostrongylus* predicted as being most abundant in all cultures.

To provide an independent comparison of LC and PCR, we conducted a routine TWC on 30 sheep (representing animals randomly-selected from each of the four groups). Because test-positive results in LC and PCR are dependent on the presence of eggs in faeces, TWCs related to the numbers of adult female worms in individual sheep, although worms of both sexes were counted (see Table 3). TWC data revealed the presence of females of *Te. circumcincta, Trichostrongylus* spp. (*T. axei, T. vitrinus, T. colubriformis*) and *C. ovina* in 21 (70%), 16 (53%) and eight (27%) of the sheep examined, respectively (Table 3). Moreover, in group AB, all sheep harboured *Te. circumcincta* (60–7340 females), whereas just three, low intensity infections of *Trichostrongylus* (50–

Table 1. Results of coprodiagnostic testing.

	Groups[a]	Day 0					Day 10				
		ABC	AB	MPC	MP	Total (%)	ABC	AB	MPC	MP	Total (%)
Number of animals		20	19	20	20	79 (100)	20	19	20	20	79 (100)
Faecal egg count	positive	20	15	19	19	73 (92)	20	17	19	7	63 (80)
	Mean	117.5	142.1	182.5	177	–	115.5	41.1	199	5	–
	standard deviation	181.6	239.2	228.7	137.6	–	125.7	35.9	317.4	8.3	–
	Range	10–770	0–1070	0–760	0–530	–	20–530	0–120	0–1310	0–30	–
PCR positive		20	19	19	20	78 (99)	20	15	19	3	57 (72)
	H. contortus	0	0	0	0	0 (0)	0	0	0	0	0 (0)
	T. circumcincta	15	17	16	18	66 (84)	17	15	15	3	50 (63)
	Trichostrongylus	18	17	18	20	73 (92)	17	3	19	0	39 (49)
	C. ovina	10	8	12	15	45 (56)	13	0	15	0	28 (35)
	O. venulosum	0	0	0	0	0 (0)	0	0	0	0	0 (0)

Results from the testing of 158 individual faecal samples by conventional faecal egg count and species-specific PCRs using the primer pairs HC-NC2 (*Haemonchus contortus*), TEL-NC2 (*Teladorsagia circumcincta*), TRI-NC2 (*Trichostrongylus* spp.), CHO-NC2 (*Chabertia ovina*) and OEV-NC2 (*Oesophagostomum venulosum*). Shown are the number of egg count positive samples, mean eggs per gram, standard deviation, and range of strongylid egg counts recorded for the individual groups of sheep. Also shown are the number of species positive samples as determined by PCR for the different groups of sheep on days 0 and 10 of the experiment.
[a]Groups of sheep assigned as ABC (albendazole-untreated control), AB (albendazole-treated), MPC (monepantel-untreated control), MP (monepantel treated).

160 females) were found, and no *Chabertia* or *Oesophagostomum*. These results are consistent with those achieved by PCR and LC using the morphometric criteria defined by Gordon [19] and McMurtry [20].

Indeed, usually there was a close agreement between the routine TWC and PCR results achieved for each individual sheep examined using both methods. PCR analysis detected infections with *Te. circumcincta*, *Trichostrongylus* and *C. ovina* in 22 (73%), 12 (40%) and eight (27%) of the sheep examined, respectively (Table 3). Although *Te. circumcincta* was detected by PCR in three

of 20 faecal samples from group MP on day 10, no adult worms of this species were detected by TWC in two of these three sheep (i.e., nos. 1415 and 1443) for which TWC reference data were recorded. Similarly, although *Trichostrongylus* DNA was detected by PCR in a sample from sheep no. 1442 from group AB, no worms were detected by TWC in the same sheep. Nonetheless, adult females of *Te. circumcincta* and *Trichostrongylus* (i.e. *T. axei* and *T. vitrinus*) were detected by TWC in sheep no. 1330 from group ABC, but DNAs from these parasites were not detected in the faeces from this sheep by PCR on day 10. *Trichostrongylus* DNA was

Table 2. Larval culture results.

		Reference (length in µm)				
		Dikmans and Andrews	Gordon	McMurtry		
Group[a]	Genus	(797–866)	(720–880)	(700–914)	xL3[c]	PCR (Ct)
ABC	*Teladorsagia*	20	56	65	54	17/20 (22.97)
	Trichostrongylus	78	42	33	40	17/20 (23.06)
	Chabertia/Oesophagostomum	2	2	2	6	13/20 (25.30)
AB	*Teladorsagia*	18	91	98	92	15/19 (24.61)
	Trichostrongylus	82	9	2	8	3/19 (25.53)
	Chabertia/Oesophagostomum	0	0	0	0	0/19 (N/A[b])
MPC	*Teladorsagia*	16	48	54	52	15/20 (23.36)
	Trichostrongylus	76	44	38	40	19/20 (21.39)
	Chabertia/Oesophagostomum	8	8	8	8	15/20 (22.54)
MP	*Teladorsagia*	0	0	0	0	3/20 (26.18)
	Trichostrongylus	0	0	0	0	0/20 (N/A)
	Chabertia/Oesophagostomum	0	0	0	0	0/20 (N/A)

Larval culture results, following anthelmintic treatment (day 10), showing the percentage of different species (%), as determined by exsheathment and total body length measurement according to different authors [18–20]. Also shown are the numbers of species detected by PCR and mean cycle threshold value (Ct).
[a]Groups of sheep assigned as ABC (albendazole-untreated control), AB (albendazole treated), MPC (monepantel-untreated control), MP (monepantel treated).
[b]No data available.
[c]Exsheathed third-stage larvae.

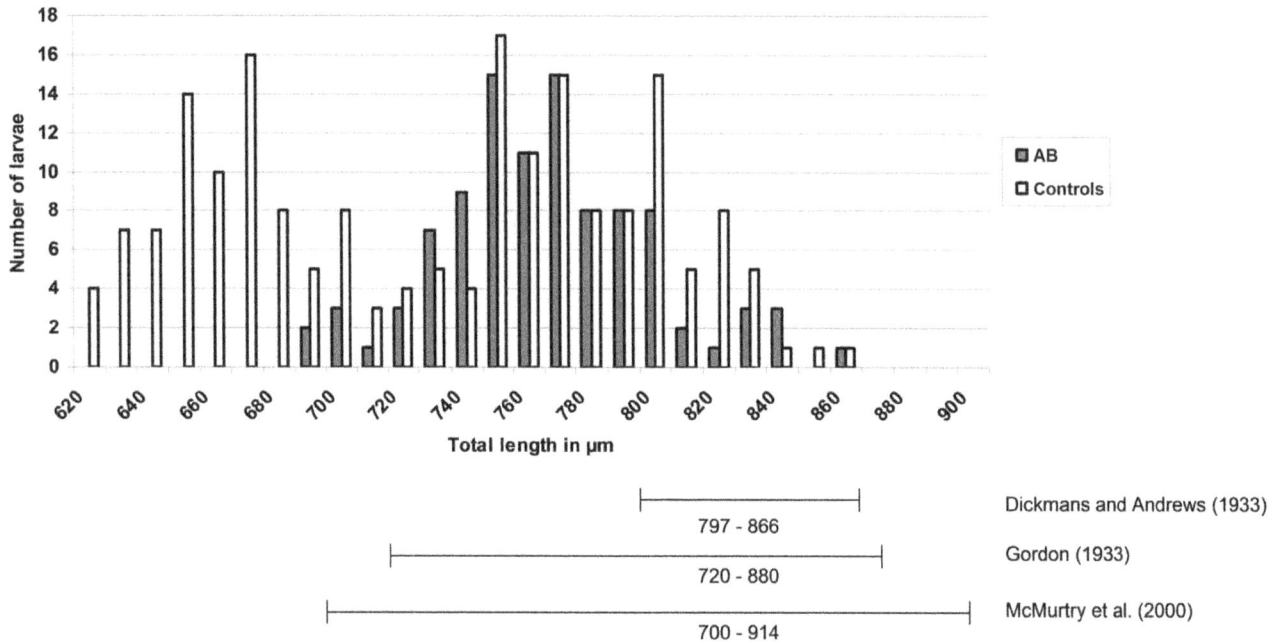

Figure 1. Histogram for the distribution of larval body-length. Distribution of the total lengths of third-stage larvae (L3) with a sheath extension of 30–40 μm, and the identification of *Teladorsagia circumcincta* L3s with respect to their total length (μm), as given by different authors [18–20].

detected by PCR in the faeces from 12 sheep with 160 to 11,850 female worms per sheep, but not in four sheep (nos. 1443, 1427, 1315 and 1443) in which <100 adult female worms per sheep were found. In spite of some differences in results between PCR and TWC, the diagnostic performance of the PCR was high. Using TWC as a reference method, PCR achieved an overall sensitivity (= the ability to detect a patent infection involving female worms of any of the species or genera being tested for) of 100%, a specificity of 87.5% and a Kappa value of 0.91 (Table 4). Kappa calculated for each PCR for each species or genus of parasite showed substantial to perfect agreement [26] with TWC results. During this study, the assay sensitivity could not be calculated for the species of *O. venulosum* and *H. contortus*, as these parasites were not detected in any of the sheep using any of the diagnostic methods employed.

Discussion

The diagnostic performance of the molecular assay assessed herein was high (sensitivity 100% and specificity 87.5%) in relation to TWC. Only for a small number of sheep there was a disagreement in the results between the two tests. Of the 136 faecal samples that contained strongylid eggs, only ten samples were test-negative by PCR (with no evidence of inhibition). Notably, for all PCR test-negative samples, EPG was <250, and all but one were collected from sheep following anthelmintic treatment. Microscopic examination revealed an abnormality in eggs and their shells from these samples, suggesting that the eggs were not viable and that DNA degradation led to these 'false-negative' PCR results. However, egg loss during flotation may also have contributed, suggesting that the direct isolation of DNA from faecal matter should be explored. Four sheep with ~100 adult female worms of *Trichostrongylus* (*T. axei* and *T. vitrinus*) were PCR-test negative for this genus. Three of these four sheep were in groups AB and MP, suggesting that anthelmintic treatment led to a reduction in fecundity or affected the ability of the female worms

to produce intact eggs, although this was not apparent upon morphological examination of these worms following TWC. Alternatively, the eggs themselves, and their DNA, may have undergone degradation in the gastrointestinal tract during or following treatment. Furthermore, the detection of low intensity infections by faecal flotation can be challenging due to the dilution and uneven distribution of eggs in the faeces of the host as well as daily variations in egg excretion [27], limiting the sensitivity of the faecal flotation approach (i.e., from a single 4 g sample collected at one time point). These latter statements are also supported by the technical limitation of FECRT, which only provides information on the effect of treatment on the reproduction of female worms rather than providing direct evidence of their effective removal [7]. It is most likely that the diagnostic sensitivity of individual assays is influenced by the reproductive potential of different species, so that eggs from highly fecund species (such as *H. contortus*, *O. venulosum* and *C. ovina*) can be more readily detected in sheep with small worm burdens than those for species with low fecundity (e.g., *Te. circumcincta* and *Trichostrongylus*) [28]. A similar restriction may apply also to the detection of parasite DNA by PCR, such that prepatent and very low-level infections might only be detectable by necropsy.

False-positive results were uncommon. In all nine cases, for which amplicons were produced from faecal samples in which no strongylid eggs were detected, subsequent sequencing confirmed, unequivocally, their specific identity, showing the limited sensitivity of the McMaster flotation method, also consistent with our previous field study [13]. In addition, in three samples found to be test-positive by PCR (and verified by direct DNA sequencing), we detected no evidence of infection based on routine total worm count (TWC). Given that TWC is based on sampling and examining sub-aliquots of gut contents, we infer this discrepancy to relate to limitations in the sensitivity of TWC rather than an issue with the PCR assay. Indeed, because only one 20-th of the total gut wash (1 litre) is examined for worms, the theoretical

Table 3. Total worm count results.

Sheep no.	Group[a]	EPG	Abomasum Teladorsagia females	all adults	L4	Ct	Small intestine Trichostrongylus females	all adults	L4	Ct	Large intestine Chabertia females	all adults	L4	Ct
1394	ABC	310	770	1960	10220	22.72	5000	8090	1200	20.72	1	1	0	27.16
1452	ABC	150	800	1200	8150	20.95	2460	3850	0	18.61	4	8	0	22.31
1338	ABC	40	200	520	1160	26.38	700	1140	0	25.34	6	7	0	24.48
1434	ABC	50	920	1620	2840	24.04	80*	100	0	40*	0	0	0	40
1353	ABC	30	300	450	11450	24.76	1460	2170	0	23.42	0	0	0	40
1330	ABC	530	850*	1300	5350	40*	6050*	9050	200	40*	3	3	0	26.82
1385	ABC	110	680	1120	1580	23.47	640	970	0	23.45	3	4	0	23.73
1429	ABC	280	3360	7200	30120	16.03	3420	4540	500	22.67	0	0	0	40
1403	ABC	120	1000	1950	7200	23.41	1506	2286	128	23.74	5	8	0	22.12
1427	AB	110	7340	11280	12500	21.91	60*	120	40	40*	0	0	0	40
1315	AB	50	1350	2200	5050	22.57	50*	100	0	40*	0	0	0	40
1390	AB	120	980	1660	600	22.4	0	20	0	40	0	0	0	40
1417	AB	60	60	80	1100	25.68	0	0	0	40	0	0	0	40
1305	AB	10	400	600	14500	25.1	160	200	440	25.51	0	0	0	40
1306	AB	40	816	1152	624	22.86	0	48	0	40	0	0	0	40
1409	AB	90	2600	4000	2250	24.5	0	0	0	40	0	0	0	40
1368	AB	30	80	160	160	24.6	0	20	0	40	0	0	0	40
1442	AB	30	200	300	5600	19.74	0*	0	0	27.03*	0	0	0	40
1313	MPC	750	1480	2640	820	18.53	10760	19880	1760	19.73	1	3	0	22.1
1345	MPC	1310	11200	17360	12460	21.92	1540	2460	0	23.66	7	11	0	22.18
1395	MPC	420	1800	3000	20850	20.94	11850	17750	1100	19.1	0	0	0	40
1387	MP	0	0	0	0	40	0	20	0	40	0	0	0	40
1415	MP	0	0*	0	0	26.14*	0	0	0	40	0	0	0	40
1443	MP	10	0*	0	0	25.5*	20*	20	0	40*	0	0	0	40
1379	MP	0	0	0	0	40	0	0	0	40	0	0	0	40
1362	MP	30	0	0	0	40	0	0	160	40	0	0	0	40
1326	MP	0	0	0	0	40	0	0	0	40	0	0	0	40
1451	MP	10	0	0	0	40	0	0	0	40	0	0	0	40
1399	MP	0	0	0	0	40	0	0	0	40	0	0	0	40
1445	MP	10	0	0	0	40	0	0	0	40	0	0	0	40

Total worm count results for 30 sheep following anthelmintic treatment. Corresponding faecal egg counts are given in eggs per gram (EPG) and PCR results, as cycle threshold values (Ct). Discrepancies between total worm count and PCR results indicated by asterisk. Negative PCR results are indicated by the number 40.
[a]Groups of sheep assigned as ABC (albendazole-untreated control), AB (albendazole-treated), MPC (monepantel-untreated control), MP (monepantel-treated).

minimum number of worms detectable using this approach is 20 (which equates to the observation of 1 worm in the aliquot examined). Moreover, although it has been shown [29] that the vast majority of trichostronglyids infecting the small intestine of sheep are usually present in the first six meters, the effect of sub-sampling from the gut wash likely compromises the accuracy of the method. This aspect has not been critically assessed to date and, thus, warrants detailed investigation. The inaccuracy related to the probability of detecting worms in a sub-sample would be particularly pronounced in sheep with low numbers of worms, potentially leading to significant over- or under-estimation of infection intensity. Acknowledging these issues, we selected TWC as the reference method, because it is recognized as the 'gold-standard' for the diagnosis of infections with gastrointestinal helminths [30].

Consistent with EPG and TWC data, the present PCR results did not show any evidence of resistance to monepantel in gastrointestinal strongylids, supporting previous reports of the efficacy of this new anthelmintic [31,32]. In contrast, the PCR assay did provide evidence of a reduced susceptibility to benzimidazoles (i.e., albendazole) in one or more nematode species in the population of sheep in this study. These results were expected, based on the history available for this farm (J. Larsen, unpublished) and also the relatively high prevalence of benzimidazole resistance in sheep in Australia [33,34], and were supported by coproscopic and TWC data. Indeed, following albendazole treatment, 17 of 19 sheep were shown to harbour strongylids based on McMaster flotation (day 10) and, despite a notable overall reduction in EPG, the number of samples with eggs increased (between days 0 and 10) from 15 to 17 in group AB. PCR-based testing detected infection/s in 15 of the 19 sheep on day 10, with

Table 4. Determined assay performance.

Parasite species	(n)	Sensitivity	[95% CI]	(n)	Specificity	[95% CI]	Kappa	[95% CI]	Female worms
Teladorsagia circumcincta	(20/21)	95.2%	[76.2–99.9]	(7/9)	77.8%	[40.0–97.2]	0.75	[0.5–1.0]	≥60
Trichostrongylus spp.	(11/16)	68.8%[a]	[41.3–89.0]	(13/14)	92.9%	[66.1–99.8]	0.61	[03–0.9]	≥20
Trichostrongylus spp.	(11/12)	91.7%	[61.5–99.8]	(17/18)	94.4%	[72.7–99.9]	0.86	[0.7–1.0]	≥100
Chabertia ovina	(8/8)	100%	[63.1–100]	(22/22)	100%	[84.6–100]	1.00	(1.0–1.0)	≥1
Oesophagostomum venulosum	(0/0)	N/A[b]	N/A	(30/30)	100%	[88.4–100]	N/A	N/A	N/A
Haemonchus contortus	(0/0)	N/A	N/A	(30/30)	100%	[88.4–100]	N/A	N/A	N/A
Total	(22/22)	100%	[84.6–100]	(7/8)	87.5	[47.4–99.7]	0.91	[0.7–1.0]	N/A

PCR assay performance and direct comparison with total worm count results. Shown are the calculated diagnostic sensitivity and specificity of the PCR, the number of cases identified as positive or negative in comparison to total worm counts (n), calculated Kappa values and their 95% confidence interval (CI). Also shown are the minimum number of species females as detected by PCR and the total diagnostic performance (the ability to detect infections involving the presence of any females of the target species by PCR).
[a]all PCR false-negative test results related to TWC results of <100 female worms per sheep.
[b]No data available.

subsequent sequencing indicating the presence of *Te. circumcincta* in all and *T. colubriformis* in three sheep with EPGs of 0–120 following treatment. Although *C. ovina* was initially detected in eight sheep in group AB (on day 0), this nematode was not detected following albendazole treatment (on day 10), providing no evidence of drug resistance in this species. Based on these data, a specific diagnosis of resistance to albendazole was possible and indicated a predominant link to *Te. circumcincta* and, to lesser extent, *T. colubriformis*.

Using the criteria defined by Gordon [19] and McMurtry [20], the LC results, following anthelmintic treatment, were similar to those achieved by PCR. Nonetheless, the morphological identification of L3 stages (based on total length and caudal morphology) is complicated by the similarity between *Teladorsagia* and *Trichostrongylus* species. Most notably, when using the criteria defined by Dikmans and Andrews [18], the majority of the L3s from LC for group AB were identified as *Trichostrongylus* rather than *Te. circumcincta*, thus leading to an entirely different diagnosis and conclusion regarding resistance. The inference that *Trichostrongylus* had the highest level of resistance to albendazole was neither supported by the PCR-test results nor the TWC data, emphasizing the problems associated with the use of LC. The limitations in the differentiation of some parasites following LC are reinforced by findings that host (e.g., immune response) and/or environmental factors (e.g., climate and/or the availability of appropriate nutrients for first- and second-stage larvae) can influence the length of the developing L3s [20], obviously, leading to further challenges for a correct diagnosis of resistance in the context of FECRT combined with LC. Because PCR relies on the use of species/genus-specific DNA markers, such factors do not adversely impact on its application and reliability. Furthermore, although PCR can detect *C. ovina* and *Oesophagostomum* and differentiate them, L3s of these parasites cannot be delineated morphologically [17]. In addition to these technical considerations, LC has significant practical limitations compared with a PCR-based method, particularly in relation to time-efficiency and the cost of testing.

In conclusion, based on the results of the present and previous studies [13,23], we have consistently demonstrated that our PCR approach, employing genetic markers in nuclear rDNA, is specific for strongylid nematodes [12,25] and achieves the sensitivity required for efficient diagnosis of naturally acquired strongylid infections in sheep. In addition, the present investigation provides strong evidence that this molecular assay can support FECRT for the detection of anthelmintic resistance in strongylid populations, thus eliminating the need for LC. A molecular assay that directly detects drug resistance, and, thus, replaces or at least reduces the need for FEC-based reduction trials altogether, would be a major, additional step forward. However, current tests are limited to the detection of benzimidazole resistance based mainly on three main mutations (linked to amino acid positions 167, 198 and 200) in the beta tubulin gene [7,35], but neither levamisole nor macrocyclic lactone resistance, which appear to be multi-faceted and polygenic [36]. Therefore, molecular assays for the direct detection of drug resistance will likely be limited until the genetics and genomics of resistance are much better understood. In contrast, coupled to current FECRT methods, our specific PCR assay provides a rapid, efficient and universally applicable tool for the diagnosis of resistance and the early detection of residual populations of worms in sheep following treatment, possibly reflecting an early emergence of resistance.

Taken together, our results show that the present PCR is useful as a rapid approach for routine *intra vitam* diagnosis of strongylid infections in sheep and, combined with conventional FECRT, for assessing the emergence of anthelmintic resistance, without the need for additional costly and time-consuming *ante mortem* (i.e., LC) or *post mortem* (TWC) analyses. Further applications of PCR might include its use for assessing the monospecificity of cultures used for a range of experimental investigations of strongylids and mechanisms of drug resistance in particular species or, for instance, to assess the status of parasitism in flocks of sheep destined for import/export. Given the broad applicability of such a molecular-diagnostic assay, our current focus is now on adapting it to a semi-automated platform for routine application in a service laboratory setting.

Acknowledgments

Sincere thanks to Ian Beveridge, Dianne Rees, Richard Martin, Robert Dobson and Abdul Jabbar for discussions and support.

Author Contributions

Conceived and designed the experiments: FR JWAL NA AJDC RBG ARJ. Performed the experiments: FR. Analyzed the data: FR NA GAA. Contributed reagents/materials/analysis tools: JWAL GAA RBG. Wrote the paper: FR RBG ARJ.

References

1. Sackett D, Holmes P (2006) Assessing the economic cost of endemic disease on the profitability of Australian beef cattle and sheep producers. Sydney. ISBN. 1741910021 p.
2. Zajac AM (2006) Gastrointestinal Nematodes of Small Ruminants: Life cycle, Anthelmintics, and Diagnosis. Vet Clin North Am Food Anim Pract 22: 529–541.
3. Dobson RJ, LeJambre L, Gill JH (1996) Management of anthelmintic resistance: inheritance of resistance and selection with persistent drugs. Int J Parasitol 26: 993–1000.
4. Wolstenholme AJ, Fairweather I, Prichard R, Samson-Himmelstjerna Gv, Sangster NC (2004) Drug resistance in veterinary helminths. Trends Parasitol 20: 469–476.
5. Kaminsky R, Ducray P, Jung M, Clover R, Rufener L, et al. (2008) A new class of anthelmintics effective against drug-resistant nematodes. Nature 452: 176–180.
6. Kaplan RM (2004) Drug resistance in nematodes of veterinary importance: a status report. Trends Parasitol 20: 477–481.
7. Taylor MA, Hunt KR, Goodyear KL (2002) Anthelmintic resistance detection methods. Vet Parasitol 103: 183–194.
8. Cabaret J, Berrag B (2004) Faecal egg count reduction test for assessing anthelmintic efficacy: average versus individually based estimations. Vet Parasitol 121: 105–113.
9. Coles GC, Jackson F, Pomroy WE, Prichard RK, Samson-Himmelstjerna Gv, et al. (2006) The detection of anthelmintic resistance in nematodes of veterinary importance. Vet Parasitol 136: 167–185.
10. Dobson RJ, Barnes EH, Birclijin SD, Gill JH (1992) The survival of *Ostertagia circumcincta* and *Trichostrongylus colubriformis* in faecal culture as a source of bias in apportioning egg counts to worm species. Int J Parasitol 22: 1005–1008.
11. Lichtenfels JR, Hoberg EP, Zarlenga DS (1997) Systematics of gastrointestinal nematodes of domestic ruminants: advances between 1992 and 1995 and proposals for future research. Vet Parasitol 72: 225–245.
12. Gasser RB, Bott NJ, Chilton NB, Hunt P, Beveridge I (2008) Toward practical, DNA-based diagnostic methods for parasitic nematodes of livestock – Bionomic and biotechnological implications. Biotechnol Adv 26: 325–334.
13. Roeber F, Jex AR, Campbell AJD, Campbell BE, Anderson GA, et al. (2011) Evaluation and application of a molecular method to assess the composition of strongylid nematode populations in sheep with naturally acquired infections. Infect, Genet Evol 11: 849–854.
14. Nielsen MK, Vidyashankar AN, Andersen UV, DeLisi K, Pilegaard K, et al. (2010) Effects of fecal collection and storage factors on strongylid egg counts in horses. Vet Parasitol 167: 55–61.
15. Whitlock HV (1948) Some modifications of the McMaster helminth egg-counting technique and apparatus. Journal of the Council for Scientific and Industrial Research, Australia 21: 177–180.
16. MAFF, ed (1986) Manual of veterinary parasitological laboratory techniques. London, UK: Her Majesty's Stationary Office. 20–27 p.
17. Wyk JAv, Cabaret J, Michael LM (2004) Morphological identification of nematode larvae of small ruminants and cattle simplified. Vet Parasitol 119: 277–306.
18. Dikmans G, Andrews JS (1933) A Comparative Morphological Study of the Infective Larvae of the Common Nematodes Parasitic in the Alimentary Tract of Sheep. T Am Microsc Soc 52: 1–25.
19. Gordon HM (1933) Differential Diagnosis of the Larvæ of Ostertagia spp. and Trichostrongylus spp. of Sheep. Aust Vet J 9: 223–227.
20. McMurtry LW, Donaghy MJ, Vlassoff A, Douch PGC (2000) Distinguishing morphological features of the third larval stage of ovine Trichostrongylus spp. Vet Parasitol 90: 73–81.
21. Anderson N (1972) Trichostrongylid infections of sheep in a winter rainfall region. I. Epizootiological studies in the Western District of Victoria, 1966–67. Aust J Agric Res 23: 1113–1129.
22. Gibbons LM, ed (2010) Keys to the Nematode Parasites of Vertebrates. Supplementary Volume. Wallingford: CAB International. 83–102 p.
23. Bott NJ, Campbell BE, Beveridge I, Chilton NB, Rees D, et al. (2009) A combined microscopic-molecular method for the diagnosis of strongylid infections in sheep. Int J Parasitol 39: 1277–1287.
24. Gasser RB, Chilton NB, Hoste H, Beveridge I (1993) Rapid sequencing of rDNA from single worms and eggs of parasitic helminths. Nucleic Acids Res 21: 2525–2526.
25. Gasser R, Hu M, Chilton N, Campbell B, Jex A, et al. (2006) Single-strand conformation polymorphism (SSCP) for the analysis of genetic variation. Nat Protoc 1: 3121–3128.
26. Conraths FJ, Schares G (2006) Validation of molecular-diagnostic techniques in the parasitological laboratory. Vet Parasitol 136: 91–98.
27. Villanua D, Perez-Rodriguez L, Gortazar C, Hofle U, Vinuela J (2006) Avoiding bias in parasite excretion estimates: the effect of sampling time and type of faeces. Parasitology 133: 251–259.
28. Gordon HMEpidemiologyofhelminthosisinsheep; (1981) Post-Graduate Committee in Veterinary Science, University of Sydney. pp 551–566.
29. Beveridge I, Barker IK (1983) Morphogenesis of Trichostrongylus rugatus and distribution during development in sheep. Vet Parasitol 13: 55–65.
30. Thrusfield M, ed (2007) Veterinary Epidemiology. Third Edition ed. Oxford: Blackwell Publishing. 312–315 p.
31. Hosking BC, Griffiths TM, Woodgate RG, Besier RB, Feuvre ASl, et al. (2009) Clinical field study to evaluate the efficacy and safety of the amino-acetonitrile derivative, monepantel, compared with registered anthelmintics against gastrointestinal nematodes of sheep in Australia. Aust Vet J 87: 455–462.
32. Hosking BC, Kaminsky R, Sager H, Rolfe PF, Seewald W (2010) A pooled analysis of the efficacy of monepantel, an amino-acetonitrile derivative against gastrointestinal nematodes of sheep. Parasitol Res 106: 529–532.
33. Besier RB, Love SCJ (2003) Anthelmintic resistance in sheep nematodes in Australia: the need for new approaches. Aus J Exp Agr 43: 1383–1391.
34. Love SCJ, Coles GC (2002) Anthelmintic resistance in sheep worms in New South Wales, Australia. Vet Rec 150: 87.
35. Samson-Himmelstjerna Gv (2006) Molecular diagnosis of anthelmintic resistance. Vet Parasitol 136: 99–107.
36. Beech RN, Skuce P, Bartley DJ, Martin RJ, Prichard RK, et al. (2011) Anthelmintic resistance: markers for resistance, or susceptibility? Parasitology 138: 160–174.

3

Saccade Generation by the Frontal Eye Fields in Rhesus Monkeys Is Separable from Visual Detection and Bottom-Up Attention Shift

Kyoung-Min Lee[1,2]*, Kyung-Ha Ahn[1], Edward L. Keller[2]

1 Department of Neurology, Seoul National University, Seoul, Republic of Korea, **2** The Smith-Kettlewell Eye Research Institute, San Francisco, California, United States of America

Abstract

The frontal eye fields (FEF), originally identified as an oculomotor cortex, have also been implicated in perceptual functions, such as constructing a visual saliency map and shifting visual attention. Further dissecting the area's role in the transformation from visual input to oculomotor command has been difficult because of spatial confounding between stimuli and responses and consequently between intermediate cognitive processes, such as attention shift and saccade preparation. Here we developed two tasks in which the visual stimulus and the saccade response were dissociated in space (the extended memory-guided saccade task), and bottom-up attention shift and saccade target selection were independent (the four-alternative delayed saccade task). Reversible inactivation of the FEF in rhesus monkeys disrupted, as expected, contralateral memory-guided saccades, but visual detection was demonstrated to be intact at the same field. Moreover, saccade behavior was impaired when a bottom-up shift of attention was not a prerequisite for saccade target selection, indicating that the inactivation effect was independent of the previously reported dysfunctions in bottom-up attention control. These findings underscore the motor aspect of the area's functions, especially in situations where saccades are generated by internal cognitive processes, including visual short-term memory and long-term associative memory.

Editor: Doug Wylie, University of Alberta, Canada

Funding: This work was supported by the National Research Foundation of Korea Grant funded by the Korean Government (MEST) (Global Research Network Project, 2008-H00004 to KML) and by the Smith-Kettlewell Eye Research Foundation. The funders had no role in study design, data collection and analysis, decision to publish, or preparation of the manuscript.

Competing Interests: The authors have declared that no competing interests exist.

* E-mail: kminlee@snu.ac.kr

Introduction

Initially recognized as an oculomotor area [1], the FEF have also been shown to play a role in much broader behavioral contexts, such as target selection [2–4], motor preparation [5], internal monitoring [6], adjustment of on-going saccades [7], inhibition of reflexive saccades [8], and shift of spatial attention [9]. Recently, numerous studies have implicated its function even in perceptual domains, such as in building and maintaining a visual saliency map [10], visual prediction [11], working memory of the visual world [12], and shifting visual attention [13–15]. Indeed, a majority of FEF neurons exhibit phasic or sustained visual responses with or without motor activity [16].

However, whether the FEF is causally involved in these various visual and cognitive functions remains unclear. While reversible or permanent lesions of the FEF lead to demonstrable errors in visuo-oculomotor tasks [17–21], it has been difficult to specify whether the lesions impinge upon visual or oculomotor functions, because the visual target and the saccade response were spatially confounded in the tasks employed in the investigations. Furthermore, visual attention was co-localized with saccade planning in most previous task paradigms: A transient visual change occurred at a position in the peripheral fields, triggering a shift of bottom-up attention as well as a saccadic movement of the eyes to the same position. Recently, a few studies have provided evidence that the

oculomotor and the attentional roles by the FEF are in fact separable: FEF inactivation disrupted covert visual search in the absence of eye movements [22]. Shifts of gaze and shifts of attention may be carried out by different cell types [23] and different dopaminergic receptors [24] in this cortical area.

Here, using reversible inactivation techniques and two novel behavioral tasks, we aimed at dissecting cognitive processes underlying the visuo-oculomotor transformation often ascribed to this area. The results suggested a distinction between visual detection and saccade generation in FEF functions, as well as between bottom-up attention shift and saccade target selection by the cortex.

Materials and Methods

Ethics Statement

All experimental procedures were approved by the Seoul National University Hospital Animal Care and Use Committee (IACUC No: 09–0166, Project Title: Neural mechanisms of saccade choice in primate frontal cortex).

Subjects and Surgical Preparation

Two adult female rhesus monkeys (*Macaca mulatta*, M9 and M10) weighing between 4 and 5 kg were used. A head-restraint post and recording cylinders were implanted under isoflurane anesthesia and sterile surgical conditions. The recording cylinders (20 mm, internal diameter) were positioned over craniotomies centered on the right arcuate sulcus in all animals.

Procedures to Minimize Animal Discomfort, Distress, Pain and Injury

Three situations existed in which a monkey might experience discomfort, distress and/or pain in our experimental protocols: a) survival surgery; b) restraint for handling or routine testing and c) training and experimental recording sessions. The following steps were taken to ameliorate animal suffering in each situation. **a) Survival surgery.** The purpose of the surgical procedures was to implant recording chambers and a head restraint device for neurophysiological experiments. All surgeries were carried out in the animal surgical suite at the Primate Center of Seoul National University Hospital. Animals were prepared with sterile, anesthetic surgical procedures. A licensed veterinarian was present throughout the surgical procedures and the recovery period for anesthetic induction and for monitoring and recording all measured physiological variables. Animals were allowed free access to water but no food the night prior to scheduled surgery. One hour before the surgery the animal was given atropine sulfate (0.08 mg/kg, I.M.) to prevent excessive salivation during the surgery. One-half hour later it was sedated with zoletil chloride (10 mg/kg, I.M.), intubated, and placed under Isofluorane anesthesia. A saline drip was maintained through an intravenous catheter placed into a leg vein. Throughout the surgery, core body temperature, heart rate, blood pressure, oxygen saturation and respiratory rate was continuously monitored. The animal was returned to its home cage after waking from the anesthesia and allowed to recover fully from the effects of surgery before behavioral training started. During the period of post-surgical recovery the animal was monitored closely and given injections of an analgesic agent (meloxicam 0.4 mg/kg I.M.) and antibiotics (cephazolin, 25/mg/kg) in consultation with the veterinarian for 3 days post-op. **b) Restraint for handling or routine testing.** Restraint for certain procedures, such as physical examination or blood sampling for health check, was accomplished with zoletil chloride (10 mg/kg, I.M.). **c) Training and experimental recording sessions.** After recovery from the surgical procedure the animal was trained to be held by the arms and moved into a large plastic primate chair. This was done by supplying the animal with rewards of fruit and juice. The chair had a perch with an adjustable height for each animal's comfort. Wastes fell into a collection pan below the animal, and thus, did not cause the animal discomfort. The animals were trained by the delivery of water or fruit juice rewards in daily sessions during which time they received their entire liquid intake in the experimental apparatus. When the animal was fully trained the experiments began. During the experimental sessions the animal's head was painlessly restrained through the use of the implanted head post which mated to a vertical rod attached to the primate chair. The animals did not show any sign of discomfort by the head restraint device: They continued to train steadily for the period of time that they were in restraint and often fell asleep as they sat in the darkened room between blocks of trials.

Behavioral Tasks

A) The extended memory-guided saccade task (Figure 1a). A trial began with illumination of a central fixation spot (a gray disc, 0.5 degree in diameter). Visual stimuli were presented 400 ms after the animal acquired fixation at the spot. When a single stimulus was briefly (200 ms) shown on either side, as in the traditional version of the task, the animal was required to remember the location, wait through a delay period ranging between 800 and 1200 ms, and make a saccade to the now-empty location as soon as the fixation spot was extinguished. More crucial for our current aim, two new conditions were added: When two stimuli, one on each side, had appeared at the same time, the animal was trained to make an upward saccade. On the other hand, a downward saccade was the correct response if no stimulus had appeared before the fixation target turned off. Notice that these two additional conditions forced the animal to detect, remember and explicitly report whether it had seen the visual stimuli or not, and that the direction of saccade response was disjoint from that of the visual stimuli. The discs were 1.0 degree in diameter with luminance of 1.24 cd/m^2, unless specified otherwise in the text, against a background luminance of 0.12 cd/m^2 (measured by a chromameter, CS-100; Minolta Photo Imaging, Mahwah, NJ). The eccentricity of the visual stimuli were adjusted to match the amplitude of saccades evoked by electrical stimulation before each muscimol injection (see below 2.4. Muscimol inactivation). However, we chose not to adjust the direction of visual stimuli, since 1) the evoked saccades were all to the upper left quadrant and the directional variation across inactivated sites was smaller than the separation between visual stimuli which was 90 degrees or more, and 2) we reasoned that the effect of inactivation would spread over time to a larger volume of tissue that included the nearest stimulus direction.

B) The four-alternative delayed saccade task (Figure 1b). Upper panel shows the pre-trained location and color association, e.g. red is associated with the upper-right visual field. The association remained the same for both monkeys throughout the experiments. Lower panel depicts the events in the task: A trial began when the animal fixated at a central gray fixation disc (0.5 degree in diameter). Soon after the fixation, four gray targets appeared in the peripheral visual field, and after 400 ms the central disc changed to one of the four colors each associated with a particular target location. After a random delay ranging between 500 and 1000 ms, the central disc disappeared, which served as the cue for the animal to make a saccade response. The discs were 1.0 degree in diameter, with luminance of 1.24 cd/m^2 against a background luminance of 0.12 cd/m^2. The colors used for the fixation spot, peripheral targets, and central cue were equiluminant and chosen based on the CIE 1976 (L*a*b*) space, which is approximately uniform in perception of color difference [25], such that the colors were at the same distance in the space from the two neighboring ones and the gray. A chromameter (CS-100; Minolta PhotoImaging, Mahwah, NJ) was used for measuring luminance and chromaticity of the colors. The eccentricity of the peripheral targets were adjusted to match the amplitude of saccades evoked by electrical stimulation before each muscimol injection (see below 2.4. Muscimol inactivation). The direction of visual stimuli were not adjusted for the reasons stated above.

Note that, since the four gray peripheral targets were indistinguishable, a bottom-up shift of attention to the targets was not prompted by the targets nor needed for performing the task. In fact, successful performance of the task required the animal to volitionally maintain top-down attention focused on the fixation point in order to detect the color change and decide on where and when to make the saccade. The target selection was based solely on pre-learned associative memory. Here we defined attention shift in the usual sense as bottom-up visual processing of salient targets in the visual field, not disputing that the act of a saccade would entail or ensue an attentional shift.

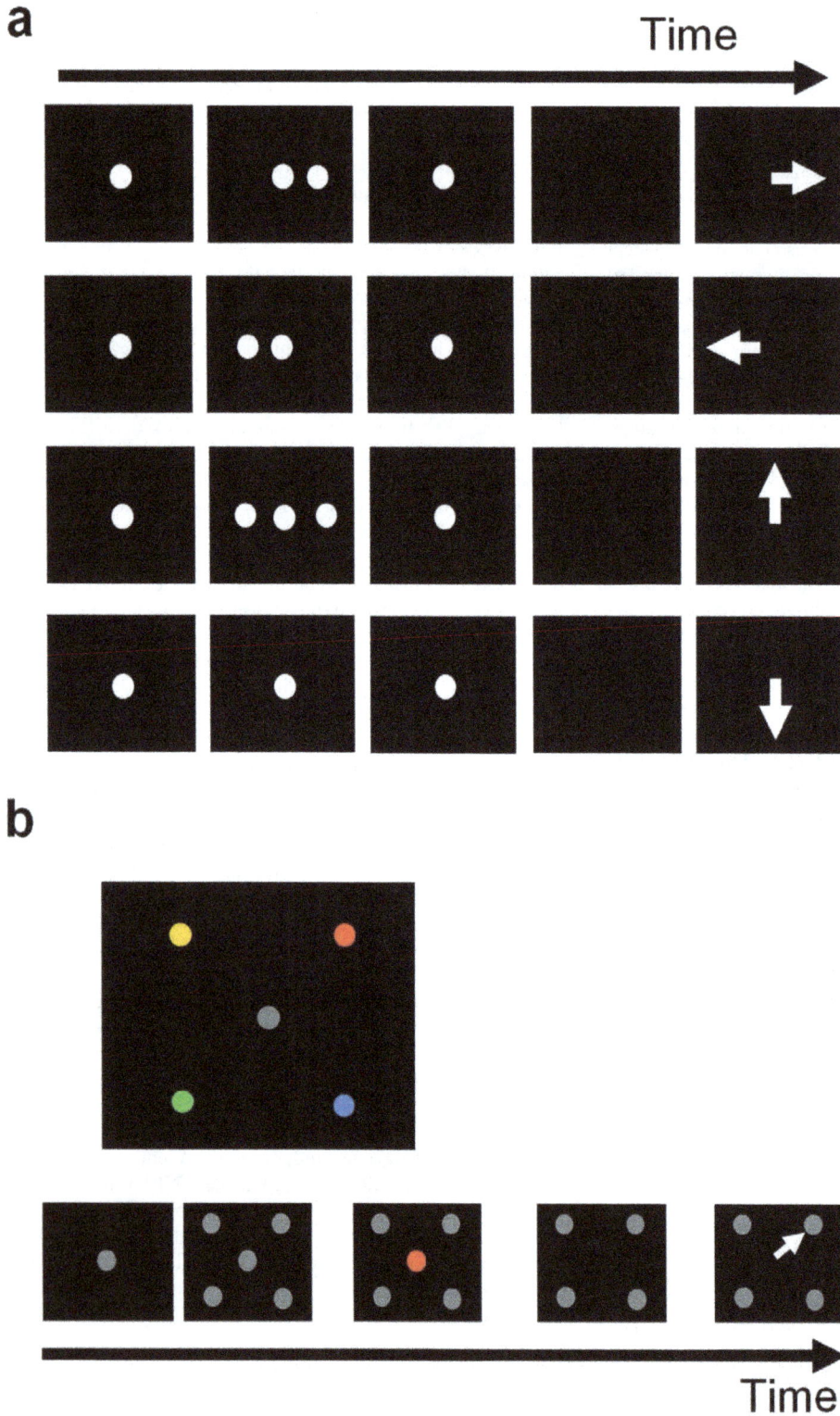

Figure 1. Two tasks used in the study are schematically depicted. a, The extended memory-guided saccade task. Visual events in task conditions are shown in rows of panels as a function of time: from the top row, two single-target conditions, bilateral stimulus condition, and no-stimulus condition. Arrows in the right-most panels indicate the correct saccade direction. **b,** The four-alternative delayed saccade task. The associations between color and spatial location shown in the top panel were pre-trained before inactivation experiments. Visual events in a trial are schematically depicted along the time line: the appearance of fixation target at the center, display of four alternative gray targets in the periphery, the onset of a color cue at the center, the color-cue turning-off signaling when to make the saccade, and the saccade to the color-matched target.

Experimental Procedures and Data Analysis

The performance in the task was monitored by infrared video-oculography with a sampling rate of 500 Hz (Eyelink2, SR Research Ltd, Kanata, Ontario, Canada). Saccade behavior was measured off-line using programs written in MATLAB (The Mathworks, Natick, MA, USA). Markers were available for all experimental events used in each task. The onset and offset of saccades were determined by velocity criteria ($30°/s$ radial velocity for onset and $10°/s$ for offset). Correct placement of these marks was checked manually and adjusted where necessary.

Forty trials of a task was presented in a block with task conditions randomly mixed (typically, 8~12 trials per condition). The two tasks alternated over a set of eight blocks, i.e., four blocks per task. This task alternation ensured that the inactivation effect which might change rather rapidly was monitored equally for both tasks. The block sets were run immediately before muscimol injection, and at approximately half-an-hour interval after the injection. The percent correct was assessed over the same task blocks in a block set. Error trials were classified as fixation error, motor error, and choice error, in a similar manner to our previous study [26].

Muscimol Inactivation

Details of the inactivation methods were the same as described previously [26]. After completing the mapping of the FEF for the low-threshold region for evoking saccades, we initiated a series of experiments using muscimol injections. In each monkey, the injection sites were selected based on the following criteria: 1) Electrical stimulation at the site evoked saccades at a current level below 70 µA with a probability higher than 50% (cathode-first bipolar pulse duration 0.2 ms, pulse frequency 200 Hz, train duration 100 ms). 2) The evoked saccades were directed contralaterally, closer to the horizontal meridian than to the vertical meridian, and with the amplitude between 5 and 20 degrees of visual angle. This criterion was applied since we fixed the direction of the visual stimuli, as explained above, and the range for eccentricity adjustment was limited. For each injection site, we first lowered a microelectrode inside a guide tube. After the electrode had penetrated the dura and eye movement-related activity began to be recorded, we applied electrical stimulation at sites separated by 1 mm of electrode advancement. We located the site associated with the lowest current threshold for evoking a saccade on each penetration. The depth of this site was carefully measured using an electronic microdrive (NAN Instruments Ltd, Nazareth, Israel), and the electrode was withdrawn leaving the guide tube in place.

A 33-gauge hypodermic cannula was inserted into the guide tube and was lowered until its tip was located at the same depth previously occupied by the tip of the stimulating electrode. Injections of muscimol were made through the cannula using pressure injection from a minipump (Aladdin 1000, World Precision Instruments, Sarasota, FL, USA). The concentration of the muscimol solution was kept constant at 5 microgram/microliter. The normal volume of solution injected was 1 microliter over a period of about 2 minutes. The amount of solution injected was monitored by watching the movement of a small bubble against fiduciary marks located on the Teflon tubing connecting the pump to the injection cannula. Following the injection, the cannula was left in place for about 10 minutes and was withdrawn. Data collection began immediately after the injection and continued up to several hours in some cases. Control data were collected on the following day, and full recovery was always noted.

In each monkey, we made at least two injections of one microliter of sterile saline in each hemifield and recorded a complete set of data to control for the possibility that any negative effects produced by muscimol inactivation might have been caused by local pressure on cortical neurons or local dilution of the extracellular fluid at the injection sites.

Results

Visual Detection is not Affected in the Field where Saccades were Impaired by FEF Inactivation

The first task that we developed to dissociate the spatial confounding of visual and saccade functions was an extension of the memory-guided saccade task (Figure 1a). During FEF inactivation, the performance was severely impaired in contralateral single stimulus trials (Figure 2b,f), consistent with observations by previous investigators [18,27]. Performance when a single target appeared in the ipsilateral field (Figure 2c,g) was nearly perfect as expected. More informatively, the inactivation had no significant impact on the bilateral- and no-stimulus conditions (Figures 2a, e and d, h, respectively). Thus, it appeared that while unable to make memory-guided saccades to contralateral visual fields, the animal showed no difficulty in monitoring visual events in the fields and reporting the brief appearance or absence of a stimulus during the delay period. These findings were consistent over six and four injection experiments in M10 and M9, respectively. Two-way analysis-of-variance test was performed on the percent correct data pooled over all injections in each monkey. The post-injection time was set as a continuous independent variable and the injection type (muscimol vs. saline) as the other discrete independent variable. The interaction between the two main effects indicated whether there was a significant difference between the injection types in the change of performance over time. The interaction was significant ($p<0.05$) in the case of the contralateral single stimulus condition, whereas it failed to reach significance in other conditions (p value given in each panel of Figure 2).

The direction of saccades in error trials were analyzed for further insights on the effects of FEF inactivation. The animals made error responses in a small portion of bilateral stimulus trials, which grew worse over time after muscimol or saline injections (Figures 2a, e). Most of the errors arose in target selection, rather than in saccade execution, in that the end-points were not deviated much from the target locations. The selection errors were distributed comparably between the right or left targets in both animals (two hours after muscimol injections, rightward error saccades occurred in 44.1% of total error trials and leftward ones in 39.3% in M9; 35.7% rightward and 42.7% in M10). Thus, there was no sign of propensity toward the rightward errors in this condition which would have suggested a perceptual deficit in the inactivated field. Furthermore, the proportion of rightward saccades over total error responses was not different between muscimol and saline injections: 44.1% and 35.7% for M9 and M10, respectively, after muscimol injections and 42.3% and 38.2% after saline injections ($p>0.05$, chi-squared test, for both animals).

With the contralateral single stimulus and two hours after muscimol injection, both monkeys made more downward errors than upward ones. Downward errors were 63.2% and 70.4% of total error trials in M9 and M10, respectively. (They never made erroneous rightward saccades in the left stimulus trials.) The downward bias of error responses might by itself be interpreted as a sign of perceptual or mnemonic disruption by FEF inactivation: That is, the animal responded as if they did not see or remember the left stimulus. However, this interpretation contradicted with

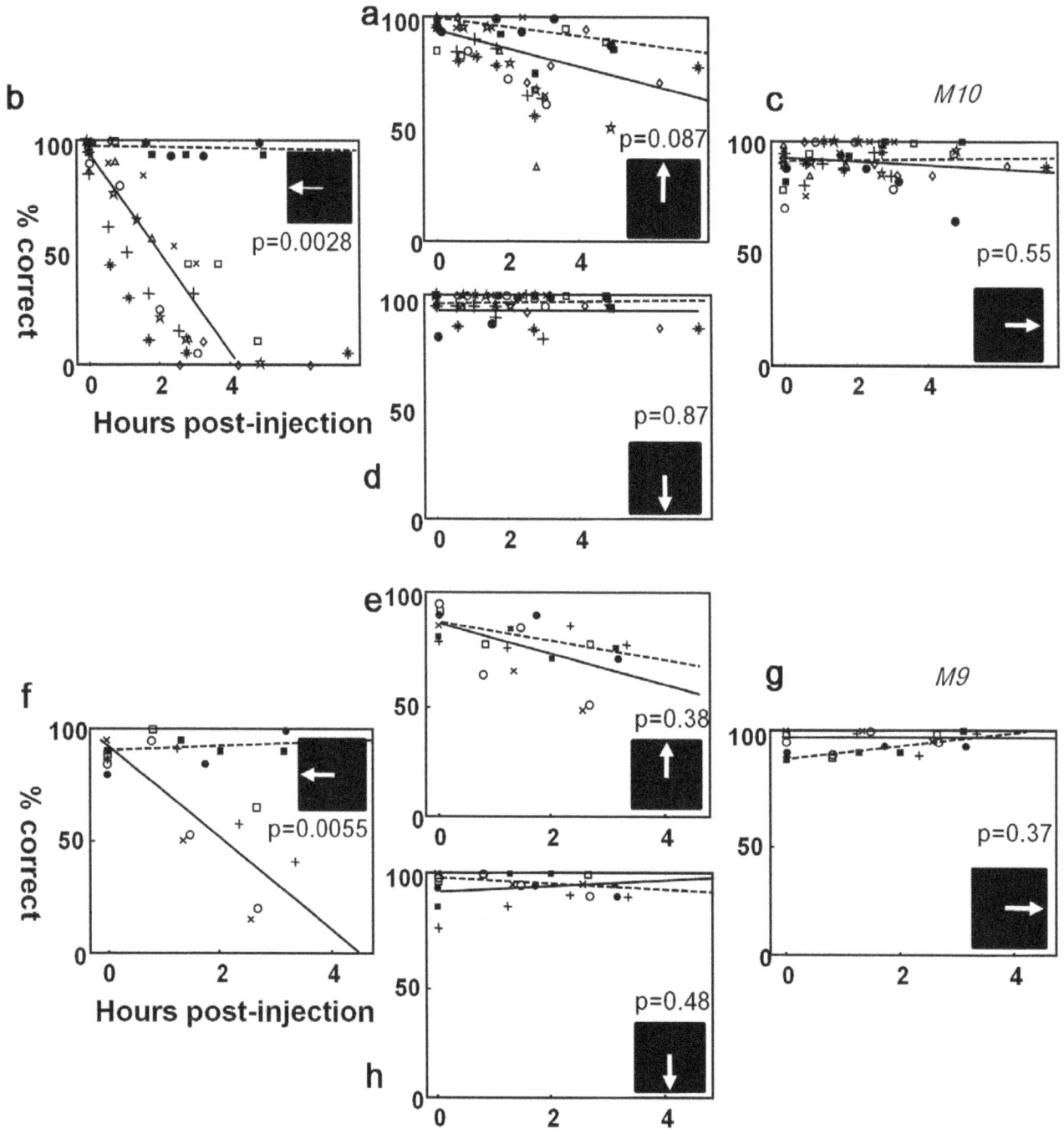

Figure 2. The effect of FEF inactivation on the extended memory-guided saccade task is shown. Changes in performance on the task by M10 (**a–d**) and M9 (**e–h**) are plotted as a function of time after muscimol injection into the FEF on the right side. Each data point was the percent correct out of 36 to 45 trials. Data points of a marker type were from the same inactivation session. Six inactivation experiments were performed in M10 and four in M9. Two control experiments with normal saline injection were performed in each animal with the data indicated by filled markers (circles and squares). The solid and broken lines indicate the regression over the pooled data with muscimol and saline injections, respectively. The p values are for the interaction between time-after-injection and injection type (muscimol vs. saline) in two-way ANOVA. The small icon in each panel indicate the correct saccade direction for the task condition.

the preserved performance in the bilateral condition and no rightward biasing in the error trials as stated above.

We therefore tested the visual threshold more directly by dimming the bilateral stimuli in three experiments with M10 (Figure 3). We reasoned that if the detection threshold were affected by the inactivation, the animal, having not perceived one

stimulus, would act as if the trial were an ipsilateral single-stimulus condition, and make an incorrect, rightward saccade. The performance in the bilateral stimulus condition would then decline during the inactivation. However, the percent correct in the bilateral stimulus condition did not change significantly from what had been before inactivation. Nor did we observe changes in the direction of error saccades: When the luminance of stimuli was low, the monkey made downward saccades as if they had seen no targets at all, rather than rightward ones which would have increased if the detection threshold was elevated only in the inactivated field. No rightward saccade was observed with or without FEF inactivation at the lowest luminance level (0.5 cd/m^2). The proportions of downward saccades in total error trials with the luminance at 0.74 cd/m^2 were 74.3% and 76.5% before and two hours after muscimol injections, respectively, while the proportion of rightward errors were 12.8% and 10.2% in the same sessions. Evidently then, although the performance got worse at lower luminance levels, the visual threshold remained the same in both hemi-fields, before and after muscimol injection.

The Saccade Dysfunction during FEF Inactivation is not Secondary to Dysfunction in Bottom-up Attention Shift

Given the results above that elementary visual detection was unaffected by FEF inactivation and previous reports that the FEF contributed to covert visual search [22,28], we asked whether the inactivation primarily interfered with high-level visual processing, such as the spatial deployment of attention, and led to the impairment of memory-guided saccades as a secondary effect to the high-level visual dysfunction.

Perhaps the oculomotor function of FEF is tightly linked to and therefore conditional on its role in bottom-up shift of visual attention [9]. In other words, the impact of FEF inactivation may be specific to situations where a saccade is preceded and mediated by an exogenous attentional shift to a peripheral visual stimulus. According to this idea, it may be argued that no deficit is observed in the bilateral stimulus condition in our first task, because visual attention is not lateralized or attracted toward one side, first by the bottom-up processing of visual stimuli.

With this possibility in mind, we trained the animals on a four-alternative delayed-saccade task. In this task, a saccade target was

chosen based on arbitrary learned associations between color and spatial location in the visual field (Figure 1b, the upper panel). Since the four peripheral targets were indistinguishably gray, a bottom-up shift of attention to the targets was not required for generating a saccade response. Instead, target selection was based solely on pre-learned associative memory. This task was similar to that used in our previous study [26], but was modified by a slight but important variation that dissociated visual attention and saccade intention: The animal was required to hold fixation at the central colored disc until it disappeared. This variation served two purposes: 1) the animal's top-down attention was required to remain focused on the central disc until a saccade response was generated; 2) the determination of the correct target and the actual response, i.e., the central color cue vs. the saccade to a peripheral target, was separated in time as well as in space, reducing even further the possibility that the saccade was triggered by a bottom-up drive from the visual transients in the peripheral fields, or by a bottom-up shift of visual attention.

After muscimol injections to FEF, the performance on the four-alternative delayed saccade task deteriorated in a spatially specific manner (Figure 4). Errors occurred only when the correct target associated with a color cue was on the contralateral side to the injected FEF. The errors were comparable in types and proportions to those reported in our previous study [26]. Two-way analysis of variance on the percent correct data with the post-injection time and the injection type (muscimol vs. saline) revealed that the interactions between the two main effects were significant only when the correct target was in the contralateral fields (p value given in each panel of Figure 4).

Discussion

Transformation of Visual Input into Saccade Command by FEF

Previous studies have shown that the detrimental effects induced by surgical or reversible chemical lesions in FEF depended on task contexts [17–21]: The impairment is severe specifically when the saccade response is made to a remembered target. Surgical removal of FEF resulted in long-term deficits in memory-guided saccades only [20,27], whereas muscimol inactivation produced deficits in both memory-guided and visually guided saccades, with a much worse effect on the former [18,26]. Such task selectivity of FEF inactivation indicates that the basic processes for visual perception and saccade execution are unaffected by the lesion. On the other hand, this selectivity has often been taken as evidence for the area's importance in high-level visual functions, such as constructing the saliency map from a visual stimulus array, or controlling visual attention based on the map [2,5,10,12,13]. A common line of thinking behind these notions is that visual input is transformed into a saccade command at the FEF, taking advantage of the co-existence of visual, visuo-movement, and movement cells with similar response fields within the same area [4].

Here, we dissected cognitive components associated with the transformation from visual input to oculomotor output, by developing two novel behavioral paradigms. Using the extended memory-guided saccade task, we spatially separated visual and motor processing, and with the four-alternative delayed saccade task, the functional linkage between bottom-up attention shift and saccadic eye movements was dissociated. Based on these cognitive dissections, we observed that the FEF inactivation did not disrupt visual detection at the affected visual fields (Figure 2). Nor was the contralateral stimulus neglected, as evidenced by the correct, up-saccade response in the bilateral stimulus condition.

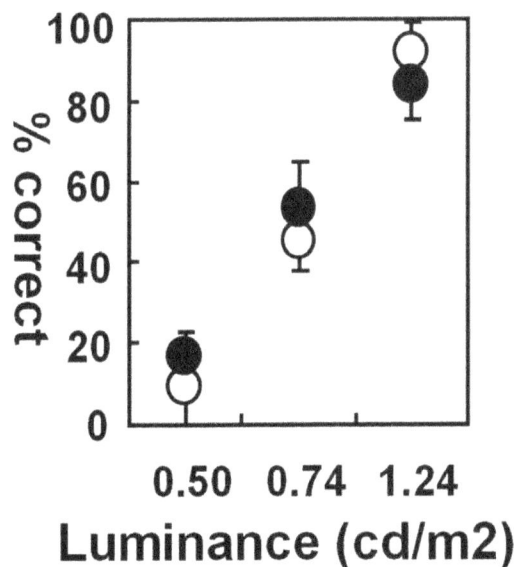

Figure 3. Performance in the bilateral-stimulus trials before and during FEF inactivation is plotted as a function of the luminance of the stimuli. The percent correct was calculated from a block of trials (n = 22~25) at the luminance, administered before muscimol injections (open circles) and about two hours after them (filled circles). The mean and standard deviation (error bar) are given for the percent correct data over three muscimol injections on M10.

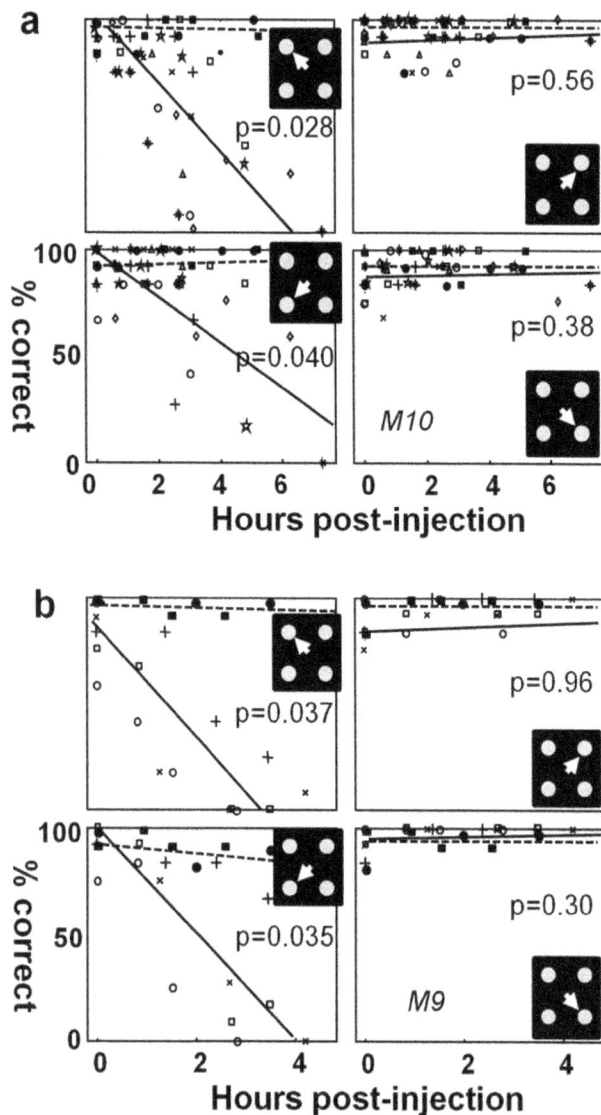

Figure 4. The effect of FEF inactivation on the four-alternative delayed saccade task is shown. Changes in performance on the task by two animals (M10 and M9 in **a** and **b**, respectively) are plotted as a function of time after muscimol injection into the FEF on the right side. Each data point was the percent correct out of 36 to 45 trials. Data points of a marker type were from the same inactivation session. Six inactivation experiments were performed in M10 and four in M9. Two control sessions with normal saline injection were performed in each animal with the data shown in filled circles and squares. The solid and broken lines indicate the regression over the pooled data with muscimol and saline injections, respectively. The p values are for the interaction between time-after-injection and injection type (muscimol vs. saline) in two-way ANOVA. The small icon in each panel indicate the direction of a correct saccade.

The reasons remain unclear to us why the animals responded with downward saccades when a single stimulus was flashed to the left, inactivated side. This finding by itself may indicate a perceptual deficit. However, given the preserved performance with bilateral stimuli, even with low luminance stimuli, we would prefer to interpret it as a manifestation of mnemonic dysfunction either of the stimulus or of the intention to move to the left. Perhaps an instability of memory trace of the left target, in conjunction with the lack of experiencing a stimulus on the intact field might have misled the animals into judging that there had been no stimulus at all.

It did not matter for saccade impairment induced by FEF inactivation which part of the visual field received information specifying a saccade target. Saccade impairment was observed regardless of whether the information was given in the periphery as in the memory-guided saccade task, or at the center as in our four-alternative delayed saccade task. This finding suggests a rather loose functional linkage between visual and movement neurons in the FEF, contrary to the view that takes the spatial co-registration between visual and saccade response fields in the FEF neurons as evidence for a direct transformation from visual information into oculomotor commands.

The Relationship between Attention and Oculomotor Functions by FEF

In this study, we also learned that a bottom-up attention shift was not a necessary pre-condition for FEF to generate a saccade (Figure 4). Therefore, the muscimol effect on saccade generation was independent of and likely additional to its effect on orienting bottom-up attention which was previously demonstrated using a covert visual search task [22].

As stated earlier, we do not dispute that the eye movements entail top-down attention shifting, nor that FEF plays a role in top-down or bottom-up attention control. Rather, our aim here was to examine how the role of FEF in attention control was related to that in saccade generation. Specifically, we asked whether the oculomotor aspect in FEF's functional role depended on its role in attention, and if saccade impairments were inducible when bottom-up attention shift was not required.

It is noteworthy that the common component of the FEF inactivation effects was an inability to generate a saccade and that the disability was specific to certain task situations. The inactivation effect seemed to hinge on the requirement that saccades be created based on memorized information regardless of the memory type, be it from the short-term spatial memory stored briefly as in the memory-guided saccade task or from the long-term associative memory as in the four-alternative delayed saccade task. We speculate, in generalization of the current findings, that the FEF is specifically required in situations where saccades are generated based on internal information and in the absence of perceptually salient external stimuli specifying the target.

This notion that the FEF is critically needed for "cognitively-driven" saccades is in keeping with previous reports that demonstrated the effects on FEF activities of the feature similarity between a target and distractors [29] and feature-based attention [30]. These studies showed correlates of visual top-down selection in FEF, without the concomitant production of a saccade, indicating that the activities indeed reflected internal cognitive information which could be used for the control of top-down attention or saccade generation.

Implications for Human Neuropsychology

Our findings demonstrate that FEF is not essential for visual detection and that the inactivation effect on saccade generation is independent of that on visual bottom-up attention. In this regard, the behavioral deficits observed in our animals resemble oculo-motor apraxia in human patients in which the formation of saccade intention is considered defective.

The pattern of deficits during FEF inactivation was also consistent with hemispatial neglect, but distinct from visual extinction. In fact, a normal performance was observed in the condition with double simultaneous stimuli, ruling out the possibility that FEF lesions underlie visual extinction. This finding is consistent with human neuropsychological data which localized the neural substrates for visual extinction to more posterior parts of the cerebral cortex [31].

References

1. Bizzi E (1967) Discharge of frontal eye field neurons during eye movements in unanesthetized monkeys. Science 157: 1588–1590.
2. Lee KM, Keller EL (2008) Neural activity in the frontal eye fields modulated by the number of alternatives in target choice. J Neurosci 28 2242–2251.
3. Schall JD, Hanes DP (1993) Neural basis of saccade target selection in frontal eye field during visual search. Nature 366: 467–469.
4. Schiller PH, Chou I (1998) The effects of frontal eye field and dorsomedial frontal cortex lesions on visually guided eye movements. Nat Neurosci 1: 248–253.
5. Bruce CJ, Goldberg ME (1984) Physiology of the frontal eye fields. Trends Neurosci 7: 436–441.
6. Sommer MA, Wurtz RH (2002) A pathway in primate brain for internal monitoring of movements. Science 296: 1480–1482.
7. Schall JD, Stuphorn V, Brown JW (2002) Monitoring and control of action by the frontal lobes. Neuron 36: 309–322.
8. Munoz DP, Everling S (2004) Look away: the anti-saccade task and the voluntary control of eye movement. Nat Rev Neurosci 5: 218–228.
9. Moore T, Fallah M (2001) Control of eye movements and spatial attention. Proc Natl Acad Sci U S A 98: 1273–1276.
10. Thompson KG, Bichot NP (2005) A visual salience map in the primate frontal eye field. Prog Brain Res 147: 251–262.
11. Umeno MM, Goldberg ME (1997) Spatial processing in the monkey frontal eye field. I. Predictive visual responses. J Neurophysiol 78: 1373–1383.
12. Umeno MM, Goldberg ME (2001) Spatial processing in the monkey frontal eye field. II. Memory responses. J Neurophysiol 86: 2344–2352.
13. Moore T, Fallah M (2004) Microstimulation of the frontal eye field and its effects on covert spatial attention. J Neurophysiol 91: 152–162.
14. Buschman TJ, Miller EK (2009) Serial, covert shifts of attention during visual search are reflected by the frontal eye fields and correlated with population oscillations. Neuron 63: 386–396.
15. Buschman TJ, Miller EK (2007) Top-down versus bottom-up control of attention in the prefrontal and posterior parietal cortices. Science 315: 1860–1862.
16. Bruce CJ, Goldberg ME (1985) Primate frontal eye fields. I. Single neurons discharging before saccades. J Neurophysiol 53: 603–635.
17. Dias EC, Kiesau M, Segraves MA (1995) Acute activation and inactivation of macaque frontal eye field with GABA-related drugs. J Neurophysiol 74: 2744–2748.
18. Dias EC, Segraves MA (1999) Muscimol-induced inactivation of monkey frontal eye field: effects on visually and memory-guided saccades. J Neurophysiol 81: 2191–2214.
19. Sommer MA, Tehovnik EJ (1997) Reversible inactivation of macaque frontal eye field. Exp Brain Res 116: 229–249.
20. Latto R, Cowey A (1971) Visual field defects after frontal eye-field lesions in monkeys. Brain Res 30: 1–24.
21. Schiller PH, True SD, Conway JL (1979) Effects of frontal eye field and superior colliculus ablations on eye movements. Science 206: 590–592.
22. Monosov IE, Thompson KG (2009) Frontal eye field activity enhances object identification during covert visual search. J Neurophysiol 102: 3656–3672.
23. Gregoriou GG, Gotts SJ, Desimone R (2012) Cell-type-specific synchronization of neural activity in FEF with V4 during attention. Neuron 73: 581–594.
24. Noudoost B, Moore T (2011) Control of visual cortical signals by prefrontal dopamine. Nature 474: 372–375.
25. Wyszecki G, Stiles WS (1982) Color Science: Concepts and Methods, Quantitative Data and Formulae. New York, NY: John Wiley & Sons, Inc. 164–169
26. Keller EL, Lee KM, Park SW, Hill JA (2008) The Effect of Inactivation of the Cortical Frontal Eye Field on Saccades Generated in a Choice Response Paradigm. J Neurophysiol 100: 2726–2737.
27. Deng SY, Goldberg ME, Segraves MA, Ungerleider LG, Mishkin M (1986) The effect of unilateral ablation of the frontal eye fields on saccadic performance in the monkey. In: Keller EL, Zee DS, editors. Adaptive Processes in the Visual and Oculomotor Systems. Oxford: Pergamon Press. 201–208.
28. Wardak C, Ibos G, Duhamel JR, Olivier E (2006) Contribution of the monkey frontal eye field to covert visual attention. J Neurosci 26: 4228–4235.
29. Bichot NP, Schall JD (1999) Effects of similarity and history on neural mechanisms of visual selection. Nat Neurosci 2: 549–554.
30. Zhou H, Desimone R (2011) Feature-based attention in the frontal eye field and area V4 during visual search. Neuron 70: 1205–1217.
31. Karnath HO, Himmelbach M, Kuker W (2003) The cortical substrate of visual extinction. Neuroreport 14: 437–442.

Author Contributions

Conceived and designed the experiments: KML ELK. Performed the experiments: KML KHA. Analyzed the data: KML KHA. Wrote the paper: KML ELK.

4

A Hidden Markov Model for Analysis of Frontline Veterinary Data for Emerging Zoonotic Disease Surveillance

Colin Robertson[1,2]*, Kate Sawford[3], Walimunige S. N. Gunawardana[4], Trisalyn A. Nelson[2], Farouk Nathoo[5], Craig Stephen[3]

1 Department of Geography and Environmental Studies, Wilfrid Laurier University, Waterloo, Ontario, Canada, 2 Spatial Pattern Analysis and Research Laboratory, Department of Geography, University of Victoria, Victoria, British Columbia, Canada, 3 Faculty of Veterinary Medicine, University of Calgary, Calgary, Alberta, Canada, 4 Faculty of Veterinary Medicine and Animal Science, University of Peradeniya, Peradeniya, Central Province, Sri Lanka, 5 Department of Mathematics and Statistics, University of Victoria, Victoria, British Columbia, Canada

Abstract

Surveillance systems tracking health patterns in animals have potential for early warning of infectious disease in humans, yet there are many challenges that remain before this can be realized. Specifically, there remains the challenge of detecting early warning signals for diseases that are not known or are not part of routine surveillance for named diseases. This paper reports on the development of a hidden Markov model for analysis of frontline veterinary sentinel surveillance data from Sri Lanka. Field veterinarians collected data on syndromes and diagnoses using mobile phones. A model for submission patterns accounts for both sentinel-related and disease-related variability. Models for commonly reported cattle diagnoses were estimated separately. Region-specific weekly average prevalence was estimated for each diagnoses and partitioned into normal and abnormal periods. Visualization of state probabilities was used to indicate areas and times of unusual disease prevalence. The analysis suggests that hidden Markov modelling is a useful approach for surveillance datasets from novel populations and/or having little historical baselines.

Editor: Corinne Ida Lasmezas, The Scripps Research Institute Scripps Florida, United States of America

Funding: Funding was provided by the Teasdale-corti Global Public Health Research Partnership Program and the Canadian National Sciences and Engineering Research Council. The funders had no role in study design, data collection and analysis, decision to publish, or preparation of the manuscript.

Competing Interests: The authors have declared that no competing interests exist.

* E-mail: crobertson@wlu.ca

Introduction

Approximately 75 percent of emerging infectious diseases (EIDs) in people are estimated to have originated in animals (i.e., zoonoses) [1–2]. Strategies to limit the impact of zoonotic EIDs can be broadly categorized as intervention at one or more of three levels: (i) controlling infections in people; (ii) blocking transmission of pathogens from animals to people; and/or (iii) preventing or controlling disease in animals [3]. Despite significant effort and funds targeting the first strategy, the global public health community continues to be caught off guard by EIDs. It is now recognized that the third strategy, control of disease in animals, may hold considerable potential for prevention of zoonotic EIDs [4]. To achieve this strategy, early detection of disease in animals is critical.

Surveillance for EIDs is confronted with the challenge of tracking something that has not yet happened. This has lead to the development of methods to track indicators of emergence or outbreaks such as risk factor surveillance and syndromic surveillance [5]. Surveillance systems using novel (pre-diagnostic) data sources that track healthcare-seeking behaviour have become widespread in human health surveillance with an aim to detect both intentional (bioterrorist) and naturally-occurring infectious disease outbreaks. Data representing early stage disease-related

behaviours (e.g., staying home from work – absenteeism data) may have predictive value and promote detection of disease at the earliest possible stage. However similar data is generally not available for animals. EID surveillance systems must rely on pre-diagnostic, syndromic, or clinical diagnoses to gather early warning signals. Syndromic surveillance for early outbreak detection often uses automated data collection and ongoing analysis for statistical signals to monitor patterns in health outcomes in near real-time to detect early signals of diseases outbreaks [6–7]. Analysis of conditions frequently seen by field veterinarians but rarely recorded or tracked can be thought of as similar to a syndromic surveillance approach, in that the data represent novel and unknown populations and may have early warning value for emerging diseases. The data presented in this study is from a system which recorded clinical diagnoses of field veterinarians [8]. This system was developed as a proto-typical complementary system to national disease reporting in Sri Lanka.

One of the drawbacks of pre-diagnostic, syndromic and clinical diagnostic data sources is that they incur an increased chance of false alarms [9]. With pre-diagnostic data sources, the data do not represent actual cases of disease, but variables related to disease - such as over-the-counter pharmaceutical sales [10], web site queries [11], or ambulance dispatch records [12]. Such data sources exhibit non-disease-related variations that need to be adjusted for in order to establish an accurate baseline level of risk. Similarly, clinical diagnoses data exhibit unknown variations that relate to how the data are collected. In many instances, making these adjustments is straightforward. For example, day of the week effects – that is, higher rates on certain days of the week - are features of many types of surveillance data. These higher rates could contribute to an outbreak signal when really the factors driving the increase are unrelated to disease, such as the greater propensity for people to visit the doctor on Mondays as compared to Fridays. With veterinary sentinel data, variability may be dependent on the sentinels themselves rather than the disease process. Therefore, with new and poorly understood surveillance data sources, developing a detailed understanding of baseline patterns (i.e., normal variation) is essential prior to conducting statistical analysis for cluster or outbreak detection.

Public health is increasingly looking towards surveillance of changing disease patterns in animals to enhance prediction and understanding of where and when EIDs in humans are likely to occur. Prediction of pre-emergence changes in pathogen dynamics in animals may hold the greatest potential of early detection in humans, and is therefore a central goal of EID surveillance [13]. A major challenge however, is the collection of appropriate data on animal health/behaviour [14]. For livestock populations, veterinarians may serve as an important source of information. However, using veterinary clinical diagnoses instead of results from diagnostic laboratory tests, the traditional data source in animal health surveillance, carries similar inherent risks to novel data sources in human surveillance systems: false alarms and unknown baseline variations.

There have been rapid advances in the development of appropriate methods of analysis for surveillance data [5,15–16]. The detection of clusters in time [17], space [18], and space-time [19–20] are now routine analysis run in many surveillance systems (e.g., Heffernan et al. [21]). The majority of methods for cluster detection can be classified as hypothesis tests that evaluate the risk of some disease or syndrome within a subset defined by space/time, against some expected value estimated to be the normal state of the process. An alternate class of methods focuses on estimation of the expected value using statistical models. A modelling approach can incorporate known demographic risk factors such as age and occupation, or environmental risks such as sources of pollution that affect disease outcomes. Models have been used widely in influenza surveillance to account for seasonal dynamics [22], as well as long-term trends in retrospective analysis of chronic diseases [23].

Hidden Markov models (HMM) have recently been developed for disease surveillance applications [24–29]. A Markov model can be used to examine the probability of transition from one state (e.g., normal variation) to another state (e.g., abnormal variation). In a hidden Markov modeling framework, the data are related to a discrete-valued unobserved Markov process, and the dynamics of this latent process are inferred from the observed data. In disease surveillance applications, it is typical to assume that the latent process is a first-order Markov chain, with the values or states of this chain relating to mixture components corresponding to separate distributions for the observed data. (e.g., counts from separately parameterized Poisson distributions). In health surveillance applications, these states can represent the overall condition of the target population such as 'endemic' and 'epidemic', or 'normal' and 'flu season'. A transition probability matrix governs transitions between the states over time. An advantage of HMMs for surveillance is that historical data are not required to train the model. Inferences about each of the states

can be learned directly from available data, and in a Bayesian setting, the prior distributions. This is an attractive feature for new surveillance systems with short durations that lack baseline data.

In the first application of HMMs to surveillance, Le Strat and Carrat [24] demonstrated a Poisson HMM for poliomyelitis that estimated weekly counts of cases at the national level as a mixture of two Poisson distributions. Recent examples of HMMs being used in disease surveillance include healthy and unhealthy states related to health services utilization from medical insurance data [28] and outbreak and non-outbreak states of influenza [25].

In this paper, we report on a study investigating baseline patterns in an animal-based infectious disease surveillance system in Sri Lanka [8]. Data were collected for a period of a year describing clinical diagnoses of cattle, buffalo and poultry, in 4 regions of Sri Lanka. Field veterinary surgeons employed by the Department of Animal Production and Health submitted surveys via mobile phone to a central database. As these data describe syndromes and diagnoses not formerly tracked in Sri Lanka, there are no validation data available. We employ a modelling approach to examine different features of the data using hidden Markov models [24]. The objectives of the current study were to determine the sources of variation in animal-based EID surveillance in Sri Lanka, establish baseline rates for overall surveys, and explore spatial and temporal variability in commonly reported cattle diseases.

Methods

Data Sources

The Infectious Disease Surveillance and Analysis System (IDSAS) was established in January 2009 as part of a collaboration between the authors and the Department of Animal Production and Health in Sri Lanka [8]. The system tracked syndromes and clinical diagnoses in cattle, buffalo, and poultry, in four districts of Sri Lanka. Forty government-employed field veterinary surgeons (FVS) from four administrative districts (Figure 1) participated as data collectors using mobile phone-based surveys coupled with global positioning systems (GPS). FVSs were instructed to submit surveys via email to a central surveillance database for every encounter with one of the target species. The data used in the present study represent the period January 1st 2009 to December 31, 2009, and the average monthly submission rate was approximately 11 surveys per month per FVS. All data obtained from farm and clinic visits made by veterinarians participating in the project remained the sole property of the Sri Lanka Department of Animal Production and Health and were used by the authors with full consent for research purposes.

Each survey submitted by a FVS represented one visit to a farm or one examination in clinic of at least one of the three species. Surveys were classified by routine visits (yes/no) and presence or absence of an animal health issue. In the case of an animal health issue, cases were given a syndrome group and a clinical diagnosis. FVSs also had the option of classifying the cause of the health issue as unknown. There were a total of 17 syndrome groups for cattle and buffalo and 11 for poultry. Options for suspected diagnoses were based on the syndromic grouping selected. For example, under "lameness", possible diagnoses included Blackquarter, Footrot, Osteomyelitis, as well as 22 others. Each FVS was responsible for one geographic area called a range, so geographic locations could be associated with each survey. Farm-level spatial data collected with GPS were not used in this analysis, as we were primarily interested in determining broad-scale sources and patterns of variation in the IDSAS data.

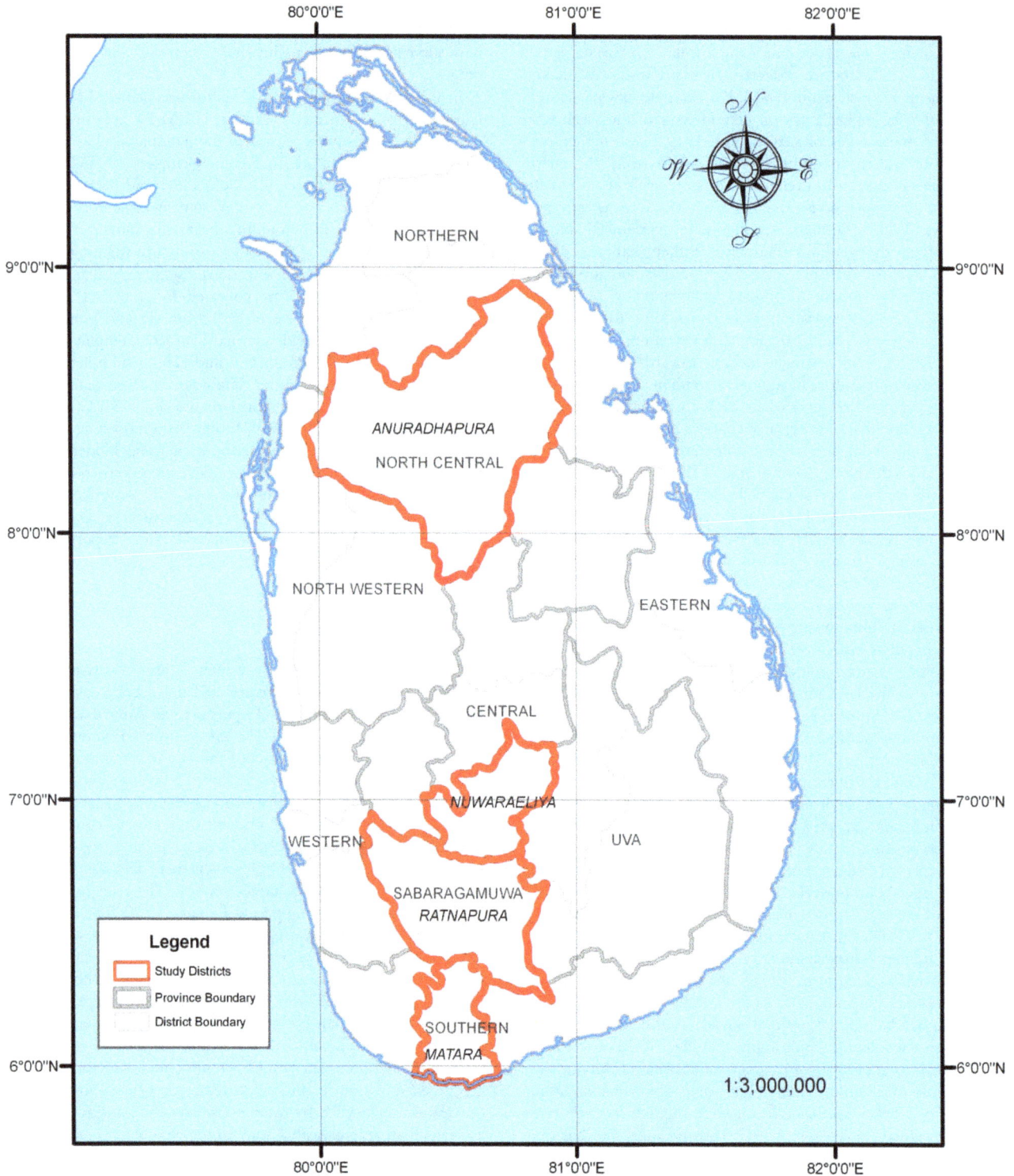

Figure 1. Study Area Map. Map of Sri Lanka and study districts that were part of the Infectious Disease Surveillance and Analysis System.

Auxiliary data were collected to help account for non-disease variation in IDSAS data. FVS-specific information such as sex and the number of years since graduation from veterinary school was collected when the FVS was enrolled in the project. There were also specific dates when re-training was conducted and indicator variables were used to represent these periods. The retraining sessions increased enthusiasm and participation levels of the FVSs as sharp increases in submissions were noted in exploratory analysis of the data [8]. These factors represent what we term a *sentinel process*; factors related to the FVS as disease sentinels, rather than disease.

We obtained monthly temperature and precipitation data as district averages from the Sri Lankan Department of Meteorology as disease patterns in animals are often seasonal and may therefore exhibit a relationship with local weather patterns or seasons.

Analysis of Surveillance Data

In this study, we model animal health conditions as seen by FVSs in Sri Lanka. We extend on the spatial Poisson HMM for disease surveillance given in Watkins et al. [29], by simultaneously accounting for covariates (described above) impacting the observed data. The data collected by IDSAS can be conceptualized as arising from two independent processes, the *sentinel process*, and the *disease process* (Figure 2). We were interested in accounting for variability related to the sentinel process, in order to learn more about variability related to disease during the study.

To formulate our model, we let Y_{it} denote the observed number of submissions to the IDSAS system during week t by FVS i. Underlying each observed count Y_{it} is a latent variable S_{it} taking one of two values, with $S_{it} = 1$ corresponding to 'normal' conditions and $S_{it} = 2$ corresponding to 'abnormal' conditions. We conceptualize 'normal' as the baseline and 'abnormal' as higher than baseline numbers of submissions. Conditioning on the latent state S_{it} we assume the data are independently drawn from a Poisson distribution

$$y_{it}|S_{it} \sim Pois(\lambda_{S_{it}}) \qquad (1)$$

with λ_1 being the mean number of submissions in the normal state, and λ_2 the mean in the abnormal state (i.e., $\lambda_2 > \lambda_1$). The sequence of states occupied by the FVS i over time is represented through the vector $\mathbf{S}_i = (S_{1i,...}\ S_{Ti})'$ and we assume each such sequence evolves from its initial state S_{1i}, according to a first-order homogeneous Markov chain so that $Pr\{S_{it}|S_{it-1}, S_{it-2},...,S_{i1}\} = Pr\{S_{it}|S_{it-1}\}$. The dynamics of this latent Markov model are governed by three unknown parameters: P_{Init} an initial state probability governing the distribution of S_{1i}, and two transition probabilities P_{12} and P_{21}, which represent the rates of transition between the normal and abnormal states. Following the parameterization in Watkins et al. [29], a Dirichlet prior

Table 1. Description of prior distributions and hyper-parameters for model parameters.

Model	Parameter	Prior Distribution	Description
HMM$_{1,2}$	μ_1	Normal(0,0.01)*	Mean state 1
HMM$_{1,2}$	μ_2	Normal(0,0.01)*	Mean state 2
HMM$_{1,2}$	P_{Init}	Dirichlet(0.5,0.5)	Initial Probability
HMM$_{1,2}$	P	Beta(0.5,0.5)	Probability transition matrix
HMM$_{1,2}$	Y	Poisson(λ)	Observed count data
HMM$_2$	X	Normal(0,0.001)*	Covariate coefficients

*Parameterized as mean and precision (1/variance, as in WinBUGS). For disease-level models, a *Normal*(0,10) prior was used to accommodate very small expected counts.

distribution for initial probabilities, and Beta prior distributions on subsequent probabilities were employed. An outline of prior distributions for model parameters is given in Table 1. In what follows we shall denote this five parameter model (λ_1, λ_2, P_{Init}, P_{12}, P_{21}) for total submissions as HMM$_1$.

This model can be extended through the incorporation of covariates and this is typically done in one of two ways. First, we can allow the covariates to model variation in the Poisson parameters corresponding to the normal and abnormal states, where stationary between-state transition probabilities are assumed. Alternatively, covariates can be incorporated into an HMM via the transition probability matrix itself [30], resulting in an inhomogeneous HMM. For example, Wall and Li [28] present a HMM for medical service utilization data where covariates relate to transitions between healthy and unhealthy states via a logistic regression. In the model here, the former approach is adopted, maintaining stationary transition probabilities. Covariates were included in the model by relating each Poisson mean to a state-dependent baseline rate $\mu_{S_{it}}$, and a vector of FVS (i.e. spatial)

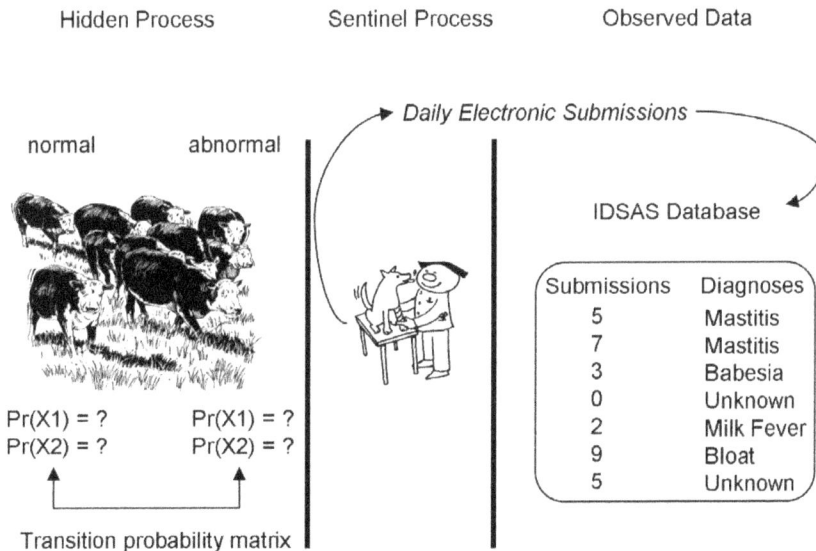

Hidden Process   Sentinel Process   Observed Data

Figure 2. Data Generating Processes. Conceptual model of data generating processes in the Infectious Disease Surveillance and Analysis System in the context of hidden markov models. The hidden states of interest are the normal or abnormal state of animal health as seen by field veterinary surgeons. Observed data may include weekly submission counts, or counts of specific reported diagnoses.

and time specific covariates X, via a log-link Poisson regression:

$$\log(\lambda_{it}) = \mu_{s_{it}} + \beta X_{it} \qquad (2)$$

where β is the corresponding vector of regression coefficients which is assumed constant between the two states. The baseline rate, or intercept, is 'switched' between the normal and abnormal states based on the current state of the Markov chain.

The inclusion of covariates allows for spatial information to be included in the model. The four districts in which IDSAS operated were selected primarily to capture variation in environment, climate, and agricultural practices. For true outbreaks of disease or changes in pattern of disease, we might expect similar submissions among FVSs in the same district. To account for similarity of conditions within district versus other districts, submissions from FVSs in common districts were summed. The count y_{it} of submissions for FVS i at time t was added to counts for all FVS in the same district.

$$y_{it}* = \sum_{\substack{j=1 \\ j \neq i}}^{40} y_{jt-1} D_{ij} \qquad (3)$$

where D_{ij} is an $n \times n$ matrix with 1 s indicating FVSs in the same district and 0 otherwise. This information was included in a temporally lagged variable, representing the count of district wide submissions in the previous time period. We report results for the model with covariates included as HMM$_2$.

All models were run on the individual submission counts to generate an understanding of the factors affecting the IDSAS data. To investigate the patterns of individual diseases, the four most frequently reported suspected diagnoses in cattle were investigated. Cattle are one of the primary livestock species assessed and treated by FVSs in Sri Lanka and as such constituted the majority of submissions. For the disease-specific models, covariate effects for sentinel-level variables were taken from estimates from the total submissions model, as we expect to these be constant factors effecting submissions equally. Disease-related variables (temperature, precipitation, and temporally lagged district-wide submissions) were estimated separately for each disease. Additionally, because natural disease prevalence varies by district, each district has separate mean rates for normal and abnormal states.

Models were implemented in a Bayesian setting with posterior distributions sampled using Markov chain Monte Carlo (MCMC) with implementation in WinBUGS [31]. Bayesian modelling is a convenient choice for developing HMMs as sensitivity to distributional assumptions can be easily assessed, and a full probability distribution is obtained for model parameters in the posterior distribution. In all analyses, two parallel MCMC chains were run for a 1000 iteration burn-in period followed by a production run of 4000 iterations. Convergence of the samplers to the corresponding stationary distributions was assessed using both visual inspection of the posterior sampling history, and the Gelman-Rubin statistic [32].

Model goodness-of-fit was evaluated using posterior predictive checking [33]. Simulated draws from the posterior distribution P(theta|Y) of model parameters were used to simulate replicate data sets Y^{rep} from the posterior predictive distribution P(Y^{rep}|Y), which were used to compute the deviance (P[Y^{rep}|theta]; computed as $-2*$ log-likelihood) for each of 999 posterior and predictive draws. The deviance was then computed for the observed data, and the proportion of pairs (P[Y|theta], P[Y^{rep}|theta]) where P[Y^{rep}|theta]>P[Y|theta] is the posterior predictive p-value. Here, extreme p-values (i.e., 0.05>p>0.95) yield evidence of a poorly fitting model.

Results for the state variable are reported for two thresholds. The posterior mean state for each FVS/week pair (a total 2080) yield values ranging from 1.0 for 'normal' to 2.0 for 'abnormal' and values in between. We set a lower threshold of 1.50 to define membership in state two, and an upper threshold of 2.00. In all modelling results reported, coefficients with 95% credible intervals covering zero are excluded.

Simulation Study

A simulation study was developed to evaluate model performance. Data from two Poisson models were simulated onto a 10×10 spatial grid representing disease-reporting units in a hypothetical surveillance system (n = 100). Three covariates were also simulated for each area. The normal state (i.e., state 1) Poisson model was as follows

$$\lambda_{it} = \exp(1.8 + 1.3X_1 + 3X_2) \qquad (4)$$

and the abnormal state model (i.e., state 2) was

$$\lambda_{it} = \exp(2.7 + 1.3X_1 + 3X_2) \qquad (5)$$

Relationships for covariates X_1 and X_2 were the same between states but the intercept shifted from 1.8 during the normal state to 2.7 in the abnormal state. The purpose of the model is to detect shifts in state based on observations and simultaneously characterize the relationships between the mean and the covariate variables. We also evaluated whether the model could determine different covariate effects in different states, by changing the abnormal state model to include a third covariate:

$$\lambda_{it} = \exp(2.7 + 1.3X_1 + 3X_2 - 1.6X_3) \qquad (6)$$

In the simulation study analysis, spatial information (neighborhood relationships) was not used, but could easily be incorporated through a conditional autoregressive random effect, pooling observations from neighbouring areas, or including region-specific dummy variables.

The normal state model was used to generate counts for 52 time periods (i.e., one year at weekly intervals) based on a normal distribution with a mean determined by Equation 4 and a standard deviation of 1. Different types of spatial patterns (outbreaks 1–5, see Figure 3) were created to establish areas where counts were replaced with counts estimated from the abnormal state model (Equation 5). Thus distinct spatial areas and time periods where counts and covariates in state two were created against a baseline of state one. In the second scenario, estimates for the abnormal state were obtained from Equation 6. Model performance was then evaluated as the percentage of correctly classified states.

Results

Simulation Study

The HMM model correctly classified 99.7% of the observations in the shifted intercept scenario. Out of 5100 (51 time periods×100 spatial units) observations (first week is not used because inference is based totally on initial values), 5088 were classified with the correct state. The 12 incorrectly classified states all occurred in outbreak five (see Figure 3), where all units were in the abnormal state, so all were errors of omission (i.e., incorrectly

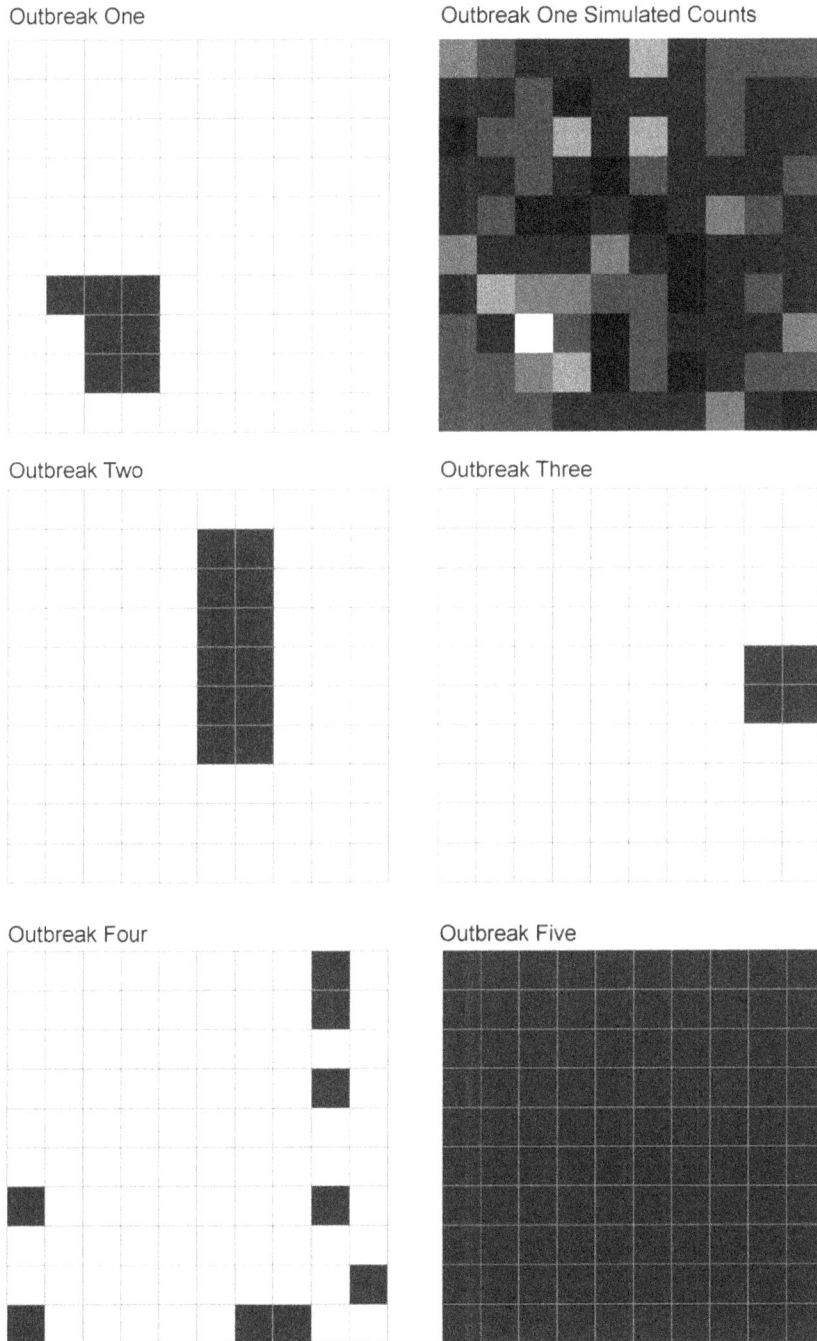

Figure 3. Simulated outbreak patterns in a hypothetical surveillance system. White cells generated under model for state one, and black cells generated under model for state two. The count data that was simulated using outbreak one is also shown: dark colours indicate low counts and lighter colours indicate high counts.

classified as normal). The coefficient estimates were similar to the true values for both variables, though the mean for the normal state was slightly underestimated (Table 2). In contrast, in the scenario with shifted mean and the addition of a third covariate effect in the abnormal state model, the model failed to converge completely. Posterior estimates for the intercept and covariate $X1$ were similar and converged (not reported), however estimates for coefficients on $X2$ and $X3$ both failed to converge. The model was run for 20,000 iterations. Convergence problems may be related to model identification issues, and these issues need further

investigation, but are not uncommon with Bayesian mixture models employing weakly-informative priors.

Animal Health Surveillance Submission Patterns

During the study period, there were a total of 5758 submissions to the IDSAS system that reported an animal health issue. The HMM_1 without covariates yielded a total of 753 abnormal events during the study period based on a posterior mean threshold of greater than 1.5. When constrained to a higher degree of certainty (posterior mean threshold of 2.00), the number of abnormal events

Table 2. Model results from simulation study for five different outbreak scenarios occurring during a 52 week simulated surveillance system.

Parameter	True value	Posterior mean (95% credible interval)
μ_1	1.80	1.73 (1.71, 1.74)
μ_2	2.70	2.66 (2.63, 2.69)
$X1$	1.30	1.42 (1.29, 1.54)
$X2$	3.00	3.13 (3.03, 3.25)

was 390 (Table 3). The mean submission rate for state one was 0.45 (sd = 0.10) submissions per FVS, per week, and in abnormal periods the mean rate was 6.72 (sd = 0.05). When covariates were added to the model (HMM$_2$), the number of abnormal events increased to 870 and 450 for the two threshold levels, while mean rates adjusted to 0.34 (sd = 0.10) and 6.65(sd = 0.10) submissions per FVS, per week for state one and two respectively. Covariate effects are reported in Table 3. Positive association with submission rates was limited to the variable indicating training periods, while covariates identifying male and less experienced FVS were negatively associated with submissions. Precipitation, temperature, and district reports had no effect in the total submissions model. The temporal patterns of abnormal events relative to all submission counts for each FVS are outlined in Figure 4. Using the upper threshold, the submission counts for state one ranged from zero to six, and from four to 103 for state two. The count densities plotted on a log scale are presented in Figure 5. Posterior predictive model checking did not reveal strong evidence indicating a lack of fit, with an overall posterior predictive p-value of 0.13 obtained for the deviance goodness-of-fit measure.

Commonly Reported Cattle Diseases

In total, there were 3943 reported cattle cases during the study period. The most commonly reported diagnoses in cattle were mastitis (543), ephemeral fever (234), babesiosis (212), and milk fever (210). Monthly cases for each of the districts are given in Figure 6, along with environmental variables maximum temperature and total monthly precipitation.

Model results for the four most common diagnoses are outlined in Table 4. As noted earlier, coefficients for sentinel-level variables were set as estimated in the total-submission model, and only covariate effects for temperature, precipitation, and district reports were estimated for disease-level models. Overall, the effects of the covariate variables in disease-level models were minimal, with rate

Table 3. Submission pattern model parameter estimates reported as rate ratios.

Parameter	Posterior mean (95% credible interval)	Standard deviation
μ_1	0.34 (0.28–0.41)	0.10
μ_2	6.65 (6.05–7.29)	0.05
Training	1.19 (1.08–1.32)	0.05
Years	0.59 (0.55–0.63)	0.03
Male	0.90 (0.84–0.96)	0.03

ratios ranging from 0.93 to 1.10. Temperature was positively associated with reported diagnoses of all diseases. Precipitation was not associated with diagnoses of any of the four diagnoses. Temporally lagged district reports were negatively associated with mastitis, babesiosis, and milk fever, and positively associated with ephemeral fever.

The posterior mean states are presented in Figure 7 for each of the four main disease categories. A possible outbreak of ephemeral fever is evident in Anuradhapura towards the end of the study period. Other periods of high submissions for babesiosis, milk fever, and mastitis are found in the Nuwara Eliya district.

Discussion

Variation was modelled in data submitted to a mobile-phone based infectious disease surveillance system in Sri Lanka. Results indicate that submission varied according sentinel level factors, and that HMMs are a convenient methodology to approach novel sources of surveillance data. The average submission rate for surveys varied by district, ranging from 0.34 surveys per week during normal periods to in 6.34 surveys per week during abnormal periods. The number of abnormally high submissions increased when covariates were added to the model. Baseline estimates for normal patterns of mastitis, babesiosis, and milk fever were highest in Nuwara Eliya, the main cattle-dairy region in Sri Lanka. The baseline estimate for the normal pattern of ephemeral fever was highest in Anuradhapura, a region that experiences seasonal droughts.

The number of new pathogens in animals and humans are increasing and known infections are changing in pattern as natural and social systems adapt to changes in climate. The role of animals in emergence of new diseases is widely recognized [4], and surveillance of EIDs via animal-based systems such as IDSAS holds potential for detection and response at an early stage, yet studying this in the absence of an actual EID is a major challenge. While detecting an EID was the goal of the IDSAS system, enhanced understanding of the pathogen distribution as seen by veterinarians in the field represents an opportunity to both establish what is normal, and subsequently detect patterns that are unusual. This alone may be enough information to develop processes to inspire further action and promote early detection [34]. Further, the improved timeliness of IDSAS data as compared to laboratory testing is another attractive feature of using clinical diagnoses data for EID surveillance.

As this analysis has demonstrated, there are complex variations driving surveillance data using novel sources such as field-based veterinary surveys. In Sri Lanka, sentinel process factors such as the sex and work experience of the submitter impacted submission rates, as did periodic disruptions due to training and/or political events. The advantage of a modelling perspective to surveillance is that these sources of variation can be partitioned out in order to generate a finer understanding of the disease process. Previous analysis [8] using a subset of this data using the cumulative sum statistic on aggregated weekly submission counts, detected 'outbreaks' during the end of July and August (~wk 30-31-38). In the model outputs here, it is evident that the high submissions during this period was confined largely to Nuwara Eliya. The model here provides greater geographical and temporal granularity while accounting for sentinel-specific non-outbreak variation. However, there is also value in learning about the sentinel process. This type of methodology could be used within ongoing surveillance systems to identify demographic characteristics more common amongst high submitters, and therefore serve to inform the sentinel selection process and ongoing sentinel inclusion or

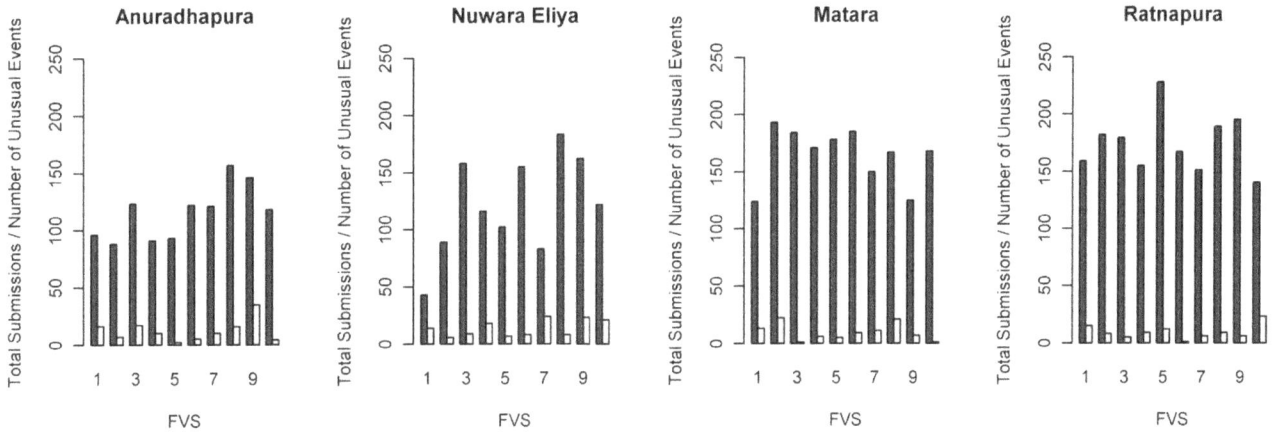

Figure 4. Submission counts and the number of unusual states per veterinarian. Total weekly submissions to the Infectious Disease Surveillance and Analysis System during the study period and the number of unusual states, by field veterinary surgeon and district. The number of weeks in state one (normal) is indicated in dark grey and the number of abnormal events in white.

exclusion. In addition, exploration of the factors driving temporal variation in submissions can help to guide sentinel retraining and electronic prompts reminding sentinels to submit data.

When examining the results of the model HMM_1 on total submissions, we note a high number of abnormal events. When variables are included in HMM_2, the overall effect of the important variables actually reduces expected mean submissions, which results in more 'unusual' events. The question becomes, what is the value of accounting for sentinel-level factors. Given that alerts generated by surveillance systems typically overwhelm the number that can actually be investigated [35], should adjustments be biased downwards? The analysis here suggests that adjustments are useful because they provide a more complete understanding of the processes generating the surveillance data. In the context of sentinels for disease surveillance, this might simply be helping to identify characteristics that predict a more engaged

Submission Density

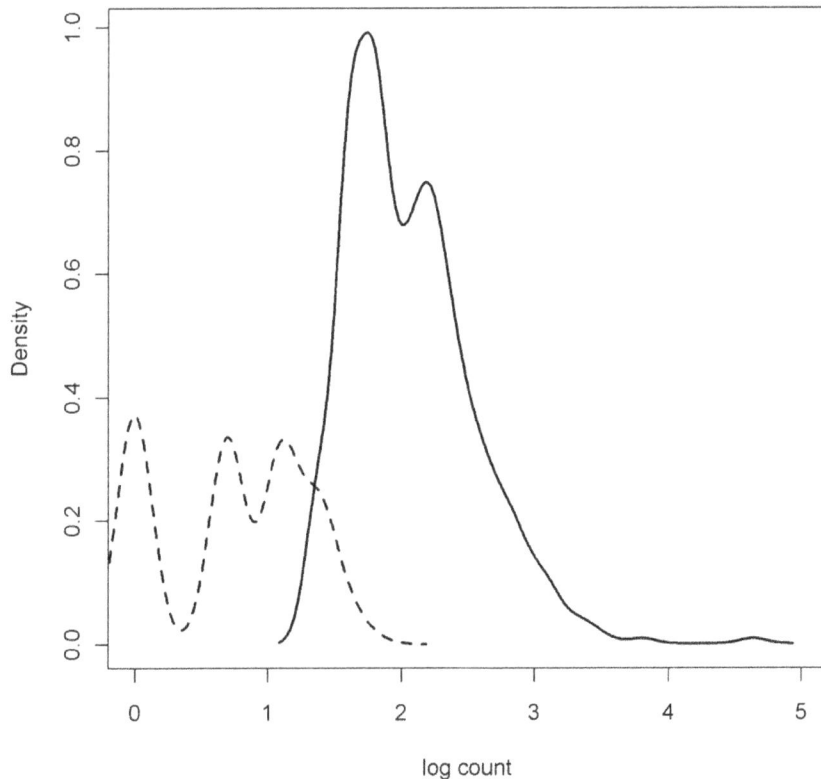

Figure 5. Submission count densities. Density of the log count of submissions in state one (dashed) and state two (solid).

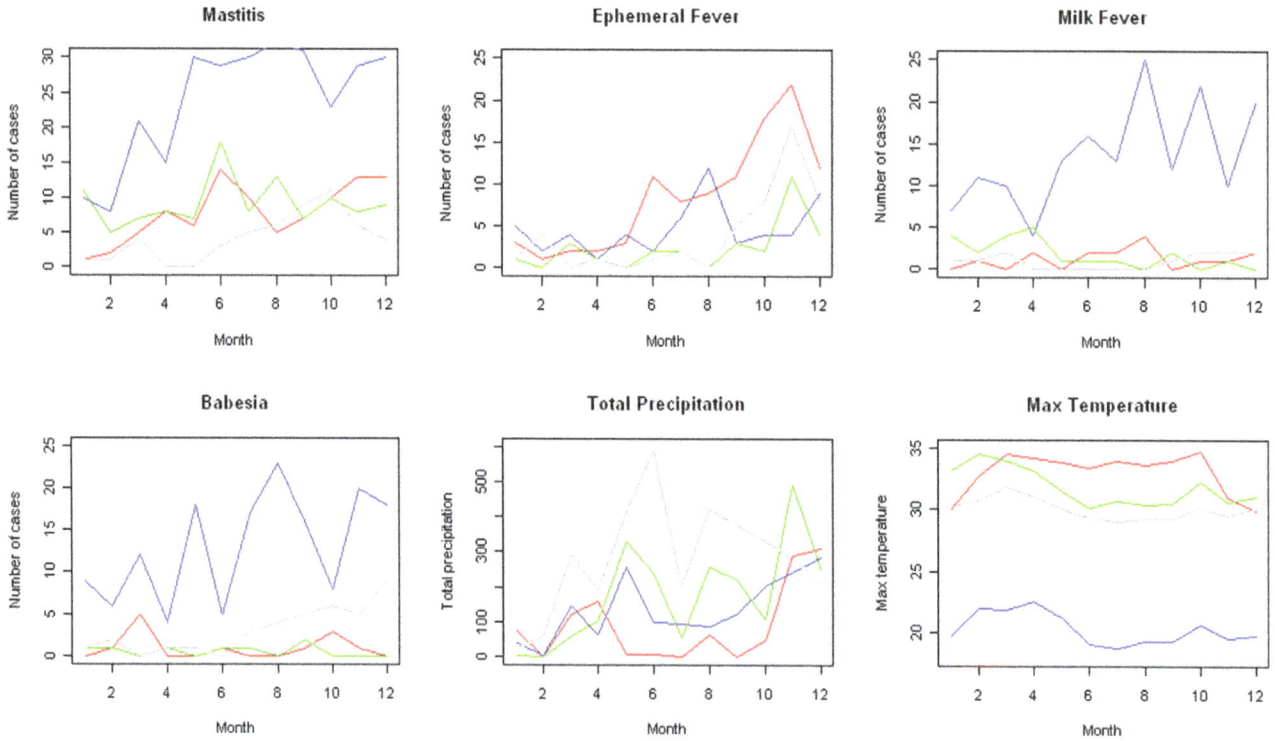

Figure 6. Monthly total cases for commonly reported diagnoses in each of the four districts. Anauradhapura (red), Nuwara Eliya (blue), Matara (green), and Ratnapura (grey). Monthly averages for district-wide total precipitation and maximum temperature.

sentinel relative to others. Another issue is that variables such as sex and experience may have an overall effect, but cannot be attributed to individuals. While states are discrete, state probabilities can be visualized across space and time as in Figure 7, providing visual evidence of gradual changes after covariates have been taken into account.

The simulation study presented here provides evidence that the model performs well under the scenario where a shift in the mean occurs and covariate effects remain fixed. In this simulation scenario, both the mean and covariate effects were recovered well by the model. This analysis lends support to the results obtained from IDSAS data. We might therefore be able to conclude overall, the means detected for each state-district combination in the disease-level models represent baseline estimates of the weekly prevalence of these diseases as seen by FVSs based on clinical diagnoses and syndromic groupings. However, the low values for these estimates (Table 4) make interpretation somewhat

cumbersome. The state one means for all four diseases range from 0.09 for babesiosis in Anuradhapura to 0.32 for milk fever in Nuwara Eliya, while state two means ranged from 0.63 for babesiosis in Matara, to 3.51 for babesiosis in Nuwara Eliya. It is important to quantify the differences in means between the districts for the different diseases as it provides a starting point from which to understand why these differences exist. The trade off between data volume and data scale is characteristic of all statistical analysis and especially impacts analysis of surveillance data.

In developing this technique we chose to examine the four most frequently suspected diagnoses in cattle. However there are marked differences between babesiosis and mastitis in terms of epidemiology, etiology, and clinical presentation that are worth highlighting. Babesiosis is a tick-borne disease most commonly characterized by fever, inappetence, lethargy, weakness, red-tinged urine (hemoglobinuria), anemia and jaundice, though many

Table 4. Model results for four commonly reported cattle diagnoses.

Model	Anura-dhapura		Nuwara Eliya		Matara		Ratnapura		Temp-erature	Precipi-tation	District Reports
	μ_1	μ_2	μ_1	μ_2	μ_1	μ_2	μ_1	μ_2			
Mastitis	0.22	1.00	0.30	3.48	0.19	1.15	0.12	1.07	1.10	1.00	0.96
Ephemeral Fever	0.22	1.04	0.11	1.34	0.10	0.81	0.09	1.67	1.04	1.00	1.04
Babesiosis	0.09	0.79	0.24	3.51	0.08	0.63	0.13	1.05	1.10	1.00	0.93
Milk Fever	0.10	0.76	0.32	2.51	0.10	0.87	0.09	0.78	1.06	1.00	0.93

Posterior mean estimates are per week, per field veterinary surgeon, reported as rate ratios. Maximum daily temperature and total precipitation are computed for each district and month. District reports are the number of cases within the district in the previous week.

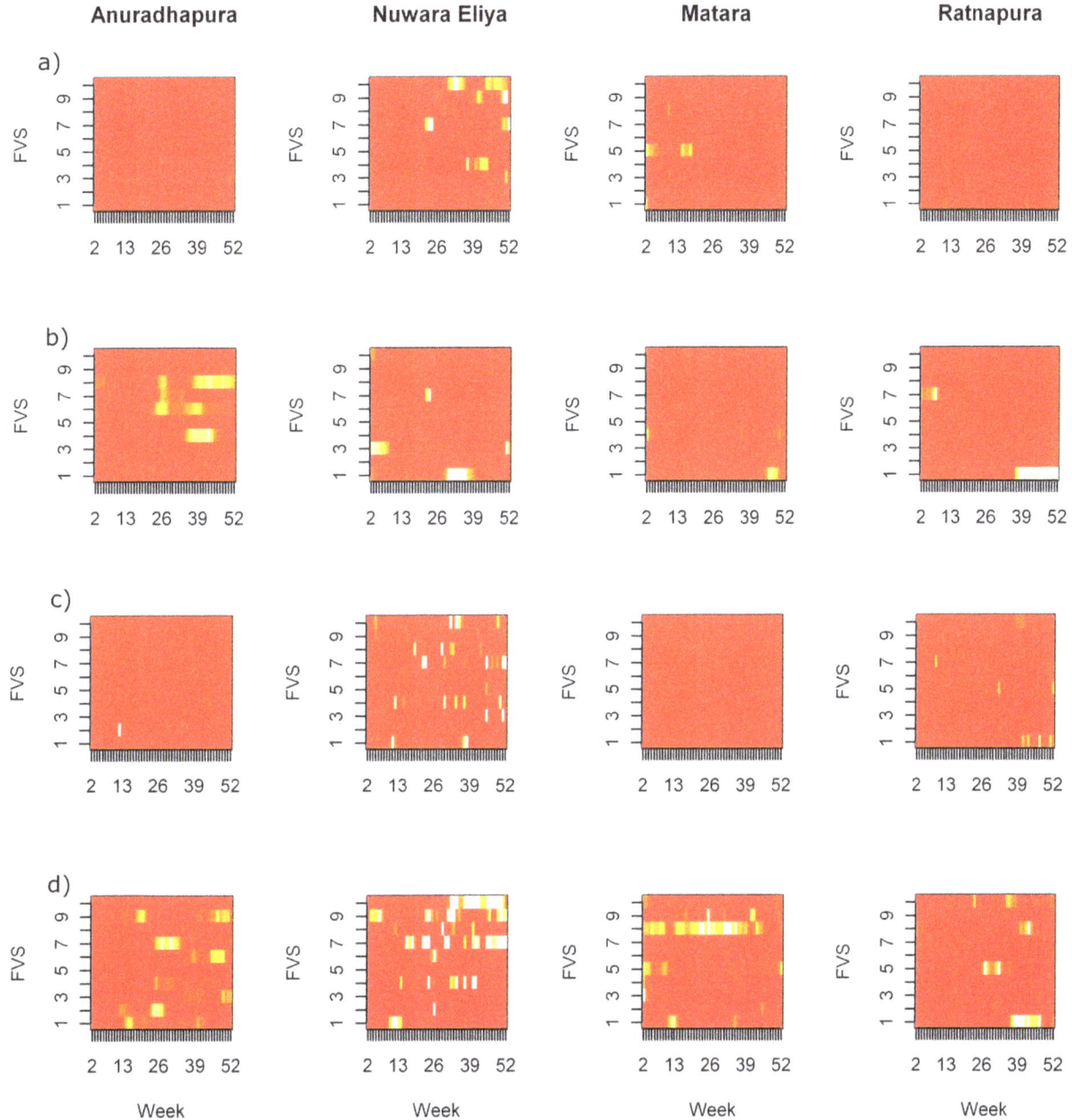

Figure 7. Posterior mean of the state variable. The model-adjusted posterior mean state for each field veterinarian surgeon by week, in each of the study districts for commonly reported cattle diagnoses. Red indicates state one and white indicates state two, and yellow intermediate values for a) Milk Fever, b) Ephemeral Fever, c) Babesiosis, and d) Mastits.

cases are asymptomatic. Recovered cases become asymptomatic carriers, and duration of infection can be up to years. There is a large degree of variability in susceptibility between cattle breeds. Transmission of babesiosis is dependent on a bite from an infected Ixodes tick, and patterns in disease prevalence in cattle are dependent in part upon the prevalence of Babesia spp. in the vector and in the prevalence of the tick species itself [36]. In contrast, mastitis, defined simply as inflammation of the udder, can be caused by a variety of bacterial and fungal pathogens. It is often characterized by a drop in milk production, and when clinically evident may be accompanied by gross changes to milk or systemic illness. It can be caused by both contagious and environmental pathogens. Incidence and prevalence is impacted

by a variety of individual animal characteristics, as well as environmental variables. Given these differences, it is worth considering whether examination of their occurrence using the same method is appropriate, and whether covariates should be fixed across suspected diagnoses.

Visualizing the probability of state two in Figure 7 on a FVS/ weekly basis provides some evidence for the stability and confidence in the model inferences. The outbreak of ephemeral fever in Anuradhapura is on face value, more unusual, than for example patterns of mastitis in Nuwara Eliya. This is because based on what we know about ephemeral fever, transmitted by biting insects and often highly correlated with periods of rain, we expect, and are more concerned with 'outbreaks', than for mastitis, which is an endemic and pervasive condition. However, outbreak levels of mastitis may in fact represent clusters which also represent another, possibly unknown pathogen. The goal is to understand and establish the normal pattern for the population, so that unusual events can be quickly spotted and explored.

The reliability of inference in a models based framework will depend on the adequacy of the modeling assumptions, in practice, there are invariably important missing variables, and relationships often change over time in unforeseen ways. There are important limitations to the study that should be noted. Firstly, there exists the possibility of selection bias in our models. As we relied on farmers to report cases to veterinarians, perceived negative repercussions of reporting a severe or unusual disease could lead to underreporting of these types of cases by farmers. This would skew our data towards common and non-epidemic diseases. A second source of potential selection bias relates to the use of government veterinarians as data providers: while FVSs are significant animal health care providers, there are also private veterinary clinics in Sri Lanka, and commercial operations sometimes employ their own veterinarians. Cases assessed by private veterinary practitioners were not captured by the IDSAS

system. Another limitation of the data is that biotic risk factors such as density dependence and interactions with wildlife were not tracked. These represent important drivers of zoonoses emergence. Going forward we hope to identify data sources that will help factor in these processes into our modelling approach.

Visualizing patterns of the state variable over time provides a quick diagnostic tool to identify changes in pattern. Also, because we are working within a Bayesian setting and have a full distribution for model parameters, we can make similar plots for the posterior uncertainty using posterior standard deviation. The modelling analysis here offers a robust framework for analysis of surveillance data with short temporal spans and multiple processes driving submissions, as is often the case with participant-generated data.

Author Contributions

Conceived and designed the experiments: CR KS FN. Performed the experiments: CR WG. Analyzed the data: CR WG. Contributed reagents/materials/analysis tools: TN CS FN. Wrote the paper: CR. Data collection: CR KS WG.

References

1. Greger M (2007) The human/animal interface: emergence and resurgence of zoonotic infectious diseases. Crit Rev Microbiol 33: 243–299.
2. Jones KE, Patel NG, Levy MA, Storeygard A, Balk D, et al. (2008) Global trends in emerging infectious diseases. Nature 451: 990–993.
3. Haydon DT, Cleaveland S, Taylor LH, Laurenson MK (2002) Identifying reservoirs of infection: a conceptual and practical challenge. Emerg Infect Dis 8: 1468–1473.
4. Rabinowitz P, MacGarr LO, Dein FJ (2008) From "us vs. them" to "shared risk": can animals help link environmental factors to human health? Eco Health 5: 224–229.
5. Lawson AB, Kleinman K, eds. Spatial and syndromic surveillance for public health. West Sussex: John Wiley. 284 p.
6. Van Metre DC, Barkey DQ, Salman MD, Morley PS (2009) Development of a syndromic surveillance system for detection of disease among livestock entering an auction market. J Am Vet Med Assoc 234: 658–664.
7. Leblond A, Hendrikx P, Sabatier P (2007) West Nile virus outbreak detection using syndromic monitoring in horses. Vector-Borne Zoonot 7: 403–410.
8. Robertson C, Sawford K, Daniel SLA, Nelson TA, Stephen C (2010) Mobile surveillance system, Sri Lanka. Emerg Infect Dis 15: 1524–1531.
9. Stoto MA, Schonlau M, Mariano LT (2004) Syndromic surveillance: is it worth the effort? Chance 17: 19–24.
10. Das D, Metzger K, Heffernan R, Balter S, Weiss D, et al. (2005) Monitoring over-the-counter medication sales for early detection of disease outbreaks—New York City. MMWR Morb Mortal Wkly Rep 54: 41–46.
11. Hulth A, Rydevik G, Linde A (2009) Web queries as a source for syndromic surveillance. PloS one 4: e4378.
12. Mostashari F, Fine A, Das D, Adams J, Layton M (2003) Use of ambulance dispatch data as an early warning system for communitywide influenzalike illness, New York City. J Urban Health 80: i43–i49.
13. Kahn LH (2006) Confronting zoonoses, linking human and veterinary medicine. Emerg Infect Dis 12: 556–561.
14. Vrbova L, Stephen C, Kasman N, Boehnke R, Doyle-Waters M, et al. (2010) Systematic review of surveillance systems for emerging zoonoses. Transbound Emerg Dis 57: 154–161.
15. Wagner MM, Moore AW, Aryel RM (2006) Handbook of Biosurveillance. London: Elsevier. 624 p.
16. Sonesson C, Bock D (2003) A review and discussion of prospective statistical surveillance in public health. J R Stat Soc Ser A Stat Soc 166: 5–21.
17. Naus JI (1965) The distribution of the size of the maximum cluster of points on a line. J Am Stat Assoc 60: 532–538.
18. Kulldorff M, Nagarwalla N (1995) Spatial disease clusters: detection and inference. Stat Med 14: 799–810.
19. Kulldorff M (2001) Prospective time periodic geographical disease surveillance using a scan statistic. J R Stat Soc Ser A Stat Soc 164: 61–72.
20. Kulldorff M, Heffernan R, Hartman J, Assuncao RM, Mostashari F (2005) A space-time permutation scan statistic for disease outbreak detection. PLoS Med 2: e59.
21. Heffernan R, Mostashari F, Das D, Karpati A, Kulldorff M, et al. (2004) Syndromic surveillance in public health practice, New York City. Emerg Infect Dis 10: 858–64.
22. Andersson E, Bock D, Frisen M (2008) Modeling influenza incidence for the purpose of on-line monitoring. Stat Methods Med Res 17: 421–438.
23. Xia H, Carlin BP (1998) Spatio-temporal models with errors in covariates: mapping Ohio lung cancer mortality. Stat Med 17: 2025–2043.
24. Le Strat Y, Carrat F (1999) Monitoring epidemiologic surveillance data using hidden Markov models. Stat Med 18: 3463–3478.
25. Rath T, Carreras M, Sebastiani P (2003) Automated detection of influenza epidemics with Hidden Markov Models. Cryptographic Hardware and Embedded Systems-CHES 2003. pp 521–532.
26. Madigan D (2005) Bayesian data mining for health surveillance. In: Lawson AB, Kleinman K, eds. Spatial and syndromic surveillance for public health. West Sussex: John Wiley. pp 203–221.
27. Martínez-Beneito MA, Conesa D, López-Quílez A, López-Maside A (2008) Bayesian Markov switching models for the early detection of influenza epidemics. Stat Med 27: 4455–4468.
28. Wall MM, Li R (2009) Multiple indicator hidden Markov model with an application to medical utilization data. Stat Med 28: 293–310.
29. Watkins R, Eagleson S, Veenendaal B, Wright G, Plant A (2009) Disease surveillance using a hidden Markov model. BMC Med Inform Decis Mak 9: e39.
30. Zucchini W, MacDonald IL (2009) Hidden Markov Models for Time Series: An Introduction Using R. Boca Raton: Chapman & Hall/CRC. 275 p.
31. Lunn DJ, Thomas A, Best N, Spiegelhalter D (2000) WinBUGS - A Bayesian modelling framework: Concepts, structure, and extensibility. Stat Comput 10: 325–337.
32. Gelman A, Rubin DB (1992) Inference from iterative simulation using multiple sequences. Stat Sci 7: 457–472.
33. Gelman A, Carlin JB, Stern HS, Rubin DB (2004) Bayesian data analysis. Boca Raton: Chapman & Hall/CRC. 668 p.
34. Gubernot DM, Boyer BL, Moses MS (2008) Animals as Early Detectors of Bioevents: Veterinary tools and a framework for animal-human integrated zoonotic disease surveillance. Public Health Rep 123: 300–315.
35. Fearnley L (2008) Signals come and go: syndromic surveillance and styles of biosecurity. Environ Plan A 40: 1615–1632.
36. Bock R, Jackson L, De Vos A, Jorgensen W (2004) Babesiosis of cattle. Parasitology 129: S247–S269.

5

Neutering Dogs: Effects on Joint Disorders and Cancers in Golden Retrievers

Gretel Torres de la Riva[1], Benjamin L. Hart[2]*, Thomas B. Farver[1], Anita M. Oberbauer[3], Locksley L. McV Messam[4], Neil Willits[5], Lynette A. Hart[1]

1 Department of Population Health and Reproduction, School of Veterinary Medicine, University of California-Davis, Davis, California, United States of America,, 2 Department of Anatomy, Physiology and Cell Biology, School of Veterinary Medicine, University of California-Davis, Davis, California, United States of America, 3 Department of Animal Science, College of Agriculture and Environmental Sciences, University of California-Davis, Davis, California, United States of America, 4 Department of Public Health Sciences, School of Medicine, University of California-Davis, Davis, California, United States of America, 5 Statistics Laboratory, Department of Statistics, University of California-Davis, Davis, California, United States of America

Abstract

In contrast to European countries, the overwhelming majority of dogs in the U.S. are neutered (including spaying), usually done before one year of age. Given the importance of gonadal hormones in growth and development, this cultural contrast invites an analysis of the multiple organ systems that may be adversely affected by neutering. Using a single breed-specific dataset, the objective was to examine the variables of gender and age at the time of neutering versus leaving dogs gonadally intact, on all diseases occurring with sufficient frequency for statistical analyses. Given its popularity and vulnerability to various cancers and joint disorders, the Golden Retriever was chosen for this study. Veterinary hospital records of 759 client-owned, intact and neutered female and male dogs, 1–8 years old, were examined for diagnoses of hip dysplasia (HD), cranial cruciate ligament tear (CCL), lymphosarcoma (LSA), hemangiosarcoma (HSA), and mast cell tumor (MCT). Patients were classified as intact, or neutered early (<12 mo) or late (≥12 mo). Statistical analyses involved survival analyses and incidence rate comparisons. Outcomes at the 5 percent level of significance are reported. Of early-neutered males, 10 percent were diagnosed with HD, double the occurrence in intact males. There were no cases of CCL diagnosed in intact males or females, but in early-neutered males and females the occurrences were 5 percent and 8 percent, respectively. Almost 10 percent of early-neutered males were diagnosed with LSA, 3 times more than intact males. The percentage of HSA cases in late-neutered females (about 8 percent) was 4 times more than intact and early-neutered females. There were no cases of MCT in intact females, but the occurrence was nearly 6 percent in late-neutered females. The results have health implications for Golden Retriever companion and service dogs, and for oncologists using dogs as models of cancers that occur in humans.

Editor: Bart O. Williams, Van Andel Institute, United States of America

Funding: Supported by the Canine Health Foundation (#01488-A) and the Center for Companion 330 Animal Health University of California, Davis (# 2009-54-F/M). The funders had no role in study design, data collection and analysis, decision to publish, or preparation of the manuscript.

Competing Interests: The authors have declared that no competing interests exist.

* E-mail: blhart@ucdavis.edu

Introduction

The overwhelming majority of companion dogs maintained in the U.S. are spayed or castrated (both referred to herein as neutered) [1]. Increasingly in the U.S. neutering is being performed early, demarcated in the present study as prior to one year of age. The impetus for this widespread practice is presumably pet population control, and is generally considered responsible pet ownership. However, this societal practice in the U.S. contrasts with the general attitudes in many European countries, where neutering is commonly avoided and not generally promoted by animal health authorities. For example, a study of 461 dogs in Sweden reported that 99 percent of the dogs were gonadally intact [2], and an intact rate of 57 percent was reported in a Hungarian study [3]. In the United Kingdom, a 46 percent intact rate was reported [4].

In the last decade, studies have pointed to some of the adverse effects of neutering in dogs on several health parameters by looking at one disease syndrome in one breed or in pooling data from several breeds. With regard to cancers, a study on osteosarcoma (OSA) in several breeds found a 2-fold increase in occurrence in neutered dogs relative to intact dogs [5]. Another study on OSA, to explore the use of Rottweilers as a model for OSA in humans, found that neutering prior to 1 year of age was associated with an increased occurrence of OSA; 3–4 times that of intacts [6].

Hemangiosarcoma is a cancer that is affected by neutering in females. A study of cardiac tumors in dogs found that cardiac HSA for spayed females was greater than 4 times that of intact females [7]. A study on splenic HSA found the spayed females had more than 2 times the risk of developing this tumor as intact females [8]. Neither of these studies separated early- versus late-spayed females with regard to increased risk, and neither focused on just one breed. A study on the epidemiology of LSA (lymphoma) in dogs, for comparison with human lymphoma, found that intact females had a significantly lower risk of developing this cancer than neutered females or neutered males or intact males [9]. Another cancer of concern is prostate cancer, which occurs in neutered males about four times as frequently as in intact males [10]. A study on cutaneous mast cell tumors (MCT) in several dog breeds, including the Golden Retriever, examined risk factors such as breed, size, and neuter status. Although early versus late neutering was not considered, the results showed a significant increase in frequency of MCT in neutered females; four times greater than that of intact females [11].

In contrast to the rather strong evidence for neutering males and/or females as a risk factor for OSA, HSA, LSA, MCT, and prostate cancer, evidence for neutering as protection against a dog acquiring one or more cancers is weak. The most frequently mentioned is mammary cancer (MC) [12]. However, a recent systematic review of published work on neutering and mammary tumors found the evidence that neutering reduces the risk of mammary neoplasia to be weak, at best [13].

With regard to joint disorders affected by neutering, one study documents a 3-fold increase in excessive tibial plateau angle – a known risk factor for development of CCL – in large dogs [14]. A paper on CCL found that, across all breeds, neutered males and females were 2 to 3 times more likely than intact dogs to have this disorder [15]. In this study, with sexes combined, neutering significantly increased the likelihood of HD by 17 percent over that of intact dogs.

Given the widespread practice of neutering in the U.S., especially with public campaigns promoting early neutering, and the contrast with neutering practices in other developed countries, the objective of this project was to retrospectively examine the effects of neutering on the risks of several diseases in the same breed, distinguishing between males and females and early or late neutering versus remaining intact using a single hospital database. Because neutering can be expected to disrupt the normal physiological developmental role of gonadal hormones on multiple organ systems, one can envision the occurrence of disease syndromes, including those listed below, to possibly be affected by neutering as a function of gender and the age at which neutering is performed. The study focused on the Golden Retriever, which is one of the most popular breeds in the U.S. and Europe. In this breed, HD, CCL, LSA, HSA, MCT, OSA, and elbow dysplasia (ED) are listed as being of particular concern [16].

Methods

Ethics Statement

No animal care and use committee approval was required because, in conformity with campus policy, the only data used were from retrospective veterinary hospital records. Upon approval, faculty from the University of California, Davis (UCD), School of Veterinary Medicine, are allowed restricted use of the record system for research purposes. The final dataset used for statistical analyses is available to qualified investigators, upon request, from the corresponding author.

Data Collection

The dataset used in this study was obtained from the computerized hospital record system (Veterinary Medical and Administrative Computer System) of the Veterinary Medical Teaching Hospital (VMTH) at UCD. The subjects included were gonadally intact and neutered female and male Golden Retrievers, 1 to 8 years of age and admitted to the hospital between January 1, 2000 and December 31, 2009. Data from patients less than 12 months of age and 9 years or older were not considered. Additional inclusion criteria were requirements for complete information on date of birth, date of neutering (if neutered) and date of diagnosis (or onset) of the joint disorder or cancer. Patients were classified as intact or neutered; the neutering was subclassified as "early" if done before 12 months of age and "late" if done at 12 months of age or older. For all neutered patients, the neuter status at the time of each visit was reviewed to ensure that neutering occurred prior to onset of the first clinical signs or diagnosis of any disease of interest.

While the study set out to estimate incidence rates related to age at the time of neutering, patients were diagnosed at different ages and with differing durations of the disease as well as varying years of exposure to the effects of gonadal hormone removal. For those intact, early-neutered and late-neutered dogs diagnosed with a disease, the age of diagnosis was recorded. Follow-up times were recorded for each patient and determined by age of the dog at the initial clinical signs or diagnosis, minus the age of the dog when first included in the study. For dogs with no disease, follow-up times were the age at the last visit to the VMTH minus the age when the dog was first included in the study.

With the goal of obtaining a sample size sufficiently large for statistical analysis, the database records were initially screened using disease-related keywords to evaluate the frequency of occurrence of HD, CCL, HSA, LSA, MCT, ED, OSA, and MC. Extensive reviews of patient records were then performed for specific evidence and information on each joint disorder or cancer for every patient included in the study. Only diseases with at least 15 cases found using this screening were included in the study.

For all patients where age at time of neutering was not available in the record, an effort was made to obtain the information by telephone from the referring veterinarian. At the same time, age of onset of the disease in question was also sought. If the information was not available from the referring veterinarian, an attempt was made to reach the dog owner for this information. In order to optimize success in obtaining information, these efforts were focused on patients born in 2000, or later, and that were admitted to the VMTH between January 1, 2005 and December 31, 2009.

Table 1 defines the categories of diagnoses based on information in the record of each case. A patient was considered as having a disease of interest if the diagnosis was made at the VMTH or by a referring veterinarian and later confirmed at the VMTH. Patients clinically diagnosed with HD and/or CCL presented with clinical signs such as difficulty standing up, lameness, or joint pain; diagnosis was confirmed with radiographic evidence and/or orthopedic physical examination. Clinical diagnoses of the various cancers were accompanied by clinical signs such as enlarged lymph nodes, lumps on the skin or presence of masses, and confirmed by imaging, appropriate blood cell analyses, chemical panels, histopathology and cytology. When a diagnosis was suspected based on clinical signs, but the diagnostic tests were inconclusive or not done, telephone calls were made to referring veterinarians and owners to confirm the diagnosis. Lacking a conclusive confirmation, the case was excluded from the analysis for that specific joint disorder or cancer. Finally, body condition scores (BCS), ranging from 1 to 9 and obtained from the patient records (when available) were taken into account because BCS, as an indication of weight on the joints, is considered to play a role in the onset of these joint disorders [17,18]. Also, neutering has been implicated in an increase in body weight, especially as indicated by body condition score [18].

Statistical Analyses

Kaplan-Meier survival analysis (K-M) [19] was used to estimate survival curves for each disease and neuter status by gender, and then log-rank and generalized Wilcoxon tests were used for post

Table 1. Categories used in determining diagnosis for joint disorders and cancers of interest in Golden Retrievers (1–8 years old) admitted to the Veterinary Medical Hospital, University of California, Davis, from 2000–2009.

Classification	Definition
No disease	No evidence of a joint disorder or cancer of interest in the medical records
VMTH	Diagnosed at the VMTH
Referring Veterinarian/VMTH	Diagnosed by referring veterinarian and confirmed at the VMTH
Referring Veterinarian	Diagnosed by referring veterinarian but no diagnostic tests done at the VMTH
Suspected	Diagnosis was suspected based on clinical signs, but diagnostic tests were inconclusive or not done, telephone calls were then made to referring veterinarians and owners to confirm diagnosis, unconfirmed cases were excluded from analysis for the suspected joint disorder or cancer
Invalid	Diagnosed prior to January 2000 or after December 2009 and before 1 year of age or 9 years of age and older were excluded from analysis for the specific joint disorder or cancer

hoc comparisons between a set of two curves and thus to evaluate differences in occurrence of the diseases of interest in each comparison group. Incidence rate estimates (IR) [20] were used to evaluate the rates of disease onset using time-at-risk of the disease, in this case, dog-years at risk. Time-at-risk for a disease is the duration of time each patient was observed prior to the disease occurrence. For late-neutered dogs, time-at-risk prior to neutering was used in the IR estimation for intact dogs and time observed after neutering was used in the IR estimate for late-neutered dogs. For each disease, rate ratios (RR) and their corresponding 95 percent confidence intervals (95% CI) were used to compare the rates of acquiring each disease with regard to neuter status (i.e., intact vs. early neutered, intact vs. late-neutered, and early- vs. late-neutered). To examine the role of BCS in the development of HD and CCL, Cox proportional hazard (CPH) models were used, in which both BCS and age at the time of neutering were included as predictors. The resulting tests of the neutering effect are adjusted for differences in BCS among the groups. Statistical level of significance was set at the 5 percent level for all analyses.

Results

Table 2 presents the sample size for each joint disorder or cancer of patients meeting all inclusion criteria, separately for males and females according to neuter status classification as to intact, early-neutered, and late-neutered. The number of subjects available for analyses of each disease varied because a patient could be excluded from the analyses for one disease, if for example, the diagnosis was made prior to one year of age or after 8 years, but would be included for analyses of all other diseases that may occur within the ages 1 to 8 years. A case could be considered as intact for one disease if onset was prior to neutering and as late-neutered for another disease that may have occurred after neutering. Meeting all inclusion criteria were 145 intact males, 178 early-neutered males, 72 late-neutered males, 122 intact females, 172 early-neutered females, and 70 late-neutered females (Table 2). The overall percentages of cases in the sample for the five diseases affected by early and/or late neutering considered for statistical analyses are presented in Figure 1 for males and in Figure 2 for females. Mean follow-up times for all the diseases of interest in intact, early-neutered and late-neutered dogs are listed in Table 3.

As shown in Table 4, K-M survival analysis revealed that early neutering was associated with an increased occurrence of HD, CCL, and LSA. As shown in this table, comparisons of the IR analyses reveal that late neutering was associated with the subsequent occurrence of MCT and HSA in females. After the initial screening, ED, OSA, and MC occurred in such low numbers that statistical analyses were not feasible. MC was diagnosed in only two cases in the total number of 364 females, both in late-neutered females.

Hip Dysplasia

Perusal of Figure 1 and Table 4 reveals that HD in early-neutered males, affecting 10.3 percent, was more than double the proportion of intact males with the disorder, which was 5.1 percent, a significant difference (K-M: p<0.01). There was also a significant difference between early and late neutering in males (K-M: $p<0.05$). The mean ages of HD onset for intact, early-neutered, and late-neutered male dogs were 4.4, 3.6, and 4.7 years, respectively. No difference was found between early-neutered dogs with and without HD when compared with respect to their BCS, (means 6.1 and 5.7, respectively; CPH: p = 0.22). No other comparisons of HD occurrence were significant; HD was not increased in occurrence by early or later neutering in females (Figure 2).

Cranial Cruciate Ligament Tear

As revealed in Figures 1 and 2, there was no occurrence of CCL in either intact male or intact female dogs, or in late-neutered females. However, in early-neutered dogs, the occurrence reached 5.1 percent in males and 7.7 percent in females, representing significant differences in occurrence from both intact and late-neutered dogs (K-M: p<0.05, Table 4). The mean age of CCL onset in early-neutered males was 3.6 years and the single late-neutered male dog diagnosed with CCL was 7.4 years. The mean age of onset of CCL for early-neutered female dogs was 4.8 years. For CCL, no differences were found between neutered males with and without CCL with regards to their BCS (means 5.8 and 5.8 respectively; CPH: p = 0.48). Likewise, no differences in mean BCS were found between neutered females with and without CCL (means 5.8 and 5.8 respectively; CHP: p = 0.26).

Lymphosarcoma

Although the rates of occurrence of this disease were lower in both male and female intact dogs, than in the early-neutered dogs, the difference was statistically significant only in males. Early-neutered males had nearly 3 times the occurrence of LSA as intact males and no cases of LSA were observed in the late-neutered males (K-M: p<0.05, Table 4, Figure 1). The mean ages of LSA onset for intact and early-neutered male dogs were 5.3 and 5.8 years respectively.

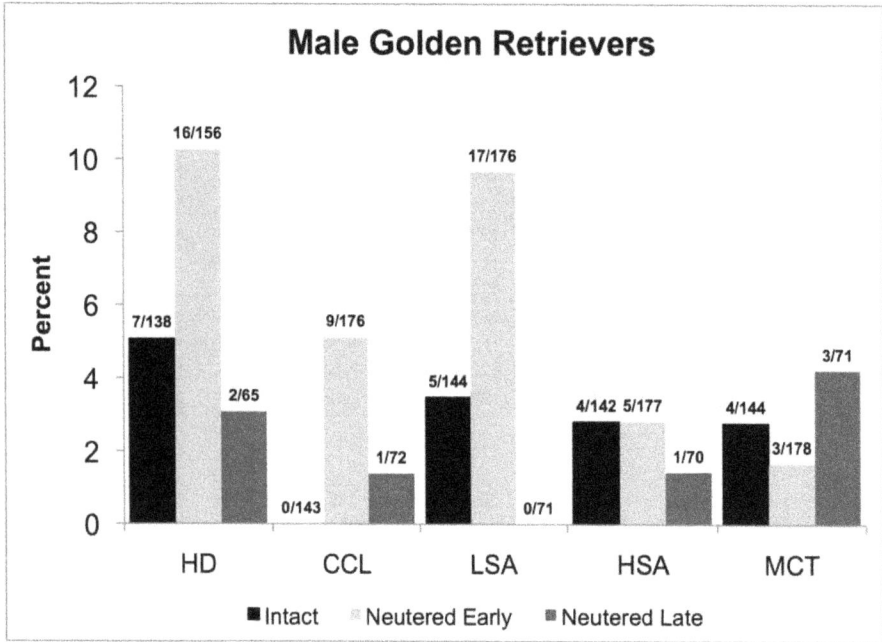

Figure 1. Percentages and number of cases over the total sample size for each neutering status group; intact and neutered early or late for male Golden Retrievers (1–8 years old) diagnosed with hip dysplasia (HD), cranial cruciate ligament tear (CCL), lymphosarcoma (LSA), hemangiosarcoma (HSA), and/or mast cell tumor (MCT) at the Veterinary Medical Teaching Hospital of the University of California, Davis, from 2000–2009. For HD and LSA, the differences between early-neutered and intact or late-neutered groups were statistically significant (K-M), as were differences for CCL between intact and early-neutered groups.

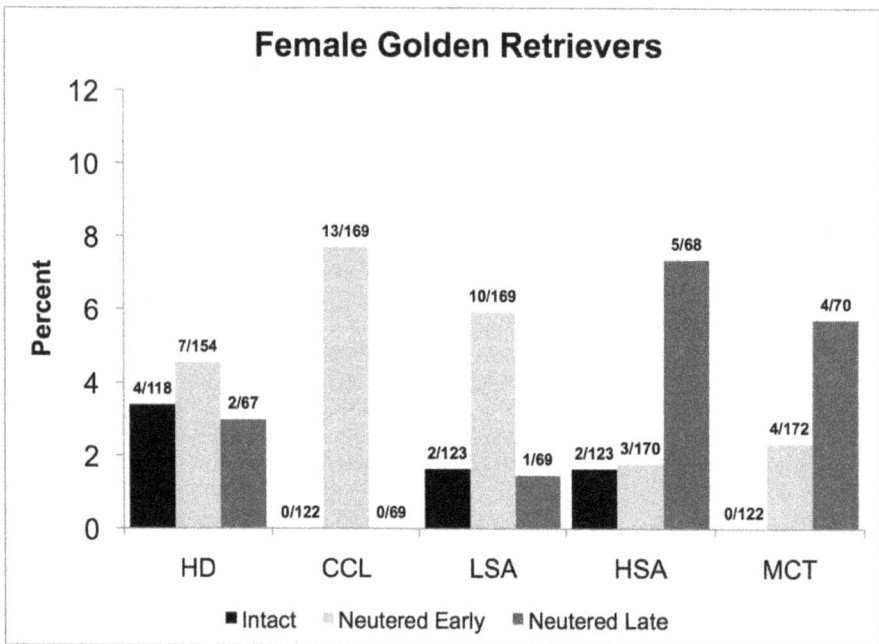

Figure 2. Percentages and number of cases over the total sample size for each neutering status group; intact and neutered early or late for female Golden Retrievers (1–8 years old) diagnosed with hip dysplasia (HD), cranial cruciate ligament tear (CCL), lymphosarcoma (LSA), hemangiosarcoma (HSA), and/or mast cell tumor (MCT) at the Veterinary Medical Teaching Hospital of the University of California, Davis, from 2000–2009. For CCL the difference between intact and early-neutered was statistically significant (K-M). For HSA, the differences between early and late-neutered and intact and late-neutered groups were statistically significant (RR), as were differences for MCT between early and late-neutered groups. A similar statistical comparison for late neutering and intact groups was not possible for MCT because there were 0 cases in the intact group.

Table 2. Total sample sizes obtained for male and female Golden Retrievers (1–8 years old) admitted to the Veterinary Medical Hospital, University of California, Davis, from 2000–2009 according to neuter status classification: intact, early-neutered, and late-neutered.

Disease	Total	Intact	Neutered Early	Neutered Late
Males				
HD	359	138	156	65
CCL	391	143	176	72
LSA	391	144	176	71
HAS	389	142	177	70
MCT	393	144	178	71
Total*	395	145	178	72
Females				
HD	339	118	154	67
CCL	360	122	169	69
LSA	361	123**	169	69
HAS	361	123**	170	68
MCT	364	122	172	70
Total*	364	122	172	70

*Total number of dogs meeting all inclusion criteria.
**Includes patients that were diagnosed with a disease of interest prior to eventual late neutering.

Table 3. Mean follow-up times for male and female Golden Retrievers (1–8 years old) admitted to the Veterinary Medical Hospital, University of California, Davis, from 2000–2009 by disease status for each neuter category.

Disease	Intact	Early Neutered	Late Neutered
Males			
No Disease	2.12	3.16	1.77
HD	2.61	2.11	0.99
CCL	NA	3.37	NA
LSA	3.36	3.67	NA
MCT	3.45	3.53	2.98
HAS	3.05	4.57	NA
Females			
No Disease	1.48	2.48	1.40
HD	1.12	2.13	0.05
CCL	NA	3.16	NA
LSA	3.62	4.99	NA
MCT	5.70	4.44	2.28
HAS	5.37	2.70	3.23

NA = Not applicable because there were no cases of the specific joint disorder or cancer in that neuter category.

Hemangiosarcoma

Figure 2 reveals that late-neutered females at 7.4 percent were diagnosed with HSA over 4 times more frequently than intact females with 1.6 percent and early-neutered females with 1.8 percent, both significant differences (RR = 6.10, 95% CI = 1.18, 31.37 and RR = 7.48, 95% CI = 1.79, 31.30). The mean ages of HSA onset for intact, early-neutered, and late-neutered female dogs were 6.4, 7.6, and 3.2 years, respectively. No differences were apparent in males with regard to neutering and the occurrence of HSA (Figure 1).

Mast Cell Tumor

Figure 2 portrays the findings regarding MCT in female dogs, which did not occur in intact females, but was diagnosed in 2.3 percent of early-neutered females and 5.7 percent of late-neutered females. The RR cannot be estimated when disease occurrence is zero in one comparison group, as in the intact females. However, the wide difference in MCT occurrence between intact and late-neutered females was meaningful, given that the MCT occurrence in late neutered females and early neutered females was significant (RR = 4.46, 95% CI = 1.11, 17.82). The mean ages of MCT onset for the early-neutered and late-neutered female dogs were 6.2 and 6.5 years, respectively. No differences were found in the occurrence of MCT in male Golden Retrievers (Figure 1).

Discussion

This is the first study of the effects of neutering on an array of joint disorders and cancers in the same breed of dog, using a single database and examining the variables of gender and early and late neutering versus leaving the dogs gonadally intact. No cases of MC were diagnosed in intact females in this study. This finding is partially explained by the relatively low frequency in which MC is diagnosed in Golden Retrievers [16]. While this finding contrasts with the general concern expressed about the risk of MC in gonadally intact females [12,21,22], it is consistent with the recent findings from a systematic meta-analysis finding a weak link, if any, between neutering and reduced risk of MC [13].

For all five diseases analyzed in the present study, the disease rates in males and/or females were significantly increased when neutering was performed early and/or late. When a disease occurred in intact dogs, the occurrence was typically one-fourth to one-half that of early- and/or late-neutered dogs. When no intact dogs were diagnosed with a disease, such as with CCL in both sexes and MCT in females, the occurrence in early- and/or late-neutered dogs ranged between 4 and 8 percent of the sample.

The results are consistent with all of the previously reported findings, mentioned in the introduction, of neutering in males and/or females in increasing the likelihood of HSA, LSA, MCT and CCL by about the same degree. However, this is the first study to specifically report an effect of late neutering on MCT and HSA. In the case of HD, which was doubled in the early-neutered males in the present study, the previous study reported a significant increase by only 17 percent in neutered dogs grouped together [15]. These contrasting differences with the effects of neutering on HD profile the value of the approach of the present study in focusing on just one breed and separating out the effects of gender and early versus late neutering.

An important point to make is that the results of this study, being breed-specific, with regard to the effects of early and late neutering cannot be extrapolated to other breeds, or dogs in general. Because of breed-specific vulnerabilities, certain diseases being affected by neutering in Golden Retrievers may not occur in other breeds. By the same token, different joint disorders or cancers may be increased in likelihood in a different breed. A full understanding of the disease conditions affected by neutering across an array of different breeds will require several more breed-specific studies.

A logical question to ask with regard to the joint disorders of HD and CCL is if those neutered dogs diagnosed with the disorder

Table 4. Summary of some Kaplan-Meier post hoc comparisons using log-rank (LR) and generalized Wilcoxon (W) tests for male and female Golden Retrievers (1–8 years old) admitted to the Veterinary Medical Hospital, University of California, Davis, from 2000–2009.

Disease	Gender	Test type	p (early vs. intact)	p (early vs. late)	p (late vs. intact)
Males					
HD		LR	0.04	NS	NS
		W	0.01	0.04	NS
CCL		LR	0.003	0.02	NS
		W	0.004	0.01	NS
LSA		LR	0.01	0.002	NS
		W	0.04	0.01	NS
Females					
CCL		LR	0.001	0.001	NS
		W	0.006	0.004	NS

NS = Statistically non significant.

were carrying relatively more weight on their joints, which may have predisposed them to the disorder. Therefore, once an effect of early neutering was found with regard to HD (males) and CCL (males and females), the CPH model was applied to reexamine the effect of early neutering, after adjusting for differences in BCS. While neutering is expected to lead to a greater gain in body weight than in intact dogs [17,18], the BCS of early-neutered dogs with the disorders and the early neutered comparison groups without the disorders were not significantly different – and, in fact quite similar – indicating that weight on the joint was not a major determinant in the occurrence of these joint disorders. Using the CPH model to compare early-neutered with intact dogs, for both HD and CCL, neither neutering status nor BCS was significant, indicating that the two factors are fairly highly confounded. This implies that the occurrence of HD and CCL in early-neutered dogs is a combined function of the effect of neutering on growth plates, as well as the increase in weight on the joints brought on by neutering. As mentioned, when only early-neutered dogs with and without HD or CCL were compared with respect to their BCS, no differences were found between early-neutered males with and without these joint disorders.

As for the pathophysiological reasons for the joint disorders, one can point to the role of gonadal hormones in controlling the closure of bone growth plates [23,24]. An atypical growth plate closure, resulting from the absence of gonadal hormones, may increase the chance of a clinically apparent joint disorder, such as HD, CCL, and possibly ED. Confounding factors that may influence the nature of a neuter-related joint disorder are the breed-specific gender vulnerabilities, including growth rate differences, as well as the timing of growth plate closure, which occurs more quickly in males than in females. In the males of this study, the occurrence of HD was doubled in the cases with early androgen removal as compared with intact males, but in females, removal of the ovaries did not appear to be associated with an increased likelihood of HD. This presumably reflects the effect of gender on growth-plate development. However, growth-plate disturbance in both males and females seems to have played a role in the occurrence of CCL in early-neutered dogs. This joint disorder was not diagnosed in either intact males or females. The mean age of CCL onset was later in life than in HD (about 4 years and 2 years, respectively).

The role of gonadal hormone removal in the occurrence of various cancers appears to be more complicated. The effects of early neutering on the increased rate of LSA, especially in males, contrast with the effects of late neutering in females on MCT and HSA. The effects of late neutering associated with the occurrence of MCT and HSA in females bring up the issue of the role of timing of estrogen alteration. One possibility is suggested by the role of estrogen removal and microsatellite instability in colon cancer development in women. Based on clinical findings, it is speculated that estrogen secretion may sensitize the pathways involved in microsatellite instability. While estrogen remains in the system, it is protective against microsatellite instability-positive cancer cell activation and reduces the risk of colon cancer. However, upon estrogen removal, microsatellite instability-positive cancer cells become activated resulting in an increased occurrence of colon cancer [25].

Applying this concept to the role of neutering on HSA and MCT in female dogs, this study suggests that with early neutering, before an estrous period, the cells that could become neoplastic are not sensitized to estrogen and neutering would not affect disease occurrence. However, after exposure to estrogen through several estrous cycles, potentially neoplastic cells could be sensitized, but as long as the female is left intact, the estrogen is protective. Then, if neutered after several estrous cycles, the estrogen-sensitized cells could become neoplastic, hence a higher rate of HSA and especially MCT in late-neutered than early-neutered females. Obviously, much remains to be learned that could be explored with a large database with regard to the specific effects of estrogen in these cancers.

The findings presented here are clinically relevant in two realms. For dog owners and service dogs trainers and caretakers using the popular Golden Retriever as the service dog, the study points to the importance of acquiring information needed for deciding upon if and when to neuter. Specifically for Golden Retrievers, neutering males well beyond puberty should avoid the problems of increased rates of occurrence of HD, CCL, and LSA and should not bring on any major increase in the rates of HSA and MCT (at least before nine years of age). However, the possibility that age-related cognitive decline could be accelerated by neutering should be noted [26]. For females, the timing of neutering is more problematical because early neutering significantly increases the incidence rate of CCL from near zero to almost 8 percent, and late neutering increases the rates of HSA to 4 times that of the 1.6 percent rate for intact females and to 5.7 percent for MCT, which was not diagnosed in intact females.

The findings of this study also have important implications for investigators looking for canine models for research on various forms of cancer [27,28]. For some cancers of interest, not only may breeds vary in predisposition but also the possibility of interactions between gender, gonadal hormone influences, and timing of gonadal hormone alteration (if any), should be taken into account in selecting the model and in investigating causal factors to be explored.

Acknowledgments

Special thanks are extended to Marty Bryant, Abigail Thigpen, Alexandra Brindle, Katherine Sylwester and Alisha Tran.

Author Contributions

Interpreting results and editing manuscript: AMO. Conceived and designed the experiments: BLH LAH GT. Performed the experiments: GT LAH BLH. Analyzed the data: GT TBF LLM NW. Wrote the paper: GT BLH LAH.

References

1. Trevejo R, Yang M, Lund EM (2011) Epidemiology of surgical castration of dogs and cats in the United States. J Am Vet Med Assoc 238: 898–904.
2. Sallander M, Hedhammer A, Rundgren M, Lindberg JE (2001) Demographic data of population of insured Swedish dogs measured in a questionnaire study. Acta Vet Scand 71–80.
3. Kubinyi E, Turcsan B, Miklosi A (2009) Dog and owner demographic characteristicsand dog personality trait associations. Behav Processes 81: 392–401.
4. Diesel G, Brodbelt D, Laurence C (2010) Survey of veterinary practice policies andopinions on neutering dogs. Vet Rec 166: 455–458.
5. Ru G, Terracini B, Glickman LT (1998) Host related risk factors for canine osteosarcoma. Vet J 156: 31–39.
6. Cooley DM, Beranek BC, Schlittler DL, Glickman MW, Glickman LT, et al. (2002) Endogenous gonadal hormone exposure and bone sarcoma risk. Cancer Epidemiol Biomarkers Prevent 11: 1434–1440.
7. Ware WA, Hopper DL (1999) Cardiac tumors in dogs: 1982–1995. J Vet Intern Med 13: 95–103.
8. Prymak C, McKee IJ, Goldschmidt MH, Glickman LT (1988) Epidemiologic, clinical, pathologic, and prognostic characteristics of splenic hemangiosarcoma and splenic hematoma in dogs: 217 cases (1985). J Am Vet Med Assoc 193: 706–712.
9. Villamil JA, Henry CJ, Hahn AW, Bryan JN, Tyler JW, et al. (2009) Hormonal and sex impact on the epidemiology of canine lymphoma. J Cancer Epidemiol 2009: 1–7. doi:10.1155/2009/591753
10. Teske E, Naan EC, van Dijk E, Van Garderen E, Schalken JA (2002) Canine prostate carcinoma: epidemiological evidence of an increased risk in castrated dogs. Mol Cell Endocrinol 197: 251–255.
11. White CR, Hohenhaus AE, Kelsey J, Procter-Grey E (2011) Cutaneous MCTs: Associations with spay/neuter status, breed, body size, and phylogenetic cluster. J Am Anim Hosp Assoc 47: 210–216.
12. Root Kustritz MV (2007) Determining the optimal age for gonadectomy of dogs and cats. J Am Vet Med Assoc 231: 1665–1675.
13. Beauvais W, Cardwell JM, Brodbelt DC (2012) The effect of neutering on the risk of mammary tumours in dogs – a systematic review. J Small Anim Pract 53: 314–322.
14. Duerr FM, Duncan CG, Savicky RS, Park RD, Egger EL, et al. (2007) Risk factors for excessive tibial plateau angle in large-breed dogs with cranial cruciate disease. J Am Vet Med Assoc 231: 1688–1691.
15. Witsberger TH, Villamil JA, Schultz LG, Hahn AW, Cook JL (2008) Prevalence of, and risk factors for, hip dysplasia and cranial cruciate ligament deficiency in dogs. J Am Vet Med Assoc 232: 1818–1824.
16. Glickman L (1998–1999) Golden Retriever Club of America National Health Survey. Golden Retriever Club of America.
17. Kasström H (1975) Nutrition, weight gain and development of hip dysplasia. An experimental investigation in growing dogs with special reference to the effect of feeding intensity. Acta Radiologica 344: 135–179, Supplementum.
18. Duval JM, Budsberg SC, Flo GL, Sammarco Jl (1999) Breed, sex, and body weight as risk factors for rupture of the cranial cruciate ligament in young dogs. J Am Vet Med Assoc 215: 811–814.
19. Kaplan EL, Meier P (1958) Nonparametric estimation from incomplete observations. J Am Stat Assoc 53: 457–481.
20. Rothman KJ and Greenland S (1998) Modern Epidemiology. Philadelphia: Lippincott Williams & Wilkins.
21. Egenvall A, Bonnett BN, Ohagen P, Olson P, Hedhamar A, et al. (2005) Incidence of, and survival after, mammary tumors in a population of over 80,000 insured female dogs in Sweden from 1995 to 2002. Prevent Vet Med 69: 109–127.
22. Zatlouka J, Lorenzova J, Tichy F, Necas A, Kecova H, et al. (2005) Breed and age as risk factors for canine mammary tumours. Acta Vet Brno 74: 103–109.
23. Salmeri KR, Bloomberg MS, Scruggs SL, Shille V (1991) Gonadectomy in immature dogs: Effects on skeletal, physical, and behavioral development. J Am Vet Med Assoc 198: 1193–1203.
24. Grumbach M (2000) Estrogen, bone growth and sex: a sea of change in conventional wisdom. J Ped Endocrinol Metab 13: 1439–1455.
25. Slattery ML, Potter JD, Curtin K, Edwards S, Ma K, et al. (2001) Estrogens reduce and withdrawal of estrogens increase risk of microsatellite instability-positive colon cancer. Cancer Res 61: 126–130.
26. Hart BL (2001) Effects of gonadectomy on subsequent development of age-related cognitive impairment in dogs. J Am Vet Med Assoc 219: 51–56.
27. Vail DM, MacEwen EG (2002) Spontaneously occurring tumors of companion animals as models for human cancer. Cancer Invest 18: 781–792.
28. Khanna C, Lindblad-Toh K, Vail D, London C, Bergman P, et al. (2006) The dog as a cancer model. Nat Biotechnol 24: 1065–1066.

6

Does Pet Arrival Trigger Prosocial Behaviors in Individuals with Autism?

Marine Grandgeorge[1,2]*, **Sylvie Tordjman**[3], **Alain Lazartigues**[1], **Eric Lemonnier**[1], **Michel Deleau**[4], **Martine Hausberger**[2]

1 CHRU de Brest, Hôpital de Bohars, Centre de Ressources Autisme, Bohars, France, 2 UMR-CNRS 6552, Laboratoire Ethologie Animale et Humaine, Rennes, France, 3 CHRU Guillaume Régnier, Rennes, France, 4 Centre de recherches en psychologie, cognition et communication, Rennes, France

Abstract

Alteration of social interactions especially prosocial behaviors – an important aspect of development – is one of the characteristics of autistic disorders. Numerous strategies or therapies are used to improve communication skills or at least to reduce social impairments. Animal-assisted therapies are used widely but their relevant benefits have never been scientifically evaluated. In the present study, we evaluated the association between the presence or the arrival of pets in families with an individual with autism and the changes in his or her prosocial behaviors. Of 260 individuals with autism - on the basis of presence or absence of pets - two groups of 12 individuals and two groups of 8 individuals were assigned to: study 1 (pet arrival after age of 5 *versus* no pet) and study 2 (pet *versus* no pet), respectively. Evaluation of social impairment was assessed at two time periods using the 36-items ADI-R algorithm and a parental questionnaire about their child-pet relationships. The results showed that 2 of the 36 items changed positively between the age of 4 to 5 (t_0) and time of assessment (t_1) in the pet arrival group (study 1): "offering to share" and "offering comfort". Interestingly, these two items reflect prosocial behaviors. There seemed to be no significant changes in any item for the three other groups. The interactions between individuals with autism and their pets were more – qualitatively and quantitatively - reported in the situation of pet arrival than pet presence since birth. These findings open further lines of research on the impact of pet's presence or arrival in families with an individual with autism. Given the potential ability of individuals with autism to develop prosocial behaviors, related studies are needed to better understand the mechanisms involved in the development of such child-pet relationship.

Editor: Liane Young, Boston College, United States of America

Funding: The Adrienne and Pierre Sommer Foundation gave the financial support for this study. The funders had no role in study design, data collection and analysis, decision to publish, or preparation of the manuscript. The authors declare that they have no financial interests.

Competing Interests: The authors have declared that no competing interests exist.

* E-mail: marine.grandgeorge@chu-brest.fr

Introduction

Impairments of social development associated with communication deficits, restricted interests and repetitive behaviors constitute the triad of autistic disorders [1,2]. Individuals with autism have difficulty interacting with others as well as using and interpreting nonverbal communication. Social impairments have been regarded as primary deficits by several authors [3,4] since they are among the first symptoms of autistic disorders (e.g. difficulty in participating in imitative or pretend play [5,6]). Individuals with autism appear to have problems recognizing, understanding and expressing both feelings and intentions, which may be due to a lack of "theory of mind" [7]. These individuals fail to infer mental states and display impairment of abilities to understand and manage emotions (i.e. understand the other's feelings and display appropriate behavior or response [4,8]).

Many strategies, supports or therapies have been aimed at improving the everyday lives and social interactions of individuals with autism [9,10] For example, peer-mediated interventions have proved to be useful through increasing the communicative interactions and stimulating the development of joint attention [11]. Complementary and alternative interventions are also proposed: relaxation, music or activities with animals [12]. Indeed,

since early findings by Levinson's reporting that a dog could help in therapy [13], animal assisted therapies (AAT) have been used largely. Sessions with dogs, horses or dolphins are proposed, and considered overall as beneficial to improve prosocial behaviors [14–17]. However, to date, there is no scientific evaluation of their relevant benefit [18,19]. Moreover, the context in which AAT occur must be accounted for. The impact of having a pet in a therapeutic or home setting seems to be different when encountering humans [20].

More broadly, beneficial effects of having a pet at home have been reported for improvement of health or well-being of elderly, isolated women, adults and children [21–26]. It is considered as a source of non judgmental and positive affection [27,28]. Several studies suggest that children learn prosocial behaviors through their interactions with pets [29–31]. These prosocial behaviors constitute an important aspect of a child's development. They are triggered by pet's presence under certain circumstances (e.g. if a strong bond is formed, if the pet lives at home or if the human partner is younger than 6 years old [32–34]). Thus, bonding with a pet may help with developing some prosocial behaviors. This hypothesis seems to be consistent with the results of other studies about the reciprocal behavior that leads an animal to exceptional learning (e.g. Alex the parrot [35], Hoover the seal [36], Kanzi the chimpanzee [37]).

In the present study, we hypothesized that a pet at home might help individuals with autism to develop some prosocial behaviors. For this, we compared three situations: never owned a pet, owned a pet since birth (i.e. pet has been part of the individual's environment) or owned a pet after the age of 5. The age of 4 to 5 is considered as a "key age" in autistic disorders [38] because it seems to be representative of the period when the severity of autism is the most important. Indeed, older subjects might outgrow some of the major impairments. Accordingly, there is a need to avoid focusing on the basis of behavior in childhood. Consequently, the Autism Diagnostic Interview-Revised (ADI-R) explains that the most satisfactory compromise is to consider the age of 4 to 5 as the key age to evaluate the individual's behavior.

The arrival of a pet in a family has been shown to increase the level of interactions between family members: they spend more time together and share joint attention on the new family member [39]. The new arrival of a pet potentially elicits more attention in individuals with autism thus leading to a greater chance of bonding with the pet. We further hypothesized that the arrival of a pet when the human partner was old enough to "realize this change" would increase the chances of improving the human's prosocial behaviors. For this, we evaluated the individual's impairments using the ADI-R [38], to compare two time periods (i.e. t_0 at the age of 4 to 5 and t_1 at the time of assessment), and a parental questionnaire about the child-pet relationship. Since direct questioning of individuals with autism can be complicated, we only used parental reports in this study. According to the literature, individuals with autism display delays and deficits in the acquisition of language (e.g. complete absence of functional communication, impairments in conversation) [40,41]. Parents are a reliable source of information in regard to the evaluation of their child's developmental problems [42,43]. For example, in a previous study, Siegel et al. [44] found that parental reports about typical daily behaviors of their children with autism confirmed observations made during diagnostic play sessions by trained professionals. In addition, parental reports concerning both their pets and their child's behaviors are more reliable than children's interviews [45].

Methods

Participants

All the individuals with autism (n = 260; 59♀/191♂; mean age, 15±7.5 years old, range from 6 to 34 years old) in this study, came from the "Centre de Ressources sur l'Autisme de Bretagne" (Bohars, France) or the child day-care facilities controlled by the Bicêtre and Reims University Hospitals (France). The cognitive and behavioral assessments were approved by the ethics committee of Bicêtre hospital (the committee was not specific to this study). It is worth mentioning that the present research was non-invasive and did not involve pharmacological interventions. Hence, in accordance to the ethics committee, parents (or guardians) gave a simple verbal consent. All individuals met DSM-IV criteria for autistic disorders [1]. As part of a routine follow-up of individuals with autism, the same psychiatrists did the diagnosis and the ADI-R [38] assessment to confirm the diagnosis.

Cognitive and Behavioral Assessments

The cognitive functioning of individuals with autism from child day-care facilities of the University Hospitals of Bicêtre and Reims (n = 70) was assessed by two psychologists using the age-appropriate Weschler intelligence scale and the Kaufman K-

ABC [46]. All assessed individuals with autism were cognitively impaired (mean full scale IQ ± S.D: 42.1±3.4, with a range of 40–58; mean verbal IQ ± S.D: 45.2±2.3, with a range of 45–57; mean performance IQ ± S.D: 45.2±4.4, with a range of 45–80).

ADI-R was used to assess the behavior of 260 participants with autism [38]. ADI-R, an extensive, semi-structured parental interview, was conducted by trained psychiatrists (EL, ST). The structuring lies in the details of the predetermined codings for each behavioral item. The interview schedule specifies a variety of screening questions, the purpose of which is to guide the interviewer on the content of the response (yes or no responses from the informant, i.e. parents or guardians, were inadequate). Behavioral descriptions are coded. The codings have been devised with the aim of differentiating developmental delay from deviance. Thus, for each section of the interview, there is an initial compulsory probe printing. The interviewer should then continue to ask further questions until he/she is able to make the coding for each item, for example, using different supplementary probes proposed in the ADI-R. The ADI-R scale assessed the three major domains of autistic impairments: (1) reciprocal social interactions, (2) verbal and non-verbal communication and (3) stereotyped behavior and restricted interests. The presence of verbal language is defined as daily, functional and comprehensible use of spontaneous phrases of at least three words, including at least sometimes, a verb [38].

The ADI-R algorithm is validated to assess the behavior and is based on the 4-to-5-year-old period of life. To reveal possible variations, we compared the ratings at the current period (t_1) of the subset of ADI-R to those at the age of 4 to 5 (t_0) [47]. The severity of behavioral impairments was scored using the subset of ADI-R items included in the ADI-R algorithm, following the procedure previously described [48]. We give below the mean score for each main domain: (1) total reciprocal social interaction (15 items), (2) total verbal communication and total non-verbal communication (13 items for non verbal patients, the score was based on 9 items), (3) total stereotypics (8 items). A score for the combined domain (social/communication/stereotypies) was calculated and regarded as a global score of autism severity (Table 1).

Based on direct clinical observation for each participant by an independent psychiatrist, a diagnosis of autistic disorder was made according to DSM-IV [1] and ICD-10 [49] criteria and was confirmed by the ADI-R ratings. We didn't perform an Autistic Diagnostic Observation Schedule [50] assessment. It has not been a routine practice in France before 2008 [51].

Questionnaires on Human-pet Relationships

Parents were interviewed by phone by one of the investigators (MG) not involved in the ADI-R scoring (i.e. was not aware of the data values). They were asked to answer a short standardised questionnaire about the child-pet relationship. No further information was given before the beginning of the questionnaire. Verbal informed consent was given by the parents (or guardians) when the questionnaire on human-pet relationships was filled in. The consent form explained that the questionnaire and ADI-R data will be used together. ADI-R evaluation was performed by the psychiatrist who was not aware of our project. Therefore, neither parents nor evaluators were influenced by the potential expectations of the pet's impact. The interval between the ADI-R assessment and the questionnaire phase was less than one year. The data from parental questionnaire were collected between winter 2006 and winter 2007.

The questionnaire was about the presence (or absence) of pets in the family at t_0 (i.e. at the individual's age of 4 to 5) and at t_1 (i.e. at the time of ADI-R assessment). If one or more pets were present,

Table 1. Demographic and behavioral characteristics of study groups (G_{0A} and G_{0B} never owned pet; G_{alw} always owned a pet; G_{pet} didn't own a pet before the age of 5, but owned at least one at the time of assessment).

	G_{OA} (n = 12)	G_{pet} (n = 12)	G_{OB} (n = 8)	G_{alw} (n = 8)
Gender (M/F)	9/3	9/3	4/4	4/4
Age (months; mean ± SD; range)	122.8±52.3 (87–180)	137.1±60.6 (80–185)	137.2±42.7 (73–201)	128.6±44.4 (75–200)
Overall level of language[1]	9/3	9/3	2/6	2/6
Epilepsy (yes/no)	8/0	8/0	1/11	0/12
ADI-R at t_0 (mean ± SD)				
Total	44.5±5.3	44.6±4.5	45.8±1.7	43.1±3.0
Reciprocal social interactions	23.2±3.1	22.1±3.6	25.0±1.9	21.9±2.1
Non verbal Communication	10.3±2.2	11.0±1.7	10.9±0.6	9.9±1.5
Verbal Communication[2]	15.9±2.6	16.9±1.0	17.3±0.6	13.5±1.8
Restricted and repetitive behaviors	5.4±1.1	5.6±0.9	7.8±1.3	9.9±1.0
ADI-R at t_1 (mean ± SD)				
Total	38.7±4.5	38.6±5.0	39.8±7.0	38.8±5.9
Reciprocal social interactions	22.1±3.6	18.8±3.5	18.6±4.5	19.1±3.6
Non verbal Communication	7.1±2.0	10.3±1.9	10.3±2.9	7.5±2.8
Verbal Communication[2]	11.5±1.9	14.9±1.5	14.5±2.0	10.4±2.2
Restricted and repetitive behaviors	5.1±1.2	4.8±0.9	6.6±1.4	9.3±1.5
Mann Whitney U-test at t_0	U	p-value	U	p-value
Total	152	0.931	81.5	0.170
Reciprocal social interactions	157	0.707	81	0.189
Non verbal Communication	138.5	0.521	74	0.564
Verbal Communication[2]	133.5	0.353	72	0.554
Restricted and repetitive behaviors	148	0.931	74	0.560

[1]Absence/presence of verbal language as defined according to the ADI-R criteria.
[2]Scores corresponded to children who had a verbal language according to the ADI-R criteria.

parents gave information on the species and the pet ownership duration, as well as their child-pet relationship. The following data were gathered (yes or no answers): tactile interactions, visual interactions, play, care (*e.g.* feeding, walking with the pet, brushing the pet), time spent with and any privileged relationship. The above data helped us to evaluate the individual-pet bond. Moreover, parents specified whether the pet was specially acquired for their child with autism. Pets were dogs, cats and/or little furry animals. Half of the pets were acquired for the individuals with autism.

Study 1: Arrival of a Pet between the Age of 4 to 5 and the Time of ADI-R Assessment

From the initial pool of 260 participants, we selected two groups. The first group, G_{pet}, did not own a pet before t_0 but owned at least one afterwards (n = 12; pets were dogs, cats and one hamster). The G_{pet} individuals were matched with control individuals – who never owned a pet (G_{0A}, n = 12) - for sex, age, overall level of language (absence/presence of verbal language as defined by ADI-R criteria in the following section) and history of epilepsy (Table 1; all chi-square tests and Mann Whitney U-tests p>0.05). Both the total score and the sub-scores of the ADI-R were not significantly different (all Mann-Whitney U-tests, p>0.05; Table 1). The G_{pet} and G_{0A} mean age was 10.8±2.3 years old at t_1. On the average, we obtained the G_{pet} parents

responses to the questionnaire 79±29 months after the pet's arrival.

Study 2: Owned a Pet since Birth

We investigated whether the arrival (or presence) *per se* of pets was associated with changes in any of the ADI-R social items. We selected two groups from the initial pool of 260 participants. The first group, G_{alw}, owned at least one pet at home since birth (n = 8; pets were dogs, cats and one rabbit). Among the G_{alw} individuals, three owned two pets. These G_{alw} individuals were matched with control individuals - who never owned a pet (G_{0B}, n = 8) - for the same individual's characteristics as in study 1 (all chi-square and Mann Whitney U-tests p>0.05; Table 1). Both the total score and the sub-scores of the ADI-R were not significantly different (all Mann-Whitney U-tests, p>0.05; Table 1). The G_{alw} and G_{0B} mean age was 11.1±1.9 years old at t_1.

Statistical Analyses

Changes between item scores at t_0 and at t_1 in each group (G_{pet}, G_{alw}, G_{0A} and G_{0B}) were evaluated using Wilcoxon's matched-pairs signed rank test. When a significant effect was observed, Mann-Whitney test was then applied to evaluate whether or not the change could be associated with the following variables:

- individual's gender
- reasons for obtaining the pet(s)

• presence of different pets
• type of human-pet interactions (including privileged relationship)
• life setting (i.e. urban or rural)

Spearman's rank order correlation assessed the correlation between the individual's age or IQ score and his or her ADI-R item score. Since 36 tests were performed at both t_0 and t_1, in order to avoid false positive due to chance, Bonferroni correction for multiple comparison was applied systematically ($p < 0.0014$).

Results

Study 1

Comparison of ADI-R assessment between t_0 and t_1 revealed significant changes in two of the 36 items in the G_{pet}. Thus, G_{pet} had a lower deficit score for the items "offering to share", e.g. sharing food or toys with parents or other children (Wilcoxon test: $Z_{Gpet} = 21$ $p < 0.0014$; Fig. 1) and "offering comfort", e.g. reassuring parents or peers who were sad or hurt (Wilcoxon test: $Z_{Gpet} = 21$ $p < 0.0014$; Fig. 2). No changes were observed for the control individuals (Wilcoxon tests: $Z_{G0A} = 3$, $Z_{G0A} = 6$ $p > 0.05$ in both cases; Fig. 1, Fig. 2). In G_{pet} and G_{0A}, neither the total scores of ADI-R at t_0 and t_1 (Wilcoxon tests: $Z_{Gpet} = 4$ $p = 0.011$; $Z_{G0A} = 15$ $p = 0.065$) nor the sub-scores in the main domains (all Wilcoxon tests: $p > 0.0014$) were statistically different at $p < 0.0014$.

Score differences between t_0 and t_1 were neither correlated with individual's age (all Spearman's rank order correlation $p > 0.05$) nor affected by gender, life setting, presence of different pets, and type of human-pet interaction (all Mann Whitney U-tests $p > 0.05$). Interestingly, whether the parents had acquired the animal for their child or for the family revealed no significant difference in ADI-R scores (Mann Whitney U-test $= 53.5$ $p > 0.05$), indicating that the results were not influenced by the parents expectations on the pet's impact. In addition, communication and non-social aspects (e.g. scores for repetitive behavior and stereotyped patterns) were not affected by the pet's arrival (all Wilcoxon tests $p > 0.05$). No significant correlation (Spearman's rank order correlation, $p > 0.05$) between the items "offering comfort" or "offering to share" and IQ scores (verbal IQ, performance IQ and full IQ) was observed.

Parental questionnaire offered some information about the interaction type G_{pet} individual had with his or her pet (Table 2). Tactile interactions were the most reported (i.e. 75%; n = 9), followed by time spent with the pet (n = 8), play (n = 7) and visual interactions (n = 7). Care was the least reported item (n = 6). Thus, seven G_{pet} individuals were considered by their parents as having a privileged relationship with their pets. Among the five remaining individuals, three owned a cat and two owned a dog.

Study 2

No significant change was observed for individuals with autism who owned a pet since birth or for control individuals (G_{alw} and G_{OB}; all Wilcoxon test $p > 0.05$; Fig. 1, Fig. 2). In G_{alw} and G_{OB}, neither the total scores of ADI-R at t_0 and t_1 (Wilcoxon tests: $Z_{Galw} = 9$ $p = 0.447$; $Z_{G0B} = 11$ $p = 0.363$) nor the sub-scores in the four domains (all Wilcoxon tests: $p > 0.05$) were statistically different at $p < 0.0014$.

Here again, an exploration of the parental questionnaire offered some information about the interaction type G_{alw} individual had with his or her pet (Table 2). Care and play were not mentioned. Two individuals spent time with their pet, four had tactile interactions and five had visual interactions. Only three G_{alw} individuals were considered by their parents as having privileged relationships with

their pets (i.e. three dogs). However, two of the three individuals who owned the same pet since birth, neither interacted nor bonded with it (i.e. all items were reported as absent).

Discussion

Comparison of ADI-R assessment between G_{pet} and G_{alw} at two different time periods revealed significant changes in ADI-R scores only in the group experiencing the pet arrival in their homes. However, these changes were limited to two ADI-R items, "offering to share" and "offering comfort". These findings suggest an improvement in prosocial behaviors of the individuals with autism. These prosocial behaviors are mainly impaired in individuals with autism [1,52]. The absence of a significant correlation with IQ scores might imply that these changes were not related to the level of cognitive functioning. Interestingly, the individual-pet interactions (i.e. bonding) were more - qualitatively and quantitatively - reported in the case of pet arrival than pet presence since birth. To our knowledge, this is the first study showing an association between pet arrival and changes in prosocial behaviors. Our study follows the footsteps of the human-pet reports on the improvement of prosocial behaviors in individuals with typical development [53,54].

On the Significance of Changes

On the one hand, two main possible explanations could account for these findings.

First, parents may have acquired a pet because they believed that it would improve the prosocial behaviors of their children with autism. In this case, their responses to the ADI-R could be biased. The following findings strongly suggest that this was not the case:

1. Only 6 pets (of the 15 pets in Gpet) were acquired especially for the individuals with autism; the others were acquired for another family member. Changes in the prosocial behaviors were observed in both cases. Thus, these changes were not related to parental expectations.

2. This "pet study" (and its related questionnaire) began after the ADI-R completion. This suggests that the parents were not aware of the possible pet impact at t1.

3. Improvement was found only for two of the 36 items, further indicating the non-bias character of parent's responses.

The second explanation is that the arrival of a pet may have triggered a change in the individuals' "perception of the social world". Pets are supposed to enhance different skills in children with typical development such as self-esteem, socio-emotional development and empathy [32,33,54]. According to several authors, children with typical development seem to learn prosocial behaviors through their interactions with pets (e.g. sharing with and stroking the pet) [30,55]. Could this also be the case for individuals with autism? Only observational studies can reveal how individuals with autism interact with their pet and whether somehow they develop skills to understand pet's behaviors or needs [56].

On the other hand, it is not very surprising that other ADI-R items did not change, not even those related to the prosocial behaviors. Since verbal exchanges with pets are excluded, we would expect no changes in language skills whereas parents can indeed influence such skills [57]. Moreover, other studies confirm that animals neither influence motor skills nor reduce restricted behaviors in children with autism [16].

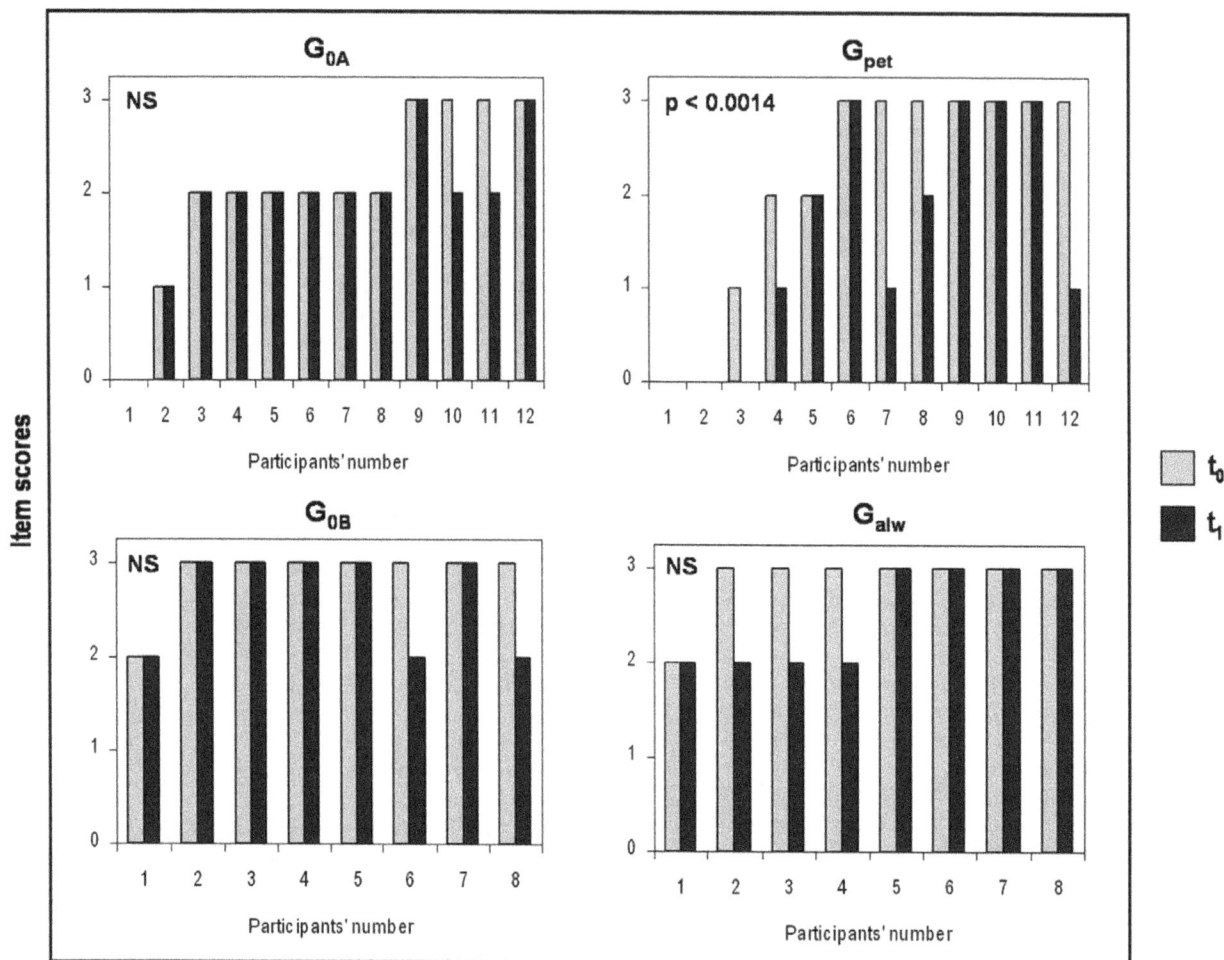

Figure 1. Item scores of "offering to share" at t_0 (4-to-5-years old; in grey) and t_1 (current period; mean age: 129.9±55.8 months old; in black) for G_{0A} (group with no pet in the family), G_{pet} (group with a pet arriving after the child's 5th birthday), G_{0B} (group with no pet in the family) and G_{alw} (group always with at least one pet at home since birth). Higher the score, more significant was the "offering to share" (e.g. sharing food or toys with parents or other children).

Potential Mechanisms

Numerous theories have been proposed to explain the pet's influence on human life (for a review, see [58]). Animals are animates, thus differ from inanimates in regard to many biological characteristics such as motion or sensory properties. Specifically, animates are beings that know, perceive, learn and think. These abilities make them appealing ([59] in [60]).

Friedman et al. [61] proposed the bio-psycho-social model that considers pets could reduce loneliness and thus could also be considered as "transitional objects" especially for the children [31,62]. Pets may also be considered as "distracters". Brickel [63] and more recently Odendaal [64] proposed to explain this phenomenon by the attention-shift theory. They stated that when a human is in a stressful situation, a pet seems to distract him/her from the anxiogenic stimulus (e.g. unknown situations in the case of people with autism). Animal's presence triggers human's attention-shift. Attention-shift offered by a pet under repeated exposure to a stressful situation, leads to a decrease in anxiety. Therefore, a family pet may also become a source and a center of attention that could be useful in individual's learning.

On the one hand, the presence of a pet can have a direct influence. When a human and a pet are interacting, each partner

uses signals emitted by the other to adjust their behavior: the behavior of one influences the response of the other (e.g. between a dog and a child [65–67]). A bond or a relationship emerges from these series of interactions where both partners have expectations on the next interaction on the basis of the previous ones [68]. Thus, as stated by Filiatre et al. [65] the pet's behavior "could contribute to the acquisition by the child of a more structured and more socially efficient behavioral repertoire". Moreover, the attitudes that children display towards pets have an impact on their prosocial and social behaviors [34,69]. On the other hand, a pet can have an indirect influence on children through the family. Indeed numerous parents state that pets can be precious tools with which they educate their children [29,70,71]. For example, Beck et al [72] showed that an increased knowledge about wild birds after a ten-week educational home-based program for feeding was associated with parental involvement.

People with autism have been shown to be less sensitive to human voices [73] or faces [74] than to other environmental stimuli. To our knowledge, little is known about how they perceive animals' characteristics, but they are quite able to classify their animal preferences based on pictures [75]. Using a task based on sorting by preference, Celani [76] showed that children with

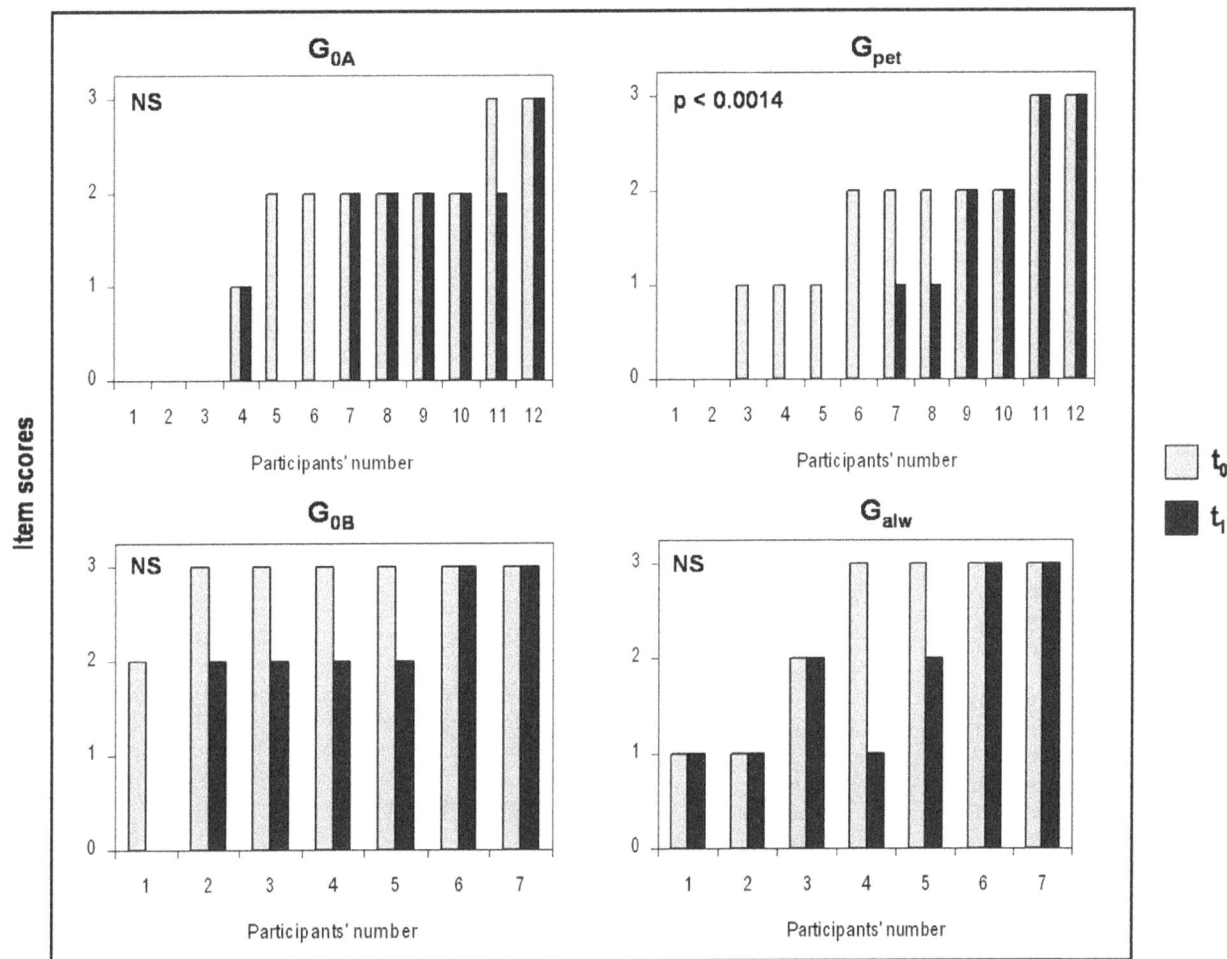

Figure 2. Item scores of "offering comfort" at t_0 (4-to-5-years old; in grey) and t_1 (current period, mean age: 129.9±55.8 months old; in black) for G_{0A} (group with no pet in the family), G_{pet} (group with a pet arriving after the child's 5th birthday), G_{0B} (group with no pet in the family) and G_{alw} (group always with at least one pet at home since birth). Higher the score, more significant was the impairment "offering comfort" (e.g. reassuring parents or peers who were sad or hurt). Comparisons were performed using Wilcoxon's matched-pairs signed ranks tests (Significant threshold: p<0.0014).

autism chose pictures with an animal (e.g. dog, cat) rather than the ones with objects. At last, some authors explained that the affinity of people with autism for pets comes from animal's multisensory

Table 2. Number of individuals with autism who display different types of relationships with their pet according to parents.

Presence of each item	G_{pet} (n = 12)	G_{alw} (n = 8)
Tactile interactions	9	2 [4]
Visual interactions	7	3 [5]
Play	7	0 [2]
Care	6	0 [0]
Time spent with pet	8	3 [3]
Privileged relationship	7	2 [2]

As three individuals of G_{alw} owned two pets, the first number showed the first pet's answer and the second number in brackets showed the second pet's answer.

characteristic. In addition, according to these authors, an animal's behavior seems to be easier to decode and to predict than that of a human partner [14,17].

Pet Presence versus Arrival

One intriguing finding was that similar results were observed for the individuals who were in the presence of a pet from birth and those who never owned a pet. Changes were only observed in the group where the pet arrived after the age of 5. Different hypotheses are possible and are explored below.

When the pet was reported to be present since the individual's birth, one would expect a cumulative effect of its presence. We cannot exclude this effect even if the ADI-R did not clearly explore it here (e.g. neither a too low nor a specific effect was explored by ADI-R items). However, we proposed an alternative explanation. Individuals with autism may usually avoid unfamiliar social partners and display diminished interest in novelty [1]. But under certain circumstances, children with autism prefer new stimuli rather than familiar ones [77]. The presence of a pet may be a mere "additional" element of the environment, therefore not attracting special attention. This is consistent with our parental questionnaire revealing that few of these individuals (G_{alw}) developed a real bond with the pet in comparison to the other group (i.e. G_{pet}, pet arrival). For example, only a quarter of G_{alw} individuals had a privileged relationship with their pet. The sole presence of the pet did not confer benefit for the individuals with autism. Such situation was previously reported in the children with typical development : the quality of relationship with their own pet appears to be a direct determinant of their socio-emotional development [33] and "pet bonding" is a stronger determinant of pet-associated benefits than the sole pet ownership [78]. If we take a look at the other side, the pet may also have formed a preferential bond with another member of the family and therefore been less demanding on the individual with autism.

The other non-exclusive possibility is that the arrival of a pet strengthens the cohesion of the family and increases the levels of interactions between their members. Pet's arrival plays an even more important role in the lives of children who have inadequate or destructive family and social environments [79]. Most families acquiring a pet experienced an increase in quantity and quality of time spent together and felt happier after pet's arrival [39]. This situation might be due to the collective attention on the new pet. This new pet arrival might induce an increased interest of the individuals towards the pet and/or their involvement in the family's interactions. Cain [39] talked about the "triangling" process initiated by the pet (i.e. structuring and promoting interactions between two humans).

In our study, playing with the pet was reported by seven of the parents in G_{pet} whereas only two of the parents in G_{alw} noticed it. This behavior is a powerful means by which children master skills that are important for their development [80]. Playing with a pet is a complex behavior, sometimes involving object manipulation as a means for practice and mastery of action schemas (i.e. sensorimotor play) or child's ability for mental representation. Thus, it provides a child with means of practicing and understanding the events of his or her social world (i.e. pretend play) [81]. These behaviors are not only observed in humans but also in human-pet interactions [55,82]. Such interactions may have some positive outcome: playing with a dog during pet therapy had beneficial impact on hospitalized children [83]. This implies that playing with a pet may be beneficial to individuals with autism.

Interestingly, in our study, taking care of the pet was reported by half of the parents in G_{pet} whereas none of the parents in G_{alw} noticed it. Our finding infers the positive influence of pet arrival on parental support in the development of individuals with autism. Previous studies have shown that parents use pets to teach their children how to take care of pets by giving them age-appropriate tasks [29]. With parental support, the child involvement towards a pet may influence his/her socio-emotional development [84].

Finally individuals with autism may be sensitive to an overall change in their social sphere. Therefore the changes may be related merely to the overall family functioning rather than the sole pet arrival. This however would not explain why only two precise items were affected and not the others.

Conclusion

This study reveals that in individuals with autism, pet arrival in the family setting may bring about changes in specific aspects of their socio-emotional development. It suggests the improvement of some prosocial behaviors in such individuals under certain circumstances. Thus, it offers a "window of opportunity" to future longitudinal developmental studies to further confirm these findings and explain their underlying mechanisms. Given the current state of knowledge, we suggest further research exploring our hypothesis on the association between the arrival of a new pet and the change in a family dynamic to evaluate the impact of another child's arrival.

Our study has limitations that need to be noted. Both our study design and its lack of power (40 individuals from an initial cohort of 260 participants) didn't allow us to clarify the exact role of pets in the families who already owned pets. Nevertheless these first results open interesting lines of research exploring the efficacy of animals employed in AAT settings. Further studies with larger sample sizes (e.g. including more control groups) are needed to clarify the exact role of pets in this context.

Acknowledgments

We are thankful to Dr. Ann Cloarec, researcher, Ethos laboratory and Zarrin Alavi, (for her pertinent advice) medical writer and translator, Brest University Hospital, Department of Internal Medicine and Chest Diseases; INSERM CIC 0502, to Pr Michel Botbol, CHRU Brest, to families for their participation, to the Fondation Sommer for their support and the French GIS CCS (Groupe d'Intérêt Scientifique - Comportement Cerveau et Société)

Author Contributions

Conceived and designed the experiments: MG MH AL ST MD EL. Performed the experiments: MG MH EL. Analyzed the data: MG MH EL. Contributed reagents/materials/analysis tools: MG MH EL. Wrote the paper: MG MH ST EL.

References

1. American Psychiatric Association (1994) Diagnostic and Statistical Manual of Mental Disorders. Washington.
2. Wing L, Gould J (1979) Severe impairements of social interaction and associated abnormalities in children: Epidemiology and classication. Journal of Autism and Developmental Disorders 9: 11–29.
3. Baron-Cohen S (1995) Mindblindness: An Essay on Autism and Theory of Mind. Cambridge: MIT Press. 197 p.
4. Mundy P (1995) Joint attention and social-emotional approach behavior in children with autism. Development and Psychopathology 7: 63–82.
5. Osterling JA, Dawson G, Munson JA (2002) Early recognition of 1-year-old infants with autism spectrum disorder versus mental retardation. Development and Psychopathology 14: 239–251.
6. Baranek GT (1999) Autism during infancy: A retrospective video analysis of sensory-motor and social behaviors at 9–12 months of age. Journal of Autism and Developmental Disorders 29: 213–224.
7. Baron-Cohen S, Leslie AM, Frith U (1985) Does the autistic-child have a theory of mind. Cognition 21: 37–46.
8. Kasari C, Sigman M, Mundy P, Yirmiya N (1990) Affective sharing in the context of joint attention interactions of normal, autistic, and mentally-retarded children. Journal of Autism and Developmental Disorders 20: 87–100.
9. McConnell SR (2002) Interventions to facilitate social interaction for young children with autism: Review of available research and recommendations for educational intervention and future research. Journal of Autism and Developmental Disorders 32: 351–372.
10. Wong HHL, Smith RG (2006) Patterns of complementary and alternative medical therapy use in children diagnosed with autism spectrum disorders. Journal of Autism and Developmental Disorders 36: 901–909.
11. Pierce K, Schreibman L (1997) Multiple peer use of pivotal response training to increase social behaviors of classmates with autism: Results from trained and untrained peers. Journal of Applied Behavior Analysis 30: 157–160.
12. Gasalberti D (2006) Alternative Therapies for Children and Youth With Special Health Care Needs. Journal of Pediatric Health Care 20: 133–136.
13. Levinson BM (1962) The dog as a "co-therapist". Mental Hygiene 179: 46–59.
14. Redefer LA, Goodman JF (1989) Pet-facilitated therapy with autistic children. Journal of Autism and Developmental Disorders 19: 461–467.
15. Nathanson DE, DeFaria S (1993) Cognitive improvement of children in water with and without dolphins. Anthrozoös 65: 17–29.
16. Bass M, Duchowny C, Llabre M (2009) The Effect of Therapeutic Horseback Riding on Social Functioning in Children with Autism. Journal of Autism and Developmental Disorders 39: 1261–1267.
17. Martin F, Farnum J (2002) Animal-assisted therapy for children with pervasive developmental disorders. Western Journal of Nursing Research 24: 657–670.

18. Barker SB, Wolen AR (2008) The Benefits of Human-Companion Animal Interaction: A Review. West Lafayette, IN. Univ Toronto Press Inc. pp.487–495.

19. Katcher A (2000) The future of education and research on the human-animal bond and animal-assisted therapy Part B: Animal-assisted therapy and the study of human-animal relationships: Discipline or bondage? Context or transitional object? In: A F, editor. Handbook on animal-assisted therapy: Theoretical foundations for guidelines and practice. San Diego: Academic Press. pp.461–473.

20. Burrows KE, Adams CL, Spiers J (2008) Sentinels of Safety: Service Dogs Ensure Safety and Enhance Freedom and Well-Being for Families With Autistic Children. Qualitative Health Research 18: 1642–1649.

21. Anderson WP, Reid CM, Jennings GL (1992) Pet Ownership And Risk-Factors For Cardiovascular-Disease. Medical Journal of Australia 157: 298–301.

22. Friedmann E, Katcher AH, Lynch JJ, Thomas SA (1980) Animal companions and one-year survival after discharge from a coronary-care unit. Public Health Reports 95: 307–312.

23. Turner DC, Rieger G, Gygax L (2003) Spouses and cats and their effects on human mood. Anthrozoos 16: 213–228.

24. Beck AM, Meyers NM (1996) Health enhancement and companion animal ownership. Annual Review of Public Health 17: 247–257.

25. Serpell JA (1991) Beneficial-effects of pet ownership on some aspects of human health and behavior. Journal of the Royal Society of Medicine 84: 717–720.

26. Paul ES, Serpell JA (1996) Obtaining a new pet dog: Effects on middle childhood children and their families. Applied Animal Behaviour Science 47: 17–29.

27. Beck AM, Katcher AH (1984) A new look at pet-facilitated therapy. Journal of the American Veterinary Medical Association 184: 414–421.

28. Bryant BK (1990) The richness of the child pet relationship: A consideration of both benefits and costs of pets to children. Anthrozoos 3: 253–261.

29. Endenburg N, Baarda B (1996) The Role of Pets in Enhancing Human Well-being: Effects on Child Development. In: Robinson I, editor. The Waltham Book of Human-Animal Interactions: Benefits and Responsibilities of Pet Ownership. pp.7–17.

30. Filiatre JC, Millot JL, Montagner H., Eckerlin A, Gagnon AC (1988) Advances in the study of the relationship between children and their pet dogs. Anthrozöos 2: 22–32.

31. George H (1988) Child therapy and animals. In: CE S, editor. Innovative interventions in child and adolescent therapy. New York: John Wiley. pp.400–418.

32. Kidd AH, Kidd RM (1985) Children's attitudes toward their pets. Psychological Reports 57: 15–31.

33. Melson GF (1991) Children's attachment to their pets: Links to socio-emotional development. Children's Environments Quarterly 82: 55–65.

34. Bailey C (1988) Exposure of Preschool Children to Companion Animals: Impact on Role Taking Skills. Dissertation Abstracts International 48: 1976.

35. epperberg IM, Brezinsky MV (1991) Acquisition of a relative class concept by an african grey parrot (Psittacus erithacus) - Discriminations based on relative size. Journal of Comparative Psychology 105: 286–294.

36. Ralls K, Fiorelli P, Gish S (1985) Vocalizations and vocal mimicry in captive harbor seals, Phoca vitulina. Canadian Journal of Zoology 63: 1050–1056.

37. Savage-Rumbaugh S, Lewin R (1994) Kanzi: The Ape at the Brink of the Human Mind: John Wiley & Sons Inc. 299 pages p.

38. Lord C, Rutter M, Le Couteur A (1994) Autism Diagnostic Interview-Revised: a revised version of a diagnostic interview for caregivers of individuals with possible pervasive developmental disorders. J Autism Dev Disord 24: 659–685.

39. Cain AO (1985) Pets as family members. Marriage & Family Review 8: 5–10.

40. Tager-Flusberg H (2000) Understanding the Language and Communicative Impairments in Autism. New York: Academic Press.

41. Tager-Flusberg H, Caronna E (2007) Language disorders: Autism and other pervasive developmental disorders. Pediatric Clinics of North America 54: 469–+.

42. Glascoe FP, Foster M, Wolraich ML (1997) An economic analysis of developmental detection methods. Pediatrics 99: 830–837.

43. Glascoe FP (2005) Screening for developmental and behavioral problems. Mental Retardation and Developmental Disabilities Research Reviews 11: 173–179.

44. Siegel B, Anders TF, Ciaranello RD, Bienenstock B, Kraemer HC (1986) Empirically derived subclassification of the autistic syndrome. Journal of Autism and Developmental Disorders 16: 275–293.

45. Bryant B (1986) The relevance of family and neighborhood animals to social-emotional development in middle childhood. Boston.

46. Anastasi A (1988) Psychological Testing. New York: Macmillan. 818 p.

47. Lord C, Pickles A, McLennan J, Rutter M, Bregman J, et al. (1997) Diagnosing autism: Analyses of data from the autism diagnostic interview. Journal of Autism and Developmental Disorders 27: 501–517.

48. Tordjman S, Gutknecht L, Carlier M, Spitz E, Antoine C, et al. (2001) Role of the serotonin transporter gene in the behavioral expression of autism. Molecular Psychiatry 6: 434–439.

49. World Health Organization (1994) The composite international diagnostic interview, Version 1.1. Geneva: Researcher's manual.

50. Lord C, Rutter M, Goode S, Heemsbergen J, Jordan H, et al. (1989) Autism diagnostic observation schedule: a standardized observation of communicative and social behavior. Journal of Autism and Developmental Disorders 19: 185–212.

51. Rogé B, Fombonne E, Fremolle J, Arti E (2009) Adaptation française de l'ADOS: Echelle d'observation pour le diagnostic de l'autisme: Editions Hogrefe.

52. Travis LL, Sigman M (1998) Social deficits and interpersonal relationships in autism. Mental Retardation and Developmental Disabilities Research Reviews 4: 65–72.

53. Furman W (1989) The development of children's social networks. In: Belle D, editor. Children's Social Networks and Social Support. New-York: Wiley. 151–172.

54. Hills A (1995) Empathy and belief in the mental experience of animals. Anthrozoös 8: 132–142.

55. Melson GF (2005) Why the wild things are; animals in the lives of children: Harvard University Press. 236p.

56. Grandgeorge M (2010) Could the bond to an animal allow social and cognitive recovery in children with autism? Rennes: University Rennes 2. 357p.

57. Grandgeorge M, Hausberger M, Tordjman S, Deleau M, Lazartigues A, et al. (2009) Environmental Factors Influence Language Development in Children with Autism Spectrum Disorders. PLoS ONE 4: e4683.

58. Maurer M, Delfour F, Trudel M, Adrien JL (2011) L'enfant avec un autisme et l'animal dans un lien signifiant : des possibilités d'interventions thérapeutiques. La psychiatrie de l'enfant 54: 575–609.

59. Gelman R, Spelke ES (1981) The development of thoughts about animate and inanimate objects: Implications for research on social cognition. In: JH Flavell, L Ross, editors. Social cognition. New York: Academic. pp.43–66.

60. Poulin-Dubois D, Frenkiel-Fishman S, Nayer S, Johnson S (2006) Infants' Inductive Generalization of Bodily, Motion, and Sensory Properties to Animals and People. Journal of cognition and development 7: 431–453.

61. Friedmann E, Katcher AH, Thomas SA, Lynch JJ, Messent PR (1983) Social-Interaction And Blood-Pressure - Influence Of Animal Companions. Journal of Nervous and Mental Disease 171: 461–465.

62. Triebenbacher SL (1998) Pets as transitional objects: Their role in children's emotional development. Psychological Reports 82: 191–200.

63. Brickel CM (1982) Pet-Facilitated Psychotherapy - A Theoretical Explanation Via Attention Shifts. Psychological Reports 50: 71–74.

64. Odendaal JSJ (2000) Animal-assisted therapy - magic or medicine? Journal of Psychosomatic Research 49: 275–280.

65. Filiatre JC, Millot JL, Montagner H (1986) New data on communication behavior between the young-child and his pet dog. Behavioural Processes 12: 33–44.

66. Millot JL, Filiatre JC (1986) The behavioral sequences in the communication-system between the child and his pet dog. Applied Animal Behaviour Science 16: 383–390.

67. Millot JL, Filiatre JC, Gagnon AC, Eckerlin A, Montagner H (1988) Children and their pet dogs: how they communicate. Behavioural Processes 17: 1–15.

68. Hinde R (1979) Towards Understanding Relationships. London: Academic Press.

69. Poresky RH (1996) Companion animals and others factors affecting young children's development. Anthrozoos 9: 159–168.

70. Salomon A (1981) Animals and children - The role of the pets. Canadas Mental Health 29: 9–13.

71. Macdonald A (1981) The pet dog in a home: a study of interactions. In: Fogle B, editor. Interrelations between people and pets. Springfield, Illinois: Charles C. Thomas.

72. Beck AM, Melson GF, da Costa PL, Liu T (2001) The educational benefits of a ten-week home-based wild bird feeding program for children. Anthrozoos 14: 19–28.

73. Gervais H, Belin P, Boddaert N, Leboyer M, Coez A, et al. (2004) Abnormal cortical voice processing in autism. Nature Neuroscience 7: 801–802.

74. Osterling J, Dawson G (1994) Early recognition of children with autism - a study of 1st birthday home videotapes. Journal of Autism and Developmental Disorders 24: 247–257.

75. Maurer M, Delfour F, Wolff M, Adrien JL (2010) Dogs, Cats and Horses: Their Different Representations in the Minds of Typical and Clinical Populations of Children. Anthrozoos 23: 383–395.

76. Celani G (2002) Human beings, animals and inanimate objects - What do people with autism like? Autism 6: 93–102.

77. Kenzer AL, Bishop MR (2011) Evaluating preference for familiar and novel stimuli across a large group of children with autism. Research in Autism Spectrum Disorders 5: 819–825.

78. Poresky RH, Hendrix C (1989) Companion animal bonding, children's home environments and young children's social development. Kansas City.

79. Blue GF (1986) The value of pets in children's lives. Childhood Education 63: 84–90.

80. Bruner JS (1972) Nature and uses of immaturity. American Psychologist 27: 687–708.

81. Piaget J (1962) Play, dreams, and imitation in childhood. New York: Norton.

82. Montagner H (1995) L'enfant, l'animal et l'école: AFIRAC. 222 p.

83. Kaminski M, Pellino T, Wish J (2002) Play and Pets: The Physical and Emotional Impact of Child-Life and Pet Therapy on Hospitalized Children. Children's health care 31: 321–335.

84. Haggerty Davis J, Gerace L, Summers J (1989) Pet-care management in child-rearing families. Anthrozoos 2: 189–193.

7

Diagnosis of Cattle Diseases Endemic to Sub-Saharan Africa: Evaluating a Low Cost Decision Support Tool in Use by Veterinary Personnel

Mark C. Eisler[1]*, Joseph W. Magona[2], Crawford W. Revie[3]

1 School of Veterinary Sciences, Faculty of Medicine and Veterinary Medicine, University of Bristol, Bristol, United Kingdom, 2 Bulindi Zonal Agricultural Research and Development, Hoima, Uganda, 3 Atlantic Veterinary College, University of PEI, Charlottetown, Canada

Abstract

Background: Diagnosis is key to control and prevention of livestock diseases. In areas of sub-Saharan Africa where private practitioners rarely replace Government veterinary services reduced in effectiveness by structural adjustment programmes, those who remain lack resources for diagnosis and might benefit from decision support.

Methodology/Principal Findings: We evaluated whether a low-cost diagnostic decision support tool would lead to changes in clinical diagnostic practice by fifteen veterinary and animal health officers undertaking primary animal healthcare in Uganda. The eight diseases covered by the tool included 98% of all bovine diagnoses made before or after its introduction. It may therefore inform proportional morbidity in the area; breed, age and geographic location effects were consistent with current epidemiological understanding. Trypanosomosis, theileriosis, anaplasmosis, and parasitic gastroenteritis were the most common conditions among 713 bovine clinical cases diagnosed prior to introduction of the tool. Thereafter, in 747 bovine clinical cases estimated proportional morbidity of fasciolosis doubled, while theileriosis and parasitic gastroenteritis were diagnosed less commonly and the average number of clinical signs increased from 3.5 to 4.9 per case, with 28% of cases reporting six or more signs compared to 3% beforehand. Anaemia/pallor, weakness and staring coat contributed most to this increase, approximately doubling in number and were recorded in over half of all cases. Finally, although lack of a gold standard hindered objective assessment of whether the tool improved the reliability of diagnosis, informative concordance and misclassification matrices yielded useful insights into its role in the diagnostic process.

Conclusions/Significance: The diagnostic decision support tool covered the majority of diagnoses made before or after its introduction, leading to a significant increase in the number of clinical signs recorded, suggesting this as a key beneficial consequence of its use. It may also inform approximate proportional morbidity and represent a useful epidemiological tool in poorly resourced areas.

Editor: Bernhard Kaltenboeck, Auburn University, United States of America

Funding: The authors would like to thank the UK Department for International Development (DFID) for funding under RNRRS Projects R7597 and R8318. The funders had no role in study design, data collection and analysis, decision to publish, or preparation of the manuscript.

Competing Interests: The authors have declared that no competing interests exist.

* E-mail: mark.eisler@bristol.ac.uk

Introduction

Improved diagnosis is a prerequisite for effective management of endemic cattle diseases in sub-Saharan Africa. However this is currently constrained by the limited availability of suitably trained professional staff, field-level diagnostic tests and a general lack of knowledge about disease among livestock owners [1]. Moreover, under field conditions clinical diagnosis of these diseases is complicated by the occurrence of a combination of intestinal and haemoparasites, which mutually exacerbate each other's pathogenic effects [2,3]. Where multiple similar diseases occur decision support tools might facilitate differential diagnosis [4]. Current thinking in terms of veterinary service provision favours pen-side diagnostic tests and decision support technology suitable for use by farmers, extension workers and agro-veterinary traders; i.e. those who most often make the diagnosis and treatment decisions in rural African settings [1]. Recently a low cost decision

support tool has been developed to aid the diagnosis of anaplasmosis, babesiosis, cowdriosis, fasciolosis, parasitic gastro-enteritis, schistosomosis, theileriosis, and trypanosomosis in sub-Saharan Africa [5].

In this paper we describe the outcome of a study conducted to evaluate the effectiveness of the decision support tool as a diagnostic aid under field conditions by observing whether its introduction to veterinary and animal health officers undertaking primary animal health care in Uganda would lead to changes in clinical practice.

Materials and Methods

Diagnostic Decision Support Tool

The low cost decision support tool developed to aid the diagnosis of endemic bovine infectious diseases in the mixed crop–livestock production system of sub-Saharan Africa takes the form of a simple printed card that relates each of the eight diseases considered to a number of clinical signs (Figure 1). The card depicts a grid comprising eight columns, one for each disease and sixteen rows, one for each clinical sign. The cells of the grid contain the numbers 1, 2, 3 or 4, these being weightings ascribed to each sign in terms of its importance for diagnosing each disease, or are blank (representing zero weighting). Weighting values were obtained by a Delphi survey of expert opinion [5]. The numbers are accentuated by appearing on a coloured background, red for the highest weighting value of 4, orange for the next highest value, 3, yellow for 2 and grey for the lowest weighting value of 1, thereby mitigating against the likelihood of a misread weighting value. In use, the clinician sums the values in each column including only weightings in rows representing observed clinical signs; the disease associated with the column giving the highest total is considered the most likely diagnosis. In this study, the card was implemented on A5-size paper using an ordinary colour printer and laminated in sealed plastic pouches to ensure durability and re-usability under field conditions. A version of the card was also produced within the case-books designed for data recording during the study as discussed below and illustrated in Figure 1.

Study Area

The study was carried out between January and May 2005 in Iganga, Kayunga, Sironko, Soroti and Tororo Districts in the eastern region of Uganda (Figure 2). Savannah grassland is the main vegetation in the study area, which receives 1200–1500 mm of rainfall annually distributed in a bimodal manner. Interspersed between two dry seasons are two wet seasons, March to May and September to November. The overall daily mean minimum temperature is 15°C and the mean maximum 27°C. Small seasonal variations in rainfall and temperatures exist among the districts included in the study [6].

The economically important, endemic, vector-borne and parasitic diseases of cattle in this area are typical for the East African region and include: anaplasmosis caused by *Anaplasma marginale* [7,8,9]; babesiosis caused by *Babesia bigemina* [10,7,9]; cowdriosis or heartwater, caused by *Ehrlichia ruminantium*, previously called *Cowdria ruminantium*, [11,12]; fasciolosis caused by *Fasciola gigantica* [13,14]; parasitic gastroenteritis caused most severely by *Haemonchus* sp. [8,15]; schistosomiasis [16,17]; theileriosis or East Coast fever caused by *Theileria parva*, [18,19,7,8,9]; and trypanosomosis caused by *Trypanosoma brucei*, *Trypanosoma congolense* and *Trypanosoma vivax* [20,8,21].

The elevation of the study area varies from lowland swamps and marshland, which are more widespread in Kayunga, Iganga and Soroti Districts and suitable for the snail intermediate hosts of fasciolosis and schistosomiasis, to higher altitudes on the slopes of Mt Elgon in Sironko District, where levels of infestation with the tick and tsetse vectors of anaplasmosis, babesiosis, cowdriosis, theileriosis and trypanosomosis may differ from those elsewhere [7,22].

Participants and Study Design

Fifteen clinical participants undertaking primary animal health care in each of the five districts were recruited to take part in the study, including District Veterinary Officers (DVOs), Veterinary Officers and Animal Health Officers. The DVO for each district was informed that the study would involve recording of clinical signs and case data from field visits, and requested to include participants at each of these three levels of qualification. However, the final selection of participants was at the discretion of each DVO.

The study was conducted in two phases. During Phase-1 case data from five districts across Uganda were recorded in the field using a standardised form. Each participant was asked to record as many cases as possible over a two-month period while undertaking normal clinical duties. Participants were informed that a minimum of 45 cases would be required to ensure their involvement in the second phase of the study. Details associated with each case were recorded in a standard format using the right-hand portion of the layout shown in Figure 1. Phase-1 took place between January and March.

After Phase-1 had been completed all 15 participants attended a workshop at the Livestock Health Research Institute (LIRI) in Tororo, Uganda, at which the participants were introduced to the decision support tool (DST); its potential use as a diagnostic aid was explained and some practice sessions illustrating its use in the field were conducted by the authors.

This workshop was followed by Phase-2 of the study during which each participant was once again asked to record data from at least 45 cases over a two-month period. However, during this phase the participants utilised the DST as part of their routine clinical examination and recorded data using a standardised form similar to that used in the earlier phase (i.e. the full format of the case-book shown in Figure 1). Phase-2 was conducted between April and June across the same five districts.

Study approval. The study protocol was assessed and approved by the Uganda National Council for Science and Technology.

Data storage and analysis. Basic data recorded on the forms used in both Phase-1 and Phase-2 included: date of examination; location of the case; breed, sex and age of the case; presenting signs as noted by the farmer; clinical signs observed by the participant; tentative diagnosis; date of treatment, with type and amount of drug used. For most cases follow-up visits were made, at which point the date and the participant's assessment of the response to treatment were recorded. The additional information recorded during Phase-2 related to the diagnosis suggested by the DST as being the most likely. In both the case of diagnoses made by the participant and those suggested by the DST it was possible for more than one tentative diagnosis to be specified. This typically indicated either the potential of concurrent disease or that the information available at time of diagnosis was not sufficient to specify a unique diagnosis.

At the end of each phase case data were obtained from all participants and entered into an electronic format. The data were originally stored in worksheets within Microsoft Excel but were subsequently uploaded to a Microsoft Access database to allow for the more complex querying and summary required to create appropriate data structures for analytical tasks. Summary statistics were produced using Microsoft Excel, while database queries were created in Microsoft Access.

DST diagnosis calculation. To expedite analysis and remove a potential source of error, DST diagnoses were calculated from participants' clinical sign data using matrix algebra; the 8-by-16 DST matrix (Dx) was premultiplied by the transpose of an n-by-16 signs matrix (S), comprising n cases as rows and clinical signs coded 1 or 0 for presence or absence as columns ordered as on the DST, to yield an n-by-8 scores matrix (C):

$$C = S^T.Dx$$

The scores matrix was then modified to represent diagnoses using an algorithm such that the maximum value(s) in each row was replaced by a weighting value (w), and all other values by zero; where ties occurred (i.e. the DST suggested more than one

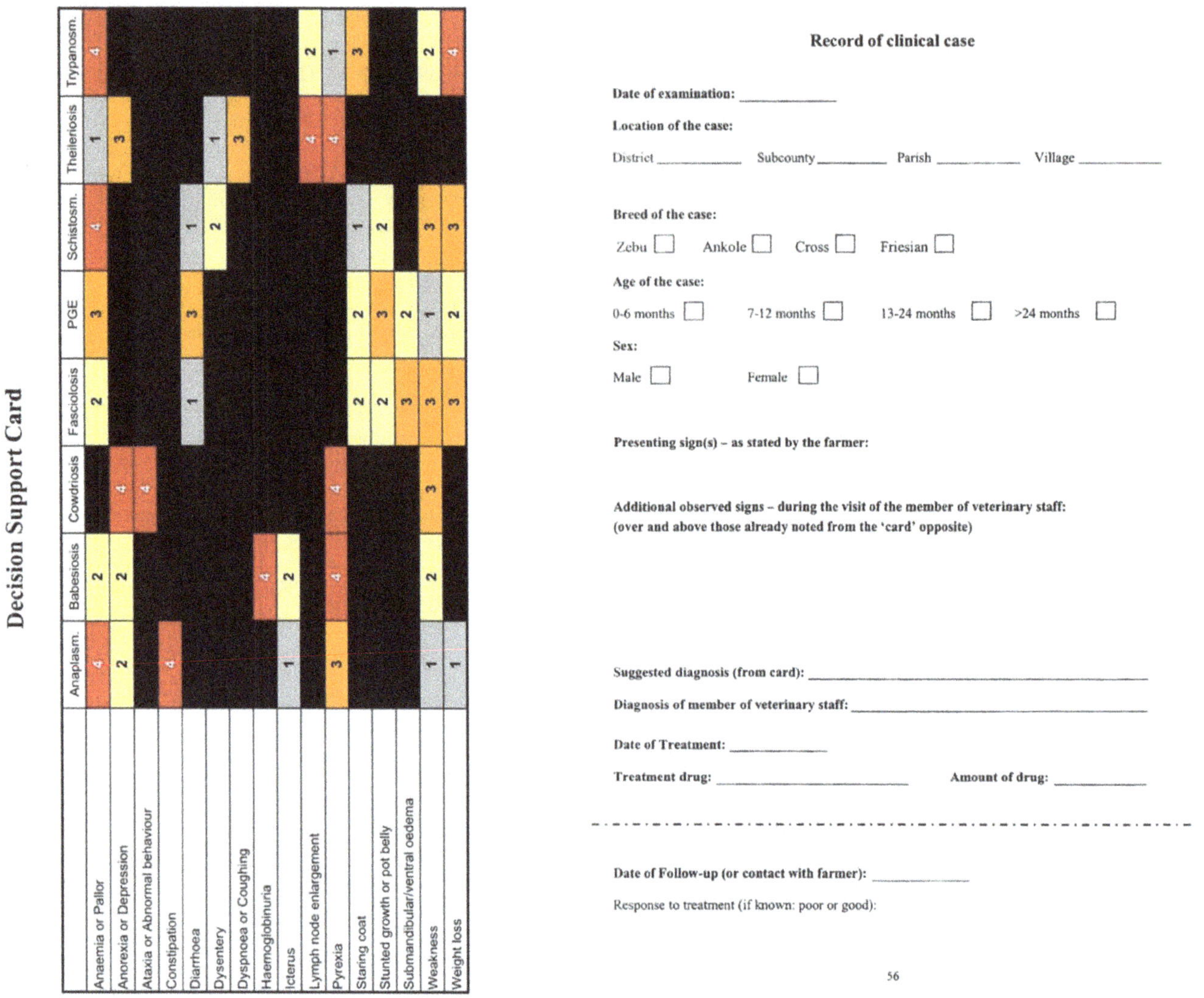

Decision Support Card

	Anaplasm.	Babesiosis	Cowdriosis	Fasciolosis	PGE	Schistosm.	Theileriosis	Trypanosm.
Anaemia or Pallor	4	2		2	3	4	1	4
Anorexia or Depression	2	2	4				3	
Ataxia or Abnormal behaviour			4					
Constipation	4							
Diarrhoea				1	3	1		
Dysentery						2	1	
Dyspnoea or Coughing							3	
Haemoglobinuria		4						
Icterus	1	2						
Lymph node enlargement							4	2
Pyrexia	3	4	4				4	1
Staring coat				2	2	1		3
Stunted growth or pot belly				2	3	2		
Submandibular/ventral oedema				3	2			
Weakness	1	2	3	3	1	3		2
Weight loss	1			3	2	3		4

Record of clinical case

Date of examination: ___________

Location of the case:

District ___________ Subcounty ___________ Parish ___________ Village ___________

Breed of the case:

Zebu ☐ Ankole ☐ Cross ☐ Friesian ☐

Age of the case:

0-6 months ☐ 7-12 months ☐ 13-24 months ☐ >24 months ☐

Sex:

Male ☐ Female ☐

Presenting sign(s) – as stated by the farmer:

Additional observed signs – during the visit of the member of veterinary staff:
(over and above those already noted from the 'card' opposite)

Suggested diagnosis (from card): ___________

Diagnosis of member of veterinary staff: ___________

Date of Treatment: ___________

Treatment drug: ___________ **Amount of drug:** ___________

Date of Follow-up (or contact with farmer): ___________

Response to treatment (if known: poor or good):

56

Figure 1. Template casebook used by participating Ugandan veterinary and animal health officers to record data in Phase-2 of the study. The template casebook was provided in the form of a printed notebook with the decision support tool appearing on each left hand page in landscape orientation so that clinical signs observed could be marked directly on it.

diagnosis), the usual weighting value (typically 12 to allow for 4 ties) was divided by the number of ties ensuring that the sum of weights for each row remained constant. Where none of the clinical signs on the DST were present, i.e. participants reported only 'other' signs, the full weighting value was recorded in an additional 9th column of the modified scores matrix representing an 'other' category that otherwise contained zeros.

Proportional morbidity. An n-by-9 matrix of participants' diagnoses (V) was constructed similarly with weights divided for multiple diagnoses as before, and diagnoses not listed on the DST in the ninth column. Proportional morbidity (P) was calculated for each of the 8 diagnoses listed on the DST plus the ninth 'other' category, as the proportion that diagnosis represented of all diagnoses by summation of the weights in each column of the n-by-9 matrix of DST or participants' diagnoses, and further dividing each sum by the grand total of all weights (n x *w*), *i.e.*

$$\textit{Proportional morbidity}: \mathbf{P}_c = \frac{\mathbf{N.C}}{w.n} \ \textit{or}\ \mathbf{P}_v = \frac{\mathbf{N.V}}{w.n}$$

where *w* is the scalar weighting value, *n* is the number of cases and N is a row vector of 1s of length *n*.

Concordance. A matrix κ representing concordance of the DST diagnoses with the participants' scores was calculated as follows:

$$\textit{Agreement}: \mathbf{A} = \frac{\mathbf{C}^{\mathbf{T}}.\mathbf{V} + [w-\mathbf{C}]^{\mathbf{T}}.[w-\mathbf{V}]}{w}.$$

$$\textit{Chance agreement}: \mathbf{Ch} = \frac{(\mathbf{N.C})^{\mathbf{T}}.(\mathbf{N.V}) + (\mathbf{N}.[w-\mathbf{C}])^{\mathbf{T}}.(\mathbf{N}.[w-\mathbf{V}])}{n.w}$$

$$\textit{Maximum agreement}: \mathbf{M} = n.w.\begin{pmatrix} 1_{1,1} & \cdots & 1_{1,9} \\ \vdots & \ddots & \vdots \\ 1_{9,1} & \cdots & 1_{9,9} \end{pmatrix}$$

$$\textit{Concordance matrix}: \boldsymbol{\kappa} = \frac{\mathbf{A}-\mathbf{Ch}}{\mathbf{M}-\mathbf{Ch}}$$

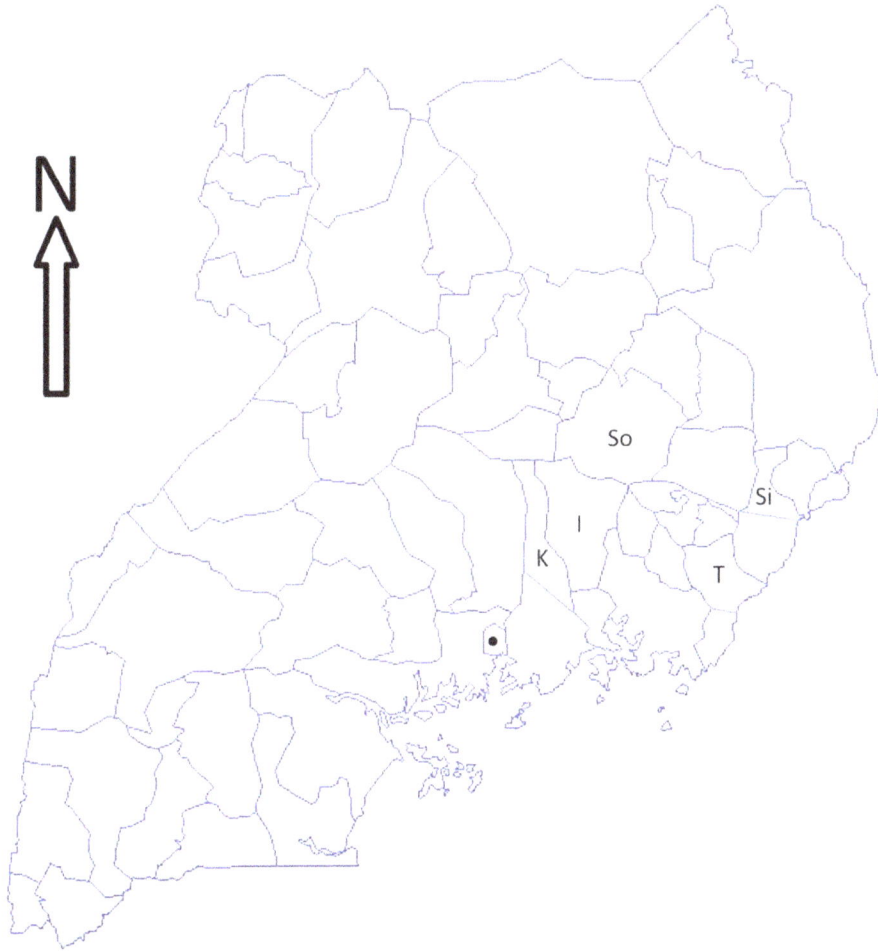

Figure 2. Map of Uganda showing the five districts in which the study was carried out. The study was carried out in Iganga (I), Kayunga (K), Sironko (Si), Soroti and Tororo (T) Districts in the eastern region of Uganda between January and May of 2005. Solid symbol is the Capital city, Kampala.

where ^{T} signifies the transpose of a matrix and the concordance matrix calculation uses element by corresponding element division of numerator by denominator 9-by-9 matrices.

Overall concordance (κ) for all nine diagnoses was calculated by summating the elements of the main diagonal, i.e. the trace (tr), of the numerator and denominator prior to division:

Overall concordance: $\kappa_{overall} = \dfrac{tr(\mathbf{A-Ch})}{tr(\mathbf{M-Ch})}$

Nomenclature when describing the relative strength of agreement associated with kappa statistics followed published recommendations [23]: <0.000, poor; 0.000–0.200, slight; 0.201–0.400, fair; 0.401–0.600, moderate; 0.601–0.800, substantial; 0.801–1.000, almost perfect.

Misclassification. A simple misclassification matrix ($\mathbf{M}$) for 'positive' agreement, uncorrected for chance, and scaled to show either participants' diagnoses in rows as a proportion of each DST diagnosis in columns ($\mathbf{M}_c$) or DST diagnoses in rows as a proportion of each participants' diagnosis in columns ($\mathbf{M}_v$), was calculated as:

Misclassification : $\mathbf{M}_c = \dfrac{\mathbf{V^T.C}}{w.\mathbf{N.C}}$ *or* $\mathbf{M}_v = \dfrac{\mathbf{C^T.V}}{w.\mathbf{N.V}}$

where each element of the numerator 9-by-9 matrix is divided by the value of the corresponding column of the denominator 1-by-9 row vector.

Differences in sign reporting and case outcomes between Phase-1 and Phase-2 were investigated using Chi-squared tests. All statistical analyses were carried out using Microsoft Excel, and MiniTab Version 14. Matrix algebra, algorithms and concordance (κ) were calculated using R version 2.14.2.

Results

Characteristics of Bovine Cases Reported by Participants

Before considering specific diseases or signs and any impact that the DST may or may not have had on diagnostic practice, it is useful to consider the breakdown of cases that were reported by the participants during the two phases of the study.

The participants reported on 713 and 751 bovine clinical cases in Phase-1 and Phase-2 respectively. The breakdown of these 1464 cases according to a number of key variables is shown in Table 1. This indicates that the composition of animals in terms of these variables remained broadly similar between the two phases. In both phases of the study, clinical examinations were conducted most often on cattle over 24-months of age, which were examined around three times more frequently than young cattle (0–6

Table 1. Breakdown of all cases (n = 1464) by key variables over the two phases of the study, pre and post-introduction of the DST.

	Phase	
	1	2
Age group		
0–6 months	13%	14%
7–12 months	25%	27%
13–24 months	22%	23%
>24 months	40%	36%
Gender		
Female	68%	62%
Male	32%	38%
District		
Iganga	17%	19%
Kayunga	19%	19%
Sironko	21%	20%
Soroti	21%	20%
Tororo	22%	22%
Participant Type		
Animal Health Officer	44%	47%
Veterinary Officer	28%	27%
District Veterinary Officer	28%	26%

months), with cattle in the intermediate age categories (7–12 and 12–24 months) falling between these two extremes.

Around twice as many female cattle were presented as were male; while Zebu cattle represented the most common breed, around half as many were identified as crossbred and much smaller proportions as Ankole and Friesian. All of the five districts in which data were recorded are roughly equally represented though the fact that all three participants from Kayunga were animal health officers rather than veterinary officers, resulted in this participant type being over-represented in the study as a whole.

Clinical Signs Recorded by Participants

There were a total of 6178 clinical signs recorded for the 1460 cases investigated by the participants over the two phases of the study. The most commonly occurring sign was anorexia or depression, seen in over 55% of cases. Weight loss, staring coat, and fever were observed in almost half of all cases, while weakness, enlarged lymph nodes, and anaemia were also present in around 40% of cases. Diarrhoea and dyspnoea or coughing were seen in around a quarter of cases, with constipation and stunted growth or a pot belly being seen in just under 20% and 15% of cases respectively. The remaining signs were observed relatively infrequently (i.e. in around 5% or fewer cases).

Of interest is whether and how the reporting of signs changed over the course of the two phases in the study. Table 2 lists signs in order of the proportional change in their observation frequency between Phase-1 and Phase-2. An increase was seen in 13 out of the 16 clinical signs, which was significant (p<0.05) for 8 signs (Table 2); significant increases were observed for anaemia or pallor, weakness, starring coat and lymph node enlargement (p<0.001); for submandibular or ventral oedema, stunted or pot

belly and weight loss (p<0.01); and for haemoglobinuria (p<0.05). There was an almost four-fold increase in the percentage of cases in which submandibular/ventral oedema was reported (p<0.01); however, as was the case for dysentery (not significant) and haemoglobinuria (p<0.05), which also saw marked increases, this was an infrequently occurring sign. The most striking changes (all highly significant; p<0.001) were observed for anaemia/pallor, weakness and staring coat. All commonly identified in around one quarter to a third of cases during Phase-1, the percentage of cases in which anaemia/pallor was observed more than doubled from under a quarter to over a half of all cases in Phase-2, while weakness and staring coat also almost doubled. In general the number of signs reported per case increased from 3.5 in the first phase to 4.9 in the second phase of the study.

The distribution of the number of clinical signs reported per clinical case during each of the two phases is shown in Figure 3, illustrating the structure of the increase in observation and reporting of clinical signs in Phase-2. In only a very few cases during Phase-1 did the participants record six or more signs for a given case; indeed, five signs were recorded in only around 100 cases during the initial phase of the study. In contrast during Phase-2, when the participants were given access to the DST, five signs were recorded in more than 200 cases, and six or more signs were observed in a similar number overall.

Participants recorded clinical signs as having been observed by themselves, by the farmer or both. The relative frequencies of individual signs identified by each group during Phases 1 and 2, are shown in Figure 4. The overall increase in mean number of signs reported per case was mostly accounted for by an increase in signs observed by participants from 2.9 to 4.7 per case, whereas those observed by farmers changed minimally from 1.4 to 1.5 signs per case. The sign most frequently reported by farmers was anorexia or depression, observed in 39.5% of cases over the two phases, and (in Phase-1) this was the one sign observed more frequently by farmers than participants. Other signs observed by farmers were weight loss, diarrhoea, weakness and staring coat in 26.8%, 16%, 13.8% and 12% of cases respectively in both phases; of these only staring coat showed an appreciable change between the two phases, more than doubling from 7.3% of cases in Phase-1 to 16.5% in Phase-2.

It should be noted that the signs participants were requested to document were not limited to those listed on the DST, and some reported additional signs. These were noted in around 19% of cases, predominantly in Phase-1 of the study. The diagnosis most commonly associated with additional signs was theileriosis (37% of all 'others' noted) followed by trypanosomosis (31%), anaplasmosis (22%) and PGE (11.4%). The remaining diagnoses were associated with fewer than 5% of 'other' signs noted. The most commonly observed specific signs not listed on the DST were lacrymation (almost 30% of the total), followed by dullness (17%) and nasal discharge (13%). Dehydration, low milk yield and corneal opacity each accounted for around 10% of the total, while a few other specific signs were observed only in a single case.

Proportional Morbidity in Bovine Cases Examined by Participants

There were four cases in Phase 2 for which participants' diagnoses were missing and so the final data set available for analysis consisted of 713 and 747 animals from Phase-1 and Phase-2 respectively. These 1460 cases were associated with a total of 1756 participants' diagnoses; in 291 (19.9%) cases participants noted that two diagnoses were likely, while in 5 cases (all in Phase-1) three possible diagnoses were reported. Where more than one diagnosis was noted, these were weighted equally in the analysis,

Table 2. Frequency with which clinical signs on the DST were observed in the two phases of the study, in decreasing order of relative change in frequency.

Clinical Sign	Phase-1		Phase-2		Relative change
	Percentage of cases in which clinical sign observed [95% CI]				(Ratio)
Submandibular or Ventral Oedema	1.5%	[0.6–2.4]	5.9%	[4.2–7.6]	3.7**
Anaemia or Pallor	22.0%	[19–25.1]	54.6%	[51–58.2]	2.4***
Dysentery	1.4%	[0.5–2.3]	3.3%	[2.1–4.6]	2.3
Haemoglobinuria	3.5%	[2.2–4.9]	7.6%	[5.7–9.5]	2.2*
Weakness	28.2%	[24.9–31.5]	54.9%	[51.3–58.5]	1.9***
Staring coat	33.0%	[29.5–36.4]	60.5%	[57–64]	1.8***
Stunted or Pot Belly	8.4%	[6.4–10.5]	15.5%	[12.9–18.1]	1.8**
Icterus	3.1%	[1.8–4.4]	4.8%	[3.3–6.4]	1.5
Lymph node enlarge	33.5%	[30.1–37]	46.3%	[42.7–49.9]	1.4***
Weight loss	43.8%	[40.1–47.4]	53.5%	[50–57.1]	1.2**
Diarrhoea	28.6%	[25.3–31.9]	32.3%	[28.9–35.6]	1.1
Anorexia or Depression	53.4%	[49.8–57.1]	57.4%	[53.9–61]	1.1
Pyrexia/Fever	43.9%	[40.3–47.5]	47.8%	[44.2–51.4]	1.1
Dyspnoea or Coughing	24.5%	[21.4–27.7]	22.6%	[19.6–25.6]	0.9
Constipation	18.0%	[15.1–20.8]	16.3%	[13.7–19]	0.9
Ataxia or Abnormal Behaviour	6.7%	[4.9–8.6]	6.0%	[4.3–7.7]	0.9
Total signs recorded	2521		3657		
Total number of cases	713		747		
Signs per case	3.5		4.9		

Statistical significance: *p<0.05,
**P<0.01,
***P<0.001.

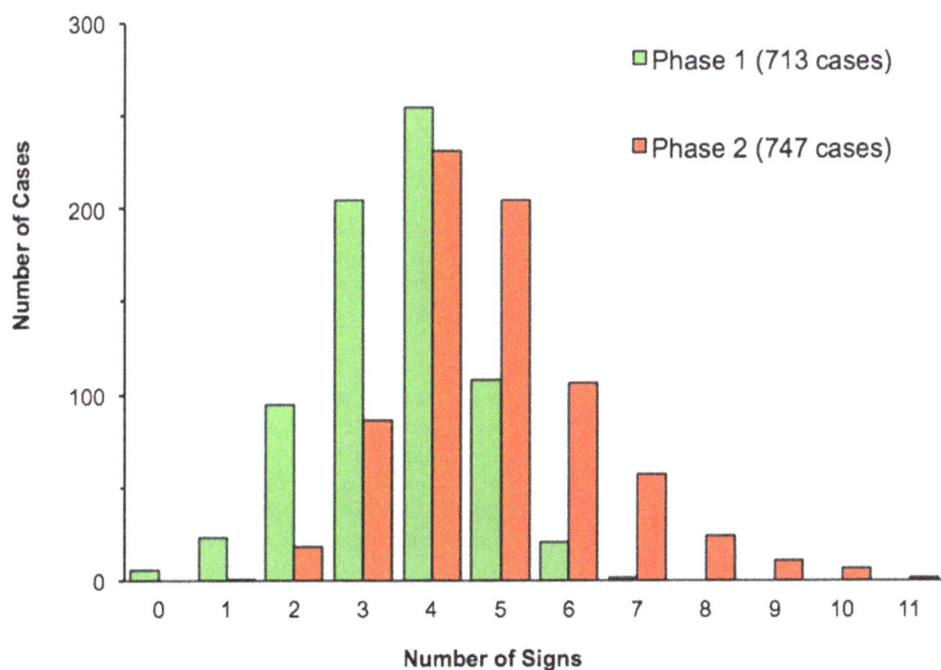

Figure 3. Frequency distribution of numbers of clinical signs recorded for bovine cases by Ugandan veterinary and animal health officers during the two phases of the study. Histogram showing the frequency distribution of number of clinical signs per case observed during each of the two phases of the study, prior to and after the introduction of the diagnostic decision support tool.

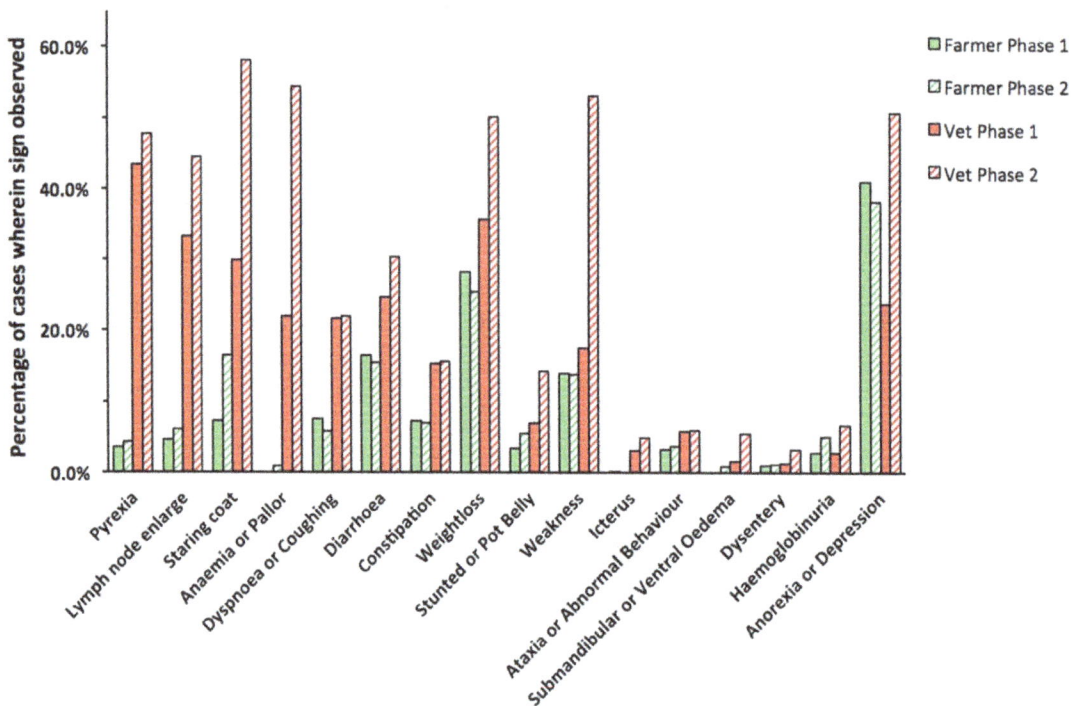

Figure 4. The percentages of bovine cases in which clinical signs were observed by Ugandan farmers and study participants (veterinary and animal health officers) during the two phases of the study. The percentages of clinical cases in which each sign was observed in cattle examined by farmers and study participants during the two phases of the study, ordered by decreasing differences between the two types of observation during Phase-1. (Phase-1, n = 713 cases; Phase-2, n = 747 cases.).

i.e. each of two diagnoses assigned to a case contributed half, and each of three one third, of the weighting assigned to singleton diagnoses.

The approximate proportional morbidity, i.e. relative frequency, of each of the eight diseases covered by the DST in each of the two study phases is illustrated in Figure 5, based on both participant's and DST diagnoses. Over the two phases combined, the most common participants' diagnoses were trypanosomosis and theileriosis, representing 23.4% and 22.5% respectively of all diagnoses, followed by anaplasmosis (16.5%), PGE (15.5%) and fasciolosis (12.0%). The proportions of participants' diagnoses for babesiosis and cowdriosis were fairly low (both less than 5%), with schistosomosis being the least frequently reported diagnosis, accounting for around 1% of all cases. A few diagnoses were made of conditions not included on the DST, these being in Phase-1 contagious bovine pleuropneumonia (5 cases), lumpy skin disease (3 cases), black quarter, mastitis (twice each), metritis, foot and mouth disease and fracture (once each), and in Phase-2 two diagnoses of lumpy skin. Categorised as 'other', these accounted for only 2.0% of all diagnoses in Phase-1, 0.2% in Phase-2 and 1.1% overall.

The participants' rates of diagnosis were assessed for departure from the null hypothesis that these were unaffected by the key variables outlined in Table 1 using Chi-squared tests. For neither sex of animal nor participant type was there evidence of difference from the expected disease profiles (p>0.5). However, breed effects were observed; while most tick-borne diseases were consistent with the null hypothesis (i.e. in proportion to the overall number of cases in each breed category) this was not the case for theileriosis, of which levels were significantly higher in crossbred and Friesian cattle and lower in Zebu (p<0.001). Conversely for both PGE

(p<0.05) and trypanosomosis (p<0.001) there were significantly higher proportions of cases in Zebu cattle.

There were also interesting departures from the null hypothesis when district was considered. Sironko had significantly higher proportions for the tick-borne diseases anaplasmosis and theileriosis (p<0.001); conversely this district appeared to have significantly lower proportions of trypanosomosis and fasciolosis (p<0.001). The proportion of PGE participants observed was significantly higher in the districts of Iganga and Tororo (p<0.001), for Tororo this elevated level predominantly during Phase-1.

For the final key variable, age group, almost all diseases except cowdriosis and schistosomosis (of which too few cases to test meaningfully for differences) differed significantly (p<0.01) from expectation under the null hypothesis that rate of diagnosis of is unaffected by age (Table 3).

Comparison of the DST with Participants' Diagnoses

Figure 5 shows the relative frequency of diagnoses suggested by participants and by the DST based on clinical signs they reported during each of the two phases of the study. Across the two phases, the DST suggested diagnoses in proportions broadly similar to those of the participants: namely a predominance of trypanosomosis (30.8% overall), this somewhat higher than for participants' diagnoses (23.4%), and theileriosis (23.2%); substantial levels of anaplasmosis (10.7%) and PGE (10.6%) albeit these proportions lower than those for participants' diagnoses (16.5% and 15.5% respectively); and rather lower levels of babesiosis and schistosomosis (both <4%). Contrastingly, the overall proportion of cowdriosis (13.6%) was considerably higher, and that of fasciolosis (3.2%) considerably lower, than those for the participants' diagnoses (4.1% and 12.0% for these two diseases respectively).

Phase 1:

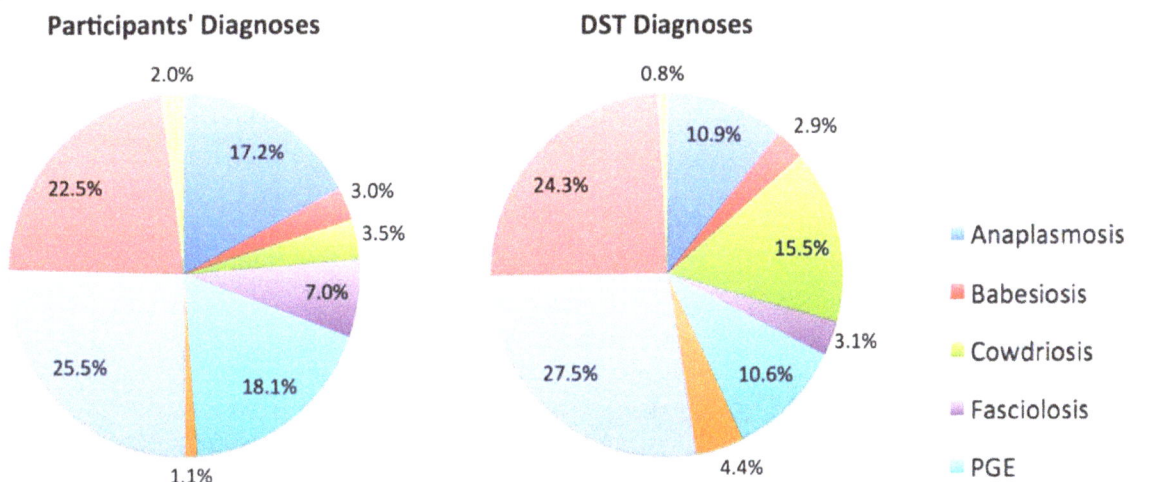

Phase 2:

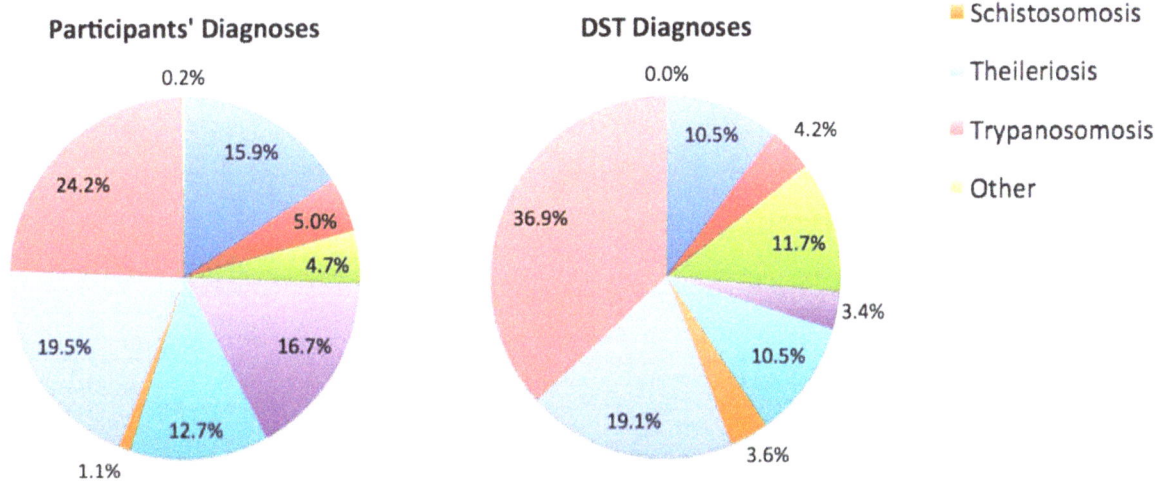

Figure 5. Approximate proportional morbidity in cattle in the eastern region of Uganda based on participating veterinary and animal health officers' diagnoses and those suggested by the DST. Numbers of individual diagnoses made in each of the two phases of the study are expressed as a proportion of all diagnoses made in that phase. Phase-1 (n = 713 cases) was prior to, and Phase-2 (n = 747 cases) after, the introduction of the diagnostic decision support tool.

Figure 5 breaks down both the DST and participants' diagnoses within each of the two phases, and further differences are apparent. Notably, whereas cowdriosis was only the fifth or sixth most common participants' diagnosis in either phase, representing fewer than 5% of the total, in Phase-1 it was the third most common diagnosis suggested by the DST, accounting for 15.5%. The DST also yielded a significantly higher proportion (P<0.001) of trypanosomosis diagnoses in Phase-2 (36.9%) than it did in

Table 3. Breakdown of participants' diagnoses by age of animal (n = 1460) across the two phases of the study.

Age group	Total	ANA*[1]	BAB*[2]	COW	FAS*[1]	PGE*[2]	THL*[2]	TRY*[2]
0–6 months	**14%**	5%	0%	6%	10%	22%	34%	2%
7–12 months	**26%**	28%	24%	20%	23%	37%	33%	15%
13–24 months	**22%**	26%	41%	29%	17%	19%	17%	26%
>24 months	**38%**	41%	35%	45%	51%	22%	16%	58%

*Differs significantly from the proportions expected under the null hypothesis that rate of diagnosis is unaffected by age: [1]p<0.01, [2]p<0.001; schistosomosis not shown as the number of cases (n = 16) was too small to meaningfully test for differences. [ANA = anaplasmosis, BAB = babesiosis, COW = Cowdriosis, FAS = Fasciolosis, PGE = parasitic gastroenteritis, THL = theileriosis, TRY = trypanosomosis.].

Table 4. Concordance matrices (κ) of participants' diagnoses and diagnoses calculated by the DST using clinical signs recorded during the study.

Participant Diagnosis	DST Diagnosis: ANA	BAB	COW	FAS	PGE	SCH	THL	TRY	Other
Phase-1									
ANA	**0.586**	−0.029	0.130	−0.055	−0.151	−0.061	−0.114	−0.212	−0.016
BAB	−0.050	**0.807**	−0.029	−0.032	−0.044	−0.037	−0.048	−0.038	−0.013
COW	−0.056	−0.032	**0.322**	−0.034	−0.056	−0.040	−0.066	−0.060	−0.014
FAS	−0.060	−0.037	−0.064	0.176	0.058	0.057	−0.110	0.103	−0.015
PGE	−0.118	−0.052	−0.052	0.102	**0.444**	0.059	−0.238	−0.002	−0.016
SCH	−0.021	−0.016	−0.004	−0.017	−0.021	**0.242**	−0.022	0.001	−0.010
THL	−0.165	−0.049	−0.083	−0.058	−0.162	−0.080	**0.733**	−0.283	0.000
TRY	−0.108	−0.051	−0.097	−0.021	−0.048	0.042	−0.237	**0.487**	−0.016
Other[1]	−0.035	0.034	−0.012	−0.025	−0.035	−0.029	0.005	−0.006	**0.432**
Phase-2									
ANA	**0.605**	−0.050	0.065	−0.030	−0.128	−0.048	−0.100	−0.178	0.000
BAB	−0.054	**0.772**	−0.049	−0.008	−0.072	−0.016	−0.061	−0.069	0.000
COW	−0.060	−0.047	**0.457**	−0.041	−0.069	−0.043	−0.060	−0.073	0.000
FAS	−0.130	−0.059	−0.113	0.082	**0.221**	0.013	−0.054	0.038	0.000
PGE	−0.078	−0.047	−0.092	0.096	**0.258**	0.117	−0.126	−0.021	0.000
SCH	−0.017	−0.017	−0.007	−0.017	−0.020	0.121	0.000	0.003	0.000
THL	−0.136	−0.069	−0.001	−0.037	−0.093	−0.043	**0.594**	−0.222	0.000
TRY	−0.132	−0.072	−0.104	−0.046	−0.097	−0.011	−0.232	**0.491**	0.000
Other[1]	−0.004	−0.004	0.019	−0.004	−0.004	−0.004	−0.004	0.000	0.000

κ-values for each DST diagnosis in columns are indicated for each participant diagnosis in rows. Main diagonal (mostly boldface numbers) indicating agreement between like diagnoses, other cells indicating possible cross-agreement between differing diagnoses. Boldface numbers indicate at least 'fair' agreement (κ ≥0.2); non-bold, positive numbers indicate slight agreement (0.2> κ >0); negative numbers indicate no cross-agreement, i.e. less than that expected by chance.
[1]Other: any participant's diagnosis other than the eight conditions listed on the DST; a DST diagnosis of 'other' resulted when none of its 16 signs was recorded for a case.
[2]SCH: schistosomosis. [Further abbreviations as Table 3.].

Phase-1 (24.3%) or participants did in either phase (23.4%); reductions in DST diagnoses of theileriosis (Phase-1, 27.5%; Phase-2, 19.1%; P<0.001) and cowdriosis (Phase-1, 15.5%, Phase-2, 11.7%; P<0.05) complemented this change. Participants diagnosed fasciolosis more than twice as frequently in Phase-2 (16.7%) as they did in Phase-1 (7.0%), a significant increase (p<0.001), and five-fold more often than did the DST in either phase (3.2% overall); complementary reductions were seen in participants diagnoses of theileriosis (Phase-1, 25.5%, Phase-2, 19.5%; p<0.05) and PGE (Phase-1, 18.1%; Phase-2, 12.7%; p<0.01).

Concordance. Concordance (κ) is a measure of agreement corrected for chance between the diagnostic outcomes (be they both presence or absence) of the two diagnostic 'arms' of the study, namely participants' diagnoses and those suggested by the DST. The concordance matrices (κ) shown in Table 4 provide this information for all possible combinations of outcomes over each of the two phases of the study. Arguably of equal interest to the levels of concordance between the DST and the participants for individual diseases as stated on the main diagonal of the κ matrix, are *cross-agreements* between results for different diseases shown by the non-diagonal entries.

A complication is that both the human participant and the DST often suggest multiple diagnoses. For example, in Phase-1 of the study, participants recorded a second diagnosis in 120 cases and a third in a further 5 cases, while in Phase-2 they recorded a second

diagnosis in 169 cases, but never a third. The DST suggested four diagnoses in 3 of the 1460 cases across the two phases, three diagnoses in 50 cases and two in 171 cases. The approach to calculating κ-values described above takes this into consideration using weighting values dependant upon the number of diagnoses per case.

Table 5 summarises the information from the main diagonals of the Phase-1 and Phase-2 concordance matrices (Table 4), together with the number of cases on which each diagnosis was based and provides the same information for the two phases combined. Concordance between outcomes of participants' diagnoses and the DSC differed markedly among diseases, and to a lesser extent between the first and second phases. Overall across both phases, the concordance of the DST with the participants was around 50% for all 1460 cases (κ = 0.486). The level of concordance was actually higher for cases seen in Phase-1 (κ = 0.519) than for those seen in Phase-2 (κ = 0.452) when the participants had the DST to hand. The individual disease having the greatest agreement was babesiosis (κ = 0.786), with similar levels in both phases of the study. Anaplasmosis, theileriosis and trypanosomosis had overall agreement levels of 0.595, 0.672 and 0.491 respectively, again with similar levels across phases, albeit theileriosis having slightly poorer agreement in Phase-2. There was least agreement by far over fasciolosis, particularly during the second phase of the study (κ = 0.082) when a significant overall increase in the proportion of cases participants reported with this diagnosis was unmatched by

Table 5. Concordance (κ) of outcomes for each of the eight diagnoses suggested by the DST with those made by participating veterinary and animal health officers.

Concordance (κ) of DST with Participants' Diagnoses (n cases with participant's diagnosis)			
Participant's Diagnosis:	**Phase-1**	**Phase-2**	**Both Phases**
All diseases	0.519(713)	0.452(747)	0.486(1460)
Babesiosis	0.807(21.5)	0.772(37)	0.786(58.5)
Theileriosis	0.733(182)	0.594(146)	0.672(328)
Anaplasmosis	0.586(122.5)	0.605(119)	0.595(241.5)
Trypanosomosis	0.487(160.7)	0.491(180.5)	0.491(341.2)
Other	0.432(14.5)	0.000(1.5)	0.406(16)
Cowdriosis	0.322(25)	0.457(35)	0.385(60)
PGE[1]	0.444(129.2)	0.258(95)	0.357(224.2)
Schistosomosis	0.242(8)	0.121(8)	0.185(16)
Fasciolosis	0.176(49.7)	0.082(125)	0.113(174.7)

NB the DST was available to participants during Phase-2 but not Phase-1.
[1]As table 3.

the number of times this diagnosis was suggested by the DST (Figure 5).

In interpreting Tables 4 and 5 it is important to consider that the concordance (κ) values indicate that portion of agreement not accounted for by chance; hence, most of the non-diagonal cells in Table 5 have trivially small or negative values, indicating no agreement. In striking contrast values in most of the diagonal cells indicate a fair to substantial level of agreement ($0.807 \geq \kappa \geq 0.242$), with the notable exceptions of fasciolosis in Phase-1 ($\kappa = 0.176$) and Phase-2 ($\kappa = 0.082$) and schistosomosis in Phase-2 ($\kappa = 0.121$) for which agreement was slight, or poor. A few further cells in the concordance matrices also have non-trivial values. For instance in Phase-1, while the DST recorded moderate concordance with participants for anaplasmosis ($\kappa = 0.586$), it also showed slight cross-agreement for that disease with participants' results for cowdriosis ($\kappa = 0.130$). Similarly in Phase-1, the (slight) agreement of the DST with participants over fasciolosis was almost equalled by a slight cross-agreement of participants' fasciolosis status with the DST's on trypanosomosis ($\kappa = 0.103$); and the moderate level of concordance ($\kappa = 0.444$) of the DST with participants over PGE was accompanied by a slight cross-agreement with fasciolosis ($\kappa = 0.102$).

Clinical signs were reported as having been observed by either the farmer or the veterinary participants themselves, and DST diagnoses could be calculated using each of these sign sets or the full, combined sign set as was used in Tables 2, 3, 4, 5 and Figure 5. A further possibility is a combined set including all signs observed by veterinary participants and a subset of those observed by farmers restricted to anorexia/depression, ataxia/abnormal behaviour, constipation, diarrhoea, dyspnoea/coughing, staring coat, weakness and weight loss; all of significance for the clinical history and though readily detected, not necessarily apparent during a brief veterinary examination. Using only signs observed by farmers in Phase-1 to calculate DST diagnoses yielded a lower overall κ-value in the 'fair' category of just 0.332, compared to the 'moderate' value of 0.519 obtained using the full sign set. Phase-1 DST diagnoses calculated using signs observed by veterinary participants alone gave a slightly higher overall κ-value of 0.541,

while complementing these signs with the restricted subset of farmers' signs gave an overall κ-value of 0.510, not appreciably different from that using the full sign set.

Other analyses using DST diagnoses derived from the full sign set in Phase-1 examined the effect of either including only one participant's diagnosis for each case (the first where more than one was recorded), which resulted in slightly better overall concordance ($\kappa = 0.567$), or restricting cases to those where both the DSC and the participant made unique diagnoses (n = 499), which led to higher still Phase-1 concordance ($\kappa = 0.641$).

Misclassification. Misclassification matrices were scaled to show either, for cases in which the participants diagnosed a particular condition (columns), the proportions of each diagnosis (rows) suggested by the DST (M_{ij}, Table 6a) or, for cases in which the DSC suggested a particular condition (columns), the proportions of each diagnosis (rows) made by participants (M_{ij}, Table 6b). These misclassification matrices enable identification of sources of discrepancy between the two diagnostic arms of the study. For instance, while cowdriosis scores highly (0.980) on the main diagonal of the Phase-1 M_{ij} matrix (Table 6a), indicating that where participants diagnosed this condition the DST suggested likewise in almost every case, the corresponding Phase-1 M_{ij} matrix (Table 6b) shows that only a modest proportion (0.221) of cases suggested as cowdriosis by the DST were diagnosed as such by participants; they also apportioned these cases among anaplasmosis (0.286), theileriosis (0.166), PGE (0.134) and trypanosomosis (0.128). This explains the 12% discrepancy between Phase-1 proportional morbidity (Figure 5) for cowdriosis derived from participants' diagnoses (3.5%) and the DST suggestions (15.5%), reassures us that virtually all of the 3.5% comprises a part of the 15.5% (there might otherwise have been no commonality between the two) and explains how the 12% difference distributes among participants' diagnoses.

Other differences between participants' and DST diagnoses manifest in Figure 5 as differences in proportional morbidity may be similarly explained using Table 6. Compared with participants, the DST apparently under-diagnosed anaplasmosis markedly in both phases; only around half (Phase-1, 0.524; Phase-2, 0.543) of cases diagnosed as anaplasmosis by participants were suggested as such by the DST, the discrepancy distributed among cowdriosis (Phase-1, 0.259; Phase-2, 0.166), theileriosis (Phase-1, 0.159; Phase-2, 0.100) trypanosomosis (Phase-1, 0.039; Phase-2, 0.140) and to a much lesser extent other conditions (Table 6a). Where the DST suggested anaplasmosis, participants agreed with a high proportion (0.825) of these diagnoses in both phases (Table 6b). With PGE, the situation was less clear-cut; while proportional morbidity was higher for participants' diagnoses (Phase-1, 18.1%; Phase-2, 12.7%) than DST suggestions (Phase-1, 10.6%; Phase-2, 10.5%), for both diagnostic arms of the study Tables 6a and b reveal misdiagnoses distributed among a number of conditions, reflecting the relatively low concordance ($\kappa = 0.357$) for this condition across both phases (Table 5). Similarly for fasciolosis, which had the lowest concordances of all in both phases and overall ($\kappa = 0.113$, Table 5), Table 6a reveals that participants' diagnoses of this condition in either phase are mostly apportioned by the DST to trypanosomosis (Phase-1, 0.450; Phase-2, 0.415), PGE (Phase-1, 0.173; Phase-2, 0.262), theileriosis (Phase-2, 0.144) or fasciolosis itself (Phase-1, 0.153), and Table 6b shows that DST-suggested diagnoses of fasciolosis are likewise mostly apportioned by participants among PGE (Phase-1, 0.513; Phase-2, 0.344), fasciolosis (Phase-1, 0.343; Phase-2, 0.397) or trypanosomosis (Phase-1, 0.143). Finally, Table 6b shows that in Phase-2, the additional proportional morbidity (Figure 5) attributed to

Table 6. Misclassification matrices, (a) M$_v$ and (b) M$_c$, of participants' diagnoses and diagnoses calculated by the DST using clinical signs recorded during the study.

(a) M$_v$ — Participant Diagnosis:

	DST Diagnosis	ANA	BAB	COW	FAS	PGE	SCH	THL	TRY	Other
Phase-1	ANA	0.524	0.000	0.000	0.039	0.027	0.000	0.009	0.040	0.000
	BAB	0.012	0.791	0.000	0.003	0.000	0.000	0.003	0.001	0.069
	COW	0.259	0.070	0.980	0.062	0.115	0.125	0.101	0.088	0.103
	FAS	0.000	0.000	0.000	0.153	0.088	0.000	0.000	0.020	0.000
	PGE	0.000	0.012	0.000	0.173	0.410	0.000	0.008	0.076	0.000
	SCH	0.008	0.000	0.000	0.087	0.077	0.625	0.000	0.067	0.000
	THL	0.159	0.047	0.000	0.034	0.041	0.000	0.835	0.077	0.310
	TRY	0.039	0.081	0.020	0.450	0.241	0.250	0.036	0.631	0.207
	Other	0.000	0.000	0.000	0.000	0.000	0.000	0.008	0.000	0.310
Phase-2	ANA	0.543	0.027	0.014	0.013	0.042	0.016	0.015	0.024	0.000
	BAB	0.013	0.725	0.000	0.008	0.013	0.000	0.003	0.003	0.000
	COW	0.166	0.041	0.864	0.035	0.039	0.078	0.116	0.052	0.667
	FAS	0.017	0.027	0.000	0.080	0.091	0.000	0.013	0.009	0.000
	PGE	0.013	0.000	0.000	0.262	0.314	0.000	0.044	0.046	0.000
	SCH	0.008	0.023	0.000	0.043	0.107	0.297	0.012	0.030	0.000
	THL	0.100	0.054	0.050	0.144	0.058	0.188	0.666	0.028	0.000
	TRY	0.140	0.104	0.071	0.415	0.335	0.422	0.131	0.809	0.333
	Other	0.000	0.000	0.000	0.000	0.000	0.000	0.000	0.000	0.000

(b) M$_c$ — DST Diagnosis:

	Participant Diagnosis	ANA	BAB	COW	FAS	PGE	SCH	THL	TRY	Other
Phase-1	ANA	0.825	0.074	0.286	0.000	0.000	0.032	0.099	0.027	0.000
	BAB	0.000	0.836	0.014	0.000	0.003	0.000	0.005	0.010	0.000
	COW	0.000	0.000	0.221	0.000	0.000	0.000	0.000	0.003	0.000
	FAS	0.025	0.008	0.028	0.343	0.114	0.139	0.008	0.129	0.000
	PGE	0.045	0.000	0.134	0.513	0.702	0.322	0.027	0.180	0.000
	SCH	0.000	0.000	0.009	0.000	0.000	0.161	0.000	0.012	0.000
	THL	0.021	0.025	0.166	0.000	0.020	0.000	0.774	0.037	0.250
	TRY	0.084	0.008	0.128	0.143	0.161	0.346	0.063	0.585	0.000
	Other	0.000	0.049	0.014	0.000	0.000	0.000	0.023	0.017	0.750
Phase-2	ANA	0.825	0.047	0.225	0.079	0.019	0.037	0.083	0.060	NA[1]
	BAB	0.013	0.850	0.017	0.040	0.000	0.031	0.014	0.014	NA
	COW	0.006	0.000	0.345	0.000	0.000	0.000	0.012	0.009	NA
	FAS	0.020	0.032	0.049	0.397	0.416	0.201	0.126	0.188	NA
	PGE	0.051	0.040	0.043	0.344	0.379	0.377	0.039	0.115	NA
	SCH	0.002	0.000	0.007	0.000	0.000	0.088	0.011	0.012	NA
	THL	0.028	0.016	0.194	0.076	0.081	0.065	0.680	0.069	NA
	TRY	0.056	0.016	0.107	0.063	0.105	0.202	0.035	0.529	NA
	Other	0.000	0.000	0.011	0.000	0.000	0.000	0.000	0.002	NA

In (a), **M$_v$**, proportions of each participant diagnosis are shown for each DST diagnosis in columns summating to 1. In (b), **M$_c$**, proportions of each DST diagnosis are shown for each participant diagnosis in columns summating to 1.
Leading diagonal indicating agreement, other cells indicating disagreement.
[1]NA: not applicable. [Other abbreviations as Table 4.].

trypanosomosis by DST diagnoses (36.9%) compared with that attributed by participants' diagnoses (24.2%) was explained by cases apportioned by participants among fasciolosis (0.188) and PGE (0.115); and Table 6a shows correspondingly that where participants diagnosed trypanosomosis in Phase-2, a high proportion of DST suggested diagnoses agreed (0.809).

Discussion

This study evaluated the effectiveness of a decision support tool as a diagnostic aid under field conditions in Uganda by observing whether its introduction to veterinary and animal health officers undertaking primary animal health care would affect their clinical practice in terms of observation of clinical signs and arrival at specific diagnoses. Fifteen participants including District Veterinary Officers, Veterinary Officers and Animal Health Officers from five districts in Uganda provided information on 1442 bovine clinical cases for which they reported a total of 6152 clinical signs. During an initial phase, participants reported clinical signs and diagnoses for 713 cases based on their usual practice, whereas in a subsequent phase clinical signs and diagnoses were reported for a further 751 cases investigated using a simple, low cost decision support tool for differentiation amongst eight common conditions. While livestock owners' perceptions of cattle diseases and their treatments have been investigated previously [1,24,25], this appears to be the first study of diagnoses by veterinary staff or animal health assistants under field conditions in the Lake Victoria Basin.

The composition of the case data sets remained broadly similar between the two phases in terms of a number of variables, namely animal age group, gender and breed, administrative district and participant type. No instructions were given to the participants in terms of case selection so we can assume that this breakdown is broadly reflective of the cattle for which they were receiving requests to carry out diagnosis. Of interest is the fact that clinical examinations were around three times as likely to involve animals in the over 24-month category than they were very young cattle (0–6 months) and that around twice as many female cattle were presented as were male, perhaps reflecting the higher perceived value of adult females in terms of reproductive potential and/or milk production; similar bias towards older animals and females was observed by Van den Bossche et al. [26] in relation to farmer use of trypanocidal drugs in cattle in Zambia.

Clinical Signs Recorded by Participants

A striking feature of this study was the increase in the average number of clinical signs per case observed following the introduction of the DST, 4.9 in Phase-2 compared with 3.5 in Phase-1. Almost 28% of Phase-2 cases showed six or more signs compared to just 3% of cases in Phase-1 (Figure 3). The individual signs contributing most to this increase were anaemia/pallor, weakness and staring coat, which all but doubled in number in Phase-2 to be seen in over half of all cases. However, while the overall number of signs reported increased in Phase-2, this increase was limited to signs listed on the DST; some other signs reported during Phase-1 but not on the DST, such as lacrymation, dullness and nasal discharge were no longer reported after its introduction. The interpretation of this may be that while the DST encourages clinical examination and recording of signs observed, this effect is limited to those signs listed on it. Finally, while dullness might be considered equivalent to anorexia/depression as listed on the DST, addition of anorexia/depression as a sign to 14 Phase-1 cases that lacked it but nevertheless reported dullness did not substantively affect the results.

Also of interest was the ability of farmers to identify clinical signs, some of which might not be manifest at the time of the veterinary staff visit, but would be reported as clinical history. Work in neighbouring Kenya showed that cattle keepers in production systems with similar disease challenge identified a number of clinical signs associated with bovine trypanosomiasis including staring coat, inappetence, weight loss, eating soil (pica),

nasal discharge, weakness, coughing, constipation, salivation, dullness, lameness, diarrhoea, reluctance to drink, swollen lymph nodes and tooth grinding [1]. In the present work, farmers were shown to identify some signs more frequently than others, and in the case of anorexia or depression more frequently than veterinary staff, at least prior to the introduction of the DST (Figure 3). It can be envisaged that the DST might be helpful to farmers in diagnosing endemic disease in their cattle, and the results obtained here support earlier work in confirming they are able to identify at least some clinical signs, but also suggest that they would benefit from additional training to facilitate this.

Proportional Morbidity

Given that the participants' diagnoses were available for both the first and second phases of the study, we initially used these to characterise the disease status of the animals examined as a measure of proportional morbidity in the population under the clinical care of the participants. The eight diseases covered by the DST included over 98% of the putative diagnoses made by the participants for cases they attended throughout the study period, and hence the DST diagnoses may also provide an approximate measure of proportional morbidity in these districts of Uganda. In around 20% of cases the participants noted that more than one diagnosis was likely; primarily this was a second possible diagnosis, though in Phase-1 there were 5 cases where three possible diagnoses were reported.

The conditions most commonly diagnosed by participants in both phases were three vector-borne diseases: trypanosomosis, theileriosis, and anaplasmosis, and two helminthiasies: parasitic gastroenteritis (PGE) and fasciolosis; babesiosis, cowdriosis and schistosomosis were far less frequently diagnosed. While trypanosomosis remained the most common diagnosis through both phases, representing around a quarter of all diagnoses, theileriosis and PGE were diagnosed significantly less commonly in Phase-2, effectively being replaced by a significant increase in fasciolosis, for which proportional morbidity doubled. These diagnoses were consistent with endemic diseases reported by other studies of cattle in the region [1,24,25], and are reflected in the range of drugs stocked by agro-veterinary shops in the region and their rates of sale [27]. No significant transboundary disease epidemics occurred during the study period.

Independent measures of occurrence of diseases within the target population, i.e. cattle under the primary animal health care of the veterinary and animal health officers participating in the study, would be of interest in evaluating the impact and performance of the DST, but there are few formal studies and reliable contemporary prevalence and incidence data are not available. Hence, while possible confounding and various uncontrolled sources of bias suggest that care must be taken not to over-interpret these results, it is interesting to comment on the observed rates of diagnosis (proportional morbidity), and compare these to values expected under the null hypothesis that rates were unaffected by the key variables outlined in Table 1. Specifically, there appeared to be predisposition towards diagnosis of theileriosis in Friesian and crossbred cattle, as compared with Zebu, whereas Ankole appeared to have greater likelihood of diagnosis of trypanosomosis than other breeds, observations consistent with known breed susceptibilities [28]. Similarly, some district level effects were observed, such as lower proportional morbidity due to trypanosomosis and fasciolosis in Sironko District, consistent with its higher elevation on the slopes of Mount Elgon, and that most diagnoses of schistosomosis in were made in Kayunga District, but it was difficult to draw any firm conclusions from these effects. The results reported here are based on data collected over two specific periods in a single year across the areas under consideration. To obtain insight into seasonal and annual variation it would be necessary to utilise the DST as an on-going diagnosis/monitoring tool.

Age effects on proportional morbidity were possibly of greater interest (Table 3). In this area of Uganda, there appears to be clear evidence that diagnosis of PGE is primarily associated with young animals while the opposite appears to be the case with trypanosomosis (significantly fewer cases in the two age classes of animals under one year and significantly more in those cattle of two years or older). However, it is arguably the age distributions for cases diagnosed with tick-borne diseases that are most interesting. For three of these (anaplasmosis, babesiosis and cowdriosis) there is evidence that the presence of disease in young animals (less than 6 months old) was significantly lower than would be expected based purely on proportions of cattle in each age group, consistent with the concept of inverse age immunity for these diseases [29]. However, this was clearly not the case for theileriosis for which the proportion with the disease was significantly higher than expected in younger and significantly lower in older animals, consistent with observations by David Bruce et al. almost 100 years earlier [18].

Comparison of the DST with Participants' Diagnoses

Previous attempts at evaluating expert systems for animal disease diagnosis have used selected test cases [5,30], whereas the present study was based on naturally occurring disease. Hence, one challenge in evaluating the performance of the DST was not having an independent assessment as to which disease or diseases were truly present in each of the cases. Unfortunately provision of definitive diagnostic capability through laboratory investigations would have been prohibitively costly and beyond the scope of this study. Even if that had been feasible, detailed diagnostic investigations in remote African rural settings might have influenced interactions between farmers and veterinary partici-pants and introduced significant bias to the study. In the absence of such a 'gold standard' to evaluate whether the tool achieved the 'correct' diagnosis we made no assumption that the human participant (veterinary or animal health officer) made the correct diagnosis and but simply assessed how often the suggested diagnosis of the DST was in agreement (Tables 4 and 5). Moreover, we note that comparisons of the two types of diagnosis differ between the two phases; Phase-1 comparison was between the DST's rendition of clinical signs reported by participants not yet introduced to it and diagnoses based on their customary clinical practice, whereas in Phase-2 the comparison was between the DST's rendition of reported clinical signs and diagnoses suggested by participants using the DST as an aid to their clinical judgement.

A further complication is that both human observers and the DST may suggest multiple diagnoses. The DST may allocate the same score to multiple diseases for a given combination of clinical signs; of the 65,536 (2^{16}) possible sign combinations, 18,352 (28.0%) yield more than one diagnosis. Indeed, the concordance values reported here must be interpreted taking into consideration that neither the participants' nor the DST diagnoses returned perfect scores when compared with themselves (participants Phase-1, overall $\kappa = 0.894$; DST Phase-1, overall $\kappa = 0.886$). Within either diagnostic arm of the study, cases with more than one diagnosis may be regarded as having internal disagreement. In terms of individual diseases, this 'self-concordance' of the participants' diagnoses was in the 'almost perfect' category ($\kappa > 0.8$) for all but fasciolosis ($\kappa = 0.770$), although no particular 'cross-agreement' was evident. Likewise, self-concordance of the DST was in the

almost perfect category ($\kappa > 0.8$) for all diseases but fasciolosis ($\kappa = 0.634$) and schistosomosis ($\kappa = 0.635$), these two having a weak mutual cross-agreement ($\kappa = 0.072$).

Concordance of the DST with participants' diagnoses is best examined in detail for Phase-1, when the DST had not yet been introduced to the participants (Table 4). For example, for the DST's result with regard to cowdriosis, in addition to a 'fair' level of agreement ($\kappa = 0.322$) with veterinary participants' results for the same condition, the DST also showed slight cross-agreement ($\kappa = 0.130$) with a participant's result for anaplasmosis. This can be contrasted with the sixth column in the Phase-1 concordance matrix (Table 4), which shows the level of (cross-)agreement of participants' results for each disease with the DST's result for schistosomosis. While this indicates that the DST was in fair agreement ($\kappa = 0.242$) with the participants with regard to presence or absence of schistosomosis, the DST also cross-agreed with the participants' results for fasciolosis, PGE and trypanoso-mosis. Despite the individual values being small, schistosomosis accrued by far the highest level of cross agreements.

Additional concordance matrices (not shown) were derived using a number of alternative approaches to the data, for instance including or not including various combinations of clinical signs observed by either farmers or participating veterinary staff in calculating the DST diagnoses, or using only the first of multiple participants' diagnoses for a particular case. Generally, clinical signs observed by farmers resulted in DST diagnoses with poorer agreement with participants' diagnoses, whereas perhaps unsur-prisingly using only a single participants' diagnosis for each case improved concordance with the DSC, probably on account of 'perfect' self-concordance ($\kappa = 1.000$) achieved by having unique participants' diagnoses. The highest Phase-1 concordance ($\kappa = 0.641$) was obtained using DST diagnoses derived from the full sign set and restricting cases to those where both the DSC and participants made unique diagnoses, again perhaps unsurprising given perfect self-concordance in both arms of the study.

Both concordance and misclassification were useful in assessing the performance of the DST in relation to participants' diagnoses. While concordance is the proportion of agreement corrected for chance taking into consideration both 'positive' and 'negative' agreements, i.e. where both participants and the DST agree that the diagnosis either is or is not a particular condition, misclassi-fication more simply represents positive agreements uncorrected for chance. Hence while concordance is a better measure of whether there was agreement between the two diagnostic arms of the study, it gives only limited indication of where disagreements lie. The misclassification matrices are less informative about agreement between the two but enable, for each ('positive') diagnosis made by one study arm, assessment of what proportion of ('positive') diagnoses were allocated to that diagnosis or alternative diagnoses by the other arm. Misclassification matrices were particularly useful in establishing how observed differences in proportional mortality between the two arms could be explained in terms of the breakdown of individual disease diagnoses.

Clearly because of the complication of multiple diagnoses these results could not easily be reduced to simple dichotomous outcomes (matched or not) from which specificity and sensitivity scores could be estimated on the basis of one or other diagnosis as 'gold standard'. The authors feel that the full concordance and misclassification matrices shown in Tables 4 and 6 are more informative and suggest these as a useful approach to the evaluation of this type of low-cost diagnostic decision support tool.

Finally, in addition to diagnoses, participants in this study also reported on the outcome of clinical cases, these being described as 'good' (as opposed to 'poor' or 'fair') in 88.4% of cases over both phases of the study although outcomes assessed by the participating clinician and not by an independent observer cannot be regarded as unbiased. Indeed, this success rate may seem rather optimistic in the face of such severe endemic disease challenge, but it was nevertheless interesting to note that there was a small but statistically significant increase (p<0.001) in the percentage of cases with a good outcome from 85.5% in Phase-1 to 92.1% in Phase-2; further studies would be required to assess whether this increase on the introduction of the DST held with unbiased observation.

Conclusion

In this study is was possible to compare the diagnostic performance of veterinary and animal health officers undertaking primary animal health care in Uganda before and after the introduction of a decision support tool and investigate changes in clinical practice in terms of observation of clinical signs and arrival at specific diagnoses. The decision support tool was shown to be highly relevant to the study area in that it covered the vast majority of diagnoses made before or after its introduction. The diagnoses suggested by the decision support tool were broadly consistent with those made by veterinary and animal health officers, but there was variation across diseases with some individual diagnoses (fasciolosis, schistosomosis and PGE) showing

less consistency. Concordance and misclassification matrices were useful in establishing levels of agreement and details of where differences lay. Importantly, the introduction of the diagnostic decision support tool led to a significant increase in the number of clinical signs recorded by the participants, suggesting this as an key beneficial consequence of its use over and above any improvement of the diagnosis made using a given sign set. In this regard one of the benefits of the DST can be regarded somewhat similar to how use of diagnostic "checklists" in human hospitals can increase efficiency and reduce missed clinical signs or mistaken diagnoses [31].

Acknowledgments

We wish to thank District Veterinary Officers (DVO), Veterinary Officers and Animal Health Officers from Iganga, Kayunga, Sironko, Soroti and Tororo Districts, Uganda that who participated in the study. We also thank the Director and staff of the Livestock Health Research Institute, Tororo Uganda, and to Dr Andrew Brownlow for logistical support.

Author Contributions

Conceived and designed the experiments: MCE. Performed the experiments: JWM. Analyzed the data: MCE CWR. Wrote the paper: MCE CRW.

References

1. Machila N, Wanyangu SW, McDermott J, Welburn SC, Maudlin I, et al. (2003) Cattle owners' perception of African bovine trypanosomosis and its control in Busia and Kwale Districts of Kenya. Acta Trop 86: 25–34.
2. Dwinger RH, Agyemang K, Kaufmann J, Grieve AS, Bah ML (1994) Effects of trypanosome and helminth infections on health and production parameters of village N'Dama cattle in The Gambia. Vet Parasitol 54: 353–365.
3. Goossens B, Osaer S, Kora S, Jaitner J, Ndao M, et al. (1997) The interaction of Trypanosoma congolense and Haemonchus contortus in Djallonké sheep. Int J Parasitol 27: 1579–1584.
4. Magona JW, Walubengo J, Olaho-Mukani W, Revie CW, Jonsson NN, et al. (2004) A Delphi survey on expert opinion on key signs for clinical diagnosis of bovine trypanosomosis, tick-borne diseases and helminthoses. Bull Anim Hlth Prod Afr 52: 130–140.
5. Eisler MC, Magona JW, Jonsson NN, Revie CW (2007) A low cost decision support tool for the diagnosis of endemic bovine infectious diseases in the mixed crop-livestock production system of sub-Saharan Africa. Epidemiol Infect 135: 67–75.
6. Ford J, Katondo J (1976) The description of climatic conditions in Uganda. Atlas of Uganda (6th Ed.). Uganda: Department of Lands and Surveys. 16–21.
7. Rubaire-Akiiki C, Okello-Onen J, Nasinyama GW, Vaarst M, Kabagambe EK, et al. (2004) The prevalence of serum antibodies to tick-borne infections in Mbale district, Uganda: the effect of agro-ecological zone, grazing management and age of cattle. J Insect Sci 4: 8. Available: http://www.insectscience.org/4.8 via the Internet. Accessed 30 Dec 2011.
8. Magona JW, Mayende JSP (2002) Occurrence of concurrent trypanosomosis, theileriosis, anaplasmosis and helminthosis in Friesian, Zebu and Sahiwal cattle in Uganda. Onderstepoort J Vet Res 69: 133–140.
9. Magona JW, Walubengo J, Olaho-Mukani W, Jonsson NN, Welburn SC, et al. (2008) Clinical features associated with seroconversion to Anaplasma marginale, Babesia bigemina and Theileria parva infections in African cattle under natural tick challenge. Vet Parasitol 155: 273–280.
10. Babeş V (1888) Sur l'haemoglobinurie bacterine des boeufs. Compte Rendue Academie de Science (Paris) 107: 692–700.
11. Cowdry EV (1925) Studies on the etiology of heartwater. I. Observations of a rickettsia, Rickettsia ruminantium (n.sp.) in the tissues of infected animals. J Exp Med 42: 231–252.
12. Uilenberg G (1981) Heartwater disease. In: Ristic M and McIntyre I, editors. Diseases of cattle in the tropics. The Hague, Netherlands: Martinus Nijhoff Publishers. 345–360.
13. Weinbren BM, Coyle TJ (1960) Uganda zebu cattle naturally infected with Fasciola gigantica with special reference to changes in the serum proteins. J Comp Pathol Therap 70: 176–181.
14. Magona JW, Olaho-Mukani W, Musisi G, Walubengo J (1999) Bovine Fasciola infection survey in Uganda. Bull Anim Hlth Prod Afr 47: 9–14.
15. Magona JW, Musisi G, Walubengo J, Olaho-Mukani W (2004) Effect of strategic deworming of village cattle in Uganda with moxidectin pour-on on faecal egg count and pasture larval counts. J S Afr Vet Assoc: 75: 189–92.

16. de Bont J, Vercruysse J (1998) Schistosomiasis in cattle. Adv Parasit 41: 285–364.
17. Makundi AE, Kassuku AA, Maselle RM, Boa ME (1998) Distribution, prevalence and intensity of Schistosoma bovis infection in cattle in Iringa district, Tanzania. Vet Parasitol 75: 59–69.
18. Bruce DB, Hamerton AE, Baterman HR, Mackie FP (1910) Amakebe: a disease of calves in Uganda. P Roy Soc Lond B, 82: 256-272.
19. Norval RAI, Perry BD, Young AS (1992) The epidemiology of theileriosis in Africa. London, Academic Press. 481 p.20.
20. Fiennes RNT-W (1970) Pathogenesis and pathology of animal trypanosomiases. In: Mulligan HW, editor. The African Trypanosomiases. London: George Allen and Unwin/Ministry of Overseas Development. 729–750.
21. Magona JW, Mayende JSP, Okiria R, Okuna NM (2004) Protective efficacy of isometamidium chloride and diminazene aceturate against natural Trypanosoma brucei, Trypanosoma congolense and Trypanosoma vivax infections in cattle under a suppressed tsetse population in Uganda. Onderstepoort J Vet Res 71: 231–237.
22. Rubaire-Akiiki C, Okello-Onen J, Musunga D, Kabagambe EK, Vaarst M, et al. (2006) Effect of agro-ecological zone and grazing system on incidence of East Coast Fever in calves in Mbale and Sironko Districts of Eastern Uganda. Prev Vet Med 75: 251–266.
23. Landis JR, Koch GG (1977). The measurement of observer agreement for categorical data. Biometrics 33: 159–174.
24. Ocaido M, Otim CP, Okuna NM, Erume J, Ssekitto C, et al. (2005) Socio-economic and livestock disease survey of agro-pastoral communities in Serere County, Soroti District, Uganda. Livestock Res Rural Dev 17: 93. Available: http://www.lrrd.org/lrrd17/8/ocai17093.htm via the Internet. Accessed 30 Dec 2011.
25. Chenyambuga SW, Waiswa C, Saimo M, Ngumi P, Gwakisa PS (2010) Knowledge and perceptions of traditional livestock keepers on tick-borne diseases and sero-prevalence of Theileria parva around Lake Victoria Basin. Livestock Res Rural Dev 22: 135. Available: http://www.lrrd.org/lrrd22/7/chen22135.htm via the Internet. Accessed 30 Dec 2011.
26. Van den Bossche P, Doran M, Connor RM (2000) An analysis of trypanocidal drug use in the Eastern Province of Zambia. Acta Trop 75: 247–258.
27. Bett B, Machila N, Gathura PB, McDermott JJ, Eisler MC (2004) Characterisation of shops selling veterinary medicines in a tsetse-infested area of Kenya. Prev Vet Med 63: 29–38.
28. Magona JW, Walubengo J, Odimim JJ (2004) Differences in susceptibility to trypanosome infection between Nkedi Zebu and Ankole cattle, under field conditions in Uganda. Ann Trop Med Parasitol. 98: 785–92.
29. Eisler MC, Torr S, Coleman PG, Morton J, Machila N (2003) Integrated control of vector-borne diseases of livestock – pyrethroids: panacea or poison? Trends Parasitol 19: 341–5.
30. Seidel M, Breslin C, Christley RM, Gettinby G, Reid SWJ, et al. (2003) Comparing diagnoses from expert systems and human experts. Agr Syst 76: 527–538.
31. Ely JW, Graber ML, Croskerry P (2011) Checklists to Reduce Diagnostic Errors. Acad Med 86: 307–313.

8

Slaughterhouse Wastewater Treatment by Combined Chemical Coagulation and Electrocoagulation Process

Edris Bazrafshan[1], Ferdos Kord Mostafapour[1], Mehdi Farzadkia[2], Kamal Aldin Ownagh[1], Amir Hossein Mahvi[2,3,4]*

1 Health Promotion Research Center, Zahedan University of Medical Sciences, Zahedan, Iran, **2** School of Public Health, Tehran University of Medical Sciences, Tehran, Iran, **3** Center for Solid Waste Research, Institute for Environmental Research, Tehran University of Medical Sciences, Tehran, Iran, **4** National Institute of Health Research, Tehran University of Medical Sciences, Tehran, Iran

Abstract

Slaughterhouse wastewater contains various and high amounts of organic matter (e.g., proteins, blood, fat and lard). In order to produce an effluent suitable for stream discharge, chemical coagulation and electrocoagulation techniques have been particularly explored at the laboratory pilot scale for organic compounds removal from slaughterhouse effluent. The purpose of this work was to investigate the feasibility of treating cattle-slaughterhouse wastewater by combined chemical coagulation and electrocoagulation process to achieve the required standards. The influence of the operating variables such as coagulant dose, electrical potential and reaction time on the removal efficiencies of major pollutants was determined. The rate of removal of pollutants linearly increased with increasing doses of PACl and applied voltage. COD and BOD$_5$ removal of more than 99% was obtained by adding 100 mg/L PACl and applied voltage 40 V. The experiments demonstrated the effectiveness of chemical and electrochemical techniques for the treatment of slaughterhouse wastewaters. Consequently, combined processes are inferred to be superior to electrocoagulation alone for the removal of both organic and inorganic compounds from cattle-slaughterhouse wastewater.

Editor: Andrew C. Marr, Queen's University Belfast, United Kingdom

Funding: The authors are grateful for the financial support of this project by the health research deputy of Zahedan University of Medical Sciences (Project No. 89-2147). The funders had no role in study design, data collection and analysis, decision to publish, or preparation of the manuscript.

Competing Interests: The authors have declared that no competing interests exist.

* E-mail: ahmahvi@yahoo.com

Introduction

Wastewater from a cattle slaughterhouse is a mixture of the processing water from both the slaughtering line and the cleaning of the guts, which causes a large variation in the concentration of organic matter. The main pollutant in slaughterhouse effluents is organic matter. The contributors of organic load to these effluents are paunch, feces, fat and lard, grease, undigested food, blood, suspended material, urine, loose meat, soluble proteins, excrement, manure, grit and colloidal particles [1,2].

Untreated slaughterhouses waste entering into a municipal sewage purification system may create severe problems, due to the very high biological oxygen demand (BOD) and chemical oxygen demand (COD) [3]. Therefore treating of slaughterhouse wastewater is very important for prevention of high organic loading to municipal wastewater treatment plants. The most common methods used for treating slaughterhouse wastewaters are fine screening, sedimentation, coagulation–flocculation, trickling filters and activated sludge processes.

The treatment of slaughterhouse wastewater by various methods such as aerobic and anaerobic biological systems [4,5,6,7] and hybrid systems [2] have been intensively studied. Aerobic treatment processes are limited by their high energy consumption needed for aeration and high sludge production. Also, the anaerobic treatment of slaughterhouse wastewater is often slowed or impaired due to the accumulation of suspended solids and floating fats in the reactor which lead to a reduction in the methanogenic activity and biomass wash-out. In addition, it is also reported that anaerobic treatment is sensitive to high organic loading rates, as a serious disadvantage [8]. Even though biological processes are effective and economical, both biological processes require long hydraulic retention time and large reactor volumes, high biomass concentration and controlling of sludge loss, to avoid the wash-out of the sludge. Among physico-chemical processes, dissolved air flotation (DAF) and coagulation–flocculation units are widely used for the removal of total suspended solids (TSS), colloids, and fats from slaughterhouse wastewaters [1].

Chemical coagulation of slaughterhouse wastewater has also been studied by adding aluminum salts and polymer compounds, and a maximum COD removal efficiency of 45–75% has been reported [9,10]. Polyaluminum chloride (PACl) is commonly used as the flocculant to coagulate small particles into larger flocs that can be efficiently removed in the subsequent separation process of sedimentation and/or filtration. Much attention has been paid to PACl in recent years because of its higher efficiency and relatively low costs compared with the traditional flocculants [11,12]. On the other hand, PACl has become one of the most effective coagulant agents in water and wastewater treatment facilities with various applications, including removal of colloids and suspended particles, organic matter, metal ions, phosphates, toxic metals and color [13].

Recently, electrochemical methods such as electrooxidation [14] and electrocoagulation have been widely used as an attractive and suitable method for the treatment of various kinds of wastewater such as poultry and cattle slaughterhouse wastewater and wastewaters contain heavy metals, by virtue of various benefits including environmental compatibility, adaptability, energy efficiency, safety, selectivity, amenability to automation, and cost effectiveness [15,16,17,18,19,20]. An examination of the chemical reactions occurring in the electrocoagulation process shows that the main reactions occurring at the electrodes (aluminum electrodes) are:

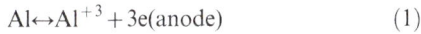

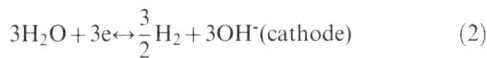

$$Al \leftrightarrow Al^{+3} + 3e(\text{anode}) \qquad (1)$$

$$3H_2O + 3e \leftrightarrow \frac{3}{2}H_2 + 3OH^-(\text{cathode}) \qquad (2)$$

In addition, Al^{3+} and OH^- ions generated at electrode surfaces react in the bulk wastewater to form aluminum hydroxide:

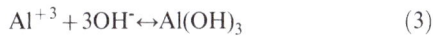

$$Al^{+3} + 3OH^- \leftrightarrow Al(OH)_3 \qquad (3)$$

The aluminum hydroxide flocs normally have large surface areas which are beneficial for a rapid adsorption of soluble organic compounds and trapping of colloidal particles [15,16,21]. Also, these flocs polymerize further and are removed easily from aqueous medium by sedimentation or/and flotation by hydrogen gas.

Chemical coagulation using PACl and electrocoagulation process with aluminum electrodes of wastewater from a cattle slaughterhouse is described in this article. The purpose of this work was to investigate the feasibility of treating cattle-slaughterhouse wastewater by combined chemical coagulation and electrocoagulation process separately to achieve the required legal direct-discharge limit of COD and BOD_5 which is 60 and 30 mg/L in

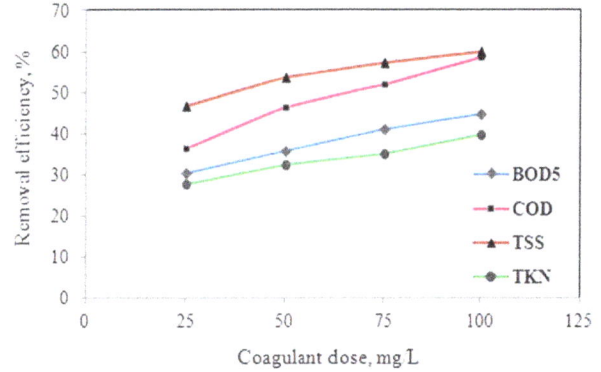

Figure 1. Effects of coagulant dose (PACl) on pollutants removal efficiency at pilot scale coagulation process.

Iran for the slaughterhouse industry effluents. The influence of the operating variables such as coagulant dose, pH, applied voltage and reaction time on the removal efficiencies of major pollutants was also determined. Information regarding the electrical energy consumption (EEC) is also included to provide an estimation of the cost of pollutants removal by an electrocoagulation system.

Results and Discussion

Wastewater characterization

Table 1 presents the slaughterhouse wastewater characteristics prior to any treatment, after 24 h settling time and the guidelines from Iran for effluent discharge in the sewage urban works. The values of the pollution parameters were lowered after 24 h of preliminary settling time. Also, the comparison of these values showed that, the COD, BOD_5, microbial indicators (Total and Fecal Coliforms) and the concentration of Oil and grease were very greater than those recommended by Iran. Consequently, the slaughterhouse effluent needed to be treated before discharge.

Table 1. Characteristics of the experimental cattle slaughterhouse wastewater.

Parameter	Raw wastewater Mean ± S.D.	24 h settled wastewater Mean ± S.D.	Permissive levels (Iran Standard for discharge to surface waters)
Number of samples	48	48	–
pH	7.31±0.12	7.44±0.16	6.5–8.5
Total COD (mg/L)	5817±473	4159±281	60
Total BOD (mg/L)	2543±362	2204±177	30
Total Suspended Solids (mg/L)	3247±845	1172±84	60
Total Kjeldhal Nitrogen (TKN) (mg/L)	137±12	92±12	–
Fat, oil, grease (mg/L)	34±9	32±7	10
Conductivity (μS/Cm)	9140±1512	9061±1400	–
Total Coliform (MPN/100 mL)	$2.8\times10^9 \pm 1.5\times10^7$	$2.3\times10^9 \pm 2.6\times10^7$	1000
Fecal Coliform (MPN/100 mL)	$1.9\times10^8 \pm 2.1\times10^6$	$1.7\times10^8 \pm 2.3\times10^6$	400

Table 2. Influence of PACl dosage on water quality parameters of coagulated mixed liquor (mean values).

PACl dosage (mg/L)	Water quality parameters of treated effluent after chemical coagulation unit					
	COD (mg/L)	BOD$_5$ (mg/L)	TSS (mg/L)	TKN (mg/L)	TC (MPN/100mL)	FC (MPN/100mL)
0	4159	2204	1172	192	2.3×10^9	1.70×10^8
25	2643	1534	623	139	2.8×10^7	3.00×10^5
50	2228	1418	544	130	1.6×10^7	2.59×10^5
75	2002	1301	501	125	2.3×10^6	2.20×10^5
100	1725	1217	470	116	1.6×10^6	1.08×10^5

Effect of preliminary settling time

Preliminary settling process is a natural treatment method that requires no chemical addition. Although some workers realized the importance of the natural settling process, there is little information available in the literature on the effect of the preliminary settling time on TSS removal capacity [22]. Most studies carried out on the treatment of slaughterhouse wastewater were based on diluted pre-settled wastewater [23].

In this study, the raw slaughterhouse wastewater was allowed to settle for 24 h in a preliminary settling tank before the addition of a coagulant. The process had an effect on BOD$_5$, COD, TSS, TKN and coliform bacteria removals on the first 24 h. TKN concentration reduced from 137 ± 12 to 92 ± 12 mg/L (on average 33% TKN removal efficiency), COD concentration reduced from 5817 ± 473 to 4159 ± 281 mg/L (approximately 28% COD removal efficiency) whereas BOD$_5$ was reduced in the wastewater from 2543 ± 362 to 2204 ± 177 mg/L (about 13% BOD$_5$ removal efficiency). Furthermore, TSS concentration was reduced to 1172 ± 84 mg/L (approximately 64% TSS removal efficiency). Similar results were reported by Amuda and Alade [10].

Also, data revealed that the effluent of the settling unit is characterized by high load of organic matter. The ratio BOD$_5$/COD of approximately 0.5, indicates that 50% of the COD of this wastewater is easily able to be degraded by biological treatment. Nevertheless, the remainder COD is high, which indicates the necessity of an efficient physicochemical treatment for this wastewater.

Effect of coagulation process (first step)

Coagulation/flocculation experiments using PACl as coagulant in the jar test were performed to investigate the effect of coagulation process in the removal efficiencies of COD, BOD$_5$, TSS, TKN and coliform bacteria. Therefore, PACl was added to the slaughterhouse wastewater to achieve particle instability and increase in the particle size, consequently achieving effective removal of organic substances present as COD and BOD$_5$. The doses of PACl as coagulant were varied between 0 and 100 mg/L to determine the optimum dose of PACl for pollutants removal. The results of jar-tests using the PACl individually are presented in Table 2 and Figure 1. It is shown that at lower doses of the PACl (25 mg/L), COD, BOD$_5$, TSS and TKN removal efficiency reached a maximum of 37%, 31%, 47% and 27%, respectively. Aguilar et al. [24] reported TKN removal efficiency 50–60% by using PACl as coagulant from slaughterhouse wastewater. Also, Amuda and Alade [10] were reported maximum removal efficiency 65% and 34% of COD and TSS using a 750 mg/L dose of alum as coagulant in abattoir wastewater treatment.

As it shown in Figure 1, the efficiency of the process increased with increasing dosages of coagulant (PACl). The curve obtained with PACl points to a considerable increase in performance from the lowest dose up to 100 mg/L. On the other hand in chemical coagulation, as seen in Figure 1, an increase in COD, BOD$_5$, TSS, TKN and other pollutants removal efficiency is noted with increasing PACl dosage, reaching nearly 40–60% for PACl dosage of 100 mg/L. Al-Mutairi et al. [9] reported that suspended solids and turbidity removal from slaughterhouse wastewater increased substantially as the alum (as coagulant) dosage is increased. Also,

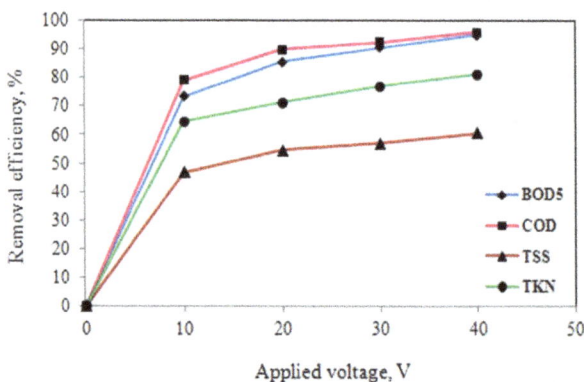

Figure 2. Effect of applied voltage on pollutants removal efficiency (coagulant dose: 25 mg/L, reaction time: 60 min).

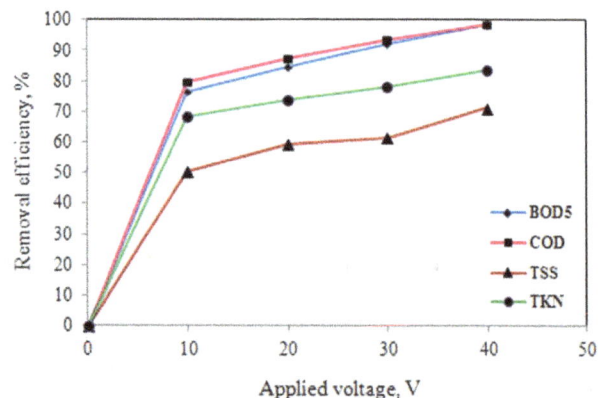

Figure 3. Effect of applied voltage on pollutants removal efficiency (coagulant dose: 50 mg/L, reaction time: 60 min).

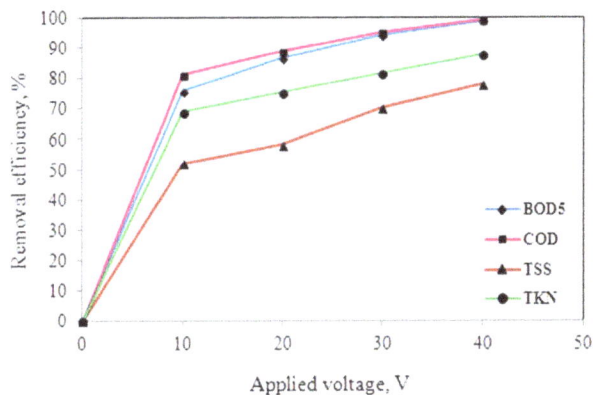

Figure 4. Effect of applied voltage on pollutants removal efficiency (coagulant dose: 75 mg/L, reaction time: 60 min).

Figure 1 shows that the TSS removal and COD and BOD5 reduction trends are similar to each other. This may be due to the high organic contents of the suspended solid particles.

Maximum TC and FC removal efficiency of >99.9% (Table 2) were obtained by using PACl at the dosage of 100 mg/L. The TC and FC reduction, increase with increase in coagulant dosage.

TC indicator of effluent with coagulant dose 25 mg/L PACl was reduced from 2.3×10^9 to 2.8×10^7 (MPN/100mL) (approximately more than 98% TC removal efficiency), and by increasing the coagulant dose to 100 mg/L, the TC indicator of effluent was decreased was reduced from 1.7×10^8 to 1.6×10^6 (MPN/100mL) (on average more than 99% TC removal efficiency) that is much more than permissible level. A similar reduction trend was determined for FC indicator. Similar results were obtained in previous reports concerning the electrocoagulation of wastewater from vegetable oil refinery wastewater using aluminum electrodes (with adding PACl as coagulant aid) [19].

According the results of this study (Table 2) it can be concluded that although the efficiency for removal of most parameters from slaughterhouse wastewater are high, but the concentration of pollutants in effluent of chemical coagulation process does not meet the effluent discharge standards to the environment. Thus, the effluent from conventional coagulation should be preceded by another treatment process to be completed. For this purpose, in this research, electrocoagulation was employed as a completion of treatment process to obtain discharge standards.

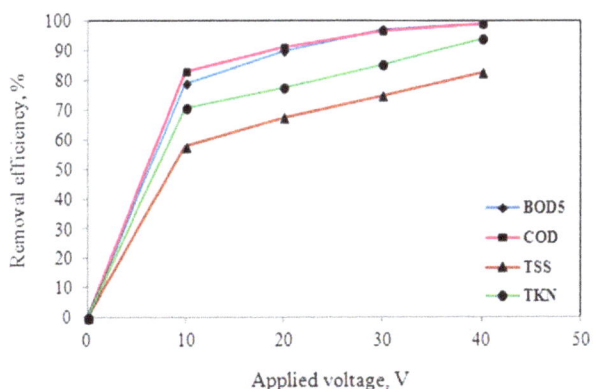

Figure 5. Effect of applied voltage on pollutants removal efficiency (coagulant dose: 100 mg/L, reaction time: 60 min).

Effect of electrocoagulation process (second step)

Electrocoagulation processes a direct current source between metal electrodes immersed in wastewater. The electrical current causes the dissolution of metal electrodes commonly iron and aluminum into wastewater. The dissolved metal ions, at an appropriate pH, can form wide ranges of coagulated species and metal hydroxides that destabilize and aggregate the suspended particles or precipitate and adsorb dissolved contaminants [25,26].

As be mentioned earlier, an examination of the chemical reactions occurring in the electrocoagulation process shows that the main reactions occurring at the aluminum electrodes are:

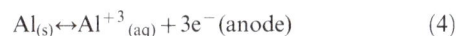

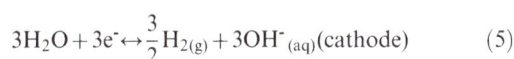

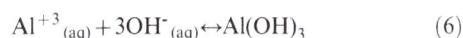

$$Al_{(s)} \leftrightarrow Al^{+3}_{(aq)} + 3e^- \text{ (anode)} \quad (4)$$

$$3H_2O + 3e^- \leftrightarrow \frac{3}{2}H_{2(g)} + 3OH^-_{(aq)} \text{(cathode)} \quad (5)$$

$$Al^{+3}_{(aq)} + 3OH^-_{(aq)} \leftrightarrow Al(OH)_3 \quad (6)$$

monomeric species such as $Al(OH)^{2+}$, $Al(OH)_2^+$, $Al_2(OH)_2^{4+}$, $Al(OH)^{1-}$ and polymeric species such as $Al_6(OH)_{15}^{3+}$, $Al_7(OH)_{17}^{4+}$, $Al_8(OH)_{20}^{4+}$, $Al_{13}O_4(OH)_{24}^{7+}$, $Al_{13}(OH)_{34}^{5+}$ are formed during the electrocoagulation process [26,27]. The aluminum hydroxide flocs act as adsorbents and/or traps for pollutants and so eliminate them from the solution [28,29].

As mentioned earlier, the performances by the two pretreatment, namely, preliminary settling and chemical coagulation, were not carried out efficiently enough to satisfy the national guideline of effluent qualities. Additional dosage of coagulant (PACl) and longer time were needed to keep the national guideline of the effluent qualities. Therefore, the electrocoagulation process was employed as the final treatment step in this study. In adopting the electrocoagulation process, it was intended to treat the pollutant efficiently as well as economically.

The effects of applied voltage and reaction time on electrocoagulation process of slaughterhouse wastewater treatment were determined. The results of the effects of operating parameters on pilot scale electrocoagulation process are shown in Table 3 and Figures 2, 3, 4, and 5.

Effect of applied voltage

One of the most important parameter influencing the performance and economy of the electrocoagulation process is the applied voltage at the electrodes [30]. To understand the effect of applied voltage on the efficiency of electrocoagulation process in treating of slaughterhouse wastewater, several voltages in the range of 10 to 40 V were applied between the electrodes in the electrocoagulation cell, and pollutants removal was determined at the conditions given in Table 3.

The applied voltage is expected to exhibit a strong effect on electrocoagulation, especially on the COD abatement: higher the current (voltage), shorter the treatment. The supply of current to the electrocoagulation system determines the amount of Al^{3+} ion released from the respective electrodes and the amount of resulting coagulant. Thus, more Al^{3+} ion get dissolved into the solution and the formation rate of $Al(OH)_3$ is increased. Also, it is well-known that electrical potential not only determines the coagulant dosage rate but also the bubble production rate and size and the flocs growth [31,32], which can influence the treatment efficiency of the electrocoagulation process.

Table 3. Influence of electrocoagulation process using aluminum electrodes on effluent quality parameters (mean values).

PACl dosage (mg/L)	Applied voltage (V)	Water quality parameters of treated effluent after electrocoagulation unit					
		COD (mg/L)	BOD mg/L	TSS (mg/L)	TKN (mg/L)	TC (MPN/100mL)	FC (MPN/100mL)
25	10	555	409	331	49	6743	1274
	20	267	223	282	40	6437	814
	30	203	146	268	32	4764	759
	40	108	79	245	26	4139	634
50	10	452	332	270	41	6274	1347
	20	283	218	221	34	5712	712
	30	145	108	209	28	4831	643
	40	29	21	156	21	4376	473
75	10	376	316	241	39	5712	785
	20	225	174	210	31	4833	531
	30	96	74	149	23	3157	375
	40	18	13	111	15	2563	114
100	10	294	254	199	34	3652	437
	20	153	125	153	26	2715	364
	30	59	33	118	17	1864	153
	40	13	10	82	7	943	72

As it can be seen from Table 3 and Figures 2, 3, 4, and 5, the removal efficiency of pollutants is very high and as expected, it appears that for a given time, the removal efficiency increased significantly with increase of electrical potential. As the results shown in Table 3 and Figures 2, 3, 4, and 5, the removal efficiencies increased as the electrical potentials are increased. As an example, COD concentration of chemical coagulation process with 25 mg/L PACl has decreased from 2643 to 555 mg/L (approximately 79% COD removal efficiency) after electrocoagulation process with electrical potential of 10 V. Again, by increasing electrical potential to 40 V, the COD concentration in the effluent decreased to 108 mg/L in 60 min (approximately 96% COD removal efficiency). In addition, the COD of effluent from chemical coagulation with 100 mg/L PACl, was decreased

to about 294 mg/L (approximately 83% COD removal efficiency) by electrocoagulation process with electrical potential of 10 V, and by increasing the electrical potential to 40 V, the COD of effluent was decreased to less than 13 mg/L (on average more than 99% COD removal efficiency) that is lower than permissible level.

According to the results of Table 3, and Figures 2, 3, 4, and 5, TKN of chemical coagulation process with 25 mg/L PACl was reduced to lower than 50 mg/L after electrocoagulation process with electrical potential of 10 V (approximately 65% TKN removal efficiency), and by increasing electrical potential to 40 V, the TKN concentration in the effluent decreased to 26 mg/L (about 81% TKN removal efficiency). Furthermore, with increase in coagulant dose to 100 mg/L and increase of applied voltage to 40 V, TKN concentration in effluent was

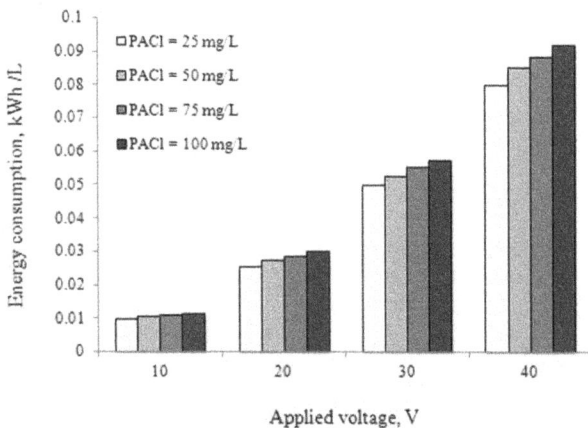

Figure 6. Electrical energy consumption during coagulation-electrocoagulation process (kWh/L).

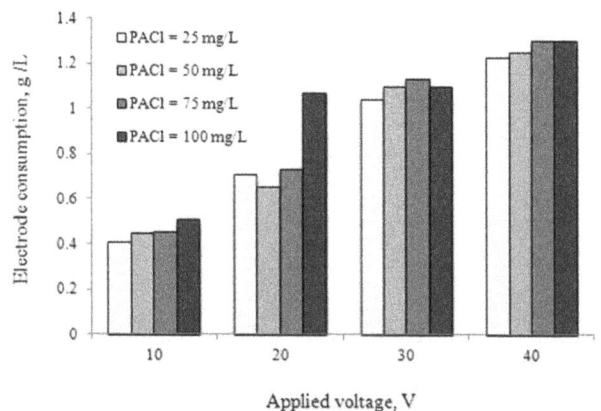

Figure 7. Electrode consumption during chemical coagulation-electrocoagulation process.

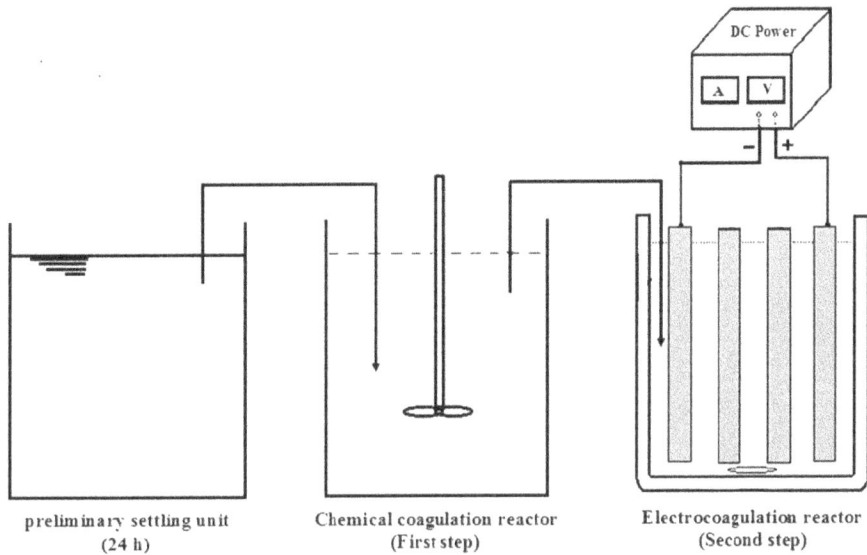

Figure 8. The schematic view of coagulation and electrocoagulation reactor.

reduced to lower than 7 mg/L (on average 94% TKN removal efficiency). A similar trend was seen for TSS and BOD$_5$ parameters.

Also, as can be seen from Table 3, the removal efficiency of bacterial indicators (TC and FC) is very high and efficiency was increased with increase in applied voltage from 10 to 40 V. Maximum removal efficiency (>99.9%) was obtained in applied voltage 40 V (coagulant dosage 100 mg/L), and thus the effluent quality was reached to permissive levels (lower than 1000 and 400 for TC and FC, respectively) and hence discharge of this effluent to environment is safe. Also, minimum removal efficiency occurred in the lowest electrical potential (10 V). This is ascribed to the fact that at high voltage, the amount of aluminum oxidized increased, resulting in a greater amount of precipitate for the removal of pollutants. In addition, it was demonstrated that bubbles density increases and their size decreases with increasing current density [33], resulting in a greater upwards flux and a faster removal of pollutants and sludge flotation. As be mentioned earlier, the main mechanisms for removal of pollutants in this process are rapid adsorption of soluble organic compounds and trapping of colloidal particles in "sweep flocs" (Al(OH)$_3$). Nevertheless, Bayar et al. [34] was reported that increase in the current density does not cause an expected removal efficiency increase; on the contrary, it can cause a relatively negative effect on it. Also, a similar trend was seen in the study of Holt et al. [32].

Electrical energy and electrode consumption

Electrical energy consumption is a very important economical parameter in the electrocoagulation process. Therefore, for the same operating conditions, after 60 min of electrocoagulation, consumption of energy and aluminum electrode is also represented in Figures 6 and 7. The electrical energy consumption was calculated using the related equations [35].

It can be understood from Figures 6 and 7 that electrical energy and electrode consumption were found to increase with increasing the applied voltage as would be expected in any other electrolytic process. An increase in applied voltage from 10 to 40 V causes an increase in energy consumption from about 0.001 to 0.08 kWh/L and from 0.011 to approximately 0.09 kWh/L for 25 and 100 mg/L of coagulant dosage (PACl), respectively. A similar

trend was seen in the study of Bayar et al. [34] on Poultry slaughterhouse wastewater treatment by electrocoagulation method.

Also, as shown in Figure 7, an increase in applied voltage from 10 to 40 V causes an increase in electrode consumption from about 0.41 to 1.23 g/L and 0.51 to 1.3 g/L of pollutants for 25 and 100 mg/L of PACl, respectively. This result is in agreement with the results obtained by Bazrafshan et al. [36,37,38].

When the applied voltage was increased from 10 V to 40 V, the COD and BOD$_5$ removal efficiency increased appreciably, to more than approximately 99%, whereas the corresponding specific energy consumption increased only slightly. Therefore, in present study, 40 V is chosen as optimum operating voltage for electrocoagulation process.

Conclusions

In this study, chemical coagulation using Polyaluminum chloride (PACl) and Electrocoagulation process using aluminum electrodes of wastewater from a cattle slaughterhouse was investigated. The effects of the different operational parameters on the removal of pollutants analyzed. The following conclusions can be reached from the results obtained in this work:

- The installation of a good fat separator prior to each biological or chemical treatment unit seemed an appropriate alternative to a chemical coagulation and electrocoagulation process.
- Preliminary settling time were investigated and found to be important operational parameter for effective treatment of slaughterhouse wastewater.
- A preliminary settling time of 24 h had an effect on the BOD$_5$, COD, TSS and TKN with removal efficiency up to 14%, 29%, 64% and 33%, respectively.
- According to the results obtained from the present experiments, the removal efficiencies increased by increasing the coagulant dose and electrical potential. At the highest applied voltage, the fastest treatment rate for pollutants (COD, BOD$_5$, TSS, TKN and microbial parameters) removal was obtained. Moreover, the energy consumption increased by increasing the applied electrical potential.

- Evaluation of the experimental results indicates that both processes (chemical coagulation and Electrocoagulation) show excellent efficiency at reducing of pollutants.

- Based on this study results, although the coagulation process had high efficiency in removing organic and microbial contaminants, but nevertheless it's not able to meet discharge standards, hence a supplemental process (such as electrocoagulation process) is essential for enhance effluent quality.

- Finally according to the results of this study, it can be concluded that the combined application of chemical coagulation and electrocoagulation processes is able to meet effluent standards for safe discharge to environment.

Materials and Methods

Slaughterhouse effluent

The effluent used throughout this study was taken from a local cattle Slaughterhouse plant with 250 cows per day capacity, located in Zahedan City in the province of Sistan and Baluchestan province (Iran), producing approximately 60 m^3 of wastewater daily. The cattle slaughterhouse effluent was sampled after the screening of coarser solids using a filter having a pore size of approximately 2.0 mm and sedimentation for 24 h. Samples were collected in polypropylene bottles, shipped cold, and kept at 4°C before use. The length of the storage before starting experiments varied from one day to six weeks. The effluent has been sampled at different times during this study and the initial characteristics varied with time (Table 1). This effluent initially contained high concentrations of soluble and undissolved organics (4159 ± 81 mg/L COD, 2204 ± 77 mg/L BOD$_5$).

Chemical treatment (coagulation) of slaughterhouse effluent

All the chemicals used in the study were of analytical reagent (AR) grade. Poly- aluminum chloride (PACl) Al$_{12}$Cl$_{12}$(OH)$_{24}$ was chosen for this study because it has been used extensively at water and wastewater treatment plants to remove solids and may function as an effective and less expensive coagulant. PACl was used in this study up to 100 mg/L (25, 50, 75 and 100 mg/L). A six-beaker jar test (flocculator) was set up at room temperature for each trial. Each of the beakers contained 2 L of settled wastewater. The coagulants were added into the beakers, and the pH values were immediately adjusted to the preset values (7 ± 0.1) using NaOH or H$_2$SO$_4$ for pH-controlled experiments. Rapid stirring at 150 rpm for 2 min was followed by gentle mixing at 50 rpm for 20 min, and the solids formed were left to settle for 30 min. Samples were taken from the water surface (supernatant) and filtered through 0.45-mm membranes. After chemical coagulation, electrocoagulation process with aluminum electrodes was performed on the supernatant.

Electrochemical treatment of slaughterhouse effluent

In each run, wastewater (supernatant) after chemical coagulation (first stage of treatment) was poured into the electrocoagulation cell. All experiments were performed in a bipolar batch

reactor (Figure 8), with four aluminum electrode connected in parallel. Only the outer electrodes were connected to the power source, and anodic and cathodic reactions occurred on each surface of the inner electrode when the current passed through the electrodes. The internal size of the cell was 15 Cm×15 Cm×25 Cm (width × length × depth) with an effective volume of 2000 Cm^3. The volume (V) of the solution of each batch was 2 L. The active area of each electrode (plate) was 14×20 Cm with a total area of 280 Cm^2. The distance between electrodes was 1.5 Cm. A power supply having an input of 220 V and variable output of 0–40 V (10, 20, 30 and 40 V) with maximum current of 5 ampere was used as direct current source. The temperature of each system was maintained at 25 ± 1°C. Different samples of 100 ml were taken at 15 min intervals for up to 1 h and filtered before being analysed to determine BOD$_5$, COD, TSS and other parameters. During the runs, the reactor unit was stirred at 150 rpm by a magnetic stirrer to allow the chemical precipitate to grow large enough for removal. During electrocoagulation, an oxide film formed at the anode. In order to overcome electrode passivation at the anode, the electrodes were rinsed in diluted HCl solution (5% v/v) after each experiment and rinsed again with tap water and finally weighted. Also the electrodes reweighted to calculate sacrificial electrode consumptions. These weights are used in the calculations of the total operating cost. In addition, the electrical energy consumed per unit volume of treated wastewater has been calculated for different experimental conditions. All analyses were conducted in duplicate for reproducibility of the experimental results, and all of the data in the Figures and Tables were the average ones.

Analytical

COD, BOD$_5$, oil-grease, conductivity, pH, total solids (TS), total suspended solids (TSS), and total Kjeldhal nitrogen (TKN) determinations were determined according to the standard methods [39]. COD was measured using COD reactor and direct reading spectrophotometer (DR/5000, HACH, USA). Five-day biological oxygen demand (BOD$_5$) was determined by the manometric method with a respirometer (BSB-Controller Model 620 T (WTW)). Oil-grease was determined with hexane extraction. The pH and conductivity were adjusted to a desirable value using NaOH or H$_2$SO$_4$, and NaCl, and measured using a pH meter model E520 (Metrohm Herisau, Switzerland) and a Conductivity Meter (Jenway Model 4200), respectively. Also the most-probable-number technique was used for the enumeration of total coliform (TC) and fecal coliform (FC) bacteria [39].

Acknowledgments

E. Bazrafshan gratefully acknowledges helpful comment from Dr. M.A. Zazouli.

Author Contributions

Conceived and designed the experiments: EB AHM. Performed the experiments: EB KAO. Analyzed the data: MF. Contributed reagents/materials/analysis tools: FKM. Wrote the paper: EB AHM.

References

1. Asselin M, Drogui P, Benmoussa H, Blais JF (2008) Effectiveness of electrocoagulation process in removing organic compounds from slaughterhouse wastewater using monopolar and bipolar electrolytic cells. Chemosphere 72: 1727–1733.
2. Tezcan Un U, Koparal AS, Bakir Ogutveren U (2009) Hybrid processes for the treatment of cattle-slaughterhouse wastewater using aluminum and iron electrodes. J Hazard Mater 164: 580–586.
3. Alvarez R, Liden G (2008) Semi-continuous co-digestion of solid slaughterhouse waste, manure, and fruit and vegetable waste. Renew Energ 33: 726–734.
4. Masse L, Masse DI (2005) Effect of soluble organic, particulate organic and hydraulic shock loads on anaerobic sequencing batch reactors treating slaughterhouse wastewater at 20C. Process Biochem 40: 1225–1232.

5. Torkian A, Eqbali A, Hashemian SJ (2003) The effect of organic loading rate on the performance of UASB reactor treating slaughterhouse effluent. Resour Conserv Recy 40: 1–11.

6. Manjunath NT, Mehrotra I, Mathur RP (2000) Treatment of wastewater from slaughterhouse by DAF-UASB system. Water Res 34: 1930–1936.

7. Palatsi J, Vinas M, Guivernau M, Fernandez B, Flotats X (2011) Anaerobic digestion of slaughterhouse waste: Main process limitations and microbial community interactions. Bioresource Technol 102: 2219–2227.

8. Cuetos MJ, Gomez X, Otero M, Moran A (2008) Anaerobic digestion of solid slaughterhouse waste (SHW) at laboratory scale: Influence of co-digestion with the organic fraction of municipal solid waste (OFMSW). Biochem Eng J 40: 99–106.

9. Al-Mutairi NZ, Hamoda MF, Al-Ghusain I (2004) Coagulant selection and sludge conditioning in a slaughterhouse wastewater treatment plant. Bioresource Technol 95: 115–119.

10. Amuda OS, Alade A (2006) Coagulation/flocculation process in the treatment of abattoir wastewater. Desalination 196: 22–31.

11. Hua Ch, Liu H, Qua J (2005) Preparation and characterization of polyaluminum chloride containing high content of Al13 and active chlorine, Colloid Surface A 260: 109–117.

12. Yan M, Wang D, Yu J, Ni J, Edwards M, et al. (2008) Enhanced coagulation with polyaluminum chlorides: Role of pH/Alkalinity and speciation. Chemosphere 71: 1665–1673.

13. Zouboulis AI, Tzoupanos N (2010) Alternative cost-effective preparation method of polyaluminium chloride (PACL) coagulant agent: Characterization and comparative application for water/wastewater treatment. Desalination 250: 339–344.

14. Tezcan Un U, Altay U, Koparal AS, Bakır Ogutveren U (2008) Complete treatment of olive mill wastewaters by electrooxidation. Chem Eng J 39: 445–452.

15. Bayramoglu M, Kobya M, Eyvaz M, Senturk E (2006) Technical and economic analysis of electrocoagulation for the treatment of poultry slaughterhouse wastewater. Sep Purif Technol 51: 404–408.

16. Bazrafshan E, Mahvi AH, Zazouli MA (2011) Removal of zinc and copper from aqueous Solutions by electrocoagulation technology using iron electrodes. Asian J Chem 23: 5506–5510.

17. Bazrafshan E, Mahvi AH, Naseri S, Mesdaghinia AR (2008) Performance evaluation of electrocoagulation process for removal of chromium (VI) from synthetic chromium solutions using iron and aluminum electrodes. Turkish J Eng Environ Sci 32: 59–66.

18. Bazrafshan E, Mahvi AH, Naseri S, Shaighi M (2007) Performance evaluation of electrocoagulation process for Diazinon removal from aqueous environment by using iron electrodes. Iran J Environ Health Sci Eng 4: 127–132.

19. Tezcan Un U, Koparal AS, Bakir Ogutveren U (2009) Electrocoagulation of vegetable oil refinery wastewater using aluminum electrodes. J Environ Manage 90: 428–433.

20. Nouri J, Mahvi AH, Bazrafshan E (2010) Application of electrocoagulation process in removal of zinc and copper from aqueous solutions by aluminum electrodes. Int J Environ Res 4: 201–208.

21. Adhoum N, Monser L, Bellakhal N, Belgaied JE (2004) Treatment of electroplating wastewater containing Cu^{2+}, Zn^{2+} and Cr (VI) by electrocoagulation. J Hazard Mater B112: 207–213.

22. Ra CS, Lo KV, Mavinic DS (1997) Swine wastewater treatment by a batch-mode 4-stage process: loading rate control using Orp. Environ Technol 18: 615–621.

23. Al-Mutairi NZ, Hamoda MF, Al-Ghusain IA (2003) Performance-based characterization of contact stabilization process for slaughterhouse wastewater. J Environ Sci Healt A 38: 2287–2300.

24. Aguilar MI, Saez J, Llorens M, Soler A, Ortuno JF (2002) Nutrient removal and sludge production in the coagulation-flocculation process. Water Res 36: 2910–2919.

25. Chen GH (2004) Electrochemical technologies in wastewater treatment. Sep Purif Technol 38: 11–41.

26. Canizares P, Carmona M, Lobato J, Martinez F, Rodrigo MA (2005) Electrodissolution of aluminum electrodes in electrocoagulation processes. Ind Eng Chem Res 44: 4178–4185.

27. Can OT, Bayramoglu M, Kobya M (2003) Decolorization of reactive dye solutions by electrocoagulation using aluminum electrodes. Ind Eng Chem Res 42: 3391–3396.

28. Cenkin VE, Belevstev AN (1985) Electrochemical treatment of industrial wastewater. Eff Water Treat J 25: 243–249.

29. Ogutveren UB, Gonen N, Koparal AS (1994) Removal of chromium from aqueous solutions and plating bath rinse by an electrochemical method. Int J Environ Stud 45: 81–87.

30. Mollah M, Schennach R, Parga JR, Cocke DL (2001) Electrocoagulation. (EC)-science and applications. J Hazard Mater B84: 29–41.

31. Letterman RD, Amirtharajah A, O. Melia CR (1999) A Handbook of Community Water Supplies. 5th Ed. AWWA, Mc Graw-Hill, N. Y. USA.

32. Holt PH, Barton GW, Wark M, Mitchell AA (2002) A quantitative comparison between chemical dosing and electrocoagulation. Colloid Surface A 211: 233–248.

33. Khosla NK, Venkachalam S, Sonrasundaram P (1991) Pulsed electrogeneration of bubbles for electroflotation. J Appl Electrochem 21: 986–990.

34. Bayar S, Sevki YY, Yilmaz AE, Irdemez S (2011) The effect of stirring speed and current density on removal efficiency of poultry slaughterhouse wastewater by electrocoagulation method. Desalination 280: 103–107

35. Martinez-Huitle CA, Brillas E (2009) Decontamination of wastewaters containing synthetic organic dyes by electrochemical methods: a general review. App Catal B Environ 87: 105–145.

36. Bazrafshan E, Biglari H, Mahvi AH (2012) Phenol removal by electrocoagulation process from aqueous solutions. Fresen Environ Bull 21: 364–371.

37. Bazrafshan E, Biglari H, Mahvi AH (2012) Application of electrocoagulation process using Iron and Aluminum electrodes for fluoride removal from aqueous environment. E-J Chem 9: 2297–2308.

38. Bazrafshan E, Biglari H, Mahvi AH (2012) Humic acid removal from aqueous environments by electrocoagulation process using iron electrodes. E-J Chem 9: 2453–2461.

39. APHA AWWA WEF (1995) Standard Methods for the Examination of Water and Wastewater, 19th Ed. Washington DC, USA.

9

Association of an MHC Class II Haplotype with Increased Risk of Polymyositis in Hungarian Vizsla Dogs

Jonathan Massey[1]*, Simon Rothwell[1], Clare Rusbridge[2], Anna Tauro[3], Diane Addicott[4], Hector Chinoy[5], Robert G. Cooper[1,5], William E. R. Ollier[1], Lorna J. Kennedy[1]

1 Centre for Integrated Genomic Medical Research (CIGMR), Institute of Population Health, Faculty of Medical and Human Sciences, The University of Manchester, Manchester, United Kingdom, 2 Stone Lion Veterinary Hospital, London, United Kingdom, 3 Alcombe Veterinary Surgery, London, United Kingdom, 4 Hungarian Vizsla Breed Club, Royal Tunbridge Wells, United Kingdom, 5 Rheumatic Diseases Centre, Manchester Academic Health Science Centre, The 6 University of Manchester, Salford Royal NHS Foundation Trust, Salford, United Kingdom

Abstract

A breed-specific polymyositis is frequently observed in the Hungarian Vizsla. Beneficial clinical response to immunosuppressive therapies has been demonstrated which points to an immune-mediated aetiology. Canine inflammatory myopathies share clinical and histological similarities with the human immune-mediated myopathies. As MHC class II associations have been reported in the human conditions we investigated whether an MHC class II association was present in the canine myopathy seen in this breed. 212 Hungarian Vizsla pedigree dogs were stratified both on disease status and degree of relatedness to an affected dog. This generated a group of 29 cases and 183 "graded" controls: 93 unaffected dogs with a first degree affected relative, 44 unaffected dogs with a second degree affected relative, and 46 unaffected dogs with no known affected relatives. Eleven DLA class II haplotypes were identified, of which, DLA-DRB1*02001/DQA1*00401/DQB1*01303, was at significantly raised frequency in cases compared to controls (OR = 1.92, p = 0.032). When only control dogs with no family history of the disease were compared to cases, the association was further strengthened (OR = 4.08, p = 0.00011). Additionally, a single copy of the risk haplotype was sufficient to increase disease risk, with the risk substantially increasing for homozygotes. There was a trend of increasing frequency of this haplotype with degree of relatedness, indicating low disease penetrance. These findings support the hypothesis of an immune-mediated aetiology for this canine myopathy and give credibility to potentially using the Hungarian Vizsla as a genetic model for comparative studies with human myositis.

Editor: Frederick Miller, National Institutes of Health, United States of America

Funding: The Hungarian Vizsla Breed Club (UK) made a donation to the research. Di Addicott is associated with this organisation and co-ordinated the sample collection and analysed the family pedigrees. The funders had no role in study design, data analysis, or decision to publish.

Competing Interests: Clare Rusbridge is affiliated with Stone Lion Veterinary Hospital and Anna Tauro with Alcombe Veterinary Surgery, both commercial companies. There are no patents, products in development or marketed products to declare.

* E-mail: jonathan.massey@manchester.ac.uk

Introduction

A polymyositis (an immune-mediated form of generalised inflammatory myopathy) with specific characteristics is being increasingly observed in the Hungarian Vizsla dog [1,2]. Affected dogs generally present with difficulty eating and drinking (dysphagia), regurgitation, and sialorrhea. Involvement of the masticatory muscle can result in marked masticatory muscle atrophy and generalised muscle involvement can lead to exercise intolerance and weakness. Definitive diagnosis is by muscle biopsy histopathology, which commonly shows endomysial and/or perimysial infiltration by lymphocytes and histiocytes [1]. In one study, using three dogs, CD4+ T-cells were found in excess of CD8+ T-cells which advocates a divergent aetiology to other cases of canine polymyositis [1]. Other diagnostic tests, such as serum creatine kinase concentration, electromyography, fluoroscopy of the oesophagus, and Magnetic Resonance Imaging (MRI) of affected muscle groups can aid in diagnosis. It is also important to rule out other neuromuscular diseases and infectious myopathies. Immunosuppressive drug therapies have been used to treat the

disease and dogs appear to respond well [3]. This has furthered support for the hypothesis of an immune-mediated aetiology for myositis in this particular breed.

Canine immune-mediated inflammatory myopathies share many clinical and histological characteristics with those in humans [4]. The human immune-mediated myopathies are broadly separated into three sub-groups: polymyositis (PM), dermatomyositis (DM) and inclusion body myositis (IBM). There are known disease risk associations with all of these human conditions with allelic variants in the Human Leukocyte Antigen (HLA) class I and class II regions [5].

The incidence of polymyositis in the general canine population is unknown. It has been described at increased frequency in Boxers and Newfoundlands [6], although this is likely a specific form of the disease, with evidence of circulating sarcolemma autoantibodies [7]. Studies in canine polymyositis have shown increased expression of Dog Leukocyte Antigen (DLA) class I and class II molecules on the surface of muscle fibres and infiltrating cells [1] but no associated alleles or haplotypes have as yet been identified.

Other forms of inflammatory myopathies in dogs include masticatory muscle myositis, which appears to be unique to this species. Like in polymyositis, increased expression of DLA class I and II expression has been shown [8]. Dermatomyositis is an inflammatory disease of the skin and muscle, and has been described at high frequency in the Shetland sheepdog and Rough collie. Genetic investigations of this condition in the Shetland sheepdog have revealed an associated linkage region on canine chromosome 35 [9], but fine-mapping studies have been lacking. Additionally, a microarray study in the Shetland sheepdog was able to identify 285 genes, many with immune function, that were differentially regulated in cases vs controls [10]. In a study of familial dermatomyositis in four litters of Rough collies and Rough collie-Labrador crossbreeds, there was an association of disease severity with the DLA class II allele DLA-DRB1*015 but no association with two DLA class I genes [11].

We have previously been able to show DLA class II associations with a range of complex immune-mediated disorders, such as hypothyroid disease and diabetes mellitus [12,13]. Building upon this we present the findings of the first DLA association study of a canine polymyositis.

Materials and Methods

Samples

Canine saliva samples (Oragene® ANIMAL, DNA Genotek Inc., Canada) or blood in ethylenediaminetetraacetic acid (EDTA) (residual blood from a diagnostic test) were submitted to the UK DNA Archive for Companion Animals, University of Manchester. Samples were submitted by veterinary surgeons and owners. In total there were 212 samples included in the study (29 cases and 183 controls), with samples selected from the UK wherever possible. However, three cases originated from New Zealand, Australia and Canada. Six control samples originated from Hungary and four from the USA.

Diagnosis of polymyositis was assigned with varying degrees of confidence, based on the presence or absence of particular criteria, summarised in Table 1. As well as the identification of consistent clinical signs [3], 12 cases had definitive histopathological confirmation by muscle biopsy and one by study at post-mortem. The most common biopsy site was the temporal muscle. Where this was the case, to rule out masticatory muscle myositis (MMM), dogs were required to be 2 M antibody negative (antibody directed against specific masticatory muscle fibres) or have an additional muscle site biopsy. A further four cases were classified as "probable" and had biopsies where 2 M antibody screening was not performed/pending but MMM was ruled out based on the presence of dysphagia and sialorrhea, features not considered typical of MMM. In these 17 cases with biopsy, myasthenia gravis (MG) was ruled out through a mixture of negative acetylcholine receptor antibody (AChR) tests, masticatory muscle atrophy, and high creatine kinase levels (>1000U/L). The remaining 12 dogs were classified as "possible" cases where biopsy was not performed but MMM and MG were ruled out based on clinical signs of dysphagia/sialorrhea and masticatory muscle atrophy, respectively.

Family history of polymyositis and the degree of relatedness between dogs were ascertained from pedigrees and owner reporting. There were 93 first degree unaffected relatives, defined as dogs showing no clinical signs of the disease that had at least one affected offspring, parent or sibling. 44 second degree unaffected relatives, defined as dogs showing no clinical signs of the disease that had at least one affected half-sibling, grandparent, grandchild, aunt, uncle, niece or nephew. 46 control dogs were selected,

defined as dogs showing no clinical signs of polymyositis (based on information from owners and clinicians) and no reported family history of polymyositis. The average age of onset in cases was 2.92 years (range 0.5–8 years), consistent with previous observations [1,2]. Dogs in the control group had an average age of 6.92 years, ranging from 0.58–13.83 years, with 17 out of 46 dogs over the age of 8 years.

DNA Extraction

DNA was extracted from blood using QIAamp® DNA Blood Midi Kit (Qiagen, Crawley, UK). DNA from the Oragene® ANIMAL saliva kit was extracted using the manufacturer's standard protocol. DNA concentration was measured using a NanoDrop® ND-1000 spectrophotometer (Wilmington, USA) and diluted in water to 5 ng/µl for PCR.

Typing of DLA Class II Loci

All dogs were characterised for three class II loci: DLA-DRB1, DLA-DQA1, and DLA-DQB1 using Sequence-Based Typing (SBT) of exon 2 of each of these genes.

PCR was performed in a 96-well plate format. A 25 µl reaction volume was used per well, which consisted of: 5 µl of genomic DNA (5 ng/µl), 2.5 µl of 10x PCR buffer (with added MgCl$_2$, 20 mM) (Roche), 0.5 µl of dNTPs (10 mM) (Roche), 0.5 µl of each forward and reverse primer, 0.13 µl FastStart Taq (5 U/µl) (Roche), and 15.87 µl of distilled water.

DRB1 primers: **DRBIn1** CCG TCC CCA CAG CAC ATT TC, **DRBIn2T7** TAA TAC GAC TCA CTA TAG GG TGT GTC ACA CAC CTC AGC ACC A. DQA1 primers: **DQAIn1** TAA GGT TCT TTT CTC CCT CT, **DQAIn2** GGA CAG ATT CAG TGA AGA GA. DQB1 primers: **DQB1BT7** TAA TAC GAC TCA CTA TAG GG CTC ACT GGC CCG GCT GTC TC, **DQBR2** CAC CTC GCC GCT GCA ACG TG. All primers are intronic and locus specific. The T7-tailed portion is underlined.

Amplification was performed using a touchdown PCR protocol on a PTC-225 tetrad cycler as follows: 95°C for 5 minutes; 14 touchdown cycles of: (95°C for 30 seconds, annealing for 1 minute starting at 62°C (DRB1) 54°C (DQA1) 73°C (DQB1) reducing by 0.5°C for each cycle, 72°C for 1 minute); 25 cycles of: (95°C for 1 minute, 55°C (DRB1) 47°C (DQA1) 66°C (DQB1) for 1 minute, 72°C for 1 minute); followed by a final elongation step of 72°C for 10 minutes. A negative control containing no DNA was included in each amplification to detect any contamination.

The presence of PCR product was assessed by running 5 µl of each reaction with 3 µl of loading buffer on a 2% agarose gel. Purification was performed by adding 4 µl of a 1in8 water dilution of USB® ExoSAP-IT® (Affymetrix, High Wycombe, UK) to 1 µl of PCR product and thermocycling at 37°C for 1 hour followed by 80°C for 15 minutes.

Sequencing (standard Sanger protocol) was performed in only one direction: reverse for DLA-DRB1 and DLA-DQA1 and forward for DLA-DQB1. The T7 primers (DRB1 and DQB1) or PCR primers (DQA1, DQAIn2) were used for sequencing. The product sizes are 303 bp for DLA-DRB1, 345 bp for DLA-DQA1 and 300 bp for DLA-DQB1. Sequencing data was analysed by *SBTengine®* (GenDx, Genome Diagnostics B.V., Utrecht, Netherlands). Briefly, the sequences were aligned to a consensus sequence and each polymorphic site was analysed either by the software or manually. The corrected sequence was then matched to a reference sequence library built into the software package (taken from http://www.ebi.ac.uk/ipd/mhc/dla/index.html).

Haplotypes were identified by first selecting the dogs that were homozygous for all three loci DLA-DRB1/DQA1/DQB1. This

Table 1. The criteria used to assign cases to a diagnostic confidence grouping.

	Diagnostic confidence grouping		
Criterion	Definite	Probable	Possible
Muscle biopsy showing inflammatory pathology	Yes	Yes	No
2 M antibody negative or additional muscle site biopsy	Yes	No	No
AChR antibody negative, high CK or MM atrophy	Yes	Yes	Yes
Dysphagia/sialorrhea	Yes	Yes	Yes
Number of dogs	13	4	12

identified several different combinations of alleles. Secondly, dogs that were homozygous for only two of the loci were selected and the previous haplotypes were confirmed and added to. The remaining dogs were examined using the haplotype information already gathered.

Statistical Analysis

Contingency tables (2×2) were used to calculate odds ratios, 95% confidence intervals (Cornfield) and p-values for each haplotype and allele. For the Chi-squared test (X^2), Yates's correction for continuity was utilised.

Ethics Statement

Collection of veterinary blood samples solely for research purposes, without a home office licence, is prohibited in the United Kingdom. However, residual blood remaining after a diagnostic test may be used for research and does not require a licence. Collecting saliva with swabs is considered a non-invasive procedure and does not require a licence. Residual blood was submitted by the attending veterinary surgeon with owner permission. Saliva was collected and submitted by the owners of the animals.

Results

DLA alleles and haplotypes were assigned to all dogs: affected dogs, unaffected first degree relatives of an affected dog, unaffected second degree relatives of an affected dog, and control dogs with no known family history of polymyositis. Within this group of Hungarian Viszlas, we identified seven haplotypes with a genotype count greater than five, plus four other less frequent haplotypes. Table 2 shows the frequencies of these haplotypes in each of the groups.

We did not identify any evidence of sex bias from our data but the small numbers make it difficult to draw definitive conclusions. In cases, there were marginally more males than females (Female: 41%, Male: 59%) while in the "graded controls" group there was a larger proportion of females compared to males (Female: 60%, Male: 40% - two dogs of unknown sex).

The most frequent haplotypes were DLA-DRB1*02001/DQA1*00401/DQB1*01303 and DLA-DRB1*00601/DQA1*005011/DQB1*00701, with 71% and 36% of all dogs, respectively, having at least one copy of this haplotype. One interesting observation is the marked frequency gradient of the DLA-DRB1*02001/DQA1*00401/DQB1*01303 haplotype with the highest frequency (60%) occurring in cases compared to 52% in unaffected first degree relatives, to 47% in unaffected second degree relatives, and to 27% in unrelated controls. This can be seen more clearly in Figure 1.

Comparison of cases against all dogs without polymyositis (including those dogs with a family history of affected animals) (n = 29 cases/183 controls), revealed a significant association of the DLA-DRB1*02001/DQA1*00401/DQB1*01303 haplotype with disease risk ($X^2 = 4.58$, OR = 1.92, 95% CI 1.05–3.5, p = 0.032). As Hungarian Vizslas are recognised as being a breed predisposed to polymyositis, we further analysed the data to ascertain whether a stronger association could be observed for this haplotype if only dogs with no family history of the disease were considered. Thus, we removed dogs that had a family history of the disease, and compared the case and control groups alone (n = 29 cases/46 controls). In this analysis, the genotypic frequency in affected dogs (60%) was over twice that in control dogs (27%) ($X^2 = 15$, OR = 4.08, 95% CI 1.92–8.74, p = 0.00011).

Given the differing levels of confidence in diagnosis amongst the 29 cases (Table 1), subgroup analyses were also conducted. In the 17 dogs with a "definite" or "probable" diagnosis, the genotypic frequency of DLA-DRB1*02001/DQA1*00401/DQB1*01303 was 64.7%. In the remaining 12 cases with a "possible" diagnosis, the frequency was 54.2%. Both of these frequencies were significantly different to the 27% frequency found in the group of 46 unrelated controls. For the "definite/probable" group this gave OR = 4.91, p = 0.00025, and for the "possible" group OR = 3.17, p = 0.024. Additionally the frequency of dogs homozygous for the risk haplotype in each subgroup was 35.3% and 33.3%, respectively.

As the age of onset in cases ranged up to 8 years, we assessed the frequency of the risk haplotype in a subset of 17 controls over the age of 8 years. This revealed a genotype frequency of 29.4%, which was significantly different compared to the frequency in affected dogs (OR 3.65, 95% CI 1.35–10.04, p = 0.0081).

Over a third of affected dogs were homozygous for DLA-DRB1*02001/DQA1*00401/DQB1*01303 (34.5%) compared to 8.7% of control dogs. Table 3 shows that when comparing genotypes, using a baseline of dogs that did not carry any copies of the risk haplotype, there is a significant effect on disease risk with heterozygote presence of the haplotype (OR = 5) and the effect is increased substantially for homozygotes (OR = 15). Homozygosity of the risk haplotype did not appear to reduce the age of onset for affected dogs; the average age of onset for dogs homozygous for the risk haplotype was 3.28 years compared to 2.83 years for other dogs.

There is some indication that the presence of DLA-DRB1*01501/DQA1*00601/DQB1*02301 is protective, with 9/46 unrelated control dogs having one copy compared to only 1/29 cases. However, this may be a reflection of the reduction in non-disease associated haplotypes in cases due the high frequency of the DLA-DRB1*02001/DQA1*00401/DQB1*01303 haplotype.

Table 2. Frequencies of the DLA haplotypes found in Hungarian Vizslas.

Haplotype			Cases		All Controls		Graded Controls					
							1st degree relatives		2nd degree relatives		Controls	
			2n = 58		2n = 366		2n = 186		2n = 88		2n = 92	
DRB1	DQA1	DQB1	n	%	n	%	n	%	n	%	n	%
02001	00401	01303	35	60.3	162	44.3	96	51.6	41	46.6	25	27.2
00601	005011	00701	12	20.7	72	19.7	35	18.8	14	15.9	23	25.0
00901	00101	008011	5	8.6	31	8.5	19	10.2	7	8.0	5	5.4
00801	00301	00401	3	5.2	44	12.0	17	9.1	12	13.6	15	16.3
02301	00301	00501	2	3.4	25	6.8	13	7.0	10	11.4	2	2.2
01501	00601	02301	1	1.7	16	4.4	5	2.7	2	2.3	9	9.8
04801	00101	008011	0	0	9	2.5	1	0.5	2	2.3	6	6.5
Other haplotypes			0	0	7	1.9	0	0	0	0	7	7.6

As there were two major haplotypes that carried DQA1*00101 and DQA1*00301, an allelic association analysis for each locus was also performed. This showed no significant differences between cases and controls carrying either allele (data not shown).

Discussion

This study provides evidence for an association between an MHC class II haplotype with the development of polymyositis in Hungarian Vizslas. In the dog population as a whole, the DLA-DRB1*02001/DQA1*00401/DQB1*01303 haplotype is relatively common with a haplotype frequency of 6.2% amongst approximately 10,000 dogs from over 200 breeds tested (LJ Kennedy, unpublished data). The limited DLA class II haplotype diversity of the Hungarian Vizsla is typical of many other breeds studied [14], including the Pug dog [15].

The DLA-DRB1*02001 allele does not match the DLA-DRB1*015 allele previously associated with increased disease risk in canine dermatomyositis [11], which supports a divergent aetiology for the two diseases. As there are other known canine inflammatory myopathies, it will be important to investigate if other MHC associations exist in these diseases and whether they share the same risk DLA haplotype as presented here. Given the previous observation of CD4+ T-cells being found in excess CD8+ T-cells in Hungarian Vizsla polymyositis biopsies, it would be particularly interesting to see if there are comparisons with canine masticatory muscle myositis, a disease where this is also a feature [1]. Furthermore, although MHC class I associations were not identified in a canine dermatomyositis [11], they have been demonstrated in human inflammatory myopathies, so it will be interesting to look for such an association in the canine conditions.

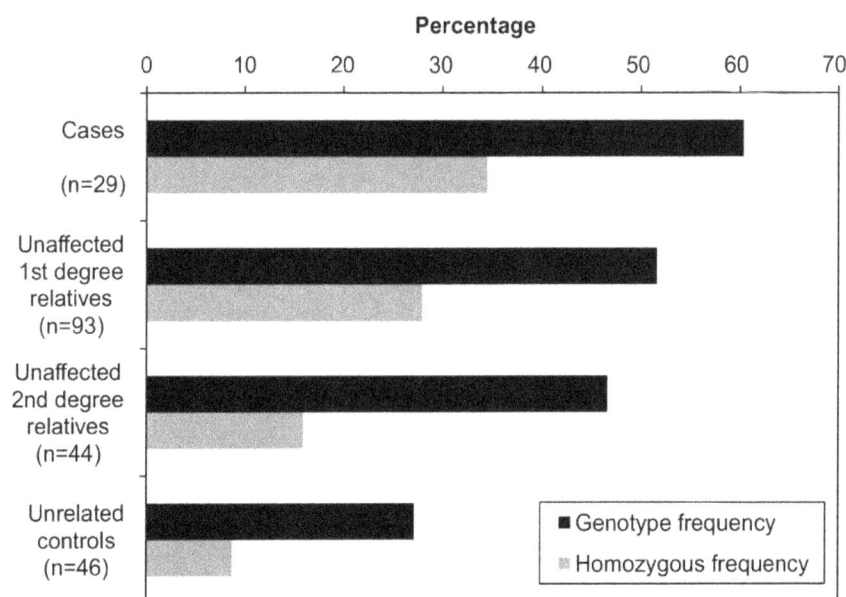

Figure 1. Haplotype and homozygous frequency of DLA-DRB1*02001/DQA1*00401/DQB1*01303 in cases and "graded controls".

Table 3. Association of the DLA-DRB1*02001/DQA1*00401/DQB1*01303 genotypes with polymyositis, relative to the disease risk in individuals who are DLA-DRB1*02001/DQA1*00401/DQB1*01303 homozygous negative.

Genotype	Cases	Controls	OR	95% CI
	n = 29	n = 46	(compared to controls)	
DRB1/DQA1/DQB1	n (%)	n (%)		
02001/00401/01303 (−/−)	4 (13.8)	24 (52.2)	1	Baseline
02001/00401/01303 (−/+)	15 (51.7)	18 (39.1)	5	1.25–21.67
02001/00401/01303 (+/+)	10 (34.5)	4 (8.7)	15	2.54–104.45

The DLA-DRB1*02001/DQA1*00401/DQB1*01303 haplotype has not previously been identified as being risk-associated in an immune-mediated disease. However, Wilbe et al. [16] found the haplotype to be protective against the immune-mediated condition of Symmetrical Lupoid Onychodystrophy (SLO) in Gordon Setters.

Carrying a single copy of the DLA-DRB1*02001/DQA1*00401/DQB1*01303 risk haplotype increases risk of polymyositis. Homozygosity of the risk haplotype further increases this risk. A possible explanation for this is that signalling through the MHC receptor requires a high threshold before a response is induced. Doubling the number of identical MHC molecules would allow this level to be reached more easily and possibly initiate autoimmunity to self-antigen. An alternative explanation could be that other susceptibility genes within the DLA region and beyond could be present on an extended haplotype [17]. This type of gene dosage effect has been shown with MHC associations in human autoimmune diseases, such as the presence of the shared epitope in rheumatoid arthritis [18] and HLA-DR2 in multiple sclerosis [17]. Homozygosity of MHC risk alleles has also been associated with increased disease risk in a canine SLE-related condition [19] and canine necrotizing meningoencephalitis [15]. It has also been associated with earlier disease onset in canine anal furunculosis [20], but this was not observed with polymyositis in this study.

The DLA-DRB1*02001/DQA1*00401/DQB1*01303 haplotype is more prevalent within pedigrees of affected Hungarian Vizsla cases, with a marked trend based on the degree of relatedness to an individual with the disease. This suggests that this haplotype has a low penetrance and provides evidence of a true association of MHC class II with polymyositis in Hungarian Vizslas; low penetrance of MHC alleles and haplotypes is expected and is a common feature in both canine and human MHC class II association studies [21]. However, this statement is not always correct and there are examples of highly penetrant MHC associations, as in the study of Pug dogs with necrotizing meningoencephalitis [15]. Although we stratified dogs based on the degree of family history of disease, the pedigree data for all controls were incomplete. Thus we were unable to model this penetrance.

Given the increased risk of polymyositis with homozygosity of the risk haplotype, it is tempting to speculate that selecting against this haplotype in the population would reduce the occurrence of the disease. However, this would reduce the diversity of an already restricted DLA repertoire and could have unintended negative consequences, such as an increased susceptibility to particular pathogens. It is also likely that polymyositis in this breed is a complex disorder, in which DLA class II genes are only part of a wider array of susceptibility loci.

The use of cases and controls from areas of the world other than the UK did not reveal any evidence of heterogeneity and thus we included the small number of these animals in the analysis. Interestingly, one haplotype was found only in three of the four control dogs from the USA, which could indicate some minor level of population stratification. However, the removal of the four samples from the USA did not change the overall results (data not shown). Given that this study was conducted within a single breed, with the majority of those dogs from UK lineages, the effects are unlikely to be due to population stratification.

Despite the differing levels of confidence in diagnosis of polymyositis in this study, we were able to show significant associations of the risk haplotype in all subgroups. However, future work will focus on improving the diagnosis of polymyositis in those dogs classified as "probable" or "possible" cases.

In conclusion, this study supports the hypothesis of an immune-mediated aetiology for this breed-specific polymyositis in the Hungarian Vizsla. The low penetrance of the risk haplotype indicates that other genetic and environmental factors will be involved. Although there are differences between the canine and human disease, mainly regarding different cellular infiltrates, the Hungarian Vizsla condition could present an important model for comparative studies. The rarity of polymyositis in humans (5–10 cases per million adults per year) [22] makes genetic association studies difficult due the problem of accruing sufficient sample sizes to gain adequate statistical power and provide replication cohorts. Pedigree dog breeds that display high predisposition for certain spontaneously occurring diseases have already proved to represent a powerful comparative genetic model for aiding in the discovery of novel genetic loci underlying analogous human conditions [23]. Reduced genetic heterogeneity and increased long-range linkage disequilibrium (LD) make the dog particularly amenable to genome-wide association studies (GWAS), with fewer individuals than would be required for an equivalent study in humans [24]. A future canine GWAS in Hungarian Vizslas could be an efficient and practical way of advancing our understanding of both the canine and human conditions of polymyositis and indeed, other inflammatory disorders.

Acknowledgments

We would like to thank the Hungarian Vizsla Breed Club (UK) for their interest and enthusiasm in providing their dog's samples for this study. Acknowledgements also go to the technical staff supporting the UK DNA Archive for Companion Animals, namely Steven Quarmby and Ezinne Ibe.

Author Contributions

Reviewed diagnosis: CR AT. Conceived and designed the experiments: JM SR CR HC RGC WERO IJK. Performed the experiments: JM SR.

Analyzed the data: JM DA IJK. Contributed reagents/materials/analysis tools: CR AT DA. Wrote the paper: JM.

References

1. Haley AC, Platt SR, Kent M, Schatzberg SJ, Durham A, et al. (2011) Breed-specific polymyositis in Hungarian Vizsla dogs. J Vet Intern Med 25: 393–397.
2. Foale RD, Whiting M, Wray JD (2008) Myositis and pharyngeal dysphagia in Hungarian vizslas. Proceedings of the 50th BSAVA Congress, Birmingham: Clinical research abstract.
3. Rusbridge C, Nicholas N, Addicott D (2011) Polymyositis and DNA collection in the Hungarian vizsla dog. Vet Rec 168: 85–86.
4. Shelton GD, Hoffman EP, Ghimbovschi S, Peters IR, Day MJ, et al. (2006) Immunopathogenic pathways in canine inflammatory myopathies resemble human myositis. Veterinary Immunology and Immunopathology 113: 200–214.
5. O'Hanlon TP, Carrick DM, Arnett FC, Reveille JD, Carrington M, et al. (2005) Immunogenetic risk and protective factors for the idiopathic inflammatory myopathies: distinct HLA-A, -B, -Cw, -DRB1 and -DQA1 allelic profiles and motifs define clinicopathologic groups in caucasians. Medicine (Baltimore) 84: 338–349.
6. Evans J, Levesque D, Shelton GD (2004) Canine inflammatory myopathies: a clinicopathologic review of 200 cases. J Vet Intern Med 18: 679–691.
7. Hankel S, Shelton GD, Engvall E (2006) Sarcolemma-specific autoantibodies in canine inflammatory myopathy. Vet Immunol Immunopathol 113: 1–10.
8. Paciello O, Shelton GD, Papparella S (2007) Expression of major histocompatibility complex class I and class II antigens in canine masticatory muscle myositis. Neuromuscul Disord 17: 313–320.
9. Clark LA, Credille KM, Murphy KE, Rees CA (2005) Linkage of dermatomyositis in the Shetland Sheepdog to chromosome 35. Vet Dermatol 16: 392–394.
10. Wahl JM, Clark LA, Skalli O, Ambrus A, Rees CA, et al. (2008) Analysis of gene transcript profiling and immunobiology in Shetland sheepdogs with dermatomyositis. Vet Dermatol 19: 52–58.
11. Hargis AM, Prieur DJ, Haupt KH, Collier LL, Evermann JF, et al. (1986) Postmortem findings in four litters of dogs with familial canine dermatomyositis. Am J Pathol 123: 480–496.
12. Kennedy LJ, Davison LJ, Barnes A, Short AD, Fretwell N, et al. (2006) Identification of susceptibility and protective major histocompatibility complex haplotypes in canine diabetes mellitus. Tissue Antigens 68: 467–476.
13. Kennedy LJ, Quarmby S, Happ GM, Barnes A, Ramsey IK, et al. (2006) Association of canine hypothyroidism with a common major histocompatibility complex DLA class II allele. Tissue Antigens 68: 82–86.
14. Kennedy LJ, Barnes A, Short A, Brown JJ, Lester S, et al. (2007) Canine DLA diversity: 1. New alleles and haplotypes. Tissue Antigens 69 Suppl 1: 272–288.
15. Greer KA, Wong AK, Liu H, Famula TR, Pedersen NC, et al. (2010) Necrotizing meningoencephalitis of Pug dogs associates with dog leukocyte antigen class II and resembles acute variant forms of multiple sclerosis. Tissue Antigens 76: 110–118.
16. Wilbe M, Ziener ML, Aronsson A, Harlos C, Sundberg K, et al. (2010) DLA class II alleles are associated with risk for canine symmetrical lupoid onychodystrophy (SLO). PLoS One 5: e12332.
17. Barcellos LF, Oksenberg JR, Begovich AB, Martin ER, Schmidt S, et al. (2003) HLA-DR2 dose effect on susceptibility to multiple sclerosis and influence on disease course. American Journal of Human Genetics 72: 710–716.
18. MacGregor A, Ollier W, Thomson W, Jawaheer D, Silman A (1995) HLA-DRB1*0401/0404 genotype and rheumatoid arthritis: increased association in men, young age at onset, and disease severity. Journal of Rheumatology 22: 1032–1036.
19. Wilbe M, Jokinen P, Hermanrud C, Kennedy LJ, Strandberg E, et al. (2009) MHC class II polymorphism is associated with a canine SLE-related disease complex. Immunogenetics 61: 557–564.
20. Kennedy LJ, O'Neill T, House A, Barnes A, Kyostila K, et al. (2008) Risk of anal furunculosis in German shepherd dogs is associated with the major histocompatibility complex. Tissue Antigens 71: 51–56.
21. Aguirre-Hernandez J, Polton G, Kennedy LJ, Sargan DR (2010) Association between anal sac gland carcinoma and dog leukocyte antigen-DQB1 in the English Cocker Spaniel. Tissue Antigens 76: 476–481.
22. Oddis CV, Conte CG, Steen VD, Medsger TA, Jr. (1990) Incidence of polymyositis-dermatomyositis: a 20-year study of hospital diagnosed cases in Allegheny County, PA 1963–1982. J Rheumatol 17: 1329–1334.
23. Wilbe M, Jokinen P, Truve K, Seppala EH, Karlsson EK, et al. (2010) Genome-wide association mapping identifies multiple loci for a canine SLE-related disease complex. Nat Genet 42: 250–254.
24. Karlsson EK, Lindblad-Toh K (2008) Leader of the pack: gene mapping in dogs and other model organisms. Nat Rev Genet 9: 713–725.

10

DLA Class II Alleles and Haplotypes Are Associated with Risk for and Protection from Chronic Hepatitis in the English Springer Spaniel

Nicholas H. Bexfield[1]*, Penny J. Watson[1], Jesús Aguirre-Hernandez[1], David R. Sargan[1], Laurence Tiley[1], Jonathan L. Heeney[1], Lorna J. Kennedy[2]

1 Department of Veterinary Medicine, University of Cambridge, Cambridge, United Kingdom, 2 Centre for Integrated Genomic Medical Research, University of Manchester, Manchester, United Kingdom

Abstract

Chronic hepatitis (CH) is common in dogs in the United Kingdom. An increased prevalence of the disease is seen in the English Springer spaniel (ESS), and this breed suffer from a severe form with young to middle aged female dogs being predisposed. The disease shares histological features with those of human viral hepatitis, although the specific aetiological agent has not yet been identified. The aim of the current study was to investigate whether dog leucocyte antigen (DLA) class II alleles and haplotypes are associated with susceptibility/resistance to CH in the ESS. Sequence-based genotyping of the polymorphic exon 2 from DLA-DRB1, -DQA1 and -DQB1 class II loci were performed in 66 ESSs with CH and 84 healthy controls. There was a significant difference in the distribution of the protective alleles DRB1*00501 (3.0% vs. 12.0%, odds ratio [OR] = 0.23, 95% confidence interval [CI] = 0.06–0.74) and DQB1*00501 (3.8% vs. 12.0%, OR = 0.29, 95% CI = 0.09–0.85) between cases and controls. The haplotype DLA-DRB1*00501/DQA1*00301/DQB1*00501 was present in 11.9% of controls and 3.0% of cases and was significantly associated with protection against disease development (OR = 0.26, 95% CI = 0.08–0.80). There was a significant difference in the distribution of the risk alleles DRB1*00601 (14.4% vs. 6.5%, OR = 2.40, 95% CI = 1.10–5.63) and DQB1*00701 (14.4% vs. 6.5%, OR = 2.40, 95% CI = 1.10–5.63) between cases and controls. A risk haplotype (DLA-DRB1*00601/DQA1*005011/DQB1*00701) was present in 14.4% of cases and 6.5% of controls and conferred an elevated risk of developing CH with an OR of 3.13 (95% CI = 1.20–8.26). These results demonstrate that DLA class II is significantly associated with risk and protection from developing CH in ESSs.

Editor: Naglaa H. Shoukry, University of Montreal, Canada

Funding: This work was supported by funding from the Wellcome Trust (grant number WT088619MA). The funders had no role in study design, data collection and analysis, decision to publish, or preparation of the manuscript.

Competing Interests: The authors have declared that no competing interests exist.

* E-mail: nb289@cam.ac.uk

Introduction

Canine chronic hepatitis (CH) is common in the United Kingdom with a prevalence of 12% at post mortem [1]. However, the aetiology of most cases of canine CH remains unknown [2]. Known causes identified in a small number of cases include canine adenovirus type I (CAV-1) [3], bacteria including leptospires [4] and *Helicobacter* spp. [5], and several toxins and drugs [6]. Defects in copper metabolism have been described in several breeds [7], and some dogs accumulate alpha-1 antitrypsin in hepatocytes leading to cell death [8]. To date, studies have failed to conclusively demonstrate a primary immune-mediated aetiology [9,10].

An increased prevalence of CH occurs in the English Springer spaniel (ESS) [11], suggesting a genetic predisposition to disease. The ESS suffers from a more aggressive form of CH than other breeds with a median survival of just over six months [11], compared to 19 months in a variety of other breeds of dog with CH [12]. The pathogenesis of the disease is incompletely elucidated, but is of suspected viral aetiology as it shares histological features with those of chronic viral hepatitis in humans [11,13,14].

The canine major histocompatibility complex (MHC), referred to as the dog leucocyte antigen (DLA) system, plays a central role in the control of the immune system and comprises of three regions known as class I, II and III. The first two regions are involved in the regulation and presentation of self and non-self antigens to the immune system. The class I region contains one highly polymorphic gene called DLA-88 plus several other genes [15,16]. The class II region includes four functional genes; DLA-DRA1 which appears monomorphic and DLA-DRB1, DQA1 and DQB1 which are highly polymorphic [15,16]. The full extent of their polymorphism has not yet been determined. There are currently 106 DLA-DRB1, 26 DLA-DQA1 and 62 DLA-DQB1 alleles identified in the dog and other closely related canids [17]. Furthermore, particular DLA class II allelic forms of each locus tend to be found together on the same chromosome, or haplotypes, more frequently than expected from their own individual gene frequencies. This linkage disequilibrium, or non-random association of alleles at adjacent MHC loci, results in conserved haplotype combinations which often have a restricted breed distribution [18]. Over 144 different three-locus, DLA-DRB1/DQA1/DQB1, haplotypes have been identified in more than 80 breeds of dog [18]. Although there is often a lack of within breed variability in MHC alleles expressed in pedigree dogs, the ESS shows a slightly above average diversity of MHC alleles [18,19]. Because dogs and humans share a similar set of orthologous genes, are affected by diseases of similar aetiology and live in the same environment, the dog is a useful model for studies on genetic diseases [20,21,22].

MHC genes, known as the human leucocyte antigens (HLA), are important in determining susceptibility to autoimmune, metabolic and infectious diseases in man [23,24,25]. For instance several studies have reported the influence of MHC genotype on the outcome of viral infections, such as reported in HIV-1 infected persons [26,27,28]. In humans there are also important associations between HLA polymorphisms and clinical outcome after infection with the hepatotrophic viruses, hepatitis B (HBV) and C (HCV). In HCV infection, the most profound association has been with natural killer cell immunoglobulin-like receptors (KIRs) that recognise HLA-C [29,30], while in HBV infected individuals HLA class II alleles have been associated with both protection from, and risk of disease progression [31,32].

To date, the role of DLA in disease susceptibility has largely been established for canine immune-mediated diseases, although an association between DLA haplotypes and other canine non immune-mediated diseases including generalised demodicosis [33], anal gland carcinoma [34], and cranial cruciate ligament rupture [35] has also been identified. Only one study has also examined the possible association between DLA class II genes and canine hepatitis in the Dobermann Pincher, a disease of suspected autoimmune aetiology [36].

The aim of this study was to determine whether DLA class II alleles and haplotypes were associated with CH in the ESS.

Results

The study cohort of dogs with CH comprised 47 females and 19 males, and the median age was three years 11 months (range, seven months to eight years one month). The median age of the control dogs was nine years eight months (range eight years to 14 years one month) and there were 55 females and 29 males.

DLA class II alleles and haplotypes were assigned to all dogs with CH and control dogs. Within this group of ESS we identified ten DLA-DRB1 alleles, six DLA-DQA1 alleles and eight DLA-DQB1 alleles (Table 1). Of the DRB1 alleles, DRB1*01501 was the most common allele with a frequency of 39.3%, and the other nine alleles had frequencies between 0.4–24.3%. 40.0% of ESSs had allele DQA1*00601 and the other alleles ranged in frequency between 1.3–33.0%. Of the DQB1 alleles, DQB1*01303 was the most common (38.3%) and the others had frequencies between 1.3–22.7%. For DLA-DRB1, there was a significant difference in the distribution of the alleles DRB1*00501 (3.0% vs. 12.0%, odds ratio [OR] = 0.23, 95% confidence interval [CI] = 0.06–0.74) and DRB1*00601 (14.4% vs. 6.5%, OR = 2.40, 95% CI = 1.10–5.63) between cases and controls. For DLA-DQB1, two alleles, namely DQB1*00501 (3.8% vs. 12.0%, OR = 0.29, 95% CI = 0.09–0.85) and DQB1*00701 (14.4% vs. 6.5%, OR = 2.40, 95% CI = 1.10–5.63) had a significantly different distribution between cases and controls.

There were a total of 11 different DLA-DRB1/DQA1/DQB1 haplotypes with frequencies >1% (Table 2). In the controls there were two haplotypes with frequencies around 25%, two with frequencies between 10–15%, three with frequencies of 6.5%, two with frequencies between 1–2% and one with a frequency of

<1%. In the affected cases there were three haplotypes with frequencies between 15–20%, three with frequencies between 8–15%, three with frequencies between 1–5%, and three with frequencies <1%. In ESSs, two haplotypes differed markedly in frequency between cases and controls (Table 2). The haplotype DLA-DRB1*00601/DQA1*005011/DQB1*00701 (haplotype four) occurred in 14.4% of the cases compared with 6.5% of the controls (OR = 3.13, 95% CI = 1.20–8.26) and was defined as a risk-haplotype. One affected and two control dogs were homozygous for this risk haplotype. A lower frequency of CH was found in ESSs carrying haplotype DLA-DRB1*00501/DQA1*00301/DQB1*00501 (haplotype eight). This haplotype was found in 11.9% of the controls and 3.0% of the cases (OR = 0.26, 95% CI = 0.08–0.80) and thus is significantly associated with protection against disease development. No affected or control dog was homozygous for this protective haplotype.

Discussion

The results of this study demonstrate a significant association between DLA class II and CH in the ESS, and moreover that this may represent an important immunological risk factor for the development, or the progression and persistence, of the disease. This apparent genetic component to CH has been previously suspected in view of the predilection of this disease to occur in particular breeds including the ESS and reports of familial occurrence [37].

The present, and the majority of previous studies, have used a candidate gene approach to examine DLA class II genes. While the typing of class II genes using a sequence-based method is relatively simple, typing of the class I genes is more difficult as it requires amplification and cloning [38]. Moreover, comparatively less is known about DLA class I genes. As a first step in understanding the genetics of CH in ESS, we therefore chose to analyse class II genes, although future studies could also study the association with class I genes. Due to the high linkage disequilibrium in the MHC class II region, and the extensive polymorphism in exon two (which encodes the antigen binding domain), genetic typing of this exon was used in an attempt to detect most of the variation in the locus. The direct sequencing of the class II region yielded the characterized DLA-DRB1/DQA1/DQB1 alleles and haplotypes [17] and was used in the investigation of disease associations [39]. Because very few dogs were homozygous, we calculated haplotype and allele frequencies, rather than the number of dogs with each haplotype or allele. When performing genetic typing, all control dogs, and all dogs with CH for whom pedigree information was available (45/66) were unrelated at the grandparent level. However, it is possible that if some of the remaining dogs in the CH group were closely related, this could lead to an overrepresentation of alleles and haplotypes in this group.

There was a significant difference in the distribution of the alleles DRB1*00501, and DQB1*00501 between cases and controls, with these alleles offering protection from disease. A third allele, DQA1*00301, also approached significance as a protective allele. Haplotype eight appeared to confer protection against CH and this was identified with a frequency of 3.0% in cases and 11.9% in controls (OR = 0.26, 95% CI = 0.08–0.80). This haplotype is relatively common in the ESS, being found in 8.3% of ESS [18]. However, this haplotype was not found in Dobermann Pinschers with hepatitis [36] nor in ESSs with IMHA [40].

There was a significant difference in the distribution of the alleles DRB1*00601 and DQB1*00701 between cases and

Table 1. Frequencies of DLA class II alleles in 66 ESSs with CH and 84 healthy controls.

DLA-DRB1	Cases (frequency %) n = 132	Controls (frequency %) n = 168	Total (frequency %) n = 300	OR	95% CI	Raw P value*
00101	11 (8.3)	11 (6.5)	22 (7.3)			
00501	**4 (3.0)**	**20 (12.0)**	**24 (8.0)**	0.23	0.06–0.74	
00601	**19 (14.4)**	**11 (6.5)**	**30 (10.0)**	2.40	1.10–5.63	
00901	1 (0.8)	3 (1.8)	4 (1.3)			
01201	30 (22.7)	43 (25.6)	73 (24.3)			
01501	50 (37.9)	68 (40.5)	118 (39.3)			
01502	2 (1.5)	0	2 (0.7)			
02001	14 (10.6)	11 (6.5)	25 (8.3)			
02301	1 (0.8)	0	1 (0.4)			
012v	0	1 (0.6)	1 (0.4)			
Clump test 1 for locus (chi squared emulation, all alleles)						0.012
Clump test 2 for locus (chi squared emulation, after grouping alleles with small values together)						0.014
DLA-DQA1	**Cases (frequency %) n = 132**	**Controls (frequency %) n = 168**	**Total (frequency %) n = 300**	**OR**	**95% CI**	**Raw P value***
00101	1 (0.8)	3 (1.8)	4 (1.3)			
00201	11 (8.3)	11 (6.5)	22 (7.3)			
00301	5 (3.8)	20 (12.0)	25 (8.3)	0.29	0.09–0.85	
00401	44 (33.3)	55 (32.7)	99 (33.0)			
00601	52 (39.4)	68 (40.5)	120 (40.0)			
005011	19 (14.4)	11 (6.5)	30 (10.0)	2.40	1.10–5.63	
Clump test 1 for locus (chi squared emulation, all alleles)						0.041 (NS)
Clump test 2 for locus (chi squared emulation, after grouping alleles with small values together)						0.033 (NS)
DLA-DQB1	**Cases (frequency %) n = 132**	**Controls (frequency %) n = 168**	**Total (frequency %) n = 300**	**OR**	**95% CI**	**Raw P value***
00301	26 (19.7)	42 (25.0)	68 (22.7)			
00501	**5 (3.8)**	**20 (12.0)**	**25 (8.3)**	0.29	0.09–0.85	
00701	**19 (14.4)**	**11 (6.5)**	**30 (10.0)**	2.40	1.10–5.63	
008011	1 (0.8)	3 (1.8)	4 (1.3)			
01303	49 (37.1)	66 (39.3)	115 (38.3)			
013017	6 (4.5)	0	6 (2.0)			
02002	23 (17.4)	24 (14.2)	47 (15.7)			
02301	3 (2.3)	2 (1.2)	5 (1.7)			
Clump test 1 for locus (chi squared emulation, all alleles)						0.003
Clump test 2 for locus (chi squared emulation, after grouping alleles with small values together)						0.010

Altogether, 10 DRB1 alleles, six DQA1 alleles and eight DQB1 alleles were found in the population. The alleles DRB1*00601 and DQB1*00701 were observed in a higher frequency in cases while the alleles DRB1*00501 and DQB1*00501 were more frequent in controls. Numbers in bold indicate a significant difference between cases and controls. NS; not significant.
*After Bonferroni adjustment, significance level would be p<0.017.

controls and these were risk alleles. A third allele, DQA1*005011, also approached significance as a risk allele. A significant association between haplotype four and the presence of CH was also observed (OR = 3.13, 95% CI = 1.20–8.26), suggesting that this haplotype is a potential risk haplotype for disease development. Only one affected dog was homozygous for the risk haplotype. Haplotype four is one of the most widespread of the DLA haplotypes across all dogs, having being found in 40 of 88 breeds [18] with a reported frequency of 8.7% [19]. While this haplotype is very common in Cocker Spaniels (>60% of chromosomes in several studies), it also reaches moderate frequency (17%) in ESSs [18]. In the present study haplotype four had a frequency of 10% in all ESSs. Haplotype four has been shown to be associated with other canine diseases, including anal

gland carcinoma in the English Cocker Spaniel [34]. In primary IMHA this haplotype was also present in 30.3% of all cases compared to 19.1% of controls and was one of two potential risk haplotypes [40]. However, when individual breeds with primary IMHA were examined, this haplotype was not increased in affected ESSs.

Two control dogs were homozygous for the risk haplotype, but had no evidence of disease. This is likely to be due to the fact that CH is a complex trait with an additional environmental insults leading to disease development. The most likely reason for the lack of homozygosity for the protective haplotype among the control dogs is the relatively limited number of animals studied. Even with a heterozygote frequency of 11.9% in the control population, one would only expect one homozygote by chance alone, with no

Table 2. Frequencies of three locus DLA class II haplotypes in 66 ESSs with CH and 84 healthy controls.

Number	DRB1	DQA1	DQB1	Cases		Controls		Odds ratio	95% CI	P-value
				Number n = 132	Frequency (%)	Number n = 168	Frequency (%)			
1	01501	00601	00301	26	19.7	42	25.0			
2	01201	00401	01303	24	18.2	43	25.6			
3	01501	00601	02002	23	17.4	24	14.3			
4	00601	005011	00701	**19**	**14.4**	**11**	**6.5**	**3.13**	**1.20–8.26**	
5	02001	00401	01303	14	10.6	11	6.5			
6	00101	00201	01303	11	8.3	11	6.5			
7	01201	00401	013017	6	4.5	0	0.0			
8	00501	00301	00501	**4**	**3.0**	**20**	**11.9**	**0.26**	**0.08–0.80**	
9	01502	00601	02301	2	1.5	0	0.0			
10	00901	00101	008011	1	0.8	3	1.8			
11	01501	00601	02301	1	0.8	2	1.2			
	Other single haplotypes			1	0.8	1	0.6			
Clump test 1: cases v controls (chi squared emulation, all haplotypes										0.0017
Clump test 2 cases v controls (chi squared emulation, after grouping haplotypes with small values together)										0.0055

A total of 11 different haplotypes with frequencies >1% were identified. DLA-DRB1*00601/DQA1*005011/DQB1*00701 (haplotype four) had an increased frequency in cases and DLA-DRB1*00501/DQA1*00301/DQB1*00501 (haplotype eight) was significantly more frequent in controls, both numbers shown in bold. A p value for significance was set at 0.05 for comparison of haplotype frequencies.

homozygotes being the second most likely outcome. However, it is also possible that there are also detrimental health implications for homozygotes, therefore removing them from the population.

MHC class II antigens mainly determine which antigenic peptides an individual is able to present to $CD4^+$ T-lymphocytes in order to stimulate an immune response [41]. Expression of MHC class II is normally restricted to professional antigen-presenting cells, but it can be induced in other cell types by autoimmune, infectious or neoplastic diseases [42]. For example, epithelium-like cells can be induced to express MHC class II molecules upon exposure to inflammatory cytokines [43,44], or viral antigens [45,46]. Human hepatocytes frequently exhibit aberrant MHC class II expression in viral hepatitis [47,48], and it has also been shown that canine hepatocytes can express MHC class II during inflammation [49]. The induction of MHC class II molecules on such cells during viral infection likely plays an important role in the protective immune response of host against the virus by lysis of infected cells. Alternatively, this may lead to the development of infection-associated immunopathology by lysis of both infected and neighbouring cells that passively acquire released viral antigen.

Polymorphisms of the human immune regulatory genes, or HLA class I and II molecules, are important in influencing the host's ability to present or react to viral antigens [50]. In the case of human viral hepatitis, certain HLA haplotypes are strongly associated with the progression of liver injury following infection with HCV, whereas other are associated with HCV clearance or a lower risk of developing liver injury [29,30,51,52,53]. There are associations between certain HLA class II alleles and clearance of HBV and also an increase in viral persistence and the development of chronic liver disease [31,32,54]. CH in the ESS is of suspected viral aetiology as it shares histological features to those of chronic viral hepatitis in humans including predominantly lymphocytic inflammation and necrosis and apoptosis in areas of inflammation [11,13,14]. The canine MHC also plays a central role in the control of the immune response to infectious agents.

Selective inbreeding has, however, led to a restriction of DLA haplotypes in most breeds, which in turn will influence the susceptibility to infectious diseases. We hypothesise that the highly polymorphic DLA genes are involved in increased or decreased susceptibility to CH in the ESS, although genetic and other environmental factors are also likely involved in disease development. Akin to humans with natural HCV infection where some individuals are not infected despite high levels of exposure [55], others clear virus following infection, and other have progressive disease resulting in CH [56], a similar outcome may occur in the ESS exposed to a putative virus. Studies utilizing modern molecular techniques to identify the novel viral agent causing CH in the ESS are ongoing [57].

The only other study to investigate the possible association between DLA class II genes and canine hepatitis was performed in the Dobermann Pinscher [36]. This study identified DLA-DRB1*00601 as a risk allele for the disease, with all affected, and 56.8% of control animals homozygous for this allele. This allele was found in combination with DLA-DQA1*00401/ DQB1*01303, and 94.6% of affected Dobermann Pinschers were homozygous for this risk haplotype. In the present study, this haplotype was not found in any affected or control ESS. However, the allele DLA-DRB1*00601 was present in 14.4% cases and 6.5% controls, always in combination with DQA1*005011/ DQB1*00701 (haplotype four). Although the aetiology of hepatitis in the Dobermann Pincher is not known, an autoimmune aetiology is postulated. A T-cell mediated response is activated in genetically predisposed individuals and affected hepatocytes express MHC class II antigens [49]. Aberrant MHC class II expression is seen in human autoimmune liver disease, although this also occurs in virally infected hepatocytes [58]. In Dobermann Pincher hepatitis, MHC class II expression has been shown to be persistent and increased on the hepatocyte membrane during disease progression [49]. Although no studies have been performed to determine if CH in the ESS has an autoimmune aetiology, features such as an abundance of plasma cells and multi nucleated giant cells, common in human autoimmune parenchymal liver disease [13], are not apparent [11]. In addition, ESS with CH exhibit a poor response to corticosteroids [59] and do not have elevated serum globulins [11], a hallmark of human autoimmune hepatitis [60].

In conclusion, we have identified two alleles and one haplotype that appear to protect against the development of CH in the ESS, and two alleles and one haplotype that appears to confer risk of disease development. However, it is likely that the disease has a complex pathogenesis, whereby multiple genetic and environmental components interact to trigger and drive continued disease progression. The fact that relatively few major human genes have been identified in several genome-wide linkage scans for bacterial, parasitic and viral infectious diseases, supports the view that the genetic susceptibility is widely distributed among numerous polygenes [61]. Further identification of additional genetic risk factors for CH in the ESS is currently being performed by genome-wide association analysis using canine high density SNP arrays [62]. The results of the present study are, however, novel and likely to be of comparative value in understanding the aetiology of CH in other breeds of dog. Moreover, our findings could be used to assist breeding practices by increasing the frequency of the protective haplotype in an effort to reduce the incidence of CH in ESSs.

Materials and Methods

Study population

Ethylenediaminetetraacetic acid (EDTA) anticoagulant blood samples from 66 ESSs with CH were collected between 2006 and 2011. Samples had been submitted for haematological analysis to the Central Diagnostic Services Laboratory, University of Cambridge from the Queen's Veterinary School Hospital and other external practices in the UK. The diagnosis of CH was based on consistent clinical signs, the presence of elevated liver enzymes and confirmed by histological examination of liver tissue using standardised criteria for diagnosis [63]. It was not possible to definitively investigate the relatedness in this population as pedigree information was not available for all dogs. Pedigree information was available for 45 dogs and all were unrelated at least to the grandparental level. Analysis of the date of birth of the remaining dogs confirmed that these animals were not siblings.

Control EDTA blood samples were obtained from residual blood samples collected from 84 ESS aged eight years or over between 2009 and 2011. Since CH occurs in young to middle aged ESSs [11], we chose older dogs to use as the control group. No dog had clinical signs of liver disease and all dogs had normal liver enzymes measured at the time of blood collection. Pedigree information was available for all control dogs and all were unrelated at least to the grandparental level. All blood was stored at $-20°C$ for subsequent analysis of DLA genes.

Ethics statement

All samples consisted of residual blood remaining after diagnostic testing and were collected in accordance with guidelines of the Royal College of Veterinary Surgeons, UK and the Veterinary Surgeons Act 1966. For this reason ethical committee approval was not required. All samples were collected with informed and written owner consent.

MHC genotyping for DLA-DRB1, DQA1 and DQB1

DNA was extracted from blood samples using the QIAamp DNA Blood Midi Kit (Qiagen, Crawley, UK) according to the manufacturer's instructions. DNA concentration was measured using a fluorescence-based method (Quant-iT PicoGreen dsDNA Assay, Life Technologies, Paisley, UK), and samples were normalised to 20 ng/µl. Dogs were characterised for three DLA class II loci using sequence based typing [64,65]. Polymerase chain reactions (PCR) amplification was performed with 25 ng genomic DNA in a 25 µl reaction containing 1× PCR buffer (Qiagen), Q solution (Qiagen), final concentration of 0.1 µM each primer, 200 µM each dNTP and 2.5units Taq polymerase (HotStar Taq, Qiagen). A negative control containing no DNA template was included in each run of amplification to identify possible contamination. The primers used for DLA-DRB1 were forward DRBIn1: CCG TCC CCA CAG CAC ATT TC and reverse DRBIn2-T7: TAA TAC GAC TCA CTA TAG GG TGT GTC ACA CAC CTC AGC ACC A. The primers used to amplify DLA-QA1 were forward DQAIn1: TAA GGT TCT TTT CTC CCT CT and reverse DQAIn2: GGA CAG ATT CAG TGA AGA GA. The primers used to amplify DLA-DQB1 were forward DQB1B-T7: TAA TAC GAC TCA CTA TAG GG CTC ACT GGC CCG GCT GTC TC and reverse DQBR2: CAC CTC GCC GCT GCA ACG TG. The T7 tails are underlined. All primers were intronic and locus specific, and the product sizes were DLA-DRB1 (303 bp), DQA1 (345 bp) and DQB1 (300 bp). A standard touchdown PCR protocol was employed for all amplifications which consisted of an initial 15 min at 95°C, 14 touchdown cycles of 95°C for 30 s, followed by 1 min annealing, starting at 62°C (DRB1), 54°C (DQA1), 73°C (DQB1) and reducing by 0.5°C each cycle, and 72°C for 1 min. Then, 20 cycles of 95°C for 30 s, 55°C (DRB1), 47°C (DQA1) and 66°C (DQB1) for 1 min, 72°C for 1 min and a final extension at 72°C for 10 min were performed.

To check for the presence of a product, 5 µl amplified PCR products were resolved by electrophoresis in a 2% agarose gel, stained with ethidium bromide and viewed under ultraviolet transillumination. Prior to sequencing, all samples were purified as follows: 2units of shrimp alkaline phosphatase (Amersham, Little Chalfont, UK), and 10units of Exo1 (New England Biolabs, Hitchin, UK) were added to 5 µl of PCR product. The mixture was incubated for 1 hour at 37°C, then for 15 min at 80°C. Cycle sequencing (using T7 for DLA-DRB1 and DQB1, and DQAIn2 for DLA-DQA1) was performed using Big Dye Terminator V3 (Life Technologies), and samples were sequenced on an Applied Biosystems 373 Genetic Analyzer. Sequencing data was analysed using SBTengine (GenDX, Netherlands).

Haplotype assignment and statistical methods

Three-locus, DLA-DRB1/DQA1/DQB1, haplotypes were identified by following a sequential analytical process. First, all dogs that were homozygous at all three loci were selected, and from these several different DLA-DRB1/DQA1/DQB1 haplotype combinations were identified. Dogs that were homozygous at only two loci were then selected. From these dogs, many of the previous haplotypes were confirmed and also several additional haplotypes were identified. The remaining dogs were examined using the haplotype data already identified, and haplotypes were assigned to each of these dogs. From these dogs further possible haplotypes were identified. Allele and haplotype frequencies in cases and controls were compared using the program Clump v22 [66], to perform chi squared emulation for 2×n contingency tables (where n is the number of alleles at each locus or the number of haplotypes being scored), using 100,000 trials at each locus or for the haplotype data. The p value used for significance was set at 0.017 for comparison of allele frequencies as there were a total of three tests per locus. A p value for significance was set at 0.05 for comparison of haplotype frequencies. Where differences were detected, OR and 95% CIs were calculated for disease association of individual alleles or haplotypes.

Acknowledgments

We are grateful to owners of ESS who gave permission for their dogs to participate in this study. We would also like to thank the English Springer Spaniel Breed Society, especially the health coordinators Louise Scott and Lesley Bloomfield for their continued support and assistance in recruiting cases. We thank the UK DNA Archive for Companion Animals for extracting DNA from some of the samples. The authors are grateful to Professor Jim Kaufman for his constructive comments on the manuscript. NHB is grateful to the Wellcome Trust for sponsorship his Fellowship.

Author Contributions

Conceived and designed the experiments: NHB PJW JA DRS LJK. Performed the experiments: NHB LJK. Analyzed the data: NHB LJK. Contributed reagents/materials/analysis tools: NHB JA LT JLH LJK. Wrote the paper: NB LJK. Sample collection: NHB PJW.

References

1. Watson PJ, Roulois AJ, Scase TJ, Irvine R, Herrtage ME (2010) Prevalence of hepatic lesions at post-mortem examination in dogs and association with pancreatitis. J Small Anim Prac 51: 566–572.
2. Poldervaart JH, Favier RP, Penning LC, van den Ingh TS, Rothuizen J (2009) Primary hepatitis in dogs: a retrospective review (2002–2006). J Vet Intern Med 23: 72–80.
3. Gocke DJ, Preisig R, Morris TQ, McKay DG, Bradley SE (1967) Experimental viral hepatitis in the dog: production of persistent disease in partially immune animals. J Clin Invest 46: 1506–1517.
4. Bishop L, Strandberg JD, Adams RJ, Brownstein DG, Patterson R (1979) Chronic active hepatitis in dogs associated with leptospires. Am J Vet Res 40: 839–844.
5. Boomkens SY, Slump E, Egberink HF, Rothuizen J, Penning LC (2005) PCR screening for candidate etiological agents of canine hepatitis. Vet Microbiol 108: 49–55.
6. Bunch SE (1993) Hepatotoxicity associated with pharmacologic agents in dogs and cats. Vet Clin North Am Small Anim Pract 23: 659–670.
7. Watson PJ (2004) Chronic hepatitis in dogs: a review of current understanding of the aetiology, progression, and treatment. Vet J 167: 228–241.
8. Sevelius E, Andersson M, Jonsson L (1994) Hepatic accumulation of alpha-1-antitrypsin in chronic liver disease in the dog. J Comp Pathol 111: 401–412.
9. Andersson M, Sevelius E (1992) Circulating autoantibodies in dogs with chronic liver disease. J Small Anim Pract 33: 389–394.
10. Weiss DJ, Armstrong PJ, Mruthyunjaya A (1995) Anti-liver membrane protein antibodies in dogs with chronic hepatitis. J Vet Intern Med 9: 267–271.
11. Bexfield NH, Andres-Abdo C, Scase TJ, Constantino-Casas F, Watson PJ (2011) Chronic hepatitis in the English springer spaniel: clinical presentation, histological description and outcome. Vet Rec 169: 415. doi:410.1136/vr.d4665.
12. Strombeck DR, Miller LM, Harrold D (1988) Effects of corticosteroid treatment on survival time in dogs with chronic hepatitis: 151 cases (1977–1985). J Am Vet Med Assoc 193: 1109–1113.
13. Ishak KG (2000) Pathologic features of chronic hepatitis. A review and update. Am J Clin Pathol 113: 40–55.
14. Bateman AC (2007) Patterns of histological change in liver disease: my approach to 'medical' liver biopsy reporting. Histopathology 51: 585–596.
15. Kennedy LJ, Altet L, Angles JM, Barnes A, Carter SD, et al. (1999) Nomenclature for factors of the dog major histocompatibility system (DLA), 1998. First report of the ISAG DLA Nomenclature Committee. International Society for Animals Genetics. Tissue Antigens 54: 312–321.
16. Kennedy LJ, Altet L, Angles JM, Barnes A, Carter SD, et al. (2000) Nomenclature for factors of the dog major histocompatibility system (DLA), 1998: first report of the ISAG DLA Nomenclature Committee. Anim Genet 31: 52–61.
17. Kennedy LJ (2007) 14th International HLA and Immunogenetics Workshop: report on joint study on canine DLA diversity. Tissue Antigens 69 Suppl 1: 269–271.
18. Kennedy LJ, Barnes A, Short A, Brown JJ, Lester S, et al. (2007) Canine DLA diversity: 1. New alleles and haplotypes. Tissue Antigens 69 Suppl 1: 272–288.
19. Kennedy LJ, Barnes A, Happ GM, Quinnell RJ, Bennett D, et al. (2002) Extensive interbreed, but minimal intrabreed, variation of DLA class II alleles and haplotypes in dogs. Tissue Antigens 59: 194–204.
20. Wilbe M, Jokinen P, Hermanrud C, Kennedy LJ, Strandberg E, et al. (2009) MHC class II polymorphism is associated with a canine SLE-related disease complex. Immunogenetics 61: 557–564.
21. Wilbe M, Ziener ML, Aronsson A, Harlos C, Sundberg K, et al. (2010) DLA class II alleles are associated with risk for canine symmetrical lupoid onychodystrophy (SLO). PLoS One 5: e12332.
22. Kennedy LJ, Davison LJ, Barnes A, Short AD, Fretwell N, et al. (2006) Identification of susceptibility and protective major histocompatibility complex haplotypes in canine diabetes mellitus. Tissue Antigens 68: 467–476.
23. Donaldson PT, Doherty DG, Hayllar KM, McFarlane IG, Johnson PJ, et al. (1991) Susceptibility to autoimmune chronic active hepatitis: human leukocyte antigens DR4 and A1-B8-DR3 are independent risk factors. Hepatology 13: 701–706.
24. Fujisawa T, Ikegami H, Kawaguchi Y, Yamato E, Takekawa K, et al. (1995) Class I HLA is associated with age-at-onset of IDDM, while class II HLA confers susceptibility to IDDM. Diabetologia 38: 1493–1495.
25. Burgner D, Jamieson SE, Blackwell JM (2006) Genetic susceptibility to infectious diseases: big is beautiful, but will bigger be even better? Lancet Infect Dis 6: 653–663.
26. Fellay J, Ge D, Shianna KV, Colombo S, Ledergerber B, et al. (2009) Common genetic variation and the control of HIV-1 in humans. PLoS Genet 5: e1000791.
27. Pereyra F, Jia X, McLaren PJ, Telenti A, de Bakker PI, et al. (2010) The major genetic determinants of HIV-1 control affect HLA class I peptide presentation. Science 330: 1551–1557.
28. Steel CM, Ludlam CA, Beatson D, Peutherer JF, Cuthbert RJ, et al. (1988) HLA haplotype A1 B8 DR3 as a risk factor for HIV-related disease. Lancet 1: 1185–1188.
29. Kuniholm MH, Kovacs A, Gao X, Xue X, Marti D, et al. (2010) Specific human leukocyte antigen class I and II alleles associated with hepatitis C virus viremia. Hepatology 51: 1514–1522.
30. Knapp S, Warshow U, Hegazy D, Brackenbury L, Guha IN, et al. (2010) Consistent beneficial effects of killer cell immunoglobulin-like receptor 2DL3 and group 1 human leukocyte antigen-C following exposure to hepatitis C virus. Hepatology 51: 1168–1175.
31. Thursz MR, Kwiatkowski D, Allsopp CE, Greenwood BM, Thomas HC, et al. (1995) Association between an MHC class II allele and clearance of hepatitis B virus in the Gambia. N Engl J Med 332: 1065–1069.
32. Thio CL, Thomas DL, Karacki P, Gao X, Marti D, et al. (2003) Comprehensive analysis of class I and class II HLA antigens and chronic hepatitis B virus infection. J Virol 77: 12083–12087.
33. It V, Barrientos L, Lopez Gappa J, Posik D, Diaz S, et al. (2010) Association of canine juvenile generalized demodicosis with the dog leukocyte antigen system. Tissue Antigens 76: 67–70.
34. Aguirre-Hernandez J, Polton G, Kennedy LJ, Sargan DR (2010) Association between anal sac gland carcinoma and dog leukocyte antigen-DQB1 in the English Cocker Spaniel. Tissue Antigens 76: 476–481.
35. Clements DN, Short AD, Barnes A, Kennedy LJ, Ferguson JF, et al. (2010) A candidate gene study of canine joint diseases. J Hered 101: 54–60.
36. Dyggve H, Kennedy LJ, Meri S, Spillmann T, Lohi H, et al. (2011) Association of Doberman hepatitis to canine major histocompatibility complex II. Tissue Antigens 77: 30–35.
37. Bexfield NH, Buxton RJ, Vicek TJ, Day MJ, Bailey SM, et al. (2012) Breed, age and gender distribution of dogs with chronic hepatitis in the United Kingdom. Vet J 10.1016/j.tvjl.2011.1011.1024.
38. Venkataraman GM, Stroup P, Graves SS, Storb R (2007) An improved method for dog leukocyte antigen 88 typing and two new major histocompatibility complex class I alleles, DLA-88*01101 and DLA-88*01201. Tissue Antigens 70: 53–57.
39. Kennedy LJ, Barnes A, Short A, Brown JJ, Seddon J, et al. (2007) Canine DLA diversity: 3. Disease studies. Tissue Antigens 69 Suppl 1: 292–296.
40. Kennedy LJ, Barnes A, Ollier WE, Day MJ (2006) Association of a common dog leucocyte antigen class II haplotype with canine primary immune-mediated haemolytic anaemia. Tissue Antigens 68: 502–508.
41. Brown JH, Jardetzky T, Saper MA, Samraoui B, Bjorkman PJ, et al. (1988) A hypothetical model of the foreign antigen binding site of class II histocompatibility molecules. Nature 332: 845–850.
42. Guardiola J, Maffei A (1993) Control of MHC class II gene expression in autoimmune, infectious, and neoplastic diseases. Crit Rev Immunol 13: 247–268.
43. Ting JP, Trowsdale J (2002) Genetic control of MHC class II expression. Cell 109 Suppl: S21–33.
44. Benoist C, Mathis D (1990) Regulation of major histocompatibility complex class-II genes: X, Y and other letters of the alphabet. Annu Rev Immunol 8: 681–715.
45. Gao J, De BP, Banerjee AK (1999) Human parainfluenza virus type 3 up-regulates major histocompatibility complex class I and II expression on respiratory epithelial cells: involvement of a STAT1- and CIITA-independent pathway. J Virol 73: 1411–1418.
46. Hanke T, Randall RE (1994) Processing of Viral-Proteins for Presentation by Molecules of the Major Histocompatibility Complex. Rev Med Virol 4: 47–61.
47. Dienes HP, Hutteroth T, Hess G, Meuer SC (1987) Immunoelectron microscopic observations on the inflammatory infiltrates and HLA antigens in hepatitis B and non-A, non-B. Hepatology 7: 1317–1325.

48. Franco A, Barnaba V, Natali P, Balsano C, Musca A, et al. (1988) Expression of class I and class II major histocompatibility complex antigens on human hepatocytes. Hepatology 8: 449–454.

49. Speeti M, Stahls A, Meri S, Westermarck E (2003) Upregulation of major histocompatibility complex class II antigens in hepatocytes in Doberman hepatitis. Vet Immunol Immunopathol 96: 1–12.

50. Germain RN (1994) MHC-dependent antigen processing and peptide presentation: providing ligands for T lymphocyte activation. Cell 76: 287–299.

51. Donaldson PT (2004) Genetics of liver disease: immunogenetics and disease pathogenesis. Gut 53: 599–608.

52. Kuzushita N, Hayashi N, Moribe T, Katayama K, Kanto T, et al. (1998) Influence of HLA haplotypes on the clinical courses of individuals infected with hepatitis C virus. Hepatology 27: 240–244.

53. Zavaglia C, Martinetti M, Silini E, Bottelli R, Daielli C, et al. (1998) Association between HLA class II alleles and protection from or susceptibility to chronic hepatitis C. J Hepatol 28: 1–7.

54. Almarri A, Batchelor JR (1994) HLA and hepatitis B infection. Lancet 344: 1194–1195.

55. Thurairajah PH, Hegazy D, Chokshi S, Shaw S, Demaine A, et al. (2008) Hepatitis C virus (HCV)-specific T cell responses in injection drug users with apparent resistance to HCV infection. J Infect Dis 198: 1749–1755.

56. Alter MJ, Margolis HS, Krawczynski K, Judson FN, Mares A, et al. (1992) The natural history of community-acquired hepatitis C in the United States. The Sentinel Counties Chronic non-A, non-B Hepatitis Study Team. N Engl J Med 327: 1899–1905.

57. Bexfield N, Kellam P (2011) Metagenomics and the molecular identification of novel viruses. Vet J 190: 191–198.

58. Herkel J, Jagemann B, Wiegard C, Lazaro JF, Lueth S, et al. (2003) MHC class II-expressing hepatocytes function as antigen-presenting cells and activate specific CD4 T lymphocyutes. Hepatology 37: 1079–1085.

59. Shawcroft A, Watson PJ, Bexfield NH, Collings AJ (2010) Effect of prednisolone treatment on survival of dogs with chronic hepatitis. Proceedings of the British Small Animal Veterinary Association Congress: 458.

60. Mieli-Vergani G, Vergani D (2011) Autoimmune hepatitis. Nat Rev Gastro-enterol Hepatol 8: 320–329.

61. Frodsham AJ, Hill AV (2004) Genetics of infectious diseases. Hum Mol Genet 13 Spec No 2: R187–194.

62. Karlsson EK, Baranowska I, Wade CM, Salmon Hillbertz NH, Zody MC, et al. (2007) Efficient mapping of mendelian traits in dogs through genome-wide association. Nat Genet 39: 1321–1328.

63. Van den Ingh TSGAM, Van Winkle TJ, Cullen JM, Charles JA, Desmet VJ (2006) Morphological classification of parenchymal disorders of the canine and feline liver: 2 Hepatocellular death, hepatitis and cirrhosis. In: Rothuizen J, Bunch SE, Charles JA, Cullen JM, Desmet VJ et al., editors. WSAVA Standards for clinical and histological diagnosis of canine and feline liver disease. 1 ed. Philadelphia, PA: Saunders Elsevier. pp. 85–102.

64. Kennedy LJ, Carter SD, Barnes A, Bell S, Bennett D, et al. (1998) Nine new dog DLA-DRB1 alleles identified by sequence-based typing. Immunogenetics 48: 296–301.

65. Kennedy LJ, Barnes A, Happ GM, Quinnell RJ, Courtenay O, et al. (2002) Evidence for extensive DLA polymorphism in different dog populations. Tissue Antigens 60: 43–52.

66. Sham PC, Curtis D (1995) Monte Carlo tests for associations between disease and alleles at highly polymorphic loci. Ann Hum Genet 59: 97–105.

11

Mites Parasitic on Australasian and African Spiders Found in the Pet Trade; a Redescription of *Ljunghia pulleinei* Womersley

Peter Masan[1,2]*, Christopher Simpson[1], M. Alejandra Perotti[3], Henk R. Braig[1]

1 School of Biological Sciences, Bangor University, Bangor, Wales, United Kingdom, **2** Institute of Zoology, Slovak Academy of Sciences, Bratislava, Slovakia, **3** School of Biological Sciences, University of Reading, Reading, United Kingdom

Abstract

Parasitic mites associated with spiders are spreading world-wide through the trade in tarantulas and other pet species. *Ljunghia pulleinei* Womersley, a mesostigmatic laelapid mite originally found in association with the mygalomorph spider *Selenocosmia stirlingi* Hogg (Theraphosidae) in Australia, is redescribed and illustrated on the basis of specimens from the African theraphosid spider *Pterinochilus chordatus* (Gerstäcker) kept in captivity in the British Isles (Wales). The mite is known from older original descriptions of Womersley in 1956; the subsequent redescription of Domrow in 1975 seems to be questionable in conspecificity of treated specimens with the type material. Some inconsistencies in both descriptions are recognised here as intraspecific variability of the studied specimens. The genus *Arachnyssus* Ma, with species *A. guangxiensis* (type) and *A. huwenae*, is not considered to be a valid genus, and is included in synonymy with *Ljunghia* Oudemans. A new key to world species of the genus *Ljunghia* is provided.

Editor: Dirk Steinke, Biodiversity Insitute of Ontario – University of Guelph, Canada

Funding: These authors have no support or funding to report.

Competing Interests: The authors have declared that no competing interests exist.

* E-mail: peter.masan@savba.sk

Introduction

Close inspection of spiders often reveals mites associated with various body parts. Although these associations are most frequently reported from tropical spider families, mites are not uncommon on temperate spider species. Deutonymphs of Astigmata mites and Heterostigmata mites can be found phoretic on spiders; larvae of the Prostigmata families Erythraedae, Trombiculidae and Trombidiidae (chigger mites) can be parasitic on spiders, while Mesostigmata mites in the family Laelapidae often occur both as immature stages and adults on spiders [1–3]. Mites on spiders go back in time at least 50 Ma. Baltic amber shows phoretic and parasitic Acari together with jumping and cell spiders [4], [5]. In addition, free-living mites (Asigmata and Mesostigmata) can become a problem for captive tarantulas when high numbers start to occlude the moist surfaces of the book lungs [6]. The large number of saprophilous and predatory Mesostigmata might overshadow the host-specific associations particularly between spider and mites of the mesostigmatic family Laelapidae. However, specific associations are well documented. For example, all life stages of *Androlaelaps pilosus* Baker (Laelapidae) can be found on the hexathelid spider *Macrothele calpeiana* (Walckenaer), the only European tarantula [7]. Here we report laelapid mites living on captive *Pterinochilus chordatus* Gerstäcker, the Kilimanjaro mustard baboon spider.

The laelapid genus *Ljunghia* includes species that have established close associations with various mygalomorph spiders in Indonesia [8,9], Malaysia [10], Australia [11–13], New Caledonia [14], Africa [15], and China [16]. It is assumed that they have developed obligatory parasitic relationships with their hosts [1]. To date, there is only one comprehensive review of *Ljunghia*, which includes a description of a new species from a Central American mygalomorph spider kept in captivity in Spain, a key for their identification and an enumeration of their host species [17].

Although there is no published record of an *Ljunghia* species from the British Isles, reports of mites parasitizing captive spiders is a common occurrence, often owing to contamination [17]. The presence of a seemingly Australian mite species on an African spider on the territory of the UK is interesting and might be either a consequence of the brisk business of tarantulas as pets including the wide-spread exchange of spiders among the breeders or an indication for a wider geographical distribution of *Ljunghia*.

The main aim of this study was a morphological redescription of *Ljunghia pulleinei*. Detailed observations of the most important morphological features of this mite allowed to discern more details than those reported in the original descriptions [11]. Generally, the original description of Womersley does not include illustrations of diagnostic morphologies as well as important metric data of some idiosomal structures and setae. There is one redescription of this species, that of Domrow [12], based on specimens that differ in some characters, e.g. distinctly shorter idiosomal setae when compared with the type specimens. Inconsistencies in the descriptions of Womersley and Domrow are another good reason for the following redescription.

Results and Discussion

Genus *Ljunghia* Oudemans

Ljunghia Oudemans, 1932: 204 [8]. Type species *Ljunghia selenocosmiae* Oudemans, 1932; by monotypy [8].

Ljunghia (Metaljunghia) Fain, 1989: 158 [9]. Type species *Ljunghia rainbowi* Domrow, 1975; by original designation [12].

Arachnyssus Ma, 2002: 8 [16]. Type species *Ljunghia guangxiensis* Ma, 2002; by original designation [16]. New synonymy.

Diagnosis (Adults). Chelicerae chelate-dentate in female, with fixed digit usually reduced in size; cheliceral digits of male subequal in length, with curved spermatodactyl slightly exceeding the tip of the movable digit. Dorsal shield entire, not covering the whole dorsal surface, and with hypotrichous setation (at most, 32 pairs of setae present). Sternal shield with three pairs of setae, metasternal shields and setae often absent. A pair of genital setae present or absent, usually placed on epignal shield. Anal shield relatively small, elongate, bearing three circum-anal setae. Leg setation holotrichous to markedly hypotrichous.

Notes on the genus. The genus *Ljunghia* was proposed by Oudemans [8], based on adults and deutonymphs collected from the theraphosid spider of the genus *Selenocosmia* Ausserer in Sumatra. Oudeman's genus *Ljunghia* has gained broad acceptance [9], [12], [15], [17], [20], mostly as a member of the subfamily Iphiopsinae within the family Laelapidae, and is currently divided into two subgenera, *Ljunghia* and *Metaljunghia*. We agree with Moraza *et al.* that this subgeneric structure is not useful, and it is not used here [17].

A new separate genus *Arachnyssus* was erected [16] to accommodate two mesostigmatic mite species associated with the mygalomorph theraphosid spider *Selenocosmia huwena* Wang, Peng & Xie (= *Haplopelma schmidti* von Wirth, based on the newest taxonomic revision [21]) in China. The most important features that define the genus *Arachnyssus*, classified within the family Macronyssidae, are: (1) entire dorsal shield; (2) idiosomal setae very long, with tips reaching far beyond the insertions of following setae; (3) anus with anterior position to adanal setae; (4) coxae I–IV not armed with spines; (5) sternal shield saddle-shaped, with posterior margin deeply concave; (6) epigynial shield short, tongue-shaped; (7) anal shield drop-shaped; (8) epigynial and anal shields well separated [16].

It is obvious that the author who erected *Arachnyssus* neglected the existence of the genus *Ljunghia* because there is no reference to this genus in his paper [16] and all of the above characters enumerated for *Arachnyssus* can be found in *Ljunghia* [17]. Therefore *Arachnyssus* is here regarded as synonymous with *Ljunghia*, and the two species, namely *A. guangxiensis* and *A. huwenae* are therefore, newly transferred to the genus *Ljunghia*.

Ljunghia pulleinei Womersley

Ljunghia pulleini Womersley, 1956: 591–593 [11].

Ljunghia pulleini – Domrow, 1975: 35–37 (in part: only specimens of the type series) [12].

Ljunghia pulleinei (emend. nov.) s. str. – Fain, 1991: 78–79 [13].

Ljunghia (Metaljunghia) pulleini – Fain, 1989: 159 [9]; Moraza *et al.*, 2009: 125 (in part) [17].

Material examined. 4 females, 2 males – on *Pterinochilus chordatus* (det. R. C. Gallon) kept in captivity in the Laboratory of Molecular Parasitology, School of Biological Sciences, Bangor University, Gwynedd, NW Wales. The mites were collected by one of the authors, MAP, following the technique described aboved; October 2006.

Description (Adults). Female. Dorsal idiosoma (Figure 1A). Idiosoma oblong, egg-shaped, 810–860 μm long and 610–635 μm wide (650 μm long and 443 μm wide in freshly moulted and poorly sclerotized specimen). Dorsal shield entire, oblong, suboval, 560–595 μm long and 320–355 μm wide nearly at level of setae z5, usually not completely covering dorsal surface, with regularly rounded posterior margin and smooth surface. The shield free of anterior sections of peritremes, anterior ends of peritremes reaching close to paravertical setae z1. Podonotal region of the shield with 15 pairs of setae (j1–j6, z1, z2, z4–z6, s1–s4), opisthonotum with reduced complement of three setal pairs (J4, Z4 and Z5). Most dorsal shield setae simple, smooth, needle-like, sinuous and considerably elongated, the longest setae up to 270 μm in length and with thread-like distal part reaching far beyond the insertions of following setae; only setae j1, z1 and J4 short. Metric data for some selected dorsal setae as follows: j1 33–44 μm, j4 220–230 μm, j5 136–153 μm, j6 230–260 μm, J4 25–31 μm, z5 170–190 μm, Z4 142–152 μm, Z5 152–162 μm, the longest setae situated on soft membranous dorsal integument 220–255 μm. Dorsolateral membranous integument with 13 pairs of setae.

Ventral idiosoma (Figure 1B). Presternal platelets absent. Sternal shield almost quadrangular, longitudinally narrowed, 30–40 μm long in midline, 120–132 μm wide at level of setae st2 and 149–158 μm at level of setae st3, smooth on surface, deeply concave posteriorly; anterolateral corners well developed, slender and obtusely acuminate; the shield bearing two pairs of lyrifissures and three pairs of setae, length of sternal shield setae slightly increasing posteriorly: st1 100–115 μm, st2 105–122 μm, st3 150–170 μm. Metasternal platelets and setae st4 absent, a pair of metasternal lyrifissures placed on soft membrane close to posterolateral corners of sternal shield. Endopodal sclerites absent. Epigynal shield tongue-shaped, elongated, slightly constricted between coxae IV, hyaline anteriorly, rounded posteriorly, 238–252 μm long, 75–83 μm wide at level of genital setae, with a pair of genital setae st5 (166–184 μm) inserted in posterior part and a pattern of weak longitudinal lines on medial surface; associate genital pores not detected. Peritrematal shields almost fully reduced, only short and narrow poststigmatic section present; peritremes well developed, long and with stigma between coxae III and IV. Exopodal sclerites absent, parapodal sclerites developed, crescent. A pair of small and suboval metapodal platelets present. Anal shield pear-shaped, rounded anteriorly and posteriorly, 74–82 μm wide, smooth, bearing rounded anus and three circum-anal setae; postanal seta (64–77 μm) shorter than adanals (80–90 μm); anus with posterior position on the shield. Ventral and ventrolateral membranous integument with 10 pairs of setae. All ventral setae similar to those on dorsal idiosoma.

Gnathosomal structures (Figures 2B, 2C, 2E). Anterior ventral part of hypostome as in Figure 2B, with three pairs of simple hypostomal setae h1–h3; posterior setae h3 longest; posterior surface bearing a pair of simple postcoxal setae. Deutosternal groove relatively narrow and difficult to examine posteriorly, with only three detectable transverse rows of denticles on its anterior section. Corniculi obscure and covered by hypertrophied, lobe-like projection. Chelicerae chelate-dentate (Figure 2C); fixed digit reduced in size, markedly shorter and thiner than movable digit, and armed with distal hook; movable digit relatively robust, with distal hook and two massive subdistal teeth. Epistome rounded and serrate on anterior margin (Figure 2D).

Legs. All legs with a well developed pretarsus and ambulacral apparatus (including pulvillus and two claws), shorter than idiosoma. Leg segments without specific projections or macrosetae, with the chaetotactic pattern as previously described. Coxae IV associated with relatively thin and long tubular structures of insemination apparatus (Figure 2F).

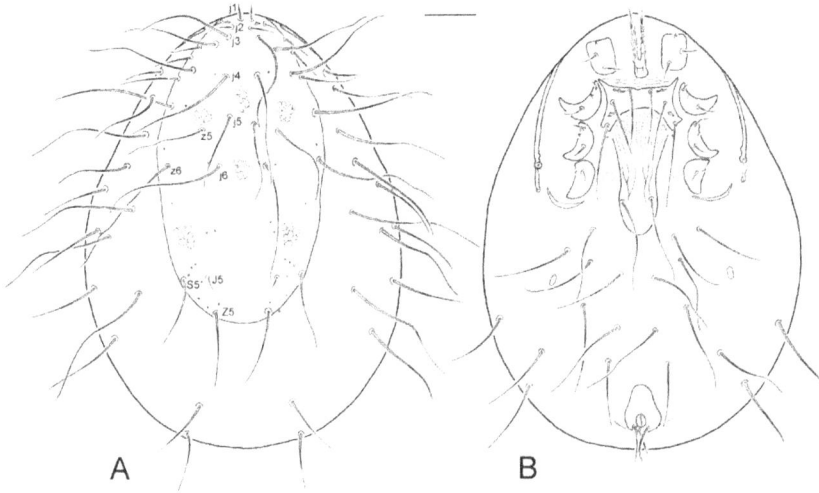

Figure 1. *Ljunghia pulleinei,* **female.** A, dorsal idiosoma (with setal notation of some dorsal setae); B, ventral idiosoma. Scale: 100 μm.

Male (Figures 2A, 2D). Idiosoma 540–590 μm long and 360–395 μm wide, dorsal shield 490–515 μm long and 285–325 μm wide. Dorsum with a compact holodorsal shield. Metric data for some selected dorsal setae as follows: j1 23–29 μm, j3 177 μm, j4 200 μm, j5 110–115 μm, J4 12–19 μm, z5 134–158 μm, z6 184–207 μm, Z4 120–126 μm, Z5 126–132 μm. Venter with separate sternogenital (Figure 2A), and anal shields. Sternogenital shield oblong, subtruncate anteriorly, rounded posteriorly, 250–270 μm long in midline, 130–138 μm wide at level of setae st3 and 94–99 μm at level of setae st5, smooth on surface; the shield bearing three pairs of lyrifissures and four pairs of setae (st1–st3, st5), length of sternogenital shield setae slightly increasing posteriorly: st1 75–81 μm, st2 99–105 μm, st3 122–141 μm, st5 150 μm.

Cheliceral digits subequal in length, without striking dentation; spermatodactyl hook-like, robust in basal part, curved distally (Figure 2D). Other characters almost identical as in female, including those on opisthogastric region.

Taxonomic notes. The original description of *Ljunghia pulleinei* was inadequately illustrated, the description itself was insufficient [11]; therefore, amendments followed in the redescription of Domrow [12], especially in the dorsal shield setation. For example, Womersley stated only 14 pairs of setae on the dorsal shield instead of 17–18 pairs documented by Domrow who examined three series of specimens: (1) the type material collected from theraphosid spider *Selenocosmia stirlingi* Hogg in South Australia; (2) specimens from a nemesiid spider of the genus

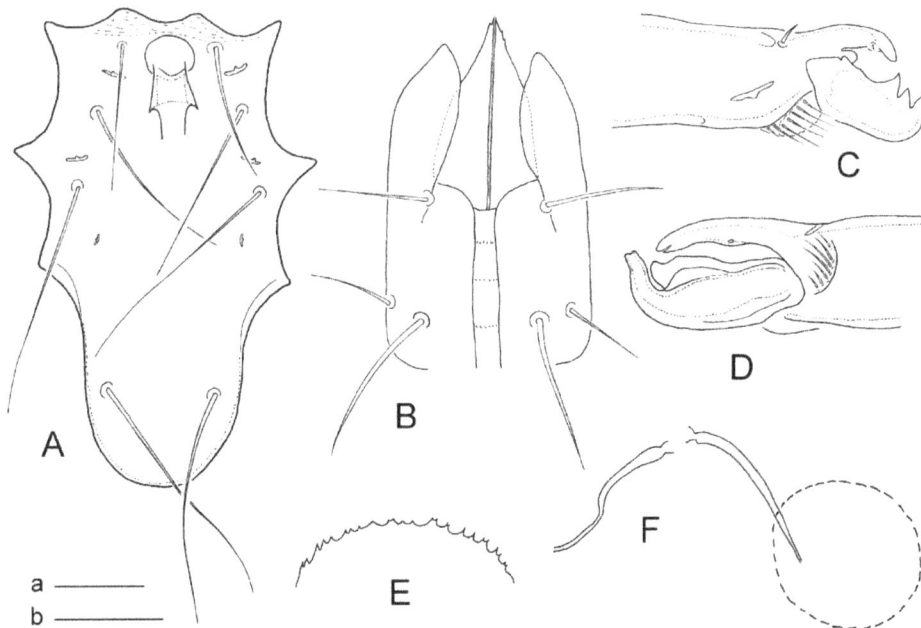

Figure 2. *Ljunghia pulleinei.* A, sternogenital shield of male; B, ventral hypostome of female (anterior part); C, cheliceral digits of female; D, cheliceral digits of male; E, epistome of female; F, tubular structures of insemination apparatus associated with coxae IV in female. Scales: a = 50 μm (Figs 2A, 2F), b = 25 μm (Figs 2B–E).

Aname L. Koch found in South Australia; (3) specimens from an unidentified diplurid spider in Queensland. All three series were keyed out together by Domrow and, despite the presence of some morphological differences, indicative of a mixture of three species, they were declared to be conspecific [12]. We now know that the specimens from the spiders of the genus *Aname*, which differ from the typical series mainly by the lack of the subterminal pair of setae on the dorsal shield, belong to the species *Ljunghia aname*, which was originally described as a new subspecies of *L. pulleinei* [13], [14]. A third unknown species is being described by Bruce Halliday (personal communication).

Unfortunately, the description and figures of adults given by Domrow [12] and of deutonymphs of *Ljunghia pulleinei* by Fain [14]) did not apply to the mites of the type series but to those of an unknown diplurid spider. The type specimens and specimens introduced by Domrow (and Fain) can be easily distinguished from each other by the length of setae situated on medial surface of the dorsal shield. They belong to two species, and show a certain degree of interspecific variability not only in the length of idiosomal setae but also in position of some dorsal shield setae (especially in J4 and Z4). So, two main patterns of chaetotaxy can be distinguished: (1) type species with longer idiosomal setae, e.g. setae j5 and z5 with tips reaching far beyond the insertions of j6, setae j6 beyond the insertions of J4, and setae z5 beyond the lateral margin of dorsal shield; (2) species illustrated by Domrow and Fain with shorter idiosomal setae, e.g. setae j5 and z5 with tips not reaching the insertions of j6, setae j6 hardly reaching to the insertions of J4, and setae z5 clearly not reaching the lateral margin of dorsal shield.

Ljunghia pulleinei bearing the longer setae cannot be reliably identified in the newest key of the genus [17]; where some statements are solely applicable to the form exhibiting short setae as described by Domrow [12]. In addition there is a mistake in their key in relation to both setal forms: "setae j4 do not reach the tips of j6". With exception of this inaccuracy and a pair of additional setae present on the opisthogastric ventral surface in our individuals, our description generally agrees with most of the published morphological characters given by Womersley and Domrow [11], [12]. In addition, we have included in our redescription new metric data for some idiosomal setae, and the shields.

Ljunghia pulleinei s. str. has here been collected from the Kilimanjaro mustard baboon spider from East Africa and previously from the common whistling spider from Australia. This is the first time that one and the same *Ljunghia* species has been associated with two different host species suggesting that *Ljunghia* species are not strictly species-specific. *Ljunghia* is well known from mygalomorph spiders but has also been reported from a more primitive liphistiid Malaysian trap door spider belonging to the Mesothelae [10]. Recently, new *Ljunghia* species have been retrieved from more liphistiid spiders from Vietnam and Thailand [22]. The female spiders showed clear bite marks of the mites on their prosomata emphasising the parasitic nature of *Ljunghia*.

Key to the species now known in *Ljunghia* Oudemans

1. Opisthonotal region of dorsal shield with strongly suppressed setation, only 2–5 pairs of setae present 2

   – Setation of opisthonotal region moderately suppressed, 7–14 pairs of setae present 7

2. Opisthonotal region with two pairs of setae, podonotal region with 14 pairs of setae . . . . *Ljunghia aname* Fain, 1991

– Opisthonotal region with at least three pairs of setae . . . 3

3. Genital setae (st5) absent; podonotal region with 20 pairs of setae, male sternogenital shield with three pairs of setae (st1–st3) . . . . *Ljunghia novaecaledoniae* Fain, 1991

   – Genital setae present; podonotal region with at most 18 pairs of setae, male sternogenital or sternogenito-ventral shield with at least four pairs of setae 4

4. Podonotal region of dorsal shield with strongly suppressed setation, only 11 pairs of setae present, opisthonotal region with 4–5 pairs of setae 5

   – Setation of podonotal region moderately suppressed, 17–18 pairs of setae present, opisthonotal region with 3 pairs of setae 6

5. Opisthonotal region with 5 pairs of setae, setae J4 absent . . . . *Ljunghia bristowi* (Finnegan, 1933)

   – Opisthonotal region with 4 pairs of setae, setae J4 present . . . . *Ljunghia rainbowi* Domrow, 1975

6. Podonotal region with 14 pairs of setae, setae j5 absent; setae j6 and z5 relatively short and subequal in length . . . . *Ljunghia africana* Fain, 1991

   – Podonotal region with 15 pairs of setae, setae j5 present; setae j6 relatively long, obviously longer than setae z5 . . . . *Ljunghia pulleinei* Womersley, 1956

7. Metasternal setae absent; opisthonotal region with 8 pairs of setae 8

   – Metasternal setae present; opisthonotal region with at least 11 pairs of setae 9

8. Podonotal region with 17 pairs of setae; setae J4 present, minute; sternal shield subrectangular; male with sternogenital shield . . . . *Ljunghia hoggi* Domrow, 1975

   – Podonotal region with 20 pairs of setae; setae J4 absent; sternal shield saddle-like, deeply concave posteriorly; male with holoventral shield . . . . *Ljunghia guangxiensis* (Ma, 2002) comb. nov.

9. Opisthonotal region with 14 pairs of setae; male with sternogenital shield bearing five pairs of setae (st1–st5) . . . . *Ljunghia minor* Fain, 1989

   – Opisthonotal region with 11 pairs of setae; male with sternogenital-ventral or holoventral shield bearing five pairs of setae together with a number of additional ventral setae 10

10. Setae J4 not modified, subequal with most of other dorsal setae; male with sternogenital-ventral shield, ventral part of the shield with 5–7 setae . . . . *Ljunghia selenocosmiae* Oudemans, 1932

    – Setae J4 reduced in length, conspicuously shorter than other dorsal setae; male with holoventral shield bearing at least 13 setae in ventral part 11

11. Podonotal region with 21 pairs of setae; setae J4 shorter, with tips not reaching the posterior margin of dorsal shield;

holoventral shield of male with 20–21 setae in ventral part
. . . .*Ljunghia luciae* Moraza, Iraola & Alemany, 2009

- – Podonotal region with 20 pairs of setae; setae J4 longer, with tips reaching beyond the posterior margin of dorsal shield; holoventral shield of male with about 13 setae in ventral part
. . . . *Ljunghia huwenae* (Ma, 2002) comb. nov.

Materials and Methods

All examined specimens of *Ljunghia pulleinei* were obtained from the mygalomorph spider *Pterinochilus chordatus* kept in captivity in Gwynedd, North Wales. *P. chordatus* is an East African theraphosid species distributed in Ethiopia, Kenya, Somalia, Sudan, Tanzania and Uganda [18].

The collection of mites was carried out on the living spider. Due to the aggressivity of the spider it was necessary to develop a technique to collect the mites attached to the dorsal parts of the cephalothorax and the abdomen. The spider was reared in a plastic container covered by a plastic lid. Small holes of 2 mm where made in the lid to allow breading but also to allow insertion of a wire to touch the mites. The tip of the wire was soaked in 100% glycerol (glycerin) and then directed inside the cage towards every single mite. Due to the sticky nature of glycerol, the mites were instantly glued to the tiny tip of the wire and extracted from the cage by slowly moving the tip out to avoid distressing the spider. Once outside the cage, the tip of the wire with a glued mite was submerged in 96% ethanol where the mites detached and became fixed and preserved for further analysis.

The mites were mounted on permanent microscope slides using Swan medium. Illustrations were made by using a high magnification microscope equipped with a drawing tube. Measurements were made from slide-mounted specimens with stage-calibrated ocular micrometers. Lengths of shields and leg segments were measured along their midlines, and widths were measured at the widest point. Dorsal setae were measured from the bases of their insertions to their tips. Measurements are mostly presented as ranges (minimum to maximum). The terminology of dorsal and ventral chaetotaxy follows Lindquist & Evans [19]. For the specific chaetotactic notation of some dorsal shield setae, see Figure 1A. The redescribed specimens are deposited at the Institute of Zoology, Slovak Academy of Sciences, Bratislava, and the Australian National Insect Collection, Canberra, Australia (2♀♀, 1♂).

Acknowledgments

We are very grateful to Bruce Halliday, of the CSIRO Ecosystem Sciences and Australian National Insect Collection, Canberra, for his review of some of our mite specimens and the very valuable discussions on *Ljunghia pulleinei* morphology.

Author Contributions

Conceived and designed the experiments: HRB MAP. Performed the experiments: MAP. Analyzed the data: PM. Contributed reagents/materials/analysis tools: HRB. Wrote the paper: PM MAP HRB. Collected and illustrated specimens examined: CS.

References

1. Welbourn W, Young OP (1988) Mites parasitic on spiders, with a description of a new species of *Eutrombidium* (Acari, Eutrombidiidae). J Arachnol 16: 373–385.
2. Baker A (1992) Acari (mites and ticks) associated with other arachnids. In: Cooper JE, Pearce-Kelly P, Williams DL, editors. Arachnida: Proceedings of a Symposium on Spiders and Their Allies. London: Chiron Press. pp. 126–131.
3. Ebermann E, Goloboff PA (2002) Association between neotropical burrowing spiders (Araneae: Nemesiidae) and mites (Acari: Heterostigmata, Scutacaridae). Acarologia 42: 173–184.
4. Wunderlich J (2004) Fossil jumping spiders (Araneae: Salticidae) in Baltic and Dominican amber, with remarks on Salticidae subfamilies. Beitr Araneol 3B: 1761–1819.
5. Dunlop JA, Wirth S, Penney D, McNeil A, Bradley RS, et al. (2012) A minute fossil phoretic mite recovered by phase-contrast X-ray computed tomography. Biol Lett 8: 457–460.
6. Pizzi R (2009) Parasites of tarantulas (Theraphosidae). J Exot Pet Med 18: 283–288.
7. Baker A (1991) A new species of the mite genus *Androlaelaps* Berlese (Parasitiformes: Laelapidae) found in association with the spider *Macrothele calpeiana* (Walckenaer) (Mygalomorphae: Hexathelidae). Bull Br Arachnol Soc 8: 219–223.
8. Oudemans AC (1932) Opus 550. Tijdschr Entomol 75: 202–210.
9. Fain A (1989) Notes on the genus *Ljunghia* Oudemans, 1932 (Acari, Mesostigmata) associated with mygalomorph spiders from the Oriental and Australian Regions. Bull Inst R Sci Nat Belg Entomol 59: 157–160.
10. Finnegan S (1933) A new species of mite parasitic of the spider *Liphistius malayanus*, from Malaya. Proc Zool Soc London 1993: 413–417.
11. Womersley H (1956) On some Acarina Mesostigmata from Australia, New Zeland and New Guinea. J Linn Soc Zool 42: 505–599.
12. Domrow R (1975) *Ljunghia* Oudemans (Acari: Dermanyssidae), a genus parasitic on mygalomorph spiders. Rec S Aust Mus 17: 31–39.
13. Fain A (1991) Notes on mites parasitic or phoretic on Australia centipedes, spiders and scorpions. Rec West Aust Mus 15: 69–82.
14. Fain A (1991) A new species of *Ljunghia* Oudemans, 1932 (Acari, Laelapidae) from a New-Caledonian spider. Bull Inst R Sci Nat Belg Entomol 61: 199–205.
15. Fain A (1991) Notes on some new parasitic mites (Acari, Mesostigmata) from Afrotropical region. Bull Inst R Sci Nat Belg Entomol 61: 183–191.
16. Ma LM (2002) A new genus and two new species of gamasid mites parasitic on spiders (Acari: Macronyssidae). Acta Arachnol Sinica 11: 8–13.
17. Moraza ML, Iraola V, Alemany C (2009) A new species of *Ljunghia* Oudemans, 1932 (Arachnida, Acari, Laelapidae) from a mygalomorph spider. Zoosystema 31: 117–126.
18. Gallon RC (2002) Revision of the African genera of *Pterinochilus* and *Eucratoscelus* (Araneae, Theraphosidae, Harpactirinae) with description of two new genera. Bull Br Arachnol Soc 12: 201–232.
19. Lindquist EE, Evans GO (1965) Taxonomic concepts in the Ascidae, with a modified setal nomenclature for the idiosoma of the Gamasina (Acarina: Mesostigmata). Mem Ent Soc Can 47: 1–64.
20. Casanueva MA (1993) Phylogenetic studies of the free-living and arthropod associated Laelapidae (Acari: Mesostigmata). Gayana Zool 57: 21–46.
21. Zhu MS, Zhang R (2008) Revision of the theraphosid spiders from China (Araneae: Mygalomorphae). J Arachnol 36: 425–447.
22. Schwendinger PJ, Ono H (2011) On two *Heptathela* species from southern Vietnam, with a discussion of copulatory organs and systematics of the Liphistiidae (Araneae: Mesothelae). Rev Suisse Zool 118: 599–637.

12

Phylogenetic Analysis of *Staphylococcus aureus* CC398 Reveals a Sub-Lineage Epidemiologically Associated with Infections in Horses

Mohamed M. H. Abdelbary[1]*, Anne Wittenberg[2], Christiane Cuny[1], Franziska Layer[1], Kevin Kurt[1], Lothar H. Wieler[2], Birgit Walther[2], Robert Skov[3], Jesper Larsen[3], Henrik Hasman[4], J. Ross Fitzgerald[5], Tara C. Smith[6], J. A. Wagenaar[7], Annalisa Pantosti[8], Marie Hallin[9¤], Marc J. Struelens[10], Giles Edwards[11], R. Böse[12], Ulrich Nübel[1], Wolfgang Witte[1]

1 Robert Koch Institute, Wernigerode, Germany, 2 Institute of Microbiology and Epizootics, Free University Berlin, Berlin, Germany, 3 Microbiology and Infection Control, Statens Serum Institut, Copenhagen, Denmark, 4 National Food Institute, Technical University of Denmark, Lyngby, Denmark, 5 The Roslin Institute, University of Edinburgh, Edinburgh, United Kingdom, 6 Department of Epidemiology, College of Public Health, the University of Iowa, Iowa City, Iowa, United States of America, 7 Department of Infectious Diseases and Immunology, Faculty of Veterinary Medicine, Utrecht University, Utrecht, the Netherlands, 8 Istituto Superiore di Sanità, Rome, Italy, 9 Centre National de Référence *Staphylococcus aureus*, Microbiology Department, Erasme University Hospital, Université Libre de Bruxelles, Brussels, Belgium, 10 European Centre for Disease Prevention and Control, Stockholm, Sweden, 11 Department of Microbiology, Scottish MRSA Reference Laboratory (SMRSARL), Glasgow Royal Infirmary, Glasgow, United Kingdom, 12 Labor Dr. Böse GmbH, Harsum, Germany

Abstract

In the early 2000s, a particular MRSA clonal complex (CC398) was found mainly in pigs and pig farmers in Europe. Since then, CC398 has been detected among a wide variety of animal species worldwide. We investigated the population structure of CC398 through mutation discovery at 97 genetic housekeeping loci, which are distributed along the CC398 chromosome within 195 CC398 isolates, collected from various countries and host species, including humans. Most of the isolates in this collection were received from collaborating microbiologists, who had preserved them over years. We discovered 96 bi-allelic polymorphisms, and phylogenetic analyses revealed that an epidemic sub-clone within CC398 (dubbed 'clade (C)') has spread within and between equine hospitals, where it causes nosocomial infections in horses and colonises the personnel. While clade (C) was strongly associated with *S. aureus* from horses in veterinary-care settings ($p = 2 \times 10^{-7}$), it remained extremely rare among *S. aureus* isolates from human infections.

Editor: Michael Otto, National Institutes of Health, United States of America

Funding: This study was supported by grant D1KI10146 from the German Federal Ministry of Education and Research. The funders had no role in study design, data collection and analysis, decision to publish, or preparation of the manuscript.

Competing Interests: One or more of the authors (R. Böse) are employed by a commercial company Labor Dr. Böse GmbH.

* E-mail: abd-el-barym@rki.de

¤ Current address: Centre de Diagnostic Moléculaire, iris-Lab, Brussels, Belgium

Introduction

Staphylococcus aureus is a frequent nasal coloniser of mammals and birds. In humans, it is a leading cause of a wide range of infections in hospitals and communities. In particular, infections caused by methicillin-resistant *S. aureus* (MRSA) are of special concern due to the limited treatment options [1]. In addition to being a major threat to human health, since the 2000s MRSA is widely disseminated as a coloniser and infectious agent in economically important livestock and companion animals including cows, sheep, goats, poultry, pigs, dogs and horses. The first sporadic reports of MRSA infections in livestock arose during the 1970s and in companion animals (dogs and cats) during the late 1980s and 1990s [2–4].

In the early 2000s, a new clonal complex of MRSA (CC398) was detected in pigs in the Netherlands [5]. Since then, CC398 has been the dominant livestock-associated MRSA (LA-MRSA) among pigs in several countries [6-11], but CC398 has also been found in various other livestock species [12–20]. The transmission of CC398 from pigs to pig farmers has been reported previously [5,6,21–24]. Hence, direct contact with livestock is considered a risk factor for human colonisation and infection with CC398 [25]. However, several studies have reported human cases of methicillin-sensitive CC398 without current contact with livestock [21,26,27].

A previous study suggested that CC398 originated in humans as MSSA and was subsequently transmitted to livestock, where it then acquired the methicillin resistance [28]. In addition to livestock, CC398 has been recovered from companion animals and other animal species [6,22,29,30]. For instance, CC398 has been isolated from horses in Austria, Belgium, Germany, the United Kingdom and the Netherlands [6,31–36]. Nosocomial spreading and infection with MRSA in veterinary hospitals have been described previously [31,37]. Several infection cases, outbreaks, and colonisations of horses and associated personnel with CC398 have been reported in equine hospitals from several countries [23,31,35,38–40].

In this study, we used mutation discovery to elucidate the population structure and evolution of MRSA CC398 from infections in horses in comparison to a collection of isolates from other host species originating from various countries in Europe and overseas. We demonstrate that a specific sub-lineage of CC398 has emerged in equine veterinary care.

Results and Discussion

Molecular typing

In this study, a convenience sample collection of 195 *S. aureus* isolates, including MSSA (n = 37) and MRSA (n = 158), was investigated (Table 1). Isolates were collected between 1993 and 2011 from twelve different host species in ten different countries (Table S1). Molecular typing of the 195 isolates revealed fourteen different *spa* types (t011, t034, t108, t571, t779, t899, t1197, t1344, t1451, t2576, t2876, t2974, t5972 and t6867) (Table S1). *Spa* types t011 and t034 were the most common, representing 45% and 40% of the isolates, respectively. Furthermore, approximately 50% of the isolates (n = 99) harboured SCC*mec* type V, while 27% of the isolates (n = 52) carried SCC*mec* type IV (Table S1).

Phylogeny

We used denaturing high-pressure liquid chromatography (dHPLC) for mutation discovery at 97 genetic housekeeping loci ($\approx$400 bp per locus) distributed along the *S. aureus* chromosome; in total, they constituted 1.4% (40,230 bp) of the CC398 genome.

Our analysis revealed 96 bi-allelic polymorphisms (i. e., polymorphic sites at which two alleles were observed) associated with 63 haplotypes. Among these polymorphisms were 34 synonymous point mutations in the protein coding genes, 58 non-synonymous point mutations, and 4 insertions or deletions ranging in size from 1 to 14 bp (Table S2). Of these, 41 polymorphisms were informative for maximum parsimony analyses. The nucleotide diversity, π (the average number of nucleotide dissimilarities per site among two isolate sequences), was 0.00008 ± 0.00001 for the coding regions. The mean nucleotide substitution rate was estimated at 5.4×10^{-6} substitutions/nucleotide site/year (95% confidence interval, 3.5×10^{-6} to 7.5×10^{-6}). This estimated mutation rate for the isolate collection is relatively

faster than a previously reported evolutionary rate for other *S. aureus* strains [41,42]. To investigate the time of the most recent common ancestor (TMRCA) of the 195 CC398 isolates, we applied a Bayesian coalescent method of phylogenetic inference as previously described [41]. According to the calculated mutation rate, the sequences variations and the isolation date (1993–2011) of our isolates dataset, we estimated that the TMRCA was $\approx$1974 (95% confidence interval, 1955 to 1991).

Based on these 96 polymorphisms, a minimum spanning tree (MST) was constructed (Figure 1). The MST demonstrated very limited diversity among the 195 investigated isolates. The ancestral node was determined by comparing concatenated sequences from the investigated loci of all investigated CC398 isolates with the concatenated sequences of N315 as an out-group. Rooting the phylogenetic tree of CC398 using N315 as an out-group revealed that isolates with *spa* type t899 (n = 2) were the most divergent group in comparison with the remaining CC398 isolates (Figure 1C). The t899 isolates had 10 mutations compared to the root (au200-2, au200-3, au201-1, au201-2, au201-3, au202-1, au202-2, au202-3, au202-4 and au202-5), which were located on the isolates chromosomes within a region of $\geq$111,139 bp (between 23,209 -134,348) (Table S2). This finding is in agreement with a study based on whole genome sequencing, which suggested that CC398 with *spa* type t899 had acquired a fragment of 123,000 bp from ST9 through horizontal gene transfer. This fragment included the *spa* gene and the SCC*mec* insertion site [28].

Correlation of certain *spa* types and SCC*mec* types with phylogenetic lineages of CC398

The MST revealed six main clades (A to F) within CC398 (Figure 1) (mutations defining each clade are listed in table S2). Mapping the 14 *spa* types and the SCC*mec* types onto the MST revealed that clade (B) consisted of isolates (n = 5) from different countries that shared the same *spa* type (t108), and four of them carried SCC*mec* type V (Figure 1C & D). Similarly, clades (A, E, and F) were composed entirely of isolates characterised by *spa* type t034, with the exception of one isolate within clade (F), which was represented by *spa* type t011 (Figure 1C). Furthermore, the Bayesian tip-association significance test (BaTS) [43] revealed that certain *spa* types (t034, t011, t571, t108, t1457, and t899), and SCC*mec* types (IV, and V) were significantly associated with phylogeny (p<0.01; Table S3). Nevertheless, our findings confirm

Table 1. Summary of the isolate collection investigated in this study.

Country of origin	Host species	Year of isolation	Colonisation/Infection
Austria (n = 17)	Bovine (n = 6)	1993 (n = 1)	Colonisation (n = 29)
Belgium (n = 6)	Cat (n = 1)	2001 (n = 1)	Infection (n = 72)
Canada (n = 1)	Chicken (n = 7)	2002 (n = 2)	Information not available (n = 94)
Denmark (n = 31)	Dog (n = 5)	2003 (n = 3)	
Germany (n = 110)	Environment (n = 1)	2004 (n = 7)	
Italy (n = 3)	Goat (n = 1)	2005 (n = 5)	
The Netherland (n = 15)	Goose (n = 2)	2006 (n = 11)	
Thailand (n = 1)	Horse (n = 53)	2007 (n = 53)	
UK (n = 5)	Human (n = 80)	2008 (n = 31)	
USA (n = 6)	Pig (n = 35)	2009 (n = 33)	
	Turkey (n = 4)	2010 (n = 12)	
		2011 (n = 38)	

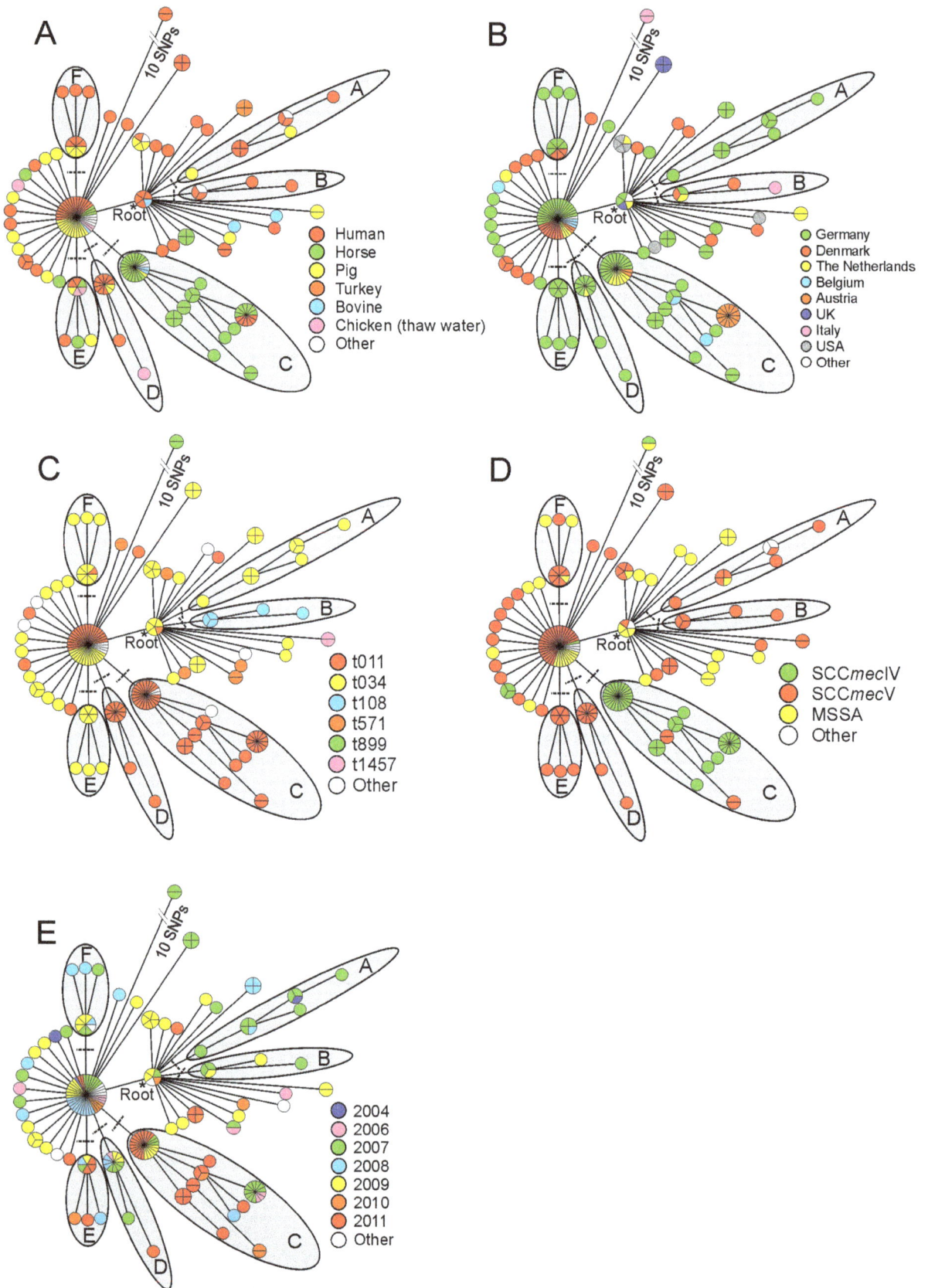

Figure 1. Minimum spanning tree (MST) represent the clustering of 195 CC398 isolates based on genome-wide SNPs; The ancestral node was determined by comparing concatenated sequences from the investigated loci of all investigated CC398 isolates with the concatenated sequences of N315 as an out-group. A) host origin of the 195 CC398 isolates, B) plotting of the geographical distribution on the

MST, C) shows the different *spa* types, D) the SCC*mec* types and the susceptibility of the 195 CC398 isolates and E) the isolation date.

that the usage of *spa* sequencing as the single typing tool for *S. aureus* might occasionally lead to misinterpretation, which is in agreement with previous observations in similar studies of other clonal complexes of *S. aureus* [28,41,44,45].

Association of host origin with phylogeny

Our analysis included CC398 isolates from 11 host species. A Bayesian statistical test (BaTS analysis; [43]) indicated that among these isolates, those from turkey meat and those from horses each displayed a significant association with phylogenetic structure within CC398 (p<0.01; Table S3). In contrast, other host species including humans were more dispersed on the phylogenetic tree (Figure 1A), not significantly different from a random distribution (p>0.1; Table S3).

The number of turkey isolates in our collection was very small (n = 4), and their geographic origins are not known with precision. Interestingly, however, we detected the φAvβ prophage in these four isolates by using targeted PCR (Table S1). This prophage was previously reported from *S. aureus* from several other bird species, suggesting CC398 in turkey may have adapted to the host through acquisition of an avian-specific prophage, similar to *S. aureus* CC5 in industrially fattened broiler chickens [46].

It is remarkable that the majority of isolates from horses under veterinary care clustered in clade (C) (41 out of 53 equine isolates total; Figure 1A). Of note, human isolates in the same clade (n = 6; 07-00334, 07-00471, 07-01238, 07-01239, 07-01335, 07-01730) were from veterinary personnel of an equine clinic in a large Austrian veterinary hospital (Stationary Care 1) who had close contact to infected horses (Table S1) [31]. Isolates in clade (C) (n = 53) had been collected from four different countries (Austria, Belgium, Germany, and the Netherlands) between 2006 and 2011 (Figure 1E), and clade (C) isolates from Germany (n = 29) had been collected from 13 equine clinics and veterinary practitioners distributed over seven different federal states (Table S1). These findings imply that clade (C) within CC398 is disseminated among hospitalised horses and veterinary personnel all over Germany and in several neighbouring European countries. At the same time, we found that clade (C) was extremely rare among *S. aureus* isolates from human infections in Germany. Among >6,700 isolates that had been submitted to the German National Reference Centre for Staphylococci and Enterococci in Robert Koch Institute between 2010 and 2011, there were 48 MRSA from human infections that displayed *spa* type t011 (Table S4). Among these, only four isolates carried the synonymous base substitution that defines clade (C) (i. e., they carried a thymidine residue at genomic position 2,533,404; SNP au309-2; Tables S2, S4), as revealed by targeted PCR and sequencing. Hence, the association of clade (C) with infections in horses is highly significant (p<0.0001; chi^2 test).

We assume that the emergence of MRSA CC398 clade (C) in horses from different European equine clinics may be due to epidemic spread, possibly comparable to several epidemic MRSA strains that rapidly spread within and between medical care hospitals and cause a large number of health-care-associated infections in humans [47–49]. A previous study based on multilocus sequence typing (MLST), *spa*-typing, and SCC*mec*-typing demonstrated that MRSA-CC398-t011-IV caused nosocomial infections in horses in an equine clinic in Switzerland [36]. The authors reported that MRSA-CC398-t011-IV was first detected in one of the personnel members who formerly worked in an equine clinic in Belgium. Later, this CC398-t011-IV was detected in infected horses and subsequently replaced ST1-t2863,

which was prevalent in wound infections in this equine clinic [36]. While samples from Switzerland were not available to us, it is well possible that the strain in this clinic was affiliated to clade (C), since the majority of clade (C) isolates in our collection also displayed *spa* type t011 (95%) and SCCmecIV (91%), respectively (Table S1, Figure S1).

One possible explanation for the spread of this CC398 subclone may be insufficient hygiene practices in veterinary settings; however, this requires further research. Several studies have reported that the nasal carriage rate of MRSA among veterinary practitioners is much greater than in medical staff in human hospitals [50–54]. In addition, the nosocomial spread of MRSA in equine clinics and between veterinary personnel was previously demonstrated [55–59]. Hence, personnel in veterinary settings may play an important role in the introduction and spread of MRSA into equine clinics. In addition, humans with frequent contact with horses can represent a reservoir for MRSA and subsequently transmit it to their household. A metapopulation model demonstrated that the occurrence of a relatively large proportion of MRSA-CC398 carriers among a susceptible human population might result in an outbreak [60].

Of note, the association of equine origin with a phylogenetic clade within CC398 observed here does not immediately indicate any specific genetic adaptation. Such adaptation is difficult to detect in general. Even for healthcare-associated MRSA, which have been studied for decades and for which abundant genome sequence data is available, it has proven extremely difficult to identify the specific adaptive traits that render these strains successful [47,61,62]. Notably, clade (C) contained isolates from other hosts (e.g. human (Stationary Care 1); calf, dog, and pig (Farm 1)) who had been in contact with horses, suggesting that genetic specialisation to the equine host may be limited or lacking.

Limitations of this study

Although our collection of *S. aureus* CC398 isolates represents the broadest host species coverage studied to date, its composition is fragmentary with respect to both, the spatial and temporal coverage of the global population of CC398. While we have taken considerable efforts to assemble a broadly representative strain collection, it includes convenience isolates that a limited number of collaborating microbiologists had considered worth to be preserved over years for various reasons. For example, even though our equine isolates had been collected in several European countries between 2006 and 2011, they by no means represent the demographics of the underlying horse population, let alone that of the more widely distributed population of *S. aureus* CC398. Several other categories (country of origin, host species) contained very few samples (e. g. only one isolate from Canada, one from a cat, etc.). In addition, very limited clinical and other meta-data was available for many of the isolates, because they initially had not been stored with the goal of any global epidemiological inferences in mind. Hence, for an in-depth investigation of the distribution of CC398 among different host species, it would be highly desirable to extend this study by including additional isolates from each of the various hosts, with an even distribution over several years and over a large geographic area, and by systematically recording epidemiological data.

The dHPLC-based mutation discovery method applied here covered 1.4% of the CC398 genome. This approach delivered improved discriminatory power compared to *spa* typing and standard MLST [44,63], and provided some novel insights into *S.*

aureus population structure. However, the resolution of analyses and the strength of any inferences would be much improved by whole-genome sequencing [42,47].

Conclusions. Our study demonstrated new insight into the phylogeny of CC398 through mutation discovery. We revealed the spread of a specific MRSA-CC398 sub-clone 'dubbed clade (C)' within equine settings, which causes infections in horses and nasal colonisation of humans. Furthermore, the spread of this sub-clone (clade (C)) can be traced through testing for the presence/absence of SNP (309-2) using diagnostic PCR followed by sequence analysis [64][65] Veterinarians play an important role in controlling the transmission of this sub-clone by taking precautions with staff hygiene, and implementation of control protocols for infections.

Materials and Methods

Bacterial isolates

In the present study, a collection of 195 *S. aureus* CC398 (MSSA; n = 37 and MRSA; n = 158) isolates was investigated (Table S1) and some of these isolates were included in previous studies [26,28,31,51,66–69]. CC398 convenience isolates were collected from nine different countries (mainly from Europe), and various hosts (humans: n = 80; animals: n = 115). The isolates investigated in this study were selected by animal species, geographical origin, and approximate period of time. Veterinary care facilities in this study were divided into stationary care (where the animals must be hospitalized for at least one night in order to receive medical treatment) or ambulatory care (medical care is provided to animals without being admitted to a hospital for treatment). MRSA isolates were chosen as follows:

[1] 10 isolates from horses were collected in Austria/Vienna. Eight of these isolates were from infected horses treated in Vienna veterinary hospital (Stationary Care 1; Table S1) from 2006 until 2007. We had previously collected and investigated isolates from nasal colonization of the veterinary personnel of this hospital, due to the emergence of CC398 over a long period in this facility, [31]. These human isolates (n = 6) were also included.

[2] 37 clinical isolates from horse were collected in Germany, from 17 different veterinary facilities (3 stationary care, 14 ambulatory care), which were distributed over 6 different German federal states (Baden-Württemberg (1), Hesse (1), Lower Saxony (3), North-Rhine-Westphalia (9), Schleswig-Holstein (2), Saxony (2), and Saarland (1)). Most of these horse isolates were sent for typing to the German Reference Centre for Staphylococci and Enterococci in Robert Koch Institute - branch Wernigerode by the Labor Dr. Boese which is providing diagnostic service for veterinarians treating horses in all the German federal states. Isolates from other animal species from Germany were also included, which originated from nasal colonization in pigs, pig farmers and their family members; colonization of posterior nares of goose, broiler chicken carcasses (thawing liquid). Isolates causing mastitis in cattle as well as various kinds of infections in humans emerging at different geographical locations in Germany were included as well (Table S1).

[3] Finally, isolates from other European countries (e.g. Belgium, Denmark, Italy, the Netherlands, UK) as well as from overseas (Canada, Thailand, USA) were included to maximize geographic distribution and range of host species. Additionally, to monitor the dissemination of one particular *S. aureus* strain among different animal species, six isolates from a Dutch farm derived from horses, dog, and cattle were included (farm 1 in Table S1).

SCC*mec*- and *spa*-typing were performed for all isolates as previously described [70]. Briefly, *spa*-typing was performed by following the Ridom Staph Type standard protocol and the *spa*-types were assigned to the Ridom database (www.ridom.org) (Ridom GmbH, Würzburg, Germany). In addition, antimicrobial susceptibility was tested using the broth dilution method according to the DIN58940 guidelines.

Mutation discovery using dHPLC

In this study, we investigated mainly metabolic housekeeping genes because polymorphisms in these genes provide the most reliable phylogenetic markers [71]. In total, we investigated 97 genetic housekeeping loci, which made up 1.4% (40,230 bp) of the CC398 genome and were scattered over the core genome of CC398. These loci had been analysed previously to investigate the population structure of other clonal complexes of *S. aureus* [41,44,72]. PCR primers were used to amplify 97 genetic housekeeping loci distributed along the 195 *S. aureus* isolate chromosomes (Table S2). Mutation discovery for the amplified gene fragments was performed using dHPLC (WaveR Nucleic Acid Fragment Analysis System, Transgenomic, Inc., Omaha, NE, USA) as described previously [44,46,72,73]. Briefly, PCR amplicon from each isolate was compared to a reference strain for detecting the heteroduplexes. Heteroduplexes result in double-stranded DNA that contains a point mutation site in comparison to the reference strain. Identified SNPs were confirmed through capillary Sanger sequencing of the PCR products from both ends using the PCR primers which are listed in Table S2.

Bacteriophage identification

For identification of phages possessing integrase group φSa3, we performed PCR using the primers int3, f2: 5′GTCAGCTTTA-GATGACGC and int3, r2: 5′AGCGCTAATGATGAACGA according to NC_00227452. For PCR demonstration of *sak*, *chp* and *scn*, we followed the protocol as described previously [74]. The presence of φAvβ prophage was determined by PCR as previously described [46].

Data analysis

Based on the discovered SNPs within the 97 genetic loci, a minimum spanning tree was constructed using Bionumerics software version 6.5 (Applied Maths, Ghent, Belgium). Additionally, sequences from the 97 housekeeping genes were concatenated for each isolate, constituting a 40,230 bp sequence alignment. A maximum likelihood tree based on this alignment was assembled using PhyML 3.1 [75]. The ancestral node was distinct by including distantly associated *S. aureus* genomic sequences. DnaSP was used to estimate the nucleotide diversity (π) and nucleotide variation (θw) and for calculating the mean pair-wise distance between alleles at synonymous (Ks) and non-synonymous (Ka) sites [76–78]. The rate of evolution and the divergence times were estimated as described previously using BEAST software (Version 1.7.5, http://beast.bio.ed.ac.uk/) [79]. The Bayesian tip-association significance test (BaTS, version 1.0) was applied to estimates of the association of the phylogeny traits with hosts, *spa* types, geographical origin, and SCC*mec* types [43].

Statistical significance of the association between SNP 309-2 and the host species was assessed using a chi-square test (http://www.r-project.org/).

Acknowledgments

We thank Christa Cuny, Annette Weller, and the staff at our central sequencing lab for excellent technical assistance. We thank Ivonne Stamm from Vet Med Labor GmbH, Germany and Franklin D. Lowy from Columbia University, USA for supplying *S. aureus* isolates. We thank Beth Hopping for reviewing and commenting the manuscript.

Author Contributions

Conceived and designed the experiments: MMHA CC UN WW. Performed the experiments: MMHA AW. Analyzed the data: MMHA AW CC FL KK UN. Contributed reagents/materials/analysis tools: LHW BW RS JL HH JRF TCS JAW AP MH MJS GE RB. Wrote the paper: MMHA UN WW.

References

1. Lowy FD (1998) Staphylococcus aureus infections. N Engl J Med 339: 520–532.
2. Devriese LA, Van Damme LR, Fameree L (1972) Methicillin (cloxacillin)-resistant Staphylococcus aureus strains isolated from bovine mastitis cases. Zentralbl Veterinarmed B 19: 598–605.
3. Scott GM, Thomson R, Malone-Lee J, Ridgway GL (1988) Cross-infection between animals and man: possible feline transmission of Staphylococcus aureus infection in humans? J Hosp Infect 12: 29–34.
4. Cefai C, Ashurst S, Owens C (1994) Human carriage of methicillin-resistant Staphylococcus aureus linked with pet dog. Lancet 344: 539–540.
5. Voss A, Loeffen F, Bakker J, Klaassen C, Wulf M (2005) Methicillin-resistant Staphylococcus aureus in pig farming. Emerg Infect Dis 11: 1965–1966.
6. Witte W, Strommenger B, Stanek C, Cuny C (2007) Methicillin-resistant Staphylococcus aureus ST398 in humans and animals, Central Europe. Emerg Infect Dis 13: 255–258.
7. Guardabassi L, Stegger M, Skov R (2007) Retrospective detection of methicillin resistant and susceptible Staphylococcus aureus ST398 in Danish slaughter pigs. Vet Microbiol 122: 384–386.
8. Smith TC, Male MJ, Harper AL, Kroeger JS, Tinkler GP, et al. (2009) Methicillin-resistant Staphylococcus aureus (MRSA) strain ST398 is present in midwestern U.S. swine and swine workers. PLoS One 4: e4258.
9. Khanna T, Friendship R, Dewey C, Weese JS (2008) Methicillin resistant Staphylococcus aureus colonization in pigs and pig farmers. Vet Microbiol 128: 298–303.
10. Pan A, Battisti A, Zoncada A, Bernieri F, Boldini M, et al. (2009) Community-acquired methicillin-resistant Staphylococcus aureus ST398 infection, Italy. Emerg Infect Dis 15: 845–847.
11. Agerso Y, Hasman H, Cavaco LM, Pedersen K, Aarestrup FM (2012) Study of methicillin resistant Staphylococcus aureus (MRSA) in Danish pigs at slaughter and in imported retail meat reveals a novel MRSA type in slaughter pigs. Vet Microbiol 157: 246–250.
12. Nemati M, Hermans K, Lipinska U, Denis O, Deplano A, et al. (2008) Antimicrobial resistance of old and recent Staphylococcus aureus isolates from poultry: first detection of livestock-associated methicillin-resistant strain ST398. Antimicrob Agents Chemother 52: 3817–3819.
13. Cuny C, Friedrich A, Kozytska S, Layer F, Nübel U, et al. (2010) Emergence of methicillin-resistant Staphylococcus aureus (MRSA) in different animal species. Int J Med Microbiol 300: 109–117.
14. Kehrenberg C, Cuny C, Strommenger B, Schwarz S, Witte W (2009) Methicillin-resistant and -susceptible Staphylococcus aureus strains of clonal lineages ST398 and ST9 from swine carry the multidrug resistance gene cfr. Antimicrob Agents Chemother 53: 779–781.
15. Tavakol M, Olde Riekerink RG, Sampimon OC, Van Wamel WJ, Van Belkum A, et al. (2012) Bovine-associated MRSA ST398 in the Netherlands. Acta Vet Scand 54: 28.
16. Monecke S, Kuhnert P, Hotzel H, Slickers P, Ehricht R (2007) Microarray based study on virulence-associated genes and resistance determinants of Staphylococcus aureus isolates from cattle. Vet Microbiol 125: 128–140.
17. Persoons D, Van Hoorebeke S, Hermans K, Butaye P, de Kruif A, et al. (2009) Methicillin-resistant Staphylococcus aureus in poultry. Emerg Infect Dis 15: 452–453.
18. Fessler AT, Olde Riekerink RG, Rothkamp A, Kadlec K, Sampimon OC, et al. (2012) Characterization of methicillin-resistant Staphylococcus aureus CC398 obtained from humans and animals on dairy farms. Vet Microbiol.
19. Fessler A, Scott C, Kadlec K, Ehricht R, Monecke S, et al. (2010) Characterization of methicillin-resistant Staphylococcus aureus ST398 from cases of bovine mastitis. J Antimicrob Chemother 65: 619–625.
20. Fessler AT, Kadlec K, Hassel M, Hauschild T, Eidam C, et al. (2011) Characterization of methicillin-resistant Staphylococcus aureus isolates from food and food products of poultry origin in Germany. Appl Environ Microbiol 77: 7151–7157.
21. Cuny C, Nathaus R, Layer F, Strommenger B, Altmann D, et al. (2009) Nasal colonization of humans with methicillin-resistant Staphylococcus aureus (MRSA) CC398 with and without exposure to pigs. PLoS One 4: e6800.
22. van Belkum A, Melles DC, Peeters JK, van Leeuwen WB, van Duijkeren E, et al. (2008) Methicillin-resistant and -susceptible Staphylococcus aureus sequence type 398 in pigs and humans. Emerg Infect Dis 14: 479–483.
23. Graveland H, Duim B, van Duijkeren E, Heederik D, Wagenaar JA (2011) Livestock-associated methicillin-resistant Staphylococcus aureus in animals and humans. Int J Med Microbiol 301: 630–634.
24. van Loo I, Huijsdens X, Tiemersma E, de Neeling A, van de Sande-Bruinsma N, et al. (2007) Emergence of methicillin-resistant Staphylococcus aureus of animal origin in humans. Emerg Infect Dis 13: 1834–1839.
25. Van den Broek, Van Cleef BA, Haenen A, Broens EM, Van der Wolf PJ, et al. (2009) Methicillin-resistant Staphylococcus aureus in people living and working in pig farms. Epidemiol Infect 137: 700–708.
26. Uhlemann AC, Porcella SF, Trivedi S, Sullivan SB, Hafer C, et al. (2012) Identification of a highly transmissible animal-independent Staphylococcus aureus ST398 clone with distinct genomic and cell adhesion properties. MBio 3.
27. van der Mee-Marquet N, Francois P, Domelier-Valentin AS, Coulomb F, Decreux C, et al. (2011) Emergence of unusual bloodstream infections associated with pig-borne-like Staphylococcus aureus ST398 in France. Clin Infect Dis 52: 152–153.
28. Price LB, Stegger M, Hasman H, Aziz M, Larsen J, et al. (2012) Staphylococcus aureus CC398: host adaptation and emergence of methicillin resistance in livestock. MBio 3.
29. van de Giessen AW, van Santen-Verheuvel MG, Hengeveld PD, Bosch T, Broens EM, et al. (2009) Occurrence of methicillin-resistant Staphylococcus aureus in rats living on pig farms. Prev Vet Med 91: 270–273.
30. Vincze S, Stamm I, Monecke S, Kopp PA, Semmler T, et al. (2013) Molecular analysis of human and canine Staphylococcus aureus strains reveals distinct extended-host-spectrum genotypes independent of their methicillin resistance. Appl Environ Microbiol 79: 655–662.
31. Cuny C, Strommenger B, Witte W, Stanek C (2008) Clusters of infections in horses with MRSA ST1, ST254, and ST398 in a veterinary hospital. Microb Drug Resist 14: 307–310.
32. Van den Eede A, Martens A, Lipinska U, Struelens M, Deplano A, et al. (2009) High occurrence of methicillin-resistant Staphylococcus aureus ST398 in equine nasal samples. Vet Microbiol 133: 138–144.
33. Loeffler A, Lloyd DH (2010) Companion animals: a reservoir for methicillin-resistant Staphylococcus aureus in the community? Epidemiol Infect 138: 595–605.
34. Loeffler A, Kearns AM, Ellington MJ, Smith LJ, Unt VE, et al. (2009) First isolation of MRSA ST398 from UK animals: a new challenge for infection control teams? J Hosp Infect 72: 269–271.
35. van Duijkeren E, Moleman M, Sloet van Oldruitenborgh-Oosterbaan MM, Multem J, Troelstra A, et al. (2010) Methicillin-resistant Staphylococcus aureus in horses and horse personnel: an investigation of several outbreaks. Vet Microbiol 141: 96–102.
36. Sieber S, Gerber V, Jandova V, Rossano A, Evison JM, et al. (2011) Evolution of multidrug-resistant Staphylococcus aureus infections in horses and colonized personnel in an equine clinic between 2005 and 2010. Microb Drug Resist 17: 471–478.
37. O'Mahony R, Abbott Y, Leonard FC, Markey BK, Quinn PJ, et al. (2005) Methicillin-resistant Staphylococcus aureus (MRSA) isolated from animals and veterinary personnel in Ireland. Vet Microbiol 109: 285–296.
38. Seguin JC, Walker RD, Caron JP, Kloos WE, George CG, et al. (1999) Methicillin-resistant Staphylococcus aureus outbreak in a veterinary teaching hospital: potential human-to-animal transmission. J Clin Microbiol 37: 1459–1463.

39. Weese JS (2010) Methicillin-resistant Staphylococcus aureus in animals. ILAR J 51: 233–244.

40. Weese JS (2005) Methicillin-resistant Staphylococcus aureus: an emerging pathogen in small animals. J Am Anim Hosp Assoc 41: 150–157.

41. Nübel U, Dordel J, Kurt K, Strommenger B, Westh H, et al. (2010) A timescale for evolution, population expansion, and spatial spread of an emerging clone of methicillin-resistant Staphylococcus aureus. PLoS Pathog 6: e1000855.

42. Harris SR, Feil EJ, Holden MT, Quail MA, Nickerson EK, et al. (2010) Evolution of MRSA during hospital transmission and intercontinental spread. Science 327: 469–474.

43. Parker J, Rambaut A, Pybus OG (2008) Correlating viral phenotypes with phylogeny: accounting for phylogenetic uncertainty. Infect Genet Evol 8: 239–246.

44. Nübel U, Roumagnac P, Feldkamp M, Song JH, Ko KS, et al. (2008) Frequent emergence and limited geographic dispersal of methicillin-resistant Staphylococcus aureus. Proc Natl Acad Sci U S A 105: 14130–14135.

45. Robinson DA, Enright MC (2004) Evolution of *Staphylococcus aureus* by large chromosomal replacements. J Bacteriol 186: 1060–1064.

46. Lowder BV, Guinane CM, Ben Zakour NL, Weinert LA, Conway-Morris A, et al. (2009) Recent human-to-poultry host jump, adaptation, and pandemic spread of Staphylococcus aureus. Proc Natl Acad Sci U S A 106: 19545–19550.

47. Holden MT, Hsu LY, Kurt K, Weinert LA, Mather AE, et al. (2013) A genomic portrait of the emergence, evolution, and global spread of a methicillin-resistant Staphylococcus aureus pandemic. Genome Res 23: 653–664.

48. Ellington MJ, Hope R, Livermore DM, Kearns AM, Henderson K, et al. (2010) Decline of EMRSA-16 amongst methicillin-resistant Staphylococcus aureus causing bacteraemias in the UK between 2001 and 2007. J Antimicrob Chemother 65: 446–448.

49. Amorim ML, Faria NA, Oliveira DC, Vasconcelos C, Cabeda JC, et al. (2007) Changes in the clonal nature and antibiotic resistance profiles of methicillin-resistant *Staphylococcus aureus* isolates associated with spread of the EMRSA-15 clone in a tertiary care Portuguese hospital. J Clin Microbiol 45: 2881–2888.

50. Nulens E, Gould I, MacKenzie F, Deplano A, Cookson B, et al. (2005) Staphylococcus aureus carriage among participants at the 13th European Congress of Clinical Microbiology and Infectious Diseases. Eur J Clin Microbiol Infect Dis 24: 145–148.

51. Wulf MW, Sorum M, van Nes A, Skov R, Melchers WJ, et al. (2008) Prevalence of methicillin-resistant Staphylococcus aureus among veterinarians: an international study. Clin Microbiol Infect 14: 29–34.

52. Wulf M, van Nes A, Eikelenboom-Boskamp A, de Vries J, Melchers W, et al. (2006) Methicillin-resistant Staphylococcus aureus in veterinary doctors and students, the Netherlands. Emerg Infect Dis 12: 1939–1941.

53. Hanselman BA, Kruth SA, Rousseau J, Low DE, Willey BM, et al. (2006) Methicillin-resistant Staphylococcus aureus colonization in veterinary personnel. Emerg Infect Dis 12: 1933–1938.

54. Moodley A, Nightingale EC, Stegger M, Nielsen SS, Skov RL, et al. (2008) High risk for nasal carriage of methicillin-resistant Staphylococcus aureus among Danish veterinary practitioners. Scand J Work Environ Health 34: 151–157.

55. Anderson ME, Lefebvre SL, Weese JS (2008) Evaluation of prevalence and risk factors for methicillin-resistant Staphylococcus aureus colonization in veterinary personnel attending an international equine veterinary conference. Vet Microbiol 129: 410–417.

56. Panchaud Y, Gerber V, Rossano A, Perreten V (2010) Bacterial infections in horses: a retrospective study at the University Equine Clinic of Bern. Schweiz Arch Tierheilkd 152: 176–182.

57. Weese JS, Lefebvre SL (2007) Risk factors for methicillin-resistant Staphylococcus aureus colonization in horses admitted to a veterinary teaching hospital. Can Vet J 48: 921–926.

58. Weese JS, Archambault M, Willey BM, Hearn P, Kreiswirth BN, et al. (2005) Methicillin-resistant Staphylococcus aureus in horses and horse personnel, 2000-2002. Emerg Infect Dis 11: 430–435.

59. Weese JS, Caldwell F, Willey BM, Kreiswirth BN, McGeer A, et al. (2006) An outbreak of methicillin-resistant Staphylococcus aureus skin infections resulting from horse to human transmission in a veterinary hospital. Vet Microbiol 114: 160–164.

60. Porphyre T, Giotis ES, Lloyd DH, Stark KD (2012) A Metapopulation Model to Assess the Capacity of Spread of Meticillin-Resistant Staphylococcus aureus ST398 in Humans. PLoS One 7: e47504.

61. Li M, Du X, Villaruz AE, Diep BA, Wang D, et al. (2012) MRSA epidemic linked to a quickly spreading colonization and virulence determinant. Nat Med 18: 816–819.

62. McAdam PR, Templeton KE, Edwards GF, Holden MT, Feil EJ, et al. (2012) Molecular tracing of the emergence, adaptation, and transmission of hospital-associated methicillin-resistant Staphylococcus aureus. Proc Natl Acad Sci U S A 109: 9107–9112.

63. Strommenger B, Bartels MD, Kurt K, Layer F, Rohde SM, et al. (2013) Evolution of methicillin-resistant Staphylococcus aureus towards increasing resistance. J Antimicrob Chemother.

64. Nübel U, Nitsche A, Layer F, Strommenger B, Witte W (2012) Single-nucleotide polymorphism genotyping identifies a locally endemic clone of methicillin-resistant *Staphylococcus aureus*. PLoS One 7: e32698.

65. Stegger M, Liu CM, Larsen J, Soldanova K, Aziz M, et al. (2013) Rapid Differentiation between Livestock-Associated and Livestock-Independent *Staphylococcus aureus* CC398 Clades. PLoS One 8: e79645.

66. Smith TC, Gebreyes WA, Abley MJ, Harper AL, Forshey BM, et al. (2013) Methicillin-resistant Staphylococcus aureus in pigs and farm workers on conventional and antibiotic-free swine farms in the USA. PLoS One 8: e63704.

67. Li S, Skov RL, Han X, Larsen AR, Larsen J, et al. (2011) Novel types of staphylococcal cassette chromosome mec elements identified in clonal complex 398 methicillin-resistant Staphylococcus aureus strains. Antimicrob Agents Chemother 55: 3046–3050.

68. McCarthy AJ, van Wamel W, Vandendriessche S, Larsen J, Denis O, et al. (2012) Staphylococcus aureus CC398 clade associated with human-to-human transmission. Appl Environ Microbiol 78: 8845–8848.

69. Hallin M, De Mendonca R, Denis O, Lefort A, El Garch F, et al. (2011) Diversity of accessory genome of human and livestock-associated ST398 methicillin resistant Staphylococcus aureus strains. Infect Genet Evol 11: 290–299.

70. Strommenger B, Braulke C, Heuck D, Schmidt C, Pasemann B, et al. (2008) spa Typing of Staphylococcus aureus as a frontline tool in epidemiological typing. J Clin Microbiol 46: 574–581.

71. Feil EJ (2004) Small change: keeping pace with microevolution. Nat Rev Microbiol 2: 483–495.

72. Kurt K, Rasigade JP, Laurent F, Goering RV, Zemlickova H, et al. (2013) Subpopulations of Staphylococcus aureus clonal complex 121 are associated with distinct clinical entities. PLoS One 8: e58155.

73. Roumagnac P, Weill FX, Dolecek C, Baker S, Brisse S, et al. (2006) Evolutionary history of *Salmonella* Typhi. Science 314: 1301–1304.

74. van Wamel WJ, Rooijakkers SH, Ruyken M, van Kessel KP, van Strijp JA (2006) The innate immune modulators staphylococcal complement inhibitor and chemotaxis inhibitory protein of Staphylococcus aureus are located on beta-hemolysin-converting bacteriophages. J Bacteriol 188: 1310–1315.

75. Guindon S, Dufayard JF, Lefort V, Anisimova M, Hordijk W, et al. (2010) New algorithms and methods to estimate maximum-likelihood phylogenies: assessing the performance of PhyML 3.0. Syst Biol 59: 307–321.

76. Rozas J (2009) DNA sequence polymorphism analysis using DnaSP. Methods Mol Biol 537: 337–350.

77. Librado P, Rozas J (2009) DnaSP v5: a software for comprehensive analysis of DNA polymorphism data. Bioinformatics 25: 1451–1452.

78. Rozas J, Sanchez-DelBarrio JC, Messeguer X, Rozas R (2003) DnaSP, DNA polymorphism analyses by the coalescent and other methods. Bioinformatics 19: 2496–2497.

79. Drummond AJ, Rambaut A (2007) BEAST: Bayesian evolutionary analysis by sampling trees. BMC Evol Biol 7: 214.

13

Vaccination with *Brucella abortus* Recombinant *In Vivo*-Induced Antigens Reduces Bacterial Load and Promotes Clearance in a Mouse Model for Infection

Jake E. Lowry[1,3]*, **Dale D. Isaak**[2], **Jack A. Leonhardt**[1], **Giulia Vernati**[1], **Jessie C. Pate**[1], **Gerard P. Andrews**[1]*

1 Department of Veterinary Sciences, University of Wyoming, Laramie, Wyoming, United States of America, 2 Department of Molecular Biology, University of Wyoming, Laramie, Wyoming, United States of America, 3 Professional Veterinary Medicine Program, College of Veterinary Medicine & Biomedical Sciences, Colorado State University, Fort Collins, Colorado, United States of America

Abstract

Current vaccines used for the prevention of brucellosis are ineffective in inducing protective immunity in animals that are chronically infected with *Brucella abortus*, such as elk. Using a gene discovery approach, in vivo-induced antigen technology (IVIAT) on *B. abortus*, we previously identified ten loci that encode products up-regulated during infection in elk and consequently may play a role in virulence. In our present study, five of the loci (D15, 0187, VirJ, Mdh, AfuA) were selected for further characterization and compared with three additional antigens with virulence potential (Hia, PrpA, MltA). All eight genes were PCR-amplified from *B. abortus* and cloned into *E. coli*. The recombinant products were then expressed, purified, adjuvanted, and delivered subcutaneously to BALB/c mice. After primary immunization and two boosts, mice were challenged i.p. with 5×10^4 CFU of *B. abortus* strain 19. Spleens from challenged animals were harvested and bacterial loads determined by colony count at various time points. While vaccination with four of the eight individual proteins appeared to have some effect on clearance kinetics, mice vaccinated with recombinant Mdh displayed the most significant reduction in bacterial colonization. Furthermore, mice immunized with Mdh maintained higher levels of IFN-γ in spleens compared to other treatment groups. Collectively, our in vivo data gathered from the S19 murine colonization model suggest that vaccination with at least three of the IVIAT antigens conferred an enhanced ability of the host to respond to infection, reinforcing the utility of this methodology for the identification of potential vaccine candidates against brucellosis. Mechanisms for immunity to one protein, Mdh, require further in vitro exploration and evaluation against wild-type *B. abortus* challenge in mice, as well as other hosts. Additional studies are being undertaken to clarify the role of Mdh and other IVI antigens in *B. abortus* virulence and induction of protective immunity.

Editor: Shan Lu, University of Massachusetts Medical Center, United States of America

Funding: This study was supported by the U.S. Department of Agriculture (USDA) Special Projects Grant, CSRE45229. The funders had no role in study design, data collection and analysis, decision to publish, or preparation of the manuscript.

Competing Interests: The authors have declared that no competing interests exist.

* E-mail: jake.lowry@colostate.edu (JEL); Gandrews@uwyo.edu (GPA)

Introduction

Brucellosis continues to be problematic to the agriculture industry world-wide, including the U.S. Furthermore, several *Brucella* spp. have been classed as category B threat list agents with the potential for use as bioterrorism weapons. Efforts to develop an effective, stable, and non-reactogenic vaccine against brucellosis have been ongoing in several laboratories, and the use of a live, attenuated platform has become the established benchmark through the use of the *B. abortus* rough strain RB51 [1]. Although moderate efficacy against *Brucella*-induced fetal abortions in domestic livestock (cattle) has been reported [2], acceptable levels of protection following immunization with RB51 has yet to be demonstrated in wildlife such as elk [3,4,5,6], and in the case of bison, results have been conflicting in terms of the vaccine's reactogenicity [7,8,9,10,11]. The exact nature of the attenuation of RB51 is also unclear, although it's rough LPS phenotype is due to at least one lesion in O-side chain biosynthesis loci [1]. A more systematic approach to the induction of active protective immunity against brucellosis has been undertaken by some laboratories

through the development of subunit vaccines [12,13,14,15,16,17]. To date, the degree of success in protecting with such vaccines depends on the ability of the candidate to drive immunity towards a Th1-type response, emphasizing the need to identify and characterize *Brucella* antigens which present T-cell epitopes to the host [18]. Despite the efforts to identify components for a next-generation subunit vaccine, formulations using recombinant *Brucella* antigens have not been thoroughly assessed for immunogenicity/efficacy. The discovery of additional *Brucella* virulence factors thus may facilitate the development of a more efficacious, less reactogenic, acellular product that may either be used as a stand-alone vaccine or used to augment primary immunization with the existing live, attenuated platform. As an example of the latter strategy, enhanced efficacy in the mouse model has been reported by over-expressing *Brucella* superoxide dismutase (SOD) in RB51 or complementing the strain's rough LPS phenotype with the O-side chain biosynthesis locus, *wboA* [19].

We previously applied the gene discovery methodology, known as in vivo-induced antigen technology (IVIAT), to identify *B. abortus* virulence genes up-regulated during infection in elk (*Cervis* elaphus), and as a result have identified ten loci with gene products potentially important to survival of the pathogen in this host [20]. Furthermore, the conserved nature of most of these gene products has led us to extend our hypothesis - that they also may be requisite virulence effectors in other *Brucella* susceptible hosts. As a preliminary approach to confirming our hypothesis, we have selected five of these in vivo-induced (IVI) products for further characterization in a surrogate murine model for *B. abortus* colonization: a conserved outer membrane protein, D15; a gluconeogenic enzyme, malate dehydrogenase (Mdh); a periplasmic component of an ABC transport system, AfuA; a component of the Type-IV secretion system (T4SS) VirJ; and a lipoprotein of unknown function BAB1_0187 (referred to as 0187). We also targeted three additional conserved gene products based on high amino acid sequence similarity with antigens identified through *Yersinia pestis* IVIAT and previous reports of a role in *Brucella* pathogenesis [21,22]: proline epimerase (PrpA), an auto-secreting (Type-V) surface antigen, Hia, and a soluble lytic transglycosylase, MltE.

Results

S19 Infection Kinetics

To establish the colonization kinetics of *B. abortus* S19 in BALB/c mice in our laboratory, thirty naive animals were infected with S19 at 5×10^4 CFU and five animals sacrificed at 7, 14, 21, 28, 42, and 70 days post-infection. Bacterial loads in spleens peaked in two weeks at 8×10^7 CFU before gradually declining to 6×10^3 CFU in 6 weeks. At 10 weeks post infection, organisms were still able to be cultured from spleens in 60% of the animals. Also, splenomegaly was observed in S19-infected mice, peaking between 14 and 21 days post-infection, and declining by day 28 (data not shown).

S19 challenge after vaccination with recombinant IVI products

In the first experiment, thirty mice were vaccinated with purified Mdh, MltE, or adjuvant-only. After hyper-immunization with the recombinant proteins, the sera were assessed for antibody. End-point titers from mice immunized with the recombinant protein ranged from a 1:1000 to 1:5000. Serum from mice receiving alhydrogel alone was non-reactive against any of the proteins.

After challenge, bacterial loads in the spleens were determined at 7, 14, 21, and 28 days post-infection. As shown in Table 1, mice vaccinated with Mdh showed a markedly significant decrease in bacterial colonization at 14 dpi, providing 2.75 log units of clearance and 2 log units of clearance at 21 days post-infection compared to adjuvant-only treated animals (p<0.001). Bacterial loads measured in MltE-immunized mice were no different than the adjuvant-only controls (not shown). Mdh-immunized animals also displayed extended splenomegaly which remained elevated relative to the adjuvant-only animals at 28 days post-infection (data not shown). By 42 days, the Mdh-immunized animals had completely cleared the infection, while S19 was still cultured from spleens of the adjuvant-only mice at the same time point (data not shown).

In a second experiment, fifteen mice each received alhydrogel only, AfuA, Hia or D15 recombinant proteins adsorbed to the adjuvant. Mice were primed and boosted twice, and serum was collected to assay for antibody titers. Reactivity of the immune sera to all three antigens was detectable out to 1:1000 for Hia and 1:5000 for D15 and AfuA (comparable to that of Mdh immunized mice). The animals were challenged as before and bacterial loads in the spleens assessed at 14, 21, and 28 days post-infection. As

Table 1. Reduction of bacterial load and more rapid clearance in a murine colonization model by immunization with recombinant *B. abortus* Mdh.

Time, Post-infection (days)	Adjuvant Only	Mdh	p value	Log reduction
0	-	-	-	-
7	2.51×10^6 $(+/- 3.34 \times 10^5)$	8.05×10^5 $(+/- 5.62 \times 10^5)$	<0.05	0.55
14	9.94×10^7 $(+/- 2.17 \times 10^7)$	2.43×10^5 $(+/- 1.12 \times 10^5)$	<0.001	2.75
21	2.64×10^6 $(+/- 8.57 \times 10^5)$	3.73×10^4 $(+/- 2.08 \times 10^4)$	<0.001	2.09
28	1.38×105 $(+/- 8.37 \times 10^4)$	1.29×10^4 $(+/- 1.00 \times 10^4)$	<0.05	1.09

shown in Table 2, in contrast to Mdh, there was no significant difference at two weeks between the adjuvant-only and antigen-immunized animal groups, however at three weeks post-infection all three experimental groups differed significantly from the adjuvant-only group with D15 showing the most pronounced effect of 1.41 log units of clearance (p<0.001). As observed with Mdh-immunized animals, splenomegaly remained consistently elevated in all test groups at 28 days post- infection relative to the adjuvant-only control animals (data not shown).

A third iteration was then conducted to evaluate VirJ, 0187, and PrpA. Following the same methods as above, antibody titers were determined to be >1:5000 (VirJ, PrpA and 0187). Mice were challenged with S19 and splenic colony counts were performed as described previously at 14 and 21 days post-infection. No significant difference was found between adjuvant-only animals and those receiving any of the three antigens (data not shown), although all immune animals displayed some degree of splenomegaly.

Mouse cytokine response to challenge with S19

Levels of IL-12p70, IL-4 and IFN-γ in the splenic homogenates were quantified from the five selected animal groups immunized with antigens which had an effect on bacterial load and/or clearance rate. No detectable IL-12p70 or IL-4 groups immunized with AfuA, Hia, D15, or adjuvant alone was observed. IL-4 was, however, detected in Mdh-vaccinated mice, although at low levels (data not shown).

IFN-γ was next assessed in vaccinated mice after challenge. As shown in Figure 1, at all sampling times, mice vaccinated with Mdh showed significantly higher levels of this cytokine (p<0.05), compared to the mice receiving AfuA, D15, or alhydrogel alone. By 21 and 28 days post-infection, IFN-γ levels among all groups had declined with the exception of the Mdh immune group, in which IFN-γ remained significantly elevated (p<0.05; Figure 1).

In Vivo assessment of IVI gene up-regulation during S19 infection in mice

"Short-unique" regions of selected IVI genes identified through IVIAT from elk infected with wild-type *B. abortus* were selected for construction of RT-PCR primers. Ten BALB/c mice were subsequently infected with S19, five of which were splenectomised at 24 and 48 hours post-infection, and bacterial mRNA isolated. Additionally, S19 was grown to mid-log phase in vitro and mRNA

Table 2. Reduction of bacterial load in a murine colonization model by immunization with recombinant B. abortus AfuA, D15, or Hia.

Time (days) Post-infection	Adjuvant Only	AfuA	D15	Hia	p value	Log reduction
0	-	-	-	-		
7	2.51×10^6 ($+/- 3.34 \times 10^5$)	ND	ND	ND		
14	9.94×10^7 ($+/- 2.17 \times 10^7$)	2.89×10^7 ($+/- 1.78 \times 10^7$)	4.40×10^7 ($+/- 2.23 \times 10^7$)	1.88×10^7 ($+/- 7.02 \times 10^6$)		
21	2.64×10^6 ($+/- 8.57 \times 10^5$)	6.53×10^4 ($+/- 5.38 \times 10^4$)	1.23×10^5 ($+/- 8.05 \times 10^4$)	4.20×10^4 ($+/- 2.81 \times 10^4$)	<0.001 (D15)	1.41
28	1.38×10^5 ($+/- 8.37 \times 10^4$)	1.59×10^4 ($+/- 9.31 \times 10^3$)	1.50×10^4 ($+/- 9.08 \times 10^3$)	2.89×10^4 ($+/- 1.27 \times 10^4$)	<0.05 (Hia)	1.91

extracted for comparison. Quantitative analysis of cDNA showed up-regulation during both 24 and 48 hours post-infection of *afuA*, *mdh*, and 0187 (Figure 2). In contrast, D15 mRNA was not detected in either the in vitro or in vivo samples, even after performing several different nested RT-PCR reactions (data not shown). While, *prpA* and *mltE* were not examined, Hia-encoding transcript was expressed at equivalent levels in vitro and during infection (data not shown).

Discussion

The use of a murine model for the characterization of *B. abortus* IVI proteins as potential protective antigens is likely not the optimal animal model for simulation of the disease state in the natural host species. Consequently, behavior of recombinant antigens and/or mutants may be different in mice than the target species. Despite this drawback, some mouse strains have been shown to be highly sensitive to the pathogen, and have been used to study *B. abortus* pathogenesis and evaluate vaccine candidates for the past two decades [23,24,25,26,27,28]. Furthermore, studies with S19 in pregnant BALB/c mice reported an identical

pathology, placentitis and septic fetal death, as with wild-type *B. abortus* infection, further supporting the applicability of this model to the simulation of disease in other host species [28,29]. The benefit of using S19 instead of wild-type *B. abortus* is reduced cost and safety, since BSL-3 small animal containment facilities are not required.

Vaccination with purified *B. abortus* Mdh resulted in significantly reduced colonization and more rapid clearance of S19 in the BALB/c mouse. Interestingly, Mdh was the only recombinant protein of the five antigens examined which facilitated some level of clearance that elicited a significant IFN-γ response, a cytokine critical for the activation of macrophages and a requisite for controlling *Brucella* infections [30]. It is therefore likely that prolonged elevated levels of IFN-γ in mice vaccinated with Mdh contribute to the reduction in the colonization by S19 in these immune animals. The nature of Mdh-induced immune-mediated enhanced clearance is unclear at present, however, it is possible that an auxiliary virulence function of the enzyme may be neutralized by a robust immune response directed toward it. The presence of IL-4 and absence of IL-12 also suggest that mice vaccinated with Mdh induce a Th2-biased response leading to

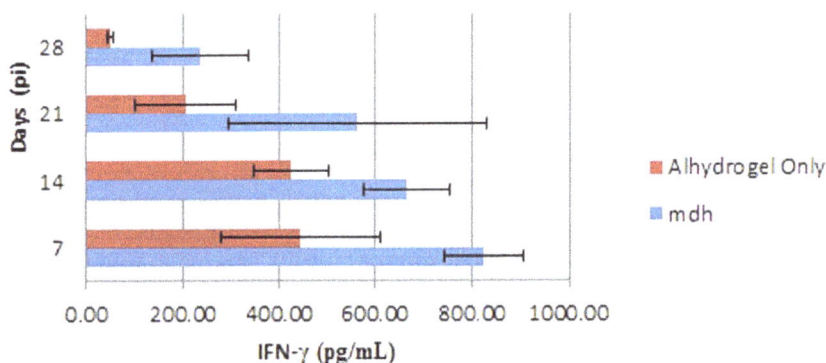

Figure 1. IFN-γ response in Mdh-immunized BALB/c mice after S19 challenge. Spleen homogenates from the five mice from each time point (7,14,21 and 28 dpi) sacrificed during the challenge studies were evaluated for IFN-γ production.

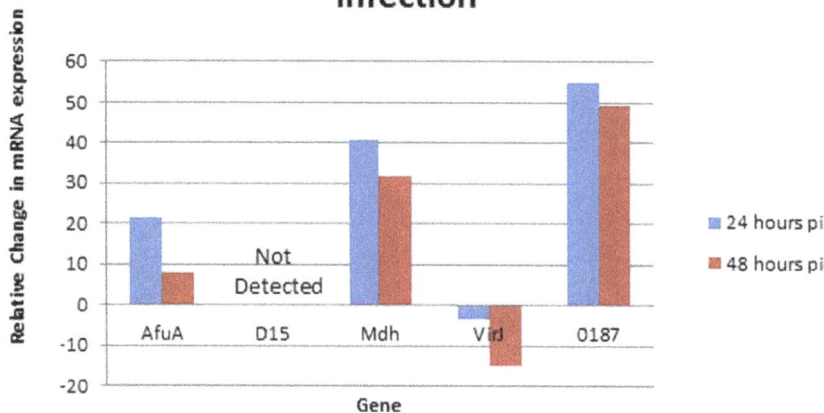

Figure 2. IVI genes upregulated in vivo during S19 infection. Average Fold change of bacterial mRNA isolated from five mice infected with S19 at each time point compared to in vitro-grown B. abortus S19.

clearance immunity mediated by antibody. In fact, a search for putative T- and B-cell epitopes across the amino acid sequence of the protein revealed only the latter (data not shown). This hypothesis may seem contrary to the traditional notion that only a Th1-biased response can reduce intracellular bacterial load in the *Brucella*-infected host. Indeed, previous experiments with other facultative intracellular pathogens such as *Yersinia pestis* have demonstrated that antibody alone can confer protection against challenge [31]. In the case of *B. abortus*, an "optimized" Th2 response might also contribute significantly to clearing infection.

Although, immunity to AfuA and D15 failed to elicit more rapid clearance of S19, bacterial loads were significantly reduced in animals immunized with either of these two proteins. In contrast to AfuA and Mdh, D15 expression was not evident early in S19 colonization, thus D15 may be relevant at a later stage of infection in the mouse. Curiously, in our previous study [20], we failed to detect antibody to Mdh and D15 in S19-immunized elk, indicating that both proteins may be regulated differently in cervids.

Hia was not identified as an IVI gene in our initial study [20], and consistent with this finding, was subsequently was found to be constitutively expressed based on our mRNA analysis (data not shown). Our selection of this gene product was based on similar homology to *Y. pestis* protein and previous reports in the literature of involvement as a virulence factor [32]. This type-V auto-secreted antigen, induced a greater level of extended splenomegaly compared to the other recombinant proteins, including Mdh. However, the increased inflammation did not correlate with heightened production of IFN-γ (data not shown). This observation suggests that perhaps immunity to Hia increases the inflammatory response during infection by mechanisms not related to IFN-γ, such as TNF-α or IL-1. Although immunization with Hia reduced bacterial load in our model comparable to D15 and AfuA, it failed to induce more rapid clearance.

As with MltE, 0187, PrpA, and VirJ failed to reduce bacterial load and/or alter clearance kinetics compared to adjuvant-only controls. 0187 is a putative lipoprotein that shares significant homology with the well characterized BA14K protein. Previous studies have demonstrated that BA14K was able to induce a Th1 response and induce IL-12 secretion [33]. We were unable to express 0187 from *B. abortus* as a full length protein but were able to stably express a truncated form shortened by 27 amino acids

from the n-terminus (data not shown). It is possible that this truncation could have resulted in conformation changes leading to an inability to induce clearance immunity.

The proline epimerase, PrpA, was described as a B-cell polyclonal activator and inducer of IL-10 [22], suggesting that immunity to this protein may promote clearance in our model based on the pivotal role IL-10 plays in *Brucella* pathogenesis [30,34]. Mice immunized with PrpA during early infection actually had splenic counts higher than animals immunized with adjuvant alone. It is possible that a secondary exposure to PrpA results in host immune dysregulation early during the course of infection.

The data from our previous study strongly suggested that the Type-IV secretion system (T4SS) accessory protein, VirJ, is up-regulated during wild type *B. abortus* infection in elk. Animals immunized with S19 however did not generate a humoral response to the protein (unpublished data), which suggests a difference in the way this secreton is utilized by S19 in cervids. Consistent with this finding, in the S19 murine colonization model, VirJ appeared to be slightly down-regulated at least during early stages of infection. A BLAST analysis upstream and downstream of the VirJ-encoding locus revealed no differences between S19, 2308 or 9-941 (Wyoming strain) DNA sequences, suggesting the involvement of a distal regulatory element(s) in controlling expression of this protein in S19. The function of VirJ, as assessed in other pathogens, is suspected to be as a periplasmic chaperone responsible for assisting substrates in associating with a "pusher" pilus before translocation through the T4SS, typically thought to be required for full virulence in this pathogen [35]. In this regard, we intend to re-evaluate VirJ in a *B. abortus* 2308 challenge model.

Data from our model system is in agreement with that previously published for S19 colonization kinetics in BALB/c mice [23]. Our vaccination efforts with a single recombinant protein, Mdh, coincide with previously reported data on mice vaccinated with RB51 in terms of the subsequent cytokine responses post-challenge [36]. IFN-γ levels peak between 6 and 7 days then begin to slowly decline, albeit remaining sustained for weeks [36]. RB51 vaccinates also lack significant production IL-12p70 or high levels of IL-4 upon challenge. [36]. This observation could be peculiar to BALB/c mice, which tend to be more biased towards humoral responses [1,30,36]. As predicted, our S19 data shows that a pro-inflammatory response is suppressed in naïve animals and behaves similarly to strain 2308 in this respect [30]. This observation suggests that a shift in cytokine production levels could be important in providing a more efficacious immune response to brucellosis.

Taken together, these data suggest the potential for use of the gluconeogenic enzyme, malate dehydrogenase, as a recombinant subunit vaccine candidate for brucellosis. AfuA, D15, and/or Hia may also represent promising subunit vaccine candidates when used together and/or in combination with Mdh. In this regard, we plan to evaluate such antigen cocktails in the near future, using wild type field isolates of *B. abortus* in mice and other host species.

Methods

Bacterial strains and growth conditions

Brucella abortus S19, was kindly provided by the Colorado Serum Company (Denver, CO), and was used exclusively for this study in the mouse colonization/infection model. Brain-heart infusion broth cultures were typically grown overnight at 37°C, serially diluted after three washes in sterile PBS, followed by plating to determine a viable cell count correlate with optical density at 600 nm.

In vivo gene expression, RNA extraction, and RT-PCR

Ten BALB/c mice were infected with 1×10^7 cfu of *B. abortus* S19 i.p. Mice were splenectomized and tissues stored in RNAlater^{TM} (Ambion, Austin, TX). Tissues were homogenized and RNA isolated with the RiboPure-Bacteria^{TM} Kit (Ambion, Austin, TX). Isolated RNA was transcribed to cDNA using RETROscript^{TM} (Ambion, Austin, TX) and cDNA targets amplified by *PfuTurbo*^{TM} DNA Polymerase (Stratagene, La Jolla, CA) in a one-step reaction. Amplification of a segment of the 16S subunit of *B. abortus* S19 was used as a positive control; negative controls were included for each gene and contained all the reaction components except reverse transcriptase. In addition a negative control was employed which lacked RNA template to confirm the absence of DNA contamination in the reaction. Concentration of PCR product in gel bands was assessed using Quantity One^{TM} 4.6 software (Bio-Rad, Hercules, CA).

Plasmid construction, recombinant protein expression, and purification

Selected IVI genes were amplified in their entirety from the *B. abortus* RB51 genome by PCR, using PfuUltra Master Mix (Stratagene, La Jolla, CA), inserted into the pET-46 Ek/LIC^{TM} system (EMD Biosciences, La Jolla, CA), and transformed into *E. coli* NovaBlue cells (EMD Biosciences, La Jolla, CA). The recombinant plasmid constructs were then purified and the insert sequence confirmed by PCR and sequencing. The recombinant plasmids were re-transformed into *E. coli* Rosetta-2[DE3] cells (EMD Biosciences, La Jolla, CA) and induced to express under 0.5 mM IPTG at 30°C. Verification of expression of recombinant products was performed by total crude protein resolution on SDS-PAGE followed by Western blot analysis using a His-tagged

Monoclonal antibody (EMD Biosciences, La Jolla, CA). Ten mls of 0.5 mM IPTG-induced cultures of recombinant *E. coli* strains were treated with BugBuster HT (EMD Biosciences, La Jolla, CA) and soluble (AfuA, Mdh, MltE, 0187) and insoluble (D15, VirJ, Hia) fractions containing recombinant histidine-tagged fusion proteins purified by the HisMag^{TM} Purification Kit (EMD Biosciences, La Jolla, CA). Insoluble fractions containing D15, VirJ, and Hia were purified under 8 M Urea, followed by dialysis against PBS. The proteins were run on a SDS-PAGE gel to confirm purity and quantified by spectral absorption at 280 nm and BCA Lowry (Pierce Chemical).

Subunit vaccine preparation

Purified proteins were mixed with a 1:7 dilution of aluminum hydroxide adjuvant (Alhydrogel^{TM}; Superfos, Denmark) in PBS and adsorbed overnight at 4°C at a concentration of 150 μg/mL.

Animal studies

All animals utilized in this study were cared for according to strict adherence to the Policies and Regulations established by the US Public Health Service "Humane Care and Use of Laboratory Animals" and an approved animal protocol from the University of Wyoming Institutional Animal Care and Use Committee (IACUC) (DHHS Assurance #A3216-1).

Ten to 30 six-week old, female BALB/c mice received 30 μg of recombinant protein subcutaneously in 200 μL of adjuvant at one site. Additional control mice were treated with adjuvant only in the same manner. Immunization regimen consisted of a prime and two boosts, 21 days apart. Retro-orbital bleeds were performed to assess antibody titers by Western blot. Animals were challenged i.p. with 5×10^4 organisms of *B. abortus* S19 at 14 days after the second boost. Five mice from each group were sacrificed at specific time points. Spleens were removed, weighed, homogenized, used to determine whole organ bacterial load following serial dilution of the homogenates in 1X Sterile PBS and plating on blood agar. The remaining homogenates were stored at −40°C for cytokine analysis.

Cytokine analysis

Supernatants from spleen homogenates were used in Quanti-Kine^{TM} ELISA Assays (R & D Systems, Minneapolis, MN) to quantify IL-12p70, IL-4, and IFN-γ cytokine levels in the spleen.

Statistics

All statistical analysis was performed with the software package SAS 9.1 Enterprise^{TM} (SAS Corporation, Cary, NC). ANOVA was used to compare means of groups and Least Significant Difference (LSD) was used to determine mean separations between the groups. $\alpha = 0.05$; p values are listed in text.

Author Contributions

Conceived and designed the experiments: JEL GPA. Performed the experiments: JEL JAL DDI JCP GPA. Analyzed the data: JEL JAL DDI GV JCP GPA. Contributed reagents/materials/analysis tools: JEL JAL DDI GV JCP GPA. Wrote the paper: JEL JCP GPA.

References

1. Schurig G, Sriranganathan N, Corbel M (2002) Brucellosis vaccines: past, present, and future. Vet Microbiol 90: 479–496.
2. Elzer PH, Enright FM, Colby L, Hagius SD, Walker JV, et al. (1998) Protection against infection and abortion induced by virulent challenge exposure after oral vaccination of cattle with *Brucella abortus* strain RB51. Am J Vet Res 59: 1575–1578.
3. Olsen SC, Fach SJ, Palmer MV, Sacco RE, Stoffregen WC, et al. (2006) Immune Responses of elk to initial and booster vaccinations with *Brucella abortus* strain RB51 or 19. Clin Vaccine Immunol 13: 1098–1103.
4. Davis, DS, Elzer, PH (2002) *Brucella* vaccines in wildlife. Veterinary Microbiology 90: 533–544.
5. Cook WE, Williams ES, Thorne ET, Kreeger TJ, Stout G, et al. (2002) *Brucella abortus* strain RB51 vaccination in elk. I. Efficacy of reduced dosage. J Wildl Dis 38: 18–26.
6. Kreeger T, Cook W, Edwards W, Elzer P, Olsen S (2002) *Brucella abortus* strain RB51 vaccination in elk. II. Failure of high dosage to prevent abortion. J Wildl Dis 38: 27–31.

7. Olsen S, Holland S (2003) Safety of re-vaccination of pregnant bison with *Brucella abortus* strain RB51. J Wildl Dis 39: 824–829.

8. Olsen SC, Boyle SM, Schurig GG, Sriranganathan NN (2009) Immune responses and protection against experimental challenge after vaccination of bison with *Brucella abortus* Strain RB51 or RB51 overexpressing superoxide dismutase and glycosyltransferase genes. Clin Vaccine Immunol 16: 535–540.

9. Elzer PH, Edmonds MD, Hagius SD, Walker JV, Gilsdorf MJ, et al. (1998) Safety of *Brucella abortus* strain RB51 in bison. J Wildl Dis 34: 825–829.

10. Olsen SC, Rhyan JC, Gidlewski T, Palmer MV, Jones AH (1999) Biosafety and antibody response of adult bison bulls after vaccination with *Brucella abortus* strain RB51. Am J Vet Res 60.

11. Palmer MV, Cheville NF, Jensen AE (1996) Experimental infection of pregnant cattle with the vaccine candidate *Brucella abortus* strain RB51: pathologic, bacteriologic, and serologic findings. Vet Pathol 33: 682–691.

12. Al-Mariri A, Tibor A, Mertens P, De Bolle X, Michel P, et al. (2001) Protection of BALB/c mice against *Brucella abortus* 544 challenge by vaccination with bacterioferritin or P39 recombinant proteins with CpG oligodeoxynucleotides as adjuvant. Infect Immun 69: 4816–4822.

13. He Y, Vemulapalli R, Schurig GG (2002) Recombinant *Ochrobactrum anthropi* expressing *Brucella abortus* Cu,Zn superoxide dismutase protects mice against *B. abortus* infection only after switching of immune responses to Th1 type. Infect Immun 70: 2535–2543.

14. Kaushik P, Singh D, Kumar S, Tiwari A, Shukla G, et al. (2010) Protection of mice against *Brucella abortus* 544 challenge by vaccination with recombinant OMP28 adjuvanted with CpG oligonucleotides. Veterinary Research Communications 34: 119–132.

15. Pasquevich KA, Estein SM, Samartino CG, Zwerdling A, Coria LM, et al. (2009) Immunization with recombinant *Brucella* Species outer membrane protein Omp16 or Omp19 in adjuvant induces specific CD4+ and CD8+ T cells as well as systemic and oral protection against *Brucella abortus* infection. Infect Immun 77: 436–445.

16. Delpino MV, Estein SM, Fossati CA, Baldi PC, Cassataro J (2007) Vaccination with *Brucella* recombinant DnaK and SurA proteins induces protection against *Brucella abortus* infection in BALB/c mice. Vaccine 25: 6721–6729.

17. Cassataro J, Velikovsky CA, Bruno L, Estein SM, de la Barrera S, et al. (2007) Improved immunogenicity of a vaccination regimen combining a DNA vaccine encoding *Brucella melitensis* outer membrane protein 31 (Omp31) and recombinant Omp31 boosting. Clin Vaccine Immunol 14: 869–874.

18. Ko J, Splitter GA (2003) Molecular host-pathogen interaction in brucellosis: current understanding and future approaches to vaccine development for mice and humans. Clin Microbiol Rev 16: 65–78.

19. Vemulapalli R, Contreras A, Sanakkayala N, Sriranganathan N, Boyle SM, et al. (2004) Enhanced efficacy of recombinant *Brucella abortus* RB51 vaccines against *B. melitensis* infection in mice. Veterinary Microbiology 102: 237–245.

20. Lowry JE, Goodridge L, Vernati G, Fluegel AM, Edwards WH, et al. (2010) Identification of *Brucella abortus* genes in elk (Cervus elaphus) using in vivo-induced antigen technology (IVIAT) reveals novel markers of infection. Veterinary Microbiology 142: 367–372.

21. Andrews GP, Vernati G, Ulrich R, Rocke TE, Edwards WH, et al. (2010) Identification of in vivo-induced conserved sequences from *Yersinia pestis* during experimental plague infection in the rabbit. Vector-Borne and Zoonotic Diseases 10(8): 749–756.

22. Spera JM, Ugalde, JE, Mucci, J, Comerci, D J, Ugalde, RA (2006) A B-lymphocyte mitogen is a *Brucella abortus* virulence factor required for persistent infection. Proc Nat Acad of Sci 103: 16514–16519.

23. Montaraz JA, Winter AJ (1986) Comparison of living and nonliving vaccines for *Brucella abortus* in BALB/c mice. Infect Immun 53: 245–251.

24. Cheers C (1984) Pathogenesis and cellular immunity in experimental murine brucellosis. Dev Biol Standard 56: 237–246.

25. Bosseray N (1992) Control methods and thresholds of acceptability for anti-*Brucella* vaccines. Dev Biol Standard 79: 121–128.

26. Bosseray N, Plommet M (1990) *Brucella suis* S2, *Brucella melitensis* Rev. 1 and *Brucella abortus* S19 living vaccines: residual virulence and immunity induced against three *Brucella* species challenge strains in mice. Vaccine 8: 462–468.

27. Baldwin CL, Winter AJ (1994) Macrophages and Brucella. Immunol Ser 60: 363–380.

28. Tobias L, Cordes DO, Schurig GG (1993) Placental pathology of the pregnant mouse inoculated with *Brucella abortus* strain 2308. Vet Pathol 30: 119–129.

29. Tobias L, Schurig GG, Cordes DO (1992) Comparative behaviour of *Brucella abortus* strains 19 and RB51 in the pregnant mouse. Res Vet Sci 53: 179–183.

30. Baldwin CL, Goenka R (2006) Host immune responses to the intracellular bacteria *Brucella*: does the bacteria instruct the host to facilitate chronic infection? Crit Rev Immunology 26: 407–442.

31. Sofer-Podesta C, Ang J, Hackett NR, Senina S, Perlin D, et al. (2009) Adenovirus-mediated delivery of an anti-V antigen monoclonal antibody protects mice against a Lethal *Yersinia pestis* challenge. Infect Immun 77: 1561–1568.

32. Alamuri P, Lower M, Hiss JA, Himpsl SD, Schneider G, et al. (2010) Adhesion,invasion, and agglutination mediated by twotrimeric autotransporters in the human uropathogen *Proteus mirabilis*. Infect Immun 78: 4882–4894.

33. Chirhart-Gilleland RL, Kovach ME, Elzer PH, Jennings SR, Roop RM, II (1998) Identification and characterization of a 14-kilodalton *Brucella abortus* protein reactive with antibodies from naturally and experimentally infected hosts and T lymphocytes from experimentally infected BALB/c mice. Infect Immun 66: 4000–4003.

34. Fernandes D, Baldwin C (1995) Interleukin-10 downregulates protective immunity to *Brucella abortus*. Infect Immun 63: 1130–1133.

35. Zhong Z, Wang Y, Qiao F, Wang Z, Du X, et al. (2009) Cytotoxicity of *Brucella* smooth strains for macrophages is mediated by increased secretion of the type-IV secretion system. Microbiology 155: 3392–3402.

36. Wang Y, Chen Z, Qiao F, Zhong Z, Xu J, et al. (2010) The type-IV secretion system affects the expression of Omp25/Omp31 and the outer membrane properties of *Brucella melitensis*. FEMS Microbiology Letters 303: 92–100.

14

Exploratory Analysis of Methods for Automated Classification of Laboratory Test Orders into Syndromic Groups in Veterinary Medicine

Fernanda C. Dórea[1]*, **C. Anne Muckle**[2], **David Kelton**[3], **J.T. McClure**[1], **Beverly J. McEwen**[4], **W. Bruce McNab**[5], **Javier Sanchez**[1], **Crawford W. Revie**[1]

1 Department of Health Management, Atlantic Veterinary College, University of Prince Edward Island, Charlottetown, Prince Edward Island, Canada, 2 Department of Pathology and Microbiology, University of Prince Edward Island, Charlottetown, Prince Edward Island, Canada, 3 Department of Population Medicine, University of Guelph, Guelph, Ontario, Canada, 4 Animal Health Laboratory, University of Guelph, Guelph, Ontario, Canada, 5 Animal Health and Welfare Branch, Ontario Ministry of Agriculture Food and Rural Affairs, Guelph, Ontario, Canada

Abstract

Background: Recent focus on earlier detection of pathogen introduction in human and animal populations has led to the development of surveillance systems based on automated monitoring of health data. Real- or near real-time monitoring of pre-diagnostic data requires automated classification of records into syndromes–syndromic surveillance–using algorithms that incorporate medical knowledge in a reliable and efficient way, while remaining comprehensible to end users.

Methods: This paper describes the application of two of machine learning (Naïve Bayes and Decision Trees) and rule-based methods to extract syndromic information from laboratory test requests submitted to a veterinary diagnostic laboratory.

Results: High performance (F_1-macro = 0.9995) was achieved through the use of a rule-based syndrome classifier, based on rule induction followed by manual modification during the construction phase, which also resulted in clear interpretability of the resulting classification process. An unmodified rule induction algorithm achieved an $F_{1-micro}$ score of 0.979 though this fell to 0.677 when performance for individual classes was averaged in an unweighted manner ($F_{1-macro}$), due to the fact that the algorithm failed to learn 3 of the 16 classes from the training set. Decision Trees showed equal interpretability to the rule-based approaches, but achieved an $F_{1-micro}$ score of 0.923 (falling to 0.311 when classes are given equal weight). A Naïve Bayes classifier learned all classes and achieved high performance ($F_{1-micro} = 0.994$ and $F_{1-macro} = .955$), however the classification process is not transparent to the domain experts.

Conclusion: The use of a manually customised rule set allowed for the development of a system for classification of laboratory tests into syndromic groups with very high performance, and high interpretability by the domain experts. Further research is required to develop internal validation rules in order to establish automated methods to update model rules without user input.

Editor: Ramin Homayouni, University of Memphis, United States of America

Funding: This project is funded by an Animal Health Strategic Investment grant (OMAFRA/AHL) (grant number 09/21) and the support of Canadian Regulatory Veterinary Epidemiology Network (CRVE-Net). The funders had no role in study design, data collection and analysis, decision to publish, or preparation of the manuscript.

Competing Interests: The authors have declared that no competing interests exist.

* E-mail: dorea.meyer@gmail.com

Introduction

Disease emergence and bioterrorism events, especially since 2001, have highlighted some of the short-comings of traditional surveillance, generally based on laboratory test results and direct reporting [1]. Focus has shifted to earlier detection of pathogen introduction in human or animal populations, leading to the implementation of new techniques using data sources upstream to those typically used in traditional surveillance [2]; especially pre-diagnosis data that are already available and automatically collected [3], such as sales of over-the-counter medicine, absences from work or school, and patients' chief complaint upon visits to an emergency center [4].

Due to the lack of sensitivity of pre-diagnostic data, surveillance systems using this information target general groups of diseases, or syndromes, and are therefore often referred to as "syndromic surveillance" [5]. Grouping pre-diagnostic data into syndromes is the first step of implementing a syndromic surveillance system [3]. Valid, reliable, and automatic classification of syndromes was an essential component of early computerized epidemic detection systems [6]. When data are structured using standardised codes, such as the Logical Observation Identifiers Names and Codes (LOINC®) used in laboratories, the International Classification of Diseases (now on its 10th revision, ICD-10), or the Systematized Nomenclature of Medicine (SNOMED®) [7], syndrome classification can be performed by mapping those codes into syndromes.

However, text mining or other machine learning tools can be invaluable when free-text or semi-structured data are being used [6]. Naïve Bayes classifiers have frequently been used in syndromic surveillance when the input data are chief complaints (free-text typed in by nurses) at emergency facilities [6,8,9,10,11].

Rule-based methods were widely used before the computational capacity of common computers made it possible for machine learning methods to be widely adopted [11]. Nevertheless, they have remained a popular choice in the health field due to their transparency and interpretability. In the 2008 challenge organized by i2b2 (Informatics for Integrating Biology to the Bedside), which consisted of automatic classification of obesity and comorbidities from discharge summaries [12], the top ten solutions were dominated by rule-based approaches, demonstrating their efficacy.

Decision trees are a third type of classification algorithm recommended when results must be delivered to a broader audience, such as health workers, as it is also an relatively simple method to interpret [13]. Other machine learning algorithms used in the medical field include: Artificial Neural Networks (ANN) [14]; and Support Vector Machines (SVM) [15]. These methods are powerful, but both adopt a "black-box" approach; so that the way in which decisions are made by the classifier is not transparent. They have been used in more complex medical tasks, such as the interpretation of radiographs and studies of drug performance [16,17,18]. However, to the authors' knowledge, the use of these algorithms to classify health data for the purposes of syndromic surveillance has not been documented in the peer-reviewed literature.

In contrast to laboratory test results, on which traditional surveillance is based, laboratory test orders can be a valuable data source for syndromic surveillance, since they are collected and stored electronically in an automated manner, but are more timely for surveillance purposes than laboratory test results. Laboratory submission data have, for example, been incorporated into CDC's BioSense Early Event Detection and Situation Awareness System [19]. Moreover, because there are fewer laboratories than sites of clinical care, the use of laboratory databases can provide more complete records and over larger areas [2]. Besides changing focus to early diagnosis, modern surveillance systems are evolving to complete *biosurveillance* systems. This term is intended to imply a broadening focus, addressing not only human health but all conditions that may threaten public health, such as a disruption in the food supply, or large social and economic disruptions resulting from outbreaks of diseases in animals [2,20]. Besides their role in the food supply and agricultural economy, animals could serve as sentinels for the detection of certain zoonotic diseases that may be recognized earlier in animals than in humans [21].

Animal data have been incorporated into a few surveillance systems for human populations, including: the Electronic Surveillance System for the Early Notification of Community-based Epidemics (ESSENCE) [22], the North Dakota Electronic Animal health Surveillance System [23] and the Multi-Hazard Threat Database (MHTD) [24]. Glickman et al (2006) [25] and Shaffer et al (2008) [26] have investigated the value of animal health data as sentinels for public health. Despite the less frequent requests for laboratory analyses made by veterinarians compared to human clinicians, the authors hypothesized that, "the consistency of test orders over time is such that increases in cases of disease will result in detectable increases in the number of test orders submitted by veterinarians that can be identified using prospective analysis" (Shaffer, 2008 [26], page2).

An overview of the development of syndromic surveillance system in the veterinary context has been provided in a recent review of the literature [27]. This review indicated that initiatives

using laboratory data had been based on establishing direct relationships between test codes and syndromic groups. The use of clinical data has typically relied on syndrome definition being provided by the veterinarian. Machine learning or rule-based methods applied to the identification of syndromes in animal health data had not been documented. This paper describes the exploratory analysis of such methods to extract syndromic information from laboratory test requests submitted to a veterinary diagnostic laboratory. These steps are part of the development of a syndromic surveillance system taking advantage of the centralized, computerized, and routinely updated sources of data provided by the Animal Health Laboratory in the province of Ontario, Canada. The initial phase of implementation, described here, focused on cattle sample submissions.

Methods

Data Source

The Animal Health Laboratory (AHL) at the University of Guelph is the primary laboratory of choice for veterinary practitioners submitting samples for diagnosis in food animals in the province of Ontario, Canada. The number of unique veterinary clients currently in the laboratory's database (2008 to 2012) is 326. The AHL has a laboratory information management system (LIMS) that is primarily used for reporting the results of diagnostic tests.

Three years of historical data from the AHL were available, from January 2008 to December 2010. Cattle were chosen as the pilot species due to high volume of submissions from dairy and beef herds in Ontario. All laboratory test orders for diagnoses in cattle were extracted from the database; all farm identification elements had been removed from these data.

Data Structure

Test requests are entered into the AHL database on a daily basis. Individual test requests are recorded as unique data entries. A common *case code* (submission number) is given to all samples from the same herd on any given day, allowing identification of samples related to the same health event. In human health, a case usually refers to one person at a time. Such that two people, with the same medical complaint, living in the same household, submitting samples on the same day would be counted as two cases. In veterinary medicine which often works in herds or flocks, samples submitted from one, two or more animals, of the same type, from the same herd ("household") with the same medical complaint on the same day, would be counted as one case.

The nature of the diagnostic sample is identified in the database by two fields: the *sample type* field, in which the laboratory staff chose from a pre-set list (blood, feces, brain tissue, etc); and the *client sample ID*, a free-text field used to enter the source animal identifier given by the client. The diagnostic tests are identified by codes pre-set in the system. All codes are textual.

Table 1 shows a sample of the data. Only the fields relevant for medical information extraction are shown. Submission numbers have been removed, but samples from the same submission are represented in the table with consecutive rows in the same shading.

Syndrome Definition

All of the historical data available were reviewed manually to identify the potential for syndromic classification at the time of sample submission. Veterinarians do not often provide detailed case history information. Therefore the identification of syndromes was based only on the type of diagnostic test requested, and the

Table 1. Sample of the data available, restricted to the fields relevant for syndrome classification.

Date	Sample ID*	Client Sample ID	Sample Type	Diagnostic test code	Diagnostic test description
2010-01-04	10-####-0001	Tulip	Milk	Beta-Lactamase_Test	**Beta-lactamase_test**
2010-01-04	10-####-0002	Plum	**Milk**	Culture_Bact	Bacterial_culture
2010-01-04	10-$$$$-0005	A517_SMALL	**Intestine**	Culture_Bact	Bacterial_culture
2010-01-04	10-$$$$-0009	B516	Tissue_Pooled	RLA	**Rotavirus_A_-_latex_agglutination**
2010-01-04	10-$$$$-0010	#517,_#516	Tissue_-_Fixed	Histopathology	Histopathology
2010-01-07	10-####-0002	139_W-H-1_-_**Pericardial**	Fluid	Culture_Bact	Bacterial_culture
2010-01-07	10-####-0004	139_W-H-1_-_**Heart**	Tissue	Culture_Bact	Bacterial_culture
2010-01-05	10-$$$$-0001	Webb/None_Given	Tissue_-_Fixed	IHC_-_Bov_Corona	**IHC_-_Bovine_coronavirus**
2010-01-05	10-$$$$-0002	Webb/None_Given	Ear_-_Notch	BVDV_Antigen_ELISA	**Bovine_viral_diarrhea_virus_-_antigen_ELISA**
2010-01-05	10-####-0001	11675_BOOSTER_110004	**Semen**	Culture_Bact	Bacterial_culture
2010-01-27	10-$$$$-0031	Black_Face_w_white_spot	Blood_-_Serum	N._caninum_ELISA	**Neospora_caninum_-_ELISA**
2010-01-27	10-####-0002	**Lung**	Tissue	Culture_Bact	Bacterial_culture
2010-01-27	10-####-0003	LuLiKiSpThTy	Tissue_Pooled	Cell_Cult_Isolation	Virus_isolation_in_cell_culture
2010-01-27	10-####-0005	**Stom._content**	Tissue	Culture_Bact	Bacterial_culture
2010-01-27	10-####-0006	**liv/spl/kid**	Tissue	Culture_Bact	Bacterial_culture

*The field containing Submission ID was removed to ensure confidentiality, and omitted in the Sample ID shown.
Samples from the same case are represented in the table with consecutive rows of the same shading. Keywords and test names relevant for classification are shown in bold.

type of sample submitted, which allowed identification of the organ system targeted for diagnosis.

A syndromic group was defined as a group of test requests that: (i) are related to diseases from the same organ system; (ii) are all diagnostic tests for the same specific disease, in cases of tests requested so frequently that their inclusion in another group would result in their being, alone, responsible for the majority of submissions; or (iii) tests that have little clinical relevance and should be filtered out (e.g., tests in environmental samples, general haematology profiles, as well as a range of "non-specific" submissions). Despite the absence of clinical information, the sample description allows identification of abortion cases through keywords such as "placenta" or "fetus". "Abortion" is therefore the only syndromic group defined based on a clinical syndrome, rather than using the three criteria listed above. Based on those criteria, an initial list of syndromic groups was compiled and then reviewed by a pathologist (BJM), a bacteriologist (CAM) and a clinician (DK). Following this review, all historical data were manually classified into syndromic groups to serve as training examples for the machine learning algorithms. Syndromic definition and manual classification were discussed until consensus was achieved among all experts.

Each submitted case (one or more test requests from a herd on a given day) could have multiple types of samples and/or multiple diagnostic tests requested. Syndromic classification was performed for each individual database entry (test request), and later collapsed by case submission numbers, eliminating repeated syndromes within the same case. As a result, a given case could be associated with multiple syndromes by virtue of clues relating to multiple organ systems found in the same submission.

Mapping of Test Codes

Based on the aforementioned list of syndromic groups, a list of all diagnostic test codes that could be mapped into a syndromic group was established. Mapping is used here to describe the direct relationship: "if test requested is X, then syndromic group is Y",

and mapping rules of this type were established for all test request codes that could be classified into only one syndromic group with certainty. This is typically the case for serological tests, where the veterinarian specifies the pathogen or disease to be confirmed, and the sample type is not informative of the organ system affected, as it is "serum" or "blood".

This mapping was built as a model in RapidMiner 5.0 (Copyright 2001–2010 by Rapid-I and contributors), an open source data mining package, which provides tools for data integration, analytical ETL (extract, transform, load), data analysis and reporting. RapidMiner includes an option to code any learned model in XML format, which can subsequently be directly manipulated.

Observations where test code was not associated with any mapping rule were assigned "Unknown" as the syndromic group at this stage in the processing. These were test requests such as "bacterial culture", which are not informative of the disease suspicion or organ system targeted by the veterinarian. These observations formed an *unmapped* subset of the data.

Algorithms for Automated Syndrome Classification

For the *unmapped* subset, text mining was used to separate all words found in the fields describing the sample type (*client sample ID* and *sample type*, Table 1) in the three years of available data. A tokenization process was applied using any non-letter character as a break point to separate words. The list of all mined words in the historical data was manually reviewed to construct a dictionary of medically relevant terms, as well as acronyms frequently used, and common misspellings. This is similar to the process described in [28] and [29].

Once the dictionary was built, all data tokenization was performed searching only for those specific tokens. For each observation being evaluated, the fields *sample type* and *client sample ID* were tokenized, and a vector was created to designate the binary occurrence of each word in the dictionary. These vectors

Table 2. Syndromic groups, defined based on an evaluation of three years of diagnostic test requests.

Syndromic group	Criteria for syndromic group creation	Number of test requests	Number of cases
Abortion	Clinical sign	559	225
Circulatory	Organ systems	57	50
Eyes and ears		37	20
GIT		8,733	2,564
Haematopoietic		231	199
Hepatic		135	119
Mastitis		49,246	6,766
Musculoskeletal		233	149
Nervous		150	129
Reproductive		857	192
Respiratory		8,501	1,452
Skin and Tegument		14	7
Systemic		3,328	700
Urinary		501	146
BSE*	Individual diseases with high number of test requests	5,306	158
BLV		34,468	3,321
BVD		12,689	2,354
Johnes disease		11,123	2,040
Neosporosis		6,198	1,467
Clinical Pathology (hematology/biochemistry)	Other types of tests	61,059	4,282
Environmental samples		655	58
Antimicrobial susceptibility		140	33
Toxicology		6,866	955
Nonspecific samples	Samples whose syndromic group could not be determined	7,708	3,374
Total		218,795	30,760**

GIT = Gastro-intestinal tract; BSE = Bovine Spongiform Encephalopathy; BLV = Bovine Leukemia Virus; BVD = Bovine Viral Diarrhea.
*BSE test requests are large compared to counts of other test submissions that can be classified as "Nervous".
**The number of cases after classification is higher than the initial number of cases because multiple syndromes can be identified within a single submission.

were then used by the classifier algorithms to learn from the training dataset and to classify test data.

The rule induction algorithm in RapidMiner [Repeated Incremental Pruning to Produce Error Reduction (RIPPER)] was used. Information gain was used as the criterion used for selecting attributes and numerical splits. The sample ratio and pureness were set at 0.9 and the minimal prune benefit 0.25. Using the XML model of rules induced by the RIPPER algorithm as a template, a manually modified set of rules was also explored.

The Naïve Bayes learner available in RapidMiner was used to develop and apply a Naïve Bayes classifier. The learner requires no parameters settings other than an indication of whether a Laplace correction should be used to prevent high influence of zero probabilities. Laplace correction was not used.

Decisions trees were constructed using gain ratio as the criterion for selecting attributes and numerical splits. The minimal size for split was set at 4, minimal leaf size 2, minimal gain 0.1, maximal depth 20, confidence 0.25, and up to 3 pre-pruning alternatives.

The XML code of the models used, as well as the set of customised rules for classification, are available upon request from the first author.

Assessing Algorithms Performance

Due to the large variability in the free-text entered by veterinarians to describe the samples submitted, it was deemed important to have a large test set, in order to assure that classification would be satisfactory once applied to new data. Manually classified historical data were split in half. After sorting sample submissions according to date and submission number, observations were alternately assigned to two different sets. Each classification algorithm was trained using one of the two sets, and then used to classify the alternative set. The process was then repeated switching training and test subsets.

Based on a comparison to the manual classification which had been carried out with the help of experts, the following performance measures were assessed for each classifier (using overall results from both test datasets): recall (the fraction of relevant instances correctly identified by the algorithm); precision (the fraction of the identified instances that were correct), and F_1-score, the harmonic mean of recall and precision; i.e. $(2 * precision * recall) * (precision+recall)^{-1}$. After computing recall, precision and F_1-score for each of the classes, these measures were averaged over all classes to give macro-averaged scores. An average weighted according to the number of records in each of the

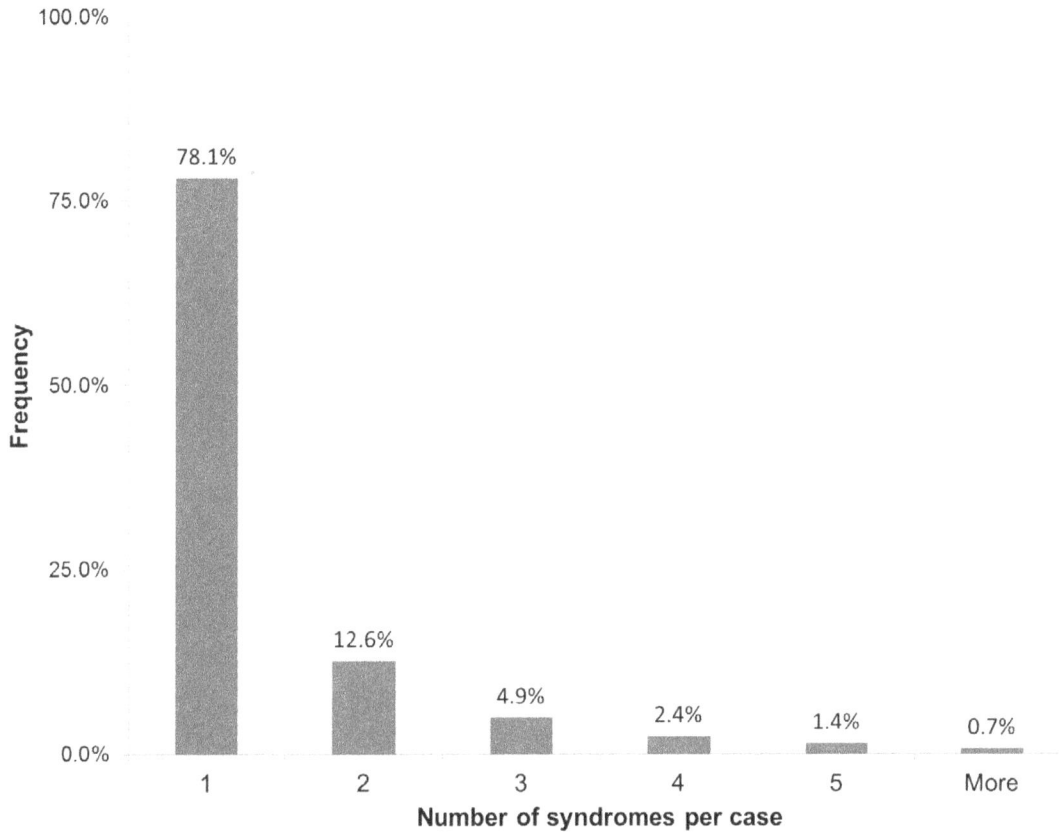

Figure 1. Number of syndromes identified in each case using information from individual test requests.

classes was also calculated; often referred to as micro-averaged scoring.

Stability was investigated by producing slightly different training subsets (for instance removing small random samples from the training set, or eliminating individual syndromic groups at a time), and assessing the resulting difference in the performance of the classifier.

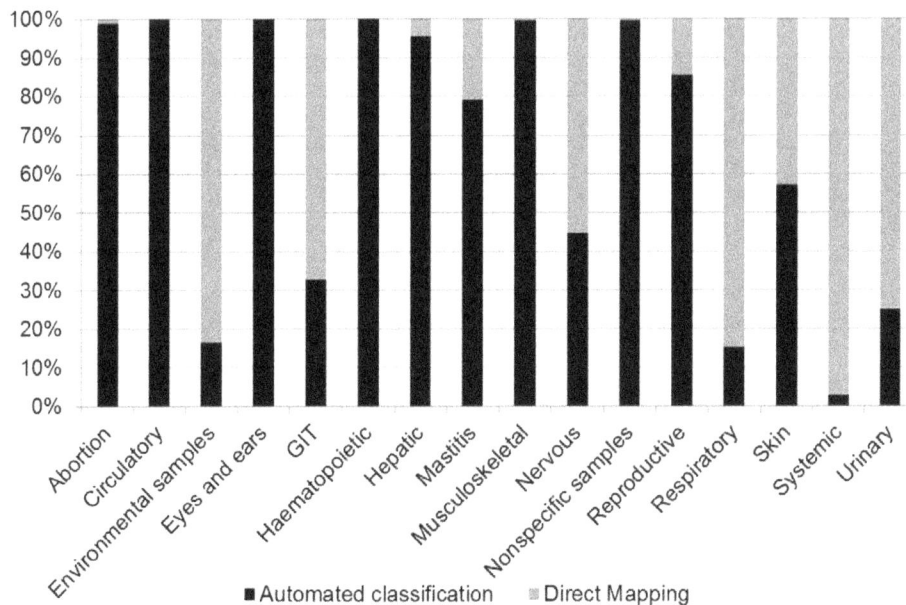

Figure 2. Percentage of test requests classified by direct mapping and automated classification.

Recent Progress in Veterinary Medicine

Table 3. Instances and syndromic groups in the *unmapped* subset of the data.

Syndromic group	Instances	Percentage of total	Cumulative percentage
Mastitis	38,934	73.26%	73.26%
Nonspecific	7,667	14.43%	87.68%
GIT	2,857	5.38%	93.06%
Respiratory	1,309	2.46%	95.52%
Reproductive	732	1.38%	96.90%
Abortion	553	1.04%	97.94%
Musculoskeletal	232	0.44%	98.38%
Haematopoietic	231	0.43%	98.81%
Hepatic	129	0.24%	99.06%
Urinary	125	0.24%	99.29%
Envir. samples	109	0.21%	99.50%
Systemic	98	0.18%	99.68%
Nervous	67	0.13%	99.81%
Circulatory	57	0.11%	99.91%
Eyes and ears	38	0.07%	99.98%
Skin and Tegument	8	0.02%	100.00%
Total	53,146		

Results

The three years of historical data contained 23,221 cases (samples from the same herd on a given day), consisting of a total of 218,795 individual test requests from cattle (i.e. bovine, dairy or beef animals of any age).

Based on an evaluation of these three years of historical data, and input from experts, the syndromic groups listed in Table 2 were defined. The table also lists the criteria for syndromic group creation and the number of test requests and cases assigned to each syndromic group following manual classification.

After classifying all sample submissions, and eliminating repeated syndromic instances within the same case, the final number of "syndromic cases" in the historical dataset was 30,760. Given that there were 23,221 initial herd investigations, this implies an average of 1.32 recorded syndromes per case. The distribution of syndromes per case is shown in Figure 1.

Of all the samples submitted, 75.7% (165,649) could be directly mapped into syndromic groups based on the test request information alone.

For the syndromic groups created based on clinical signs, nonspecific signs or specific organ systems (see Table 2), Figure 2 illustrates the percentage of test requests which could be allocated to a syndromic group via direct mapping versus those that fell into the *unmapped* subset. Around 25% (53,146) of all instances in the database could not be directly mapped into a syndromic group and these provided the material for which automated classification was explored. Although these *unmapped* instances contain 16 of the original 22 defined syndromic groups, the syndromic group "Mastitis" alone is responsible for over 70% of these instances, and three groups ("Mastitis", "Nonspecific" and "GIT") account for over 90% of the data, as shown in Table 3. For the groups Mastitis and GIT, 94% and 77% of the *unmapped* observations, respectively, refer to the test "Bacteria culture". *Unmapped* observations which are ultimately classified as "Nonspecific" contain a greater variety of test names, including the following which occur frequently: "Bacterial culture" (18%), "Histology" (27%) and "Necropsy" (18%).

The results of automated classification using different algorithms are shown in Table 4 and described in detail below.

The use of rule induction (RIPPER) achieved only moderate performance overall. Three groups with low frequency of test requests – "Environmental samples", "Skin", and Eyes and Ears" – were not included in the rules, but as shown in Table 3 these groups represent only 0.3% of all instances subjected to automated classification. The F_1-macro average was 0.677, but because the unlearned groups account for such a small proportion of the submissions, when the classes' performance is averaged accounting for the weight of each class, the $F_{1\text{-micro}}$ is 0.979 (Table 4). Upon manual review of the rules created by the algorithm, it was found that the main source of error was failure of the algorithm to establish good decision rules when multiple medically relevant words were found in the same test request. This method was easy to implement and the rules generated are transparent and easily interpreted.

The rules produced by the RIPPER algorithm were manually modified to account for some of the relationships missed, producing a set of custom rules. Running the custom rule set against the entire *unmapped* subset resulted in an $F_{1\text{-macro}}$ score of 0.997, and $F_{1\text{-micro}}$ score of 0.9995 (Table 4). The remaining errors tended to be due to use of abbreviations not common enough to have been incorporated in the rules, misspellings or the absence of a space between two words, resulting in the tokenization process failing to identify these words.

The performance of the Naïve Bayes algorithm was high ($F_{1\text{-macro}}$ of 0.955 and $F_{1\text{-micro}}$ 0.994), as shown in Table 4. The main performance issue associated with this algorithm was its instability. Slightly different datasets resulted in very different performances (results not shown). With unbalanced training and test datasets, for

Table 4. Performance measures for the algorithms implemented.

Algorithm	Class average (Macro)*			Weighted average (micro)		
	recall	precision	F-score	recall	precision	F-score
Manually modified rules	.994	1.000	.997	1.000	1.000	1.000
Rule Induction**	.626	.793	.677	.991	.981	.979
Naïve Bayes	.983	.939	.955	.994	.996	.994
Decision Trees**	.290	.416	.311	.936	.937	.923

*The total number of groups in the training data was 16, and the total number of instances 53,146.
**The Rule Induction algorithms failed to learn 3 classes, and the Decision Tree 11 classes.

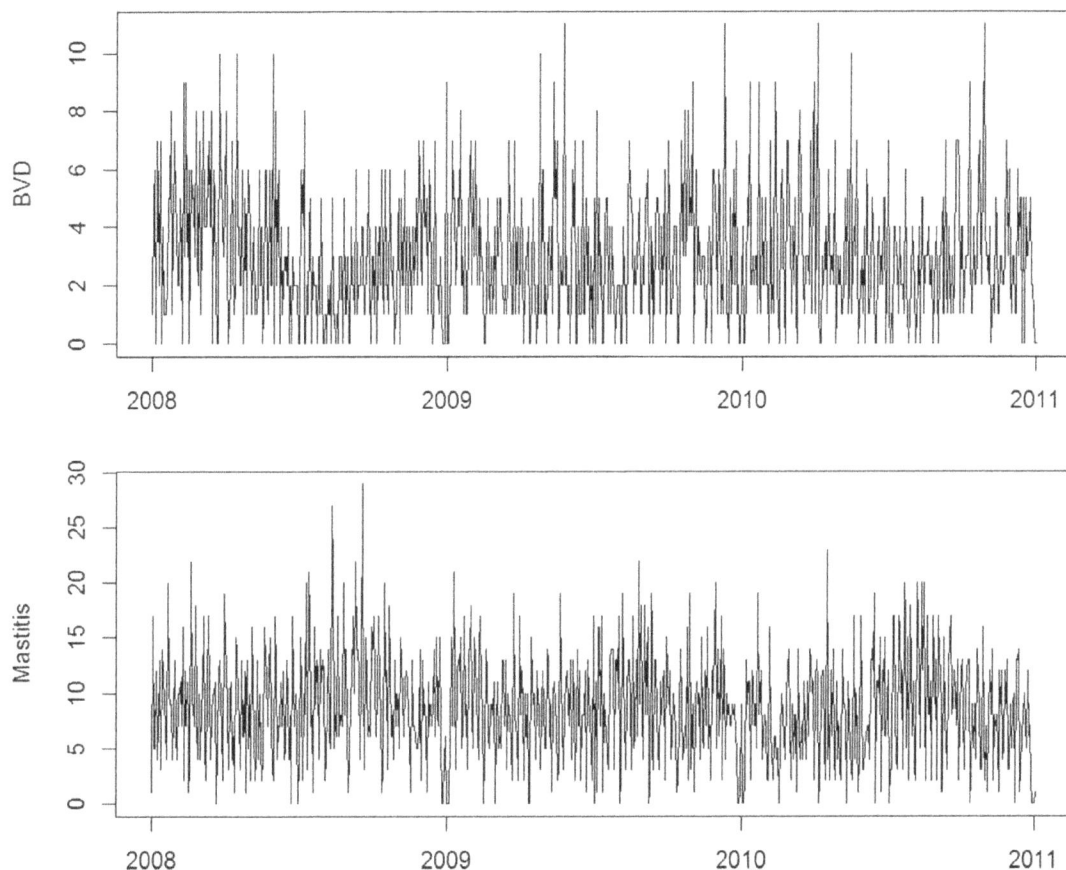

Figure 3. Daily counts of cases allocated to Bovine Viral Diarrhea (top) and Mastitis (bottom) syndromes.

instance, rather than assigning the label "Nonspecific" to samples that could not be classified, the Naïve Bayes algorithm would assign these samples, as well as misclassified samples from other groups, into one of the groups with a small number of submissions.

The classifier based on Decision Trees performed reasonably well in the micro score ($F_{1\text{-micro}}$ score of 0.923). However the classifier failed to learn 9 classes, which are biologically relevant, despite accounting for only 2% of the *unmapped* instances (which explains the high micro average). Moreover, the models appeared to be unstable: slight changes in the training data could result in a completely different 'shape' of decision tree, and a similar phenomenon was observed when the initial parameters for minimal gain and confidence where varied.

Discussion

This study evaluated the classification of structured data from animal laboratory test requests into syndromic groups for surveillance. This type of data lacks specificity not only because it precedes diagnostic results, but also due to the limited amount of clinical information provided by veterinarians. Previous work has focused on the direct mapping of specific test requests to syndromic groups [25,26]. Here the use of text-mining was explored to extract information from fields containing a description of the sample collected by the veterinarian, in order to identify the organ system(s) affected in the clinical case being investigated.

Due to the structured format of the data, the text-mining task did not need to account for sentence semantics or other contextual information. Statistical methods were sufficient to capture the

majority of medically relevant information from the fields mined. The binary occurrence of words from a manually constructed dictionary served as input to the classifier. The algorithms needed therefore to learn the relationship between these words, their co-occurrences and the target syndromic group.

Rule induction is suitable for uncovering these types of regular relations [28], and is recommended in cases when improvements in accuracy can be achieved by incorporating relationships among attributes [30]. However, upon manual review of the rules created by the algorithm, it was found that performance could be improved by including specific relationships in cases of multiple word occurrences. It was noted that the main relationships that the rule induction had failed to capture involved:

(i)   Sampling of multiple organs. For instance *heart* was associated with the "Circulatory" syndrome, and *liver* with "Gastro-intestinal", but the observation of samples from both organs in the same test request should be classified as "Systemic".

(ii)   Precedence being given to some words. "Abortion" is an actual clinical syndrome, in contrast to all other groups based on organ systems. Therefore the observation of any words related to abortion (*fetus, placenta, aborted,* etc) should result in classification of "Abortion", regardless of what fetal organ(s) was(were) collected.

(iii) The co-occurrence of words which have a different meaning than when they occur on their own. For instance *ear* is a word included in the dictionary of relevant terms and would typically be associated with the "Eyes and ears" syndrome; however, this word should be ignored when it appears in the expression *ear tag*, which refers only to animal identification within a herd.

These relationships are still simpler than typical contextual challenges associated with full textual analysis, and the set of manually modified rules exhibited high performance. The remaining issues that prevented correct classification, such as misspellings and inconsistent abbreviations relate to the quality of the data, something which often complicates the interpretation of syndromic information [31].

The rule-based algorithm using manually modified rules was considered the most suitable algorithm for the classification of the animal laboratory dataset at hand, due to its high accuracy, ease of implementation, and high interpretability/transparency. Although simple, this rule-based solution is in line with research reporting from the i2b2 Obesity Challenge. Among the top 10 performing systems, rule-based approaches were the most successful in the textual task, which required classification based on documented information [12].

Rules also have the advantage that they are transparent and can typically be easily interpreted by the collaborating health experts [28]. Their main disadvantage is the knowledge acquisition bottleneck, in the case where rules are manually created, limiting portability and flexibility [28,32]. Updates in the future to accommodate changes in the language may have to be implemented manually, rather than in an automated manner.

The Naïve Bayes classifier demonstrated high performance. The main limitation observed with the use of this algorithm was its instability when groups with low frequency were included in the dataset. This behavior has been documented elsewhere [29]. The algorithm assumes that parameters are independent [32]. In this context the parameters were the binary occurrences, within each record, of the keywords from the dictionary built. Instability was however not observed to be due to occurrence of multiple keywords; rather it was associated with groups having small numbers of training examples. Due to the fact that the Naïve Bayes approach exhibits low transparency, it was not possible to track the specific mechanisms causing the problems observed in these low frequency categories, or to instigate measures to improve the way the algorithm was recording and using relationships between samples and the classification groups.

If transparency is not a limiting issue, that is, if domain knowledge experts are not required to understand and review the way by which the classifier is making decisions and classifying each instance, the Naïve Bayes algorithm can be an alternative to manually modified rules. Besides the high performance – though not as high as the custom set of rules – its implementation was the easiest of all algorithms evaluated, and automated updates can be planned by retraining the algorithm at regular intervals.

Nonmetric methods, such as Decision Trees, provide a "natural way to incorporate prior knowledge from human experts" [30]. However, this algorithm performed very poorly when small frequency groups were present; completely missing up to nine syndromic groups. Decision Trees were also very unstable to small changes on the data. This type of behaviour, in terms of training set sensitivity, has been well documented for Decision Trees [30].

The high performance reported in this study for the rule-based classifier refers to the algorithm's ability to reproduce the manual classification of records provided by a human expert. This classification, however, is based on an active review of test orders and diagnostic specimens submitted. Clinical descriptions are not normally submitted by veterinarians, and were not available for use in the classification of records, which constitutes a limitation to the classification process. While the lack of clinical information is expected to reduce the precision and recall of the system in comparison to the actual syndromes observed by the veterinarians, the consistency of the classifier and its high accuracy in utilising the information that is available should allow the system to capture increases in the number of submissions across different syndromic groups. Figure 3 illustrates the time series of daily counts, constructed after data had been classified using the rule-based algorithm, for two syndromic groups with expected seasonal behaviour: Bovine Viral Diarrhea and Mastitis. The series reflect the expected seasonal patterns, which supports the conjecture that classified records successfully reflect real trends in the number of submissions for various syndromes.

The development of this system has been conducted at the request of the data providers and the Ontario Ministry of Agriculture Food and Rural Affairs, which is responsible for the animal surveillance activities in the province of Ontario. The system has benefited greatly from the automated extraction of surveillance information from this animal health database. As the information extraction was based on data already regularly submitted to the AHL without any requirement for passive or active collection of additional data, sustainability of the system is not expected to be an issue.

Conclusion

Real-time monitoring of animal health data depends on establishing reliable models that reflect medical knowledge and that can be applied in an automated manner. Such models should be efficient, but also comprehensible to end users.

In this study the structured format of laboratory data, and the use of standard test codes, allowed for classification of approximately 75% of test requests into syndromic groups using direct mapping. For the remainder of the data, high accuracy (F_1-macro $= 0.997$) was achieved through the use of a rule-based syndrome classifier. Induced rules were manually modified during the construction phase, but resulted in clear interpretability of decisions and resulting classification. While the use of rules was easy to implement and interpret, the construction of a dictionary of medically relevant terms and the manipulation of rules were time-consuming steps. Implementation of similar systems making use of other sources of laboratory data should be easier facilitated as standardized languages are more widely adopted in animal health laboratories, avoiding the repetition of this process for every new database.

The use of a custom rule set limits the potential for automatic revision of the classification model. Further research is required to establish internal validation rules, possibly based on the results available from historical data, in order to define automated ways to carry out model updates in the future.

Acknowledgments

The authors thank the Animal Health Laboratory for supplying the data analysed in this study.

Author Contributions

Conceived and designed the experiments: FCD JS CWR DK CAM JTM BJM WBM. Performed the experiments: FCD JS CWR. Analyzed the data: FCD JS CWR DK CAM JTM BJM WBM. Contributed reagents/materials/analysis tools: FCD JS CWR BJM WBM. Wrote the paper: FCD JS CWR DK CAM JTM BJM WBM.

References

1. Bravata DM, McDonald KM, Smith WM, Rydzak C, Szeto H, et al. (2004) Systematic review: surveillance systems for early detection of bioterrorism-related diseases. Ann Intern Med 140(11): 910–922.
2. Zeng D, Chen H, Castillo-Chavez C, Lober WB, Thurmong M (2011) Infectious Disease Informatics and Biosurveillance. New York: Springer Science+Business Media, Inc. 488 p.
3. Mandl KD, Reis B, Cassa C (2004) Measuring outbreak-detection performance by using controlled feature set simulations. MMWR Morb Mortal Wkly Rep 53 Suppl: 130–136.
4. Wagner MM, Tsui FC, Espino JU, Dato VM, Sittig DF, et al. (2001) The emerging science of very early detection of disease outbreaks. J Public Health Man 7(6): 51–59.
5. Centers for Disease Control and Prevention (CDC). Annotated Bibliography for Syndromic Surveillance; 2006. Available: http://www.cdc.gov/ncphi/disss/nndss/syndromic.htm. Accessed 2010 Jun 17.
6. Ivanov O, Wagner MM, Chapman WW, Olszewski RT (2002) Accuracy of three classifiers of acute gastrointestinal syndrome for syndromic surveillance. AMIA Ann Symp Proc: 345–349.
7. Lober WB, Trigg L, Karras B (2004) Information system architectures for syndromic surveillance. MMWR Morb Mortal Wkly Rep 53 Suppl: 203–208.
8. Chapman WW, Christensen LM, Wagner MM, Haug PJ, Ivanov O, et al. (2005) Classifying free-text triage chief complaints into syndromic categories with natural language processing. Artif Intell Med 33(1): 31–40.
9. Dara J, Dowling JN, Travers D, Cooper GF, Chapman WW (2008) Evaluation of preprocessing techniques for chief complaint classification. J Biomed Inform 41(4): 613–623.
10. Reis BY, Mandl KD (2004) Syndromic surveillance: the effects of syndrome grouping on model accuracy and outbreak detection. Ann Emerg Med 44(3): 235–241.
11. Wagner MM, Espino J, Tsui FC, Gesteland P, Chapman W, et al. (2004) Syndrome and outbreak detection using chief-complaint data–experience of the Real-Time Outbreak and Disease Surveillance project. MMWR Morb Mortal Wkly Rep Rep 53 Suppl: 28–31.
12. Uzuner O (2009) Recognizing obesity and comorbidities in sparse data. J Am Med Inform Assn 16(4): 561–570.
13. Maimon O, Rokach L (2005) Decision Trees. In: Maimon O, Rokach L, editors. Data Mining and Knowledge Discovery Handbook. New York: Springer Science+Business Media, Inc. 165–192.
14. Zhang PG. Neural Networks (2005) In:Maimon O, Rokach L, editors. Data Mining and Knowledge Discovery Handbook. New York: Springer Science+Business Media, Inc. 487–516.
15. Shmilovici A (2005) Support Vector Machines. In: Maimon O, Rokach L, editors. Data Mining and Knowledge Discovery Handbook. New York: Springer Science+Business Media, Inc. 257–276.
16. Rohatgi PK (2011) Radiological evaluation of interstitial lung disease. Curr Opin Pulm Med 17(5): 337–345.
17. Shiraishi J, Li Q, Appelbaum D, Doi K (2011) Computer-Aided Diagnosis and Artificial Intelligence in Clinical Imaging. Semin Nucl Med 41(6): 449–62.
18. Wesolowski M, Suchacz B (2012) Artificial neural networks: theoretical background and pharmaceutical applications: a review. J AOAC Int. 95(3): 652–668.
19. Ma H, Rolka H, Mandl K, Buckeridge D, Fleischauer A, et al. (2005) Implementation of laboratory order data in BioSense Early Event Detection and Situation Awareness System. MMWR Morb Mortal Wkly Rep. 54 Suppl: 27–30.
20. Kelly TK, Chalk P, Bonomo J, Parachini J, Jackson BA, et al. (2004) The Office of Science and Technology Policy Blue Ribbon Panel on the Threat of Biological Terrorism Directed Against Livestock. Washington, DC. December 8–9, 2003. ISBN: 0-8330-3633-5.
21. Davis RG (2004) The ABCs of bioterrorism for veterinarians, focusing on Category A agents. JAVMA-J Am Vet Med A. 224(7): 1084–1095.
22. Babin S, Witt C, Casper J, Wojcik RA, Lewis SLH, et al. (2003) Syndromic animal surveillance in the Electronic Surveillance System for the Early Notification of Community-based Epidemics (ESSENCE). Presented by C. Witt at the National Multi-Hazard Symposium: "One Medicine" Approach to Homeland Security, Research Triangle Park, NC, 11–12 December.
23. Goplin J, Benz M (2007) North Dakota Electronic Animal health Surveillance System. Adv Dis Surv. 4(1): 8.
24. North Carolina Department of Agriculture and Consumer Services (2010) Multi-Hazard Threat Database (MHTD). Available: http://www.ncagr.gov/oep/MHTD/index.htm. Accessed: 2010 Sep 9.
25. Glickman LT, Moore GE, Glickman NW, Caldanaro RJ, Aucoin D, et al. (2006) Purdue University-Banfield National Companion Animal Surveillance Program for emerging and zoonotic diseases. Vector-Borne Zoonot. 6(1): 14–23.
26. Shaffer LE, Funk JA, Rajala-Schultz P, Wagner MM, Wittum TE, et al. (2008) Evaluation of Microbiology Orders from a Veterinary Diagnostic Laboratory as a Potential Data Source for Early Outbreak Detection. Adv Dis Surv 6(2): 1–7.
27. Dórea FC, Sanchez J, Revie CW (2011) Veterinary syndromic surveillance: Current initiatives and potential for development. Prev Vet Med101(1–2): 1–17.
28. Solt I, Tikk D, Gál V, Kardkovács ZT (2009) Semantic classification of diseases in discharge summaries using a context-aware rule-based classifier. J Am Med Inform Assn. 16(4): 580–584.
29. Farkas R, Szarvas G, Hegedus I, Almasi A, Vincze V, et al. (2009) Semi-automated construction of decision rules to predict morbidities from clinical texts. J Am Med Inform Assn. 16(4): 601–605.
30. Duda RO, Hart PE, Stork DG (2001) Pattern Classification. New York: John Wiley and Sons, Inc.; 2001. 680p.
31. Shmueli G, Burkom H (2010) Statistical Challenges Facing Early Outbreak Detection in Biosurveillance. Technom 52: 39–51.
32. Sebastiani F (2002) Machine learning in automated text categorization. ACM Comp Surv 34(1): 1–47.

15

Local Cattle and Badger Populations Affect the Risk of Confirmed Tuberculosis in British Cattle Herds

Flavie Vial[1]*, W. Thomas Johnston[2], Christl A. Donnelly[1]

1 Department of Infectious Disease Epidemiology, MRC Centre for Outbreak Analysis and Modelling, School of Public Health, Imperial College London, London, United Kingdom, 2 Department of Health Sciences, University of York, York, United Kingdom

Abstract

Background: The control of bovine tuberculosis (bTB) remains a priority on the public health agenda in Great Britain, after launching in 1998 the Randomised Badger Culling Trial (RBCT) to evaluate the effectiveness of badger (*Meles meles*) culling as a control strategy. Our study complements previous analyses of the RBCT data (focusing on treatment effects) by presenting analyses of herd-level risks factors associated with the probability of a confirmed bTB breakdown in herds within each treatment: repeated widespread proactive culling, localized reactive culling and no culling (survey-only).

Methodology/Principal Findings: New cases of bTB breakdowns were monitored inside the RBCT areas from the end of the first proactive badger cull to one year after the last proactive cull. The risk of a herd bTB breakdown was modeled using logistic regression and proportional hazard models adjusting for local farm-level risk factors. Inside survey-only and reactive areas, increased numbers of active badger setts and cattle herds within 1500 m of a farm were associated with an increased bTB risk. Inside proactive areas, the number of *M. bovis* positive badgers initially culled within 1500 m of a farm was the strongest predictor of the risk of a confirmed bTB breakdown.

Conclusions/Significance: The use of herd-based models provide insights into how local cattle and badger populations affect the bTB breakdown risks of individual cattle herds in the absence of and in the presence of badger culling. These measures of local bTB risks could be integrated into a risk-based herd testing programme to improve the targeting of interventions aimed at reducing the risks of bTB transmission.

Editor: Anthony Fooks, Veterinary Laboratories Agency, United Kingdom

Funding: The authors gratefully acknowledge the support of the U.K. Department of Environment, Food and Rural Affairs (Defra; http://www.defra.gov.uk/index.htm) for this work. CAD thanks the U.K. Medical Research Council (MRC; http://www.mrc.ac.uk/index.htm) for Centre funding. The funders had no role in the design of the analyses, data analysis, decision to publish, or preparation (drafting, editing or finalizing) of the manuscript. The Randomised Badger Culling Trial (RBCT) was implemented by the staff of Defra and its associated agencies. Defra funds the ongoing collection and storage of routine surveillance data which were utilized in this study. Defra officials commented on a near-final draft of this manuscript.

Competing Interests: The authors have declared that no competing interests exist.

* E-mail: f.vial@imperial.ac.uk

Introduction

Bovine tuberculosis (bTB) remains an important public health concern worldwide as a result of deficiencies in preventing and/or controlling measures targeting the spread of its causative agent *Mycobacterium bovis* [1,2]. While the risk posed by *M. bovis* to human health is low in most developed countries, the main causes of concern related to *M. bovis* in industrialized countries are epizootics in domesticated and wild mammal populations [2]. Infection with *M. bovis* remains a significant livestock zoonosis in the European Union where some member states experience a reemergence of the disease despite significant historical efforts to implement eradication plans. In Great Britain, the disease was eliminated from most cattle herds by 1960, with the exception of infection hotspots in southwest England, after the implementation of a herd testing and slaughter policy [3]. However, efforts to completely eradicate bTB in Great Britain have been hampered by the maintenance of *M. bovis* in wildlife host populations, acting as reservoirs of infection, in particular badgers (*Meles meles*) [4]. Since 1979, incidence in British cattle has increased and the infection has become more geographically widespread [5]. Over 7

million cattle were tested for bovine bTB in 2009 and one in ten herds experienced bTB-related movement restrictions during the year [6] as a result of at least one member of the herd failing the tuberculin skin test or showing lesions consistent with bTB during the slaughterhouse inspection – an event known as a "herd breakdown".

Risk factors associated with bTB have been investigated in case-control studies in Europe and the USA [7,8,9,10,11,12,13,14]. Historical incidence of bTB was found to be a robust predictor of the rate of future outbreaks in both Irish [15] and British [16] herds, an indication that the source of the disease failed to be eliminated and/or that some factors in those areas make them particularly suitable for the recurrence of infection in cattle. Herd size has repeatedly been identified as one of the major bTB herd-level risk factor [16,17,18]. Large herds tend to pasture on larger areas, with higher probabilities of contiguous herds thereby facilitating cattle to cattle spread of *M. bovis* [7]. A comparative case-control study in England between 1995 and 1999 revealed that herd size was a significant predictor of both transient and persistent bTB breakdowns and associated herd size with management-related risk factors such as turnover rates, farm enterprise and feeding [10]. The same study also revealed that farms with higher stocking density showed a significantly reduced risk of a bTB breakdown [10]. Farm size, in terms of number of holdings but not total area farmed, was found to be associated with an increased bTB risk in England beyond any effect of herd size [9]. Cattle housing-type and feeding [9,10] as well as cattle purchase and movement [9,19,20] onto the farm have also been associated with an increased risk of bTB breakdown. With older animals being more likely to have been exposed to *M. bovis* than younger ones [7], dairy cattle, with their longer life expectancy tend to be more at risk of bTB than their beef counterparts [15,18,21]. Other differences in terms of management are involved such as higher production stress under intensive management conditions [13] and the twice-daily gathering of cattle during milking which increases the risk of transmission through the respiratory route [22].

M. bovis can infect a wide range of wild animals [23,24]. Brush-tail possums (*Trichosurus vulpecula*) are the primary wildlife reservoir of bovine bTB in New Zealand [25], while white-tail deer (*Odocoileus virginianus*) in Michigan [26], the wood bison in Canada (*Bison bison athabascae*) [27], the buffalo (*Syncerus caffer*) in Southern Africa [28], the wild boar (*Sus scrofa*) in Southern Europe [29,30] and badgers in Western Europe [4] have become maintenance hosts for *M. bovis*. The Randomised Badger Culling Trial (RBCT) was launched in 1998 to evaluate the effectiveness of badger culling as a control strategy for bTB in Britain [8]. The RBCT involved comparing the incidence of cattle bTB under three experimental treatments — repeated widespread ("proactive") culling, localized ("reactive") culling, and no culling ("survey-only") — each replicated ten times in large (100 km²) trial areas recruited as matched sets of three, known as "triplets". Detailed field surveys in all trial areas for which consent was obtained (see Methods) were undertaken to record the location of badger setts and other field signs of badgers such as latrines and paths. Culling in proactive areas did not start simultaneously in all triplets, with initial proactive culls ranging from December 1998 for triplet B to December 2002 for triplet D. The final proactive cull was completed in late 2005. Many earlier analyses of the RBCT have been published [9,31,32,33,34,35,36,37,38,39,40], and more details on the RBCT itself can be found in the supplementary information of [36].

In this paper, we present new analyses of spatial herd-level risks factors associated with the probability of bTB breakdowns in herds within the RBCT following the first proactive cull. We examine the extent to which proactive badger culling decreased the bTB risk for the herds involved. We also examine the impact of various local herd-level risk factors within each of the trial group (proactive, survey-only and reactive) to identify the most important bTB breakdown risk factors for herds within the RBCT areas.

Materials and Methods

Description of the dataset

The Defra animal health information system (VETNET) provided data on cattle bTB tests and herd breakdowns, distinguishing between "confirmed breakdowns" (incidents in which postmortem examination of slaughtered cattle led to detection of bTB lesions or culture of *M. bovis*) from "unconfirmed breakdowns" (incidents in which one or more cattle reacted to the tuberculin test but infection was not confirmed at postmortem or by culture). Herds with the same County Parish Holding Herd numbers (CPHH: unique herd identifier) which were registered in different treatment groups (n = 14); herds which were archived before the start of the RBCT (n = 22) and herds which showed no evidence of having had a bTB disclosing test during the RBCT (n = 745) were removed from the VETNET records; leaving us with 1306 unique herds recorded in RBCT proactive areas, 1380 unique herds recorded in RBCT survey-only areas and 1320 unique herds recorded in RBCT reactive areas.

Here our analyses were based on the number of confirmed herd breakdowns within treatment groups using information on herd location within trial areas (Table 1). In addition, a survival (or time-to-breakdown) time for each herd was calculated as the time from the end of the initial proactive cull to their first confirmed herd breakdown or to the date of the end of the trial for that triplet or to the date the herd was archived, whichever came first. In the latter case, the time-to-breakdown time was censored. Consent to survey and cull was sought from land owners in all trial areas before random allocation of the treatments and during the course of the trial (Table 2). Following treatment allocation, initial culls were conducted on all land in the proactive areas for which consent was given between 1998 and 2002. These were followed by approximately annual culls until 2005, except during 2001 when culling was suspended during the nationwide epidemic of foot-and-mouth disease. Measures of badger activity before the first proactive cull are described in detail in ref [36].

Table 1. Number of cattle herds with and without confirmed bTB breakdowns between the completion of the initial proactive cull and up to one year following the last proactive cull in each of the RBCT triplets.

Triplet	Region	Completion of initial proactive cull	Herds with no bTB breakdown	Herds with ≥1 bTB breakdown
A	Gloucestershire/Herefordshire	Jan-2000	182	114
B	North Cornwall/North Devon	Dec-1998	331	153
C	East Cornwall	Oct-1999	355	166
D	Herefordshire	Dec-2002	177	105
E	North Wiltshire	May-2000	208	108
F	West Cornwall	July-2000	433	107
G	Derby/Staffordshire	Nov-2000	417	131
H	Devon/Somerset	Dec-2000	236	85
I	Gloucestershire	Oct-2002	197	79
J	Devon	Oct-2002	316	106

Table 2. The mean number of badger setts identified during the initial survey and badgers culled during the first proactive cull on and around farms for all three treatment groups.

	% of landholders refusing access [1] (total)	Mean number of badger setts identified during the initial survey		Mean number of badgers culled during the first proactive cull (*M. bovis* +)	
		on the farms	within a 1500 m buffer	on the farms	within a 1500 m buffer
Survey-only	12% (1380)	1.90	26.76	NA	NA
Proactive	11% (1306)	2.04	29.97	1.95 (0.66)	27.27 (2.87)
Reactive	10% (1320)	2.25	28.95	NA	NA

[1]Some landholders did not consent to survey and/or cull badgers on their land.

The variables. On the basis of details recorded in the RBCT database, farms were categorized into one of three enterprise types: beef, dairy and other (a composite category including calf rearers, dealers, exempt finishing units, heifer rearers, house cows, mixed herds and stores). The median herd size was 72 animals (mean = 102, standard error = 1.7) [Supplementary Information S1]. The historic incidence of cattle bTB (number of confirmed herd breakdowns) was calculated for each trial area, for the three-year period before the initial proactive cull, except in triplets D, I and J where it was calculated for the three years prior to the start of the 2001 foot-and-mouth disease epidemic (median = 25 confirmed breakdowns, mean = 25.37, s.e. = 0.12) [Supplementary Information S1]. The median number of baseline herds in the triplets (number of herds recorded for that triplet at the time of the initial badger cull) was 124 (mean = 133.70, s.e. = 0.74). Some farms operate on more than one land parcel (defined as a discrete piece of land discontinuous with neighbouring land). Farm area was then computed as the combined area of all land parcels belonging to a particular farm. Most farms operated from two land parcels (median = 2, mean = 2.14, s.e. = 0.03, max = 16) and median farm area was estimated at 0.50 km^2 (mean = 0.69, s.e. = 0.012).

Data on the number/density of badgers culled, the number/density of *M. bovis* positive (+) badgers culled, the number/density of active badger setts and the number/density of neighbouring cattle herds within 500, 1000 and 1500 m of all the land parcels belonging to a farm were extracted from the RBCT geodatabase (ArcGIS version 9, ESRI) [Supplementary Information S1]. On land parcels for which consent to survey and/or cull was given, distinct badger and sett-related variables could be produced to reflect numbers/densities on the land parcels themselves versus numbers/densities on the buffer surrounding the parcels. When consent to cull and/or survey was not obtained (Table 2), trapping along the boundaries of the parcels for which consent was refused allowed staff to catch a proportion of the badgers residing in the no-access farm. The area of the farm and the buffer was thus used when calculating the density of badgers trapped (on both the parcels and the buffer) but not when calculating sett density (which could only be estimated inside the surveyed buffer)[Supplementary Information S1].

Statistical analyses

The significance of the following local farm-level risk factors were assessed (herd type, herd size, farm area within the triplet, the number of baseline herds, historic incidence within the trial areas, and the number of premises operated by the farm in the first instance) and subsequent models were adjusted accordingly. A distinction was made for badger-related and sett-related variables between the number of badgers culled or setts recorded on the farm's land parcels and those on the buffer surrounding the farm.

This distinction was only retained in the multivariable models if significant. The badger-related, sett-related and herd-related variables which demonstrated the most significant univariable associations with the risk of confirmed herd breakdowns were retained for multivariable model building. All models adjusted either for herd type, herd size, farm area (models A); for herd type, herd size, farm area and historic bTB incidence (models B) or for herd type, herd size, farm area and triplet [Supplementary Information S1]. Models were constructed by backward elimination, starting with a full model with quadratic terms for each non-categorical variable. Variables were eliminated on the basis of their significance in the model as well as their contribution to the variation in the data by means of an analysis of variance using a F-test (for the logistic regressions) or a likelihood ratio test (LRT) in which twice the difference in log-likelihoods was compared to a Chi-square (χ^2) distribution otherwise. An F-test was chosen for the logistic regressions as a result of overdispersion in our data. To minimize bias in the covariates, 0.5 was added before log-transforming all non-categorical variables.

Probability of confirmed bTB herd breakdown. Using the herds that did not experience any bTB breakdown during the period under study as controls, we used logistic regression to compare the probability of one or more confirmed herd bTB breakdowns for each herd recorded inside trial areas subjected to the proactive and survey-only treatments. In addition, we used logistic regression to model the probability of one or more confirmed bTB herd breakdowns during the period under study for each herd within a particular treatment (proactive, reactive or survey-only). Variables were individually screened using logistic regression controlling for local farm-level risks [Supplementary Information S1]. P-values were adjusted for overdispersion, when present, by using an inflation factor equal to the square root of the model deviance divided by the degrees of freedom. An assessment of the goodness-of-fit was obtained by examining the models' residuals.

Time to first confirmed bTB herd breakdown. Analysis of these data was undertaken using proportional hazards (PH) models, comparing the time to the first confirmed bTB breakdown for herds recorded inside trial areas subjected to the proactive and survey-only treatments. PH models were also used to predict the time to first confirmed breakdown for herds within a particular treatment group (proactive, reactive or survey-only). The badger-related, sett-related and herd-related variables which demonstrated the most significant univariable associations with time to first confirmed bTB herd breakdown were then retained for multivariable model building controlling for local farm-level risks [Supplementary Information S1]. The proportional-hazards assumption was tested for each covariate, by correlating the scaled

Schoenfeld residuals with the Kaplan-Meier estimate of the survival function [41]. Other model diagnostics included checking the martingale residuals to detect non-linearity.

Results

Data from 4006 herds were available for the analysis: 343 out of 1306 proactive herds, 408 out of 1380 survey-only herds and 403 out of 1320 reactive herds experienced a confirmed bTB breakdown between the completion of the initial proactive badger cull within their triplet and one year following their final proactive cull.

Probability of confirmed bTB herd breakdown

Overall, when comparing the probabilities of confirmed herd bTB breakdowns during the period under study between proactive and survey-only herds, we found that the best model included effects of triplet (p = 0.04), herd type, herd size, farm area and the historic bTB incidence for that trial area. The analyses of variance showed that the number of land parcels belonging to the farm (p = 0.79) and the number of baseline herds were not significant (p = 0.45). Culling treatment (p = 0.07) was also non-significant although there was a trend for reduced bTB risks among herds in proactively culled areas (OR: 1.19, 95% CI: 0.98–1.44).

Herds categorized under the "other" enterprise type, had a similar risk of bTB breakdown to that of beef herds (p = 0.75), so both types were then merged to create a "non-dairy" group. Dairy herds showed a significantly higher risk of bTB breakdown (p = 0.014) compared to non-dairy herds (OR: 1.30, 95% CI: 1.09–1.75). Larger herds (p<0.001, OR: 1.20, 95% CI: 1.13, 1.26) and bigger farms presented an increased risk of bTB breakdown (p<0.001, OR: 1.30, 95% CI: 1.22–1.39). The odds ratio here are interpreted as a doubling of the herd size or of farm area resulting in a 20% and 30% increase, respectively, in the odds of a bTB breakdown. As expected, historic bTB incidence for trial area of the herd was also a significant predictor (p<0.001) of its probability of experiencing a bTB breakdown after the initial proactive cull (OR: 2.25, 95% CI: 1.96, 2.54 corresponding to a doubling of the historic incidence).

Within survey-only areas. The number of active badger setts (both on the land parcels and outside but within 500 m) as well as the number of cattle herds within 500 m of all land parcels were the best individual predictors of the probability of a confirmed bTB breakdown for survey-only herds during the period under study [Supplementary Information S1]. Both variables remained significant predictors in the multivariable logistic model (Table 3). An increase in the number of active setts and cattle herds within the 500 m wide buffer surrounding the farm's land parcels resulted in an increased bTB risk (Table 3). Both risk factors were consistent across the 1000 m and 1500 m wide buffer [Supplementary Information S1].

Within proactive areas. The number of M. bovis positive culled badgers, the number of active badger setts (both on the land parcels and outside but within 500 m) as well as the density of cattle herds within 500 m of the land parcels were the best individual predictors of the probability of a confirmed bTB breakdown for proactive herds during the period under study [Supplementary Information S1]. The number of M. bovis positive badgers that were culled outside but within 500 m of the land parcels belonging to a farm remained the only significant predictor in the multivariable logistic model. An increase in the number of M. bovis positive badgers culled within the 500 m wide buffer surrounding the farm's land parcels resulted in an increased bTB risk (Table 3). The risk factor was consistent across the 1000 m

and 1500 m wide buffer [Supplementary Information S1]. Although non-significant, the number of active badger setts (p = 0.50, OR: 1.05, 95% CI: 0.92–1.17 corresponding to a doubling in the number of setts) and the number of cattle herds (p = 0.50, OR: 1.08, 95% CI: 0.86–1.29 corresponding to a doubling in the number of herds) outside but within 500 m of the lands parcels (risk factors indentified for the survey herds) resulted in a marginal increase in bTB risk (model B). Thus, these effects were in the same direction as those observed in survey-only areas.

Within reactive areas. The density of active badger setts (both on the land parcels and outside but within 500 m) as well as the number of cattle herds within 500 m of the land parcels were the best individual predictors of the probability of a confirmed bTB breakdown for reactive herds [Supplementary Information S1]. The number of cattle herds inside a 500 m wide buffer surrounding all land parcels belonging to a farm remained the only significant predictor in the multivariable logistic model of the probability of a confirmed bTB herd breakdown. An increase in the number of cattle herds within the 500 m wide buffer surrounding the farm's land parcels resulted in an increased bTB risk (Table 3). This risk factor was consistent across the 1000 m and 1500 m wide buffer [Supplementary Information S1]. Although non-significant, the number of active badger setts (p = 0.67, OR: 1.02, 95% CI: 0.91–1.14 corresponding to a doubling in the number of setts) outside but within 500 m of the lands parcels (risk factor indentified for the survey herds) resulted in a marginal increase in bTB risk (model B). Thus, this effect was in the same direction as those observed in survey-only areas.

Time to first confirmed bTB herd breakdown. Overall, when comparing the time to the first confirmed herd bTB breakdown between proactive and survey-only herds during the period under study, we found that the best model included effects of farm area, herd type, herd size, triplet and the historic bTB incidence within the trial area. LRT showed that the number of land parcels belonging to the farm (p = 0.90), and the number of baseline herds (p = 0.44) were not significant and removed from the model. Culling treatment (p = 0.08) was also non-significant although there was a trend for reduced bTB risks among herds in proactively culled areas (HR: 1.11, 95% CI: 0.99–1.22) (Figure 1). The variable "farm area" showed some evidence of non-proportional hazard (p = 0.04). To resolve this issue, we transformed the variable into a factor with two levels [small farms (area < median farm area) and large farms (area ≥ median farm area]. We found that such procedure had little effect on the non-proportional hazard (p = 0.06), and decided to retain "farm area" as a covariate as none of the other model diagnostics revealed violations of PH assumptions.

Dairy herds showed a significantly higher risk of bTB breakdown (p = 0.001) compared to non-dairy herds (HR: 1.33, 95% CI: 1.12–1.58). Larger herds (p<0.001, HR: 1.13, 95% CI: 1.08, 1.19) and larger farms (p<0.001, HR: 1.26, 95% CI: 1.19, 1.33) presented an increased risk of bTB breakdown. The hazard ratios here are interpreted as a doubling of the herd size or of farm area resulting in a 13% and 26% increase, respectively, in the hazard of a bTB breakdown. The triplet of the herd (p<0.001), and the historic bTB incidence for the trial area (p<0.001, HR: 2.27, 95% CI: 2.01, 2.52 corresponding to a doubling in historic incidence), were significant predictors of the herd's time to a confirmed bTB breakdown in the period under study. A Tukey's honest significance test revealed that triplet D, the last to receive proactive culling, had a significantly higher risk of bTB breakdown than all other triplets (Figure 2).

Within survey-only areas. The number of active badger setts (both on the land parcels and outside but within 500 m) as

Table 3. Multivariable models of the probability of RBCT herds experiencing a confirmed bTB breakdown during the period under study.

	Survey-only		Proactive		Reactive	
	Model A [1]	Model B	Model A	Model B	Model A	Model B
Number of *M. bovis* + badgers culled on the land parcels [2]	NA	NA	----	----	NA	NA
Number of *M. bovis* + badgers culled outside but within 500 m	NA	NA	p<0.001 OR: 1.27 (1.15–1.39)	p=0.002 OR: 1.22 (1.10–1.35)	NA	NA
Number of active setts on the land parcels [3]	----	----	----	----	NA	NA
Number of active setts outside but within 500 m	p=0.003 OR: 1.13 (1.02–1.24)	p=0.02 OR: 1.14 (1.03–1.25)	----	----	NA	NA
Density (/km²) of active setts on the land parcels	NA	NA	NA	NA	----	----
Density (/km²) of active setts outside but within 500 m	NA	NA	NA	NA	----	----
Number of cattle herds tested [4]	p=0.001 OR: 1.44 (1.22–1.66)	p=0.004 OR: 1.38 (1.16–1.61)	NA	NA	p<0.001 OR: 1.69 (1.49–1.89)	p<0.001 OR: 1.75 (1.55–1.96)
Density (/km²) of cattle herds tested	NA	NA	----	----	NA	NA
Herd type [DAIRY]	p=0.47 OR: 1.13 (0.81–1.57)	p=0.25 OR: 1.22 (0.87–1.71)	p=0.03 OR: 1.45 (1.03–1.69)	p=0.04 OR: 1.42 (1.01–2.00)	p=0.13 OR: 0.76 (0.53–1.08)	p=0.15 OR: 0.77 (0.54–1.10)
Herd size	p<0.001 OR: 1.21 (1.11–1.31)	p<0.001 OR: 1.21 (1.11–1.32)	p=0.003 OR: 1.18 (1.07–1.28)	P=0.002 OR: 1.19 (1.08–1.30)	p<0.001 OR: 1.25 (1.15–1.36)	p<0.001 OR: 1.26 (1.15–1.37)
Farm area	p=0.002 OR: 1.22 (1.09–1.35)	p<0.001 OR: 1.25 (1.12–1.38)	p<0.001 OR: 1.30 (1.17–1.43)	p<0.001 OR: 1.33 (1.20–1.46)	p=0.007 OR: 1.19 (1.07–1.32)	p=0.01 OR: 1.18 (1.04–1.31)
bTB historic incidence within trial area	NA	p<0.001 OR: 2.16 (1.74–2.58)	NA	p<0.001 OR: 2.51 (2.14–2.88)	NA	p=0.006 OR: 1.62 (1.27–1.96)

Odds ratios (OR) are quoted with their corresponding 95% confidence interval, and for covariates correspond to the change in the risk of a confirmed bTB breakdown following a doubling of the value of the covariate.

The --- means that an individual predictor was not significant and removed from the model, while NA corresponds to variables that were not included following the screening process.

[1] Models are adjusted for herd size, herd type and farm area (model A); herd size, herd type, farm area and bTB historic incidence within the trial area (model B).
[2] Relate to the badgers culled during the initial proactive cull.
[3] Relate to the badger setts identified during the initial survey.
[4] Relate to herds tested for bTB during the one year prior to the start of the initial proactive cull.

well as the number of cattle herds within 500 m of all land parcels were the best individual predictors of the time to first confirmed bTB breakdown for survey-only herds [Supplementary Information S1]. Both variables remained significant predictors in the multivariable PH model. An increase in the number of active setts and cattle herds within the 500 m wide buffer surrounding the farm's land parcels resulted in an increased bTB risk (Table 4). Both risk factors were consistent across the 1000 m and 1500 m wide buffer [Supplementary Information S1].

Within proactive areas. The number of *M. bovis* positive culled badgers, the number of active badger setts (both on the land parcels and outside but within 500 m) as well as the density of cattle herds within x meters of the land parcels were the best individual predictors of the time to first confirmed bTB breakdown for proactive herds during the period under study [Supplementary Information S1]. The number of *M. bovis* positive badgers that were culled outside but within 500 m of the land parcels belonging

to a farm remained the only significant predictor in the multivariable PH model. An increase in the number of *M. bovis* positive badgers culled within the 500 m buffer surrounding the farm's land parcels resulted in an increased bTB risk (Table 4). The risk factor was consistent across the 1000 m and 1500 m wide buffer [see Supplementary Information]. Although non-significant, the hazard ratios (model B) corresponding to the number of active badger setts (p=0.53, OR: 1.03, 95% CI: 0.94–1.12) and the number of cattle herds (p=0.65, OR: 0.97, 95% CI: 0.82–1.11) outside but within 500 m of the lands parcels are concordant with the ones derived from herds within survey-only areas.

Within reactive areas. The number of active badger setts (both on the land parcels and outside but within 500 m) as well as the number of cattle herds within 500 m of the land parcels were the best individual predictors of the time to first confirmed bTB breakdown for reactive herds [Supplementary Information S1]. Both variables remained significant predictors of the time to first

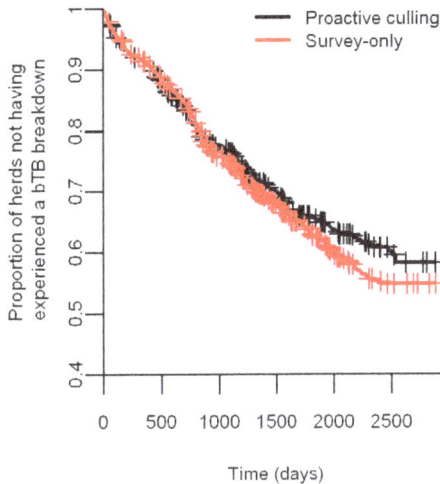

Figure 1. Effect of badger culling on time to first confirmed bTB herd breakdown. The Kaplan-Meier survival curves represent the proportion of proactive and survey-only herds not having experienced a confirmed bTB breakdown as a function of the number of days since the initial proactive cull (the Kaplan-Meier estimator is not adjusted for any other variable). The effect of proactive badger culling on the time to first breakdown is not significant.

confirmed bTB herd breakdown. An increase in the number of cattle herds and active setts within the 500 m buffer surrounding the farm's land parcels resulted in an increased bTB risk (Table 4). The risk factor associated with the number of cattle herds was consistent whether the buffer was 1000 m or 1500 m wide [Supplementary Information S1] while the number of active badger setts acted as a non-significant bTB risk factor on land over 500 m outside the farm.

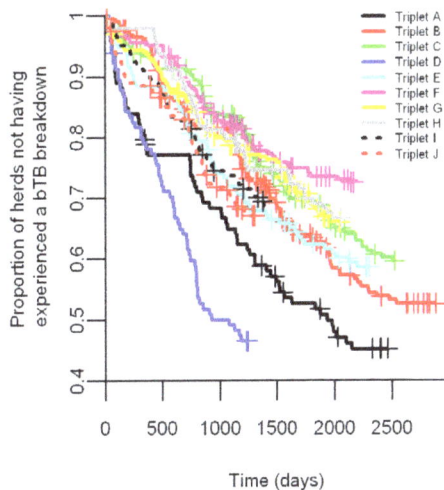

Figure 2. Time to first confirmed bTB herd breakdown for each triplet. The Kaplan-Meier survival curves represent the proportion of herds not having experienced a confirmed bTB breakdown as a function of the number of days since the initial proactive cull for each triplet (the Kaplan-Meier estimator is not adjusted for any other variable). Triplet D had a significantly higher risk of bTB breakdown than all other triplets.

Discussion

Local herd risk factors

A number of local herd-level risk factors have been identified inside all three treatment groups of the RBCT by the present analyses. Some of these risk factors had also been described for herds outside the RBCT area. Dairy herds were found to be more at risk of a confirmed bTB breakdown. Animals in dairy herds tend to have a longer life expectancy, and thus a longer exposure to bTB and increased risk of breakdown [23], than beef cattle that are slaughtered at a young age. Unlike beef farms that use a variety of breeds and crossbred animals, dairy farms in the UK predominantly use one breed of cattle (Ivan Morrison pers. comm.). A breed-related difference in susceptibility may ensue [42] although it is difficult to disentangle its potential effects from higher production stress under more intensive management conditions for dairy cattle for example [43]. Interestingly, dairy herds within the RBCT tended to be much larger than other enterprise types [Supplementary Information S1], another risk factor identified in the present study. Large herds tend to pasture on larger areas, with correspondingly higher numbers of contiguous herds and potential contact with more badgers (if badger densities were constant on all sizes of pastures) thereby facilitating cattle to cattle [7] and badger to cattle spread of *M. bovis*, respectively. Alternatively, large herd size may be associated with management practices that increase the risk of *M. bovis* transmission. Indeed, we found that herd size was positively correlated with the number of cattle movements onto the farms [Supplementary Information S1]. The arrival of an infected animal in a bTB-free herd is one of the major risk factors for herd breakdowns, as suggested by studies carried out in the UK, USA and Italy [9,17,19,44]. Another important consideration relates to the difficulty of clearing bTB from large herds by test and slaughter [45], rendering large herds more at risk of recurrent infections.

Our findings regarding the risk posed by farm area on bTB herd breakdowns were opposite to the ones described by Johnston and colleagues [9]. Total farm area, and not the number of land parcels the farm was operated on, was associated with an increased bTB risk. Larger farms, regardless of the number of land parcels, may include more active badger setts or more contiguous herds, both risk factors identified in this study. The number/density of cattle herds within 500/1000/1500 m of a farm was a significant predictor of herd breakdowns in survey-only and reactive areas. A recent study in Belgium, a country lacking a significant wildlife reservoir for bTB, showed that the larger the livestock population in an area, the higher the probability of close contacts, and bTB transmission, between them [45]. The movement and trading of animals from high bTB risk herds has been found to contribute to both the local and long-distance geographic spreading of the disease [20,46]. We found that farm area was positively correlated with the number of cattle movements onto the farm [Supplementary Information S1]. Larger farms purchased more animals, suggesting a higher probability of introducing the disease into their herd. The retention of historic bTB incidence in the multivariable models suggest that this risk factor is important in determining whether herds in a parish group are likely to experience a bTB breakdown in a particular year. Herd breakdowns tend to be recurrent [5] possibly as a result of the failure to clear the source of the disease, especially from larger herds, by test and slaughter [45]. Subsequent breakdowns could therefore arise from undetected (tuberculin-negative) infected animals. This factor is probably exacerbated for dairy herds whose turnover is less important than stores or beef enterprises. Other permanent factors (such as the

Table 4. Multivariable models of the time to first confirmed bTB breakdown for RBCT herds during the period under study.

	Survey-only		Proactive		Reactive	
	Model A [1]	Model B	Model A	Model B	Model A	Model B
Number of M. bovis + badgers culled on the land parcels [2]	NA	NA	----	----	NA	NA
Number of M. bovis + badgers culled outside but within 500 m	NA	NA	p<0.001 HR: 1.29 (1.21–1.38)	p<0.001 HR: 1.25 (1.17–1.34)	NA	NA
Number of active setts on the land parcels [3]	----	----	----	----	----	----
Number of active setts outside but within 500 m	p=0.04 HR: 1.09 (1.01–1.16)	p=0.03 HR: 1.09 (1.01–1.17)	----	----	p=0.03 HR: 1.10 (1.01–1.18)	p=0.04 HR: 1.09 (1.01–1.18)
Density (/km^2) of active setts on the land parcels	NA	NA	NA	NA	----	----
Density (/km^2) of active setts outside but within 500 m	NA	NA	NA	NA	----	----
Number of cattle herds tested [4]	p=0.002 HR: 1.30 (1.14–1.47)	p=0.01 HR: 1.26 (1.09–1.42)	NA	NA	p<0.001 HR: 1.29 (1.15–1.44)	P<0.001 HR:1 .32 (1.18–1.46)
Density (/km^2) of cattle herds tested	NA	NA	----	----	NA	NA
Herd type [DAIRY]	p=0.31 HR: 1.13 (0.89–1.44)	p=0.20 HR: 1.17 (0.91–1.48)	P=0.02 HR: 1.35 (1.05–1.73)	p=0.03 HR: 1.33 (1.22–1.57)	p=0.15 HR: 0.83 (0.65–1.07)	p=0.17 HR: 0.84 (0.65–1.08)
Herd size	p=0.02 HR: 1.10 (1.02–1.19)	p=0.02 HR: 1.11 (1.02–1.19)	p=0.04 HR: 1.10 (1.01–1.19)	p=0.04 HR: 1.09 (1.01–1.18)	p=0.001 HR: 1.15 (1.06–1.24)	p<0.001 HR: 1.16 (1.07–1.24)
Farm area	p<0.001 HR: 1.21 (1.11–1.30)	p<0.001 HR: 1.22 (1.12–1.32)	p<0.001 HR: 1.24 (1.14–1.34)	p<0.001 HR: 1.26 (1.16–1.36)	p=0.02 HR: 1.13 (1.03–1.24)	p=0.03 HR: 1.12 (1.02–1.23)
bTB historic incidence within trial area	NA	p=0.01 HR: 1.57 (1.25–1.89)	NA	p<0.001 HR: 1.87 (1.59–2.14)	NA	p<0.001 HR: 1.69 (1.43–1.95)

Hazard ratios (HR) are quoted with their corresponding 95% confidence interval, and for covariates correspond to the change in the risk of a confirmed bTB breakdown following a doubling of the value of the covariate.
Refer to other footnotes from Table 3.

presence of badgers and/or contiguous herds) may make these areas particularly prone to bTB reemergence.

The analyses of RBCT cattle incidence data using individual-herd-based models also provide insights into how local cattle herds and local badger populations affect the breakdown risks on individual cattle herds in survey-only areas (unculled areas). The presence of badgers (measured here as the number of active badger setts) was associated with an increase in bTB risk, even after adjusting for local farm-level risk factors. The higher the number of badger setts identified within 1500 m of the land parcels, the higher the probability of at least one confirmed bTB breakdown for the corresponding herd, a pattern that has also been observed in Northern Ireland [12] and the Republic of Ireland [47]. Similarly, the number of herds within 1500 m of a farm was a very significant predictor of both the probability and the time to the first bTB breakdown for that herd. The larger the cattle population surrounding a farm, the higher the number of contiguous herds that are likely to have had experienced a confirmed bTB breakdown in the past. A case-control study in Northern Ireland showed that the odds of a bTB breakdown are increased by more than two-fold if a herd has a contiguous neighbour which has experienced a confirmed bTB within the last three years [12], with a similar pattern once again observed in the Republic of Ireland [7].

Effects of badger culling on the risk of bTB herd breakdowns

Previous studies have demonstrated that the experimental reduction of badger density by culling over large ($\geq$100 km^2) tracts of land lowers the incidence of bTB inside proactively culled areas [36,48] but increases the incidence on land outside but within 2 km of the area culled [36,40]. Proactive culling has been demonstrated to reduce local densities of badgers [32], and subsequently cattle to badger contact, with benefits of culling still apparent five years after the last proactive cull [49]. Although a log-linear analysis remains the most robust approach to investigate treatment effects inside the RBCT [36], we find non-significant differences in the probability of (p=0.07) and the time to (p=0.008) a confirmed bTB herd breakdown between herds in proactive and survey-only areas during the study period, a finding consistent with previous analyses. There is a non-significant trend for herds in survey-only areas to be 19% more likely to experience a confirmed bTB breakdown than herds in areas that were proactively culled.

More importantly, our study complements previous analyses of the RBCT data by focusing on variation in bTB risk at the herd-level within trial areas (the unit of randomization). The number of culled badgers that tested positive for *M. bovis* inside the buffer surrounding the farm during the initial proactive cull remains a significant predictor of both the probability of experiencing and the time to a confirmed bTB breakdown for herds within the proactive area after the end of the initial cull. Such associations may be indicative of an underlying bTB risk for those herds which has not been eliminated by the proactive badger culling (for example higher bTB prevalence). Our findings suggest that infection in cattle and badgers are linked, and are supported by a previous study which concluded that a high degree of similarity in the *M. bovis* strain types isolated from cattle and associated badgers existed in England [33].

Reactive badger culling caused an increase in bTB incidence recorded in reactive areas [50], likely as a result of expanded badger movement patterns and increased intraspecific transmission following the cull [31,33]. In this study, we attempted to relate the herd-probability of a bTB breakdown to measures of badger presence measured prior to the start of the reactive culling. We found that the presence of badger setts (outside but within 500/1000 or 1500 m of the land parcels) is a significant predictor of the time to the first bTB breakdown (although this finding is not consistent across all analyses performed - Supplementary Information S1) but was not associated with the probability of a herd experiencing at least one confirmed bTB breakdown.

In conclusion, our findings confirm that proactive culling of badgers, whilst in operation, reduces the individual-herd probability of experiencing a herd bTB breakdown. Increased numbers of badgers carrying *M. bovis* and increased numbers of active badger setts significantly increased the probability of a breakdown for herds in proactive and survey-only/reactive areas respectively. However, given the demonstrated negative effects of proactive badger culling on bTB incidence in herds on land outside but within 2 km of the areas culled as well as its declining benefits inside trial areas once culling has stopped, detailed consideration is needed to determine whether (and where) proactive badger culling could be an effective part of bTB control in England and Wales. We also produce further evidence that the livestock population within 1500 m of a farm, but not counting the index herd, is

associated with the risk of detecting bTB. While the randomized design of the RBCT facilitates the interpretation of treatment effects (between trial areas), its principal aim was not to assess variation in bTB risk at the herd level within trial areas. Our conclusions are therefore cautious due to the observational nature of our study.

In conclusion

In the long-term, Defra is "considering the potential for a more risk-based approach to setting routine bTB testing intervals [...] (to be) in a better position to tackle the disease" [51]. On-farm surveillance for bTB is currently carried out through a programme of routine testing, with cattle herds tested every one, two, three or four years depending on the local level of risk of infection with *M. bovis* and historic incidence (risk level reviewed annually). The measures of local bTB revealed by the present analyses could be integrated into a risk-based herd testing programme to improve the targeting of interventions aimed at reducing the risks of bTB transmission to cattle herds in areas densely populated with livestock and/or badgers.

Supporting Information

Supporting Information S1 Univariable models and alternative multivariable models of herd-level bTB risk.

Acknowledgments

The RBCT was designed and overseen by the Independent Scientific Group on Cattle bTB (John Bourne (chair), Christl Donnelly (deputy chair), David Cox, George Gettinby, John McInerney, Ivan Morrison and Rosie Woodroffe) and implemented by Defra and its associated agencies. We wish to thank the many farmers and landholders in the trial areas who allowed the experimental treatments to operate on their land.

Author Contributions

Conceived and designed the experiments: CAD FV. Analyzed the data: FV WTJ. Wrote the paper: FV WTJ CAD. Interpreted the results: FV CAD. Extracted GIS data: WTJ.

References

1. Etter E, Donado P, Jori F, Caron A, Goutard F, et al. (2006) Risk Analysis and Bovine Tuberculosis, a Re-emerging Zoonosis. Annals of the New York Academy of Sciences 1081: 61–73.
2. Thoen C, LoBue P, de Kantor I (2006) The importance of Mycobacterium bovis as a zoonosis. Veterinary Microbiology 112: 339–345.
3. Proud AJ (2006) Some lessons from the history of the eradication of bovine tuberculosis in Great Britain. Government Veterinary Journal 16.
4. Cheeseman CL, Wilesmith JW, Stuart FA (1989) Tuberculosis: the disease and its epidemiology in the badger, a review. Epidemiology and Infection 103: 113–125.
5. Krebs JR, Anderson R, Clutton-Brock T, Morrison I, Young D (1997) Bovine tuberculosis in cattle and badgers. London, UK: Ministry of Agriculture, Fisheries and Food.
6. DEFRA (2009) Bovine TB statistics for Great Britain: http://www.defra.gov.uk/foodfarm/farmanimal/diseases/atoz/tb/stats/documents/09/2009gb.pdf.
7. Griffin JM, Martin SW, Thorburn MA, Eves JA, Hammond RF (1996) A case-control study on the association of selected risk factors with the occurrence of bovine tuberculosis in the Republic of Ireland. Preventive Veterinary Medicine 27: 217–229.
8. Bourne FJ, Donnelly CA, Cox DR, Gettinby G, McInerney JP, et al. (2007) Bovine TB: the scientific evidence. Final report of the Independent Scientific Group on Cattle TB. London, UK: Defra.
9. Johnston WT, Gettinby G, Cox DR, Donnelly CA, Bourne J, et al. (2005) Herd-level risk factors associated with tuberculosis breakdowns among cattle herds in England before the 2001 foot-and-mouth disease epidemic. Biology Letters 1: 53–56.
10. Reilly LA, Courtenay O (2007) Husbandry practices, badger sett density and habitat composition as risk factors for transient and persistent bovine tuberculosis on UK cattle farms. Preventive Veterinary Medicine 80: 129–142.
11. Kaneene JB, Bruning-Fann CS, Granger LM, Miller R, BA P-S (2002) Environmental and farm management factors associated with tuberculosis on cattle farms in northeastern Michigan. Journal of the American Veterinary Medical Association 221: 837–842.
12. Denny GO, Wilesmith JW (1999) Bovine tuberculosis in Northern Ireland: a case-control study of herd risk factors. Vet Rec 144: 305–310.
13. Griffin JM, Hahesy T, Lynch K, Salman MD, McCarthy J, et al. (1993) The association of cattle husbandry practices, environmental factors and farmer characteristics with the occurence of chronic bovine tuberculosis in dairy herds in the Republic of Ireland. Preventive Veterinary Medicine 17: 145–160.
14. Marangon S, Martini M, Dalla Pozza M, J. FN (1998) A case-control study on bovine tuberculosis in the Veneto Region (Italy). Preventive Veterinary Medicine 34: 87–95.
15. Olea-Popelka FJ, White PW, Collins JD, O'Keeffe J, Kelton DF, et al. (2004) Breakdown severity during a bovine tuberculosis episode as a predictor of future herd breakdowns in Ireland. Preventive Veterinary Medicine 63: 163–172.
16. White PCL, Benhin JKA (2004) Factors influencing the incidence and scale of bovine tuberculosis in cattle in southwest England. Preventive Veterinary Medicine 63: 1–7.
17. Kaneene JB, Bruning-Fann CS, Granger LM, Miller R, Porter-Spalding BA (2002) Environmental and farm management factors associated with tuberculosis on cattle farms in northeastern Michigan. Journal of the American Veterinary Medical Association 221: 837–842.

18. Porphyre T, Stevenson MA, McKenzie J (2008) Risk factors for bovine tuberculosis in New Zealand cattle farms and their relationship with possum control strategies. Preventive Veterinary Medicine 86: 93–106.

19. Gopal R, Goodchild A, Hewinson G, de la Rua Domenech R, Clifton-Hadley R (2006) Introduction of bovine tuberculosis to north-east England by bought-in cattle. Vet Rec 159: 265–271.

20. Gilbert M, Mitchell A, Bourn D, Mawdsley J, Clifton-Hadley R, et al. (2005) Cattle movements and bovine tuberculosis in Great Britain. Nature 435: 491–496.

21. Ramírez-Villaescusa AM, Medley GF, Mason S, Green LE (2010) Risk factors for herd breakdown with bovine tuberculosis in 148 cattle herds in the south west of England. Preventive Veterinary Medicine 95: 224–230.

22. Menzies FD, Neill SD (2000) Cattle-to-Cattle Transmission of Bovine Tuberculosis. The Veterinary Journal 160: 92–106.

23. Humblet MF, Boschiroli ML, Saegerman C (2009) Classification of worldwide bovine tuberculosis risk factors in cattle: a stratified approach. Veterinary Research 40.

24. O'Reilly LM, Daborn CJ (1995) The epidemiology of Mycobacterium bovis infections in animals and man: A review. Tubercle and Lung Disease 76: 1–46.

25. Coleman J, Caley P (2000) Possums as a reservoir of Bovine Tb. In: Montague TI, ed. The Brushtail Possum; Biology, Impact and Management of an Introduced Marsupial. Lincoln, New Zealand: Manaaki Whenua Press.

26. Payeur JB, Church S, Mosher L, Robinson-Dunn B, Schmitt S, et al. (2002) Bovine Tuberculosis in Michigan Wildlife. Annals of the New York Academy of Sciences 969: 259–261.

27. Nishi JS, Shury T, Elkin BT (2006) Wildlife reservoirs for bovine tuberculosis (Mycobacterium bovis) in Canada: Strategies for management and research. Veterinary Microbiology 112: 325–338.

28. Michel A, de Klerk L-M, van Pittius N, Warren R, van Helden P (2007) Bovine tuberculosis in African buffaloes: observations regarding Mycobacterium bovis shedding into water and exposure to environmental mycobacteria. BMC Veterinary Research 3: 23.

29. Richomme C, Boschiroli ML, Hars J, Casabianca F, Ducrot C (2010) Bovine Tuberculosis in Livestock and Wild Boar on the Mediterranean Island, Corsica. Journal of Wildlife Diseases 46: 627–631.

30. Naranjo V, Gortazar C, Vicente J, de la Fuente J (2008) Evidence of the role of European wild boar as a reservoir of Mycobacterium tuberculosis complex. Veterinary Microbiology 127: 1–9.

31. Woodroffe R, Donnelly CA, Cox DR, Bourne FJ, Cheeseman CL, et al. (2006) Effects of culling on badger Meles meles spatial organization: implications for the control of bovine tuberculosis. Journal of Applied Ecology 43: 1–10.

32. Woodroffe R, Gilks P, Johnston WT, Le Fevre AM, Cox DR, et al. (2008) Effects of culling on badger abundance: implications for tuberculosis control. Journal of Zoology 274: 28–37.

33. Woodroffe R, Donnelly CA, Cox DR, Gilks P, Jenkins HE, et al. (2009) Bovine tuberculosis in cattle and badgers in localized culling areas. Journal of Wildlife Diseases 45: 128–143.

34. Jenkins HE, Woodroffe R, Donnelly CA (2010) The Duration of the Effects of Repeated Widespread Badger Culling on Cattle Tuberculosis Following the Cessation of Culling. PLoS One 5: Article No.: e9090.

35. Donnelly CA, Wei G, Johnston WT, Cox DR, Woodroffe R, et al. (2007) Impacts of widespread badger culling on cattle tuberculosis: concluding analyses from a large-scale field trial. International Journal of Infectious Diseases 11: 300–308.

36. Donnelly CA, Woodroffe R, Cox DR, Bourne FJ, Cheeseman CL, et al. (2006) Positive and negative effects of widespread badger culling on tuberculosis in cattle. Nature 439: 843–846.

37. Hone J, Donnelly CA (2008) Evaluating evidence of association of bovine tuberculosis in cattle and badgers. Journal of Applied Ecology 45: 1660–1666.

38. Jenkins HE, Woodroffe R, Donnelly CA, Cox DR, Johnston WT, et al. (2007) Effects of culling on spatial associations of Mycobacterium bovis infections in badgers and cattle. Journal of Applied Ecology 44: 897–908.

39. Woodroffe R, Donnelly CA, Jenkins HE, Johnston WT, Cox DR, et al. (2006) Culling and cattle controls influence tuberculosis risk for badgers. Proceedings of the National Academy of Sciences of the United States of America 103: 14713–14717.

40. Donnelly CA, Woodroffe R, Cox DR, Bourne J, Gettinby G, et al. (2003) Impact of localized badger culling on tuberculosis incidence in British cattle. Nature 426: 834–837.

41. Schoenfeld D (1982) Partial Residuals for The Proportional Hazards Regression Model. Biometrika 69: 239–241.

42. Allen AR, Minozzi G, Glass EJ, Skuce RA, McDowell SWJ, et al. (2010) Bovine tuberculosis: the genetic basis of host susceptibility. Proceedings of the Royal Society B: Biological Sciences 277: 2737–2745.

43. Ameni G, Aseffa A, Engers H, Young D, Gordon S, et al. (2007) High Prevalence and Increased Severity of Pathology of Bovine Tuberculosis in Holsteins Compared to Zebu Breeds under Field Cattle Husbandry in Central Ethiopia. Clin Vaccine Immunol 14: 1356–1361.

44. Marangon S, Martini M, Dalla Pozza M, Ferreira Neto J (1998) A case-control study on bovine tuberculosis in the Veneto Region (Italy). Preventive Veterinary Medicine 34: 87–95.

45. Woodroffe R, Bourne FJ, Donnelly CA, Cox DR, Gettinby G, et al. (2003) Towards a sustainable policy to control TB in cattle. In: Conservation and Conflict: Mammals and Farming in Britain; Tattersall F, Manley W, eds. London, UK: Linnean Society.

46. Green LE, Cornell SJ (2005) Investigations of cattle herd breakdowns with bovine tuberculosis in four counties of England and Wales using VETNET data. Preventive Veterinary Medicine 70: 293–311.

47. Martin SW, Eves JA, Dolan LA, Hammond RF, Griffin JM, et al. (1997) The association between the bovine tuberculosis status of herds in the East Offaly Project Area, and the distance to badger setts, 1988-1993. Preventive Veterinary Medicine 31: 113–125.

48. Griffin JM, Williams DH, Kelly GE, Clegg TA, O'Boyle I, et al. (2005) The impact of badger removal on the control of tuberculosis in cattle herds in Ireland. Preventive Veterinary Medicine 67: 237–266.

49. Donnelly CA, Jenkins HE, Woodroffe RW (2010) Analysis of further data (to 2 July 2010) on the impacts on cattle TB incidence of repeated badger culling. PLoS ONE comment.

50. Le Fevre AM, Donnelly CA, Cox DR, Bourne J, Clifton-Hadley RS, et al. (2005) The impact of localised reactive badger culling versus no culling on TB incidence in British cattle: a randomised trial. Available on http://collections.europarchive.org/tna/20081027092120/http://defra.gov.uk/animalh/tb/isg/pdf/lefevre1005.pdf.

51. DEFRA (2010) Bovine Tuberculosis: The Government's approach to tackling the disease and consultation on a badger control policy. London, UK: Department for Environment, Food and Rural Affairs.

16

Contralateral Cruciate Survival in Dogs with Unilateral Non-Contact Cranial Cruciate Ligament Rupture

Peter Muir[1]*, Zeev Schwartz[1], Sarah Malek[1], Abigail Kreines[1], Sady Y. Cabrera[2], Nicole J. Buote[3], Jason A. Bleedorn[1], Susan L. Schaefer[1], Gerianne Holzman[1], Zhengling Hao[1]

1 Comparative Orthopaedic Research Laboratory, and the Department of Surgical Sciences, School of Veterinary Medicine, University of Wisconsin-Madison, Madison, Wisconsin, United States of America, 2 Department of Surgery, VCA West Los Angeles Animal Hospital, Los Angeles, California, United States of America, 3 California Animal Hospital, Los Angeles, California, United States of America

Abstract

Background: Non-contact cranial cruciate ligament rupture (CrCLR) is an important cause of lameness in client-owned dogs and typically occurs without obvious injury. There is a high incidence of bilateral rupture at presentation or subsequent contralateral rupture in affected dogs. Although stifle synovitis increases risk of contralateral CrCLR, relatively little is known about risk factors for subsequent contralateral rupture, or whether therapeutic intervention may modify this risk.

Methodology/Principal Findings: We conducted a longitudinal study examining survival of the contralateral CrCL in client-owned dogs with unilateral CrCLR in a large baseline control population (n = 380), and a group of dogs that received disease-modifying therapy with arthroscopic lavage, intra-articular hyaluronic acid and oral doxycycline (n = 16), and were followed for one year. Follow-up in treated dogs included analysis of mobility, radiographic evaluation of stifle effusion and arthritis, and quantification of biomarkers of synovial inflammation. We found that median survival of the contralateral CrCL was 947 days. Increasing tibial plateau angle decreased contralateral ligament survival, whereas increasing age at diagnosis increased survival. Contralateral ligament survival was reduced in neutered dogs. Our disease-modifying therapy did not significantly influence contralateral ligament survival. Correlative analysis of clinical and biomarker variables with development of subsequent contralateral rupture revealed few significant results. However, increased expression of T lymphocyte-associated genes in the index unstable stifle at diagnosis was significantly related to development of subsequent non-contact contralateral CrCLR.

Conclusion: Subsequent contralateral CrCLR is common in client-owned dogs, with a median ligament survival time of 947 days. In this naturally occurring model of non-contact cruciate ligament rupture, cranial tibial translation is preceded by development of synovial inflammation. However, treatment with arthroscopic lavage, intra-articular hyaluronic acid and oral doxycycline does not significantly influence contralateral CrCL survival.

Editor: Alejandro Lucia, Universidad Europea de Madrid, Spain

Funding: This work was supported by the American Kennel Club Canine Health Foundation (www.akcchf.org). The contents of this publication are solely the responsibility of the authors and do not necessarily reflect the views of the Foundation. The funders had no role in study design, data collection and analysis, decision to publish, or preparation of the manuscript.

Competing Interests: The authors have declared that no competing interests exist.

* E-mail: muirp@vetmed.wisc.edu

Introduction

Non-contact cranial cruciate ligament rupture (CrCLR) is an important cause of lameness in the dog that incurs substantial annual health-care costs [1]. It is now widely recognized that mid-substance rupture of the CrCL often occurs during normal activity, with a high incidence of bilateral rupture at the time of initial clinical presentation in the range of 11–17% [2–4]. The CrCL in dogs is anatomically equivalent to the anterior cruciate ligament (ACL) in human beings, and the dog is a widely used model for research into ACL biology and repair.

A number of studies have examined the incidence of subsequent contralateral CrCLR in dogs diagnosed with unilateral non-contact CrCLR at initial presentation. Analysis of this risk has usually been reported as an incidence after surgery (percentage of patients within the cohort). This risk is in the range of 22–54% at 6 to 17 months of

diagnosis [2,3,5–7]. One of the limitations of this approach to data analysis is that it yields little information on the pattern of subsequent contralateral rupture. It has been our clinical impression that individual dogs appear at particularly high risk of subsequent contralateral CrCLR, whereas other dogs are protected from the trait. Estimation of ligament survival over time would provide more detailed information on the pattern of subsequent contralateral CrCLR.

In the past, development of stifle arthritis was thought to occur secondary to development of joint instability associated with progressive CrCLR. However, this perspective may not be correct, since development of stifle synovitis is an early event that can often be found before fraying of the cruciate ligaments becomes arthroscopically detectable in dogs with incipient disease [8]. Ligament damage typically involves both the CrCL and the caudal cruciate ligament [9]. Development of stifle synovitis also increases the risk of subsequent contralateral CrCLR in dogs [10].

The presence of synovitis in stifle joints with incipient CrCLR suggests that immune-mediated joint degeneration is a factor in the non-contact CrCLR mechanism. The cruciate ligaments are wrapped in synovium [11]; synovial vasculature has a blood-CrCL barrier, analogous to the blood-brain barrier [12], suggesting that inflammatory changes within synovium and synovial fluid have profound effects on cruciate ligament tissue metabolism. It is also known that chronic synovitis induces marked deterioration in CrCL structural properties in a rabbit model [13]. Histologic features of lymphoplasmacytic synovitis are present in stifle joints of 51–67% affected dogs at the time of initial diagnosis [10,14]. In affected dogs, inflammatory cell populations within stifle synovium are usually mononuclear, and include T lymphocytes, B lymphocytes, major histocompatibility complex (MHC) class II⁺ dendritic cells, and activated macrophages, expressing tartrate-resistant acid phosphatase (TRAP) [15–18]. TRAP⁺ mononuclear cells are not found in normal stifle synovium of dogs [17].

At the present time, there are two hypotheses regarding the mechanism that leads to development of inflammatory stifle arthritis and eventual CrCLR: (1) cruciate fiber rupture is a consequence of a primary synovitis [8], and (2) intrinsic and extrinsic factors induce fiber rupture, with subsequent induction of synovitis by ligament matrix neoepitopes [19–21]. The immuno-logic trigger for synovitis for the first hypothesis is not known, although the presence of bacterial material within the stifle has been associated with the condition [22–24].

If development of synovitis has a significant role in the pathogenesis of progressive non-contact rupture of the cruciate ligament complex, particularly the CrCL, then disease-modifying medical therapy may block progressive stifle joint degeneration in dogs with incipient disease, and lead to a reduction in the incidence of non-contact cruciate rupture over time. In this regard, evaluation of the status of the contralateral CrCL over time in dogs with unilateral CrCLR would be one model that could be used to address this question.

The first objective of the study was to conduct a survival analysis of time to contralateral CrCLR in a large population of dogs with unilateral CrCLR presented for surgical treatment, to determine the pattern of subsequent contralateral CrCLR that is typically found in affected dogs. We hypothesized that within a large population of affected dogs, some dogs would appear protected from the risk of subsequent contralateral rupture. A secondary objective of this study was to determine whether treatment of a group of dogs with a provisional disease-modifying therapy for arthritis might ameliorate risk of subsequent contralateral rupture, and whether a biomarker for subsequent contralateral rupture risk could be identified.

Materials and Methods

Dogs

In order to determine the pattern of subsequent contralateral CrCLR in affected dogs, we performed a survival analysis of three populations of dogs from different regions of the USA; data from two of these cohorts has been previously published with limited analysis on contralateral CrCL survival [2,3]. Dogs with unilateral CrCLR that were treated surgically were studied.

In *Group 1*, a cohort of 125 dogs [2] presented to the Department of Surgery, VCA West Los Angeles Hospital, Los Angeles, CA between 2000 and 2006 was studied. In *Group 2*, a cohort of 84 Labrador retrievers [3] presented to the Animal Medical Center, New York, NY and Dallas Veterinary Surgical Center, Dallas, TX between 2000 and 2003 was studied. In *Group 3*, a cohort of 171 dogs was studied at the University of Wisconsin-

Madison, School of Veterinary Medicine, Veterinary Medical Teaching Hospital, Madison, WI. Initially, the medical records of all dogs (298 dogs) that received surgical treatment during the period 2007–2009 were reviewed for inclusion in the survival analysis. Of these records, 51 were excluded because of incomplete data or were lost to follow-up, 16 were excluded because a disease-modifying treatment with intra-articular hyaluronic acid and doxycycline was provided (see below), and 60 were excluded because the dog was found to have bilateral CrCLR on initial examination. The remaining 171 records were included in the study and examined in detail. In *Group 4*, a cohort of 16 dogs with unilateral CrCLR rupture and clinical and radiographic evidence of incipient non-contact cruciate rupture in the contralateral stifle were studied. Dogs presented to the University of Wisconsin-Madison, School of Veterinary Medicine, Veterinary Medical Teaching Hospital, Madison, WI [8] were studied, after treatment with a single intra-articular injection of hyaluronic acid (HA) and a course of oral doxycycline. Doxycycline has been previously reported to have disease-modifying effects on arthritic joints in human beings and dogs [25–27]. All procedures at the University of Wisconsin-Madison were conducted with the approval of the Animal Care & Use Committee, School of Veterinary Medicine, University of Wisconsin-Madison (V1070).

Medical records review

For inclusion in the analysis, CrCLR was confirmed during surgical treatment, with clinical follow-up of a least one year for censored cases. Breed, age, bodyweight, and gender were obtained from the medical record. Pre-operative tibial plateau angle (TPA) in the index stifle was also recorded [2,3] in all groups. If the dog developed a subsequent contralateral CrCLR during the study period, the time interval to contralateral CrCLR was recorded in days as a complete case. For dogs that did not experience a contralateral CrCLR, the time interval to clinical or telephone follow-up was recorded, as a censored case.

Follow-up information was obtained from the medical record, by telephone conversation with the owner, or telephone conversation with the attending clinician, if surgery for subsequent contralateral CrCLR had been performed at a different hospital, as previously described [2,3]. In the Groups 2 and 3, a standard questionnaire was used to obtain telephone follow-up, as previously described [3].

Provisional disease-modifying therapy for synovitis/arthritis

Initial clinical, radiographic, and arthroscopic findings in the cohort of dogs in Group 4 have been previously reported [8]. Inclusion criteria for this cohort of dogs included 1) pelvic limb lameness; 2) clinical and radiographic signs of synovial effusion and arthritis in both stifles; 3) stifle instability in the index stifle; 4) no clinically detectable instability in the contralateral stifle based on palpation and stress radiographic examination [8]; 5) no history of traumatic injury; and 6) no previous stifle surgery.

Age, weight, gender, and history were recorded. Bilateral orthogonal stifle radiographs were made immediately before surgery, at 10 weeks after surgery, and at long-term follow-up at least 12 months after surgery. Radiographs were graded for the following parameters: "overall disease severity" (0–3), "joint effusion" (0–2), "osteophytosis" (0–3) and "intraarticular miner-alization" (0–2) [28]. Radiographic grading was performed by a single observer (PM). In addition during the initial visit and at long-term follow-up, stress radiographs of the contralateral stifle were made [8]. Dogs were positioned in lateral recumbency, with the affected stifle resting on the x-ray table. The x-ray beam was centered over the stifle joint and collimated to include both the tibial and femoral diaphysis. A standard lateral view was taken with the joint in approximately 90–110 degrees of flexion (neutral view). For the tibial compression view, the stifle was maintained as the same angle of flexion, and manual stress was applied to the metatarsals to flex the hock joint maximally (stress view). Cranial tibial translation was then measured [8] by a single observer (ZS).

During surgical stabilization of the index stifle with tibial plateau leveling osteotomy (TPLO), arthoscopic examination of the unstable index and contralateral stable stifle joints was performed [8]. Pain management was supervised by a board-certified veterinary anesthesiologist. Dogs were premedicated, anesthetized, and administered an epidural or regional nerve block before surgery. No intra-articular anesthetic agents were used. Immediately after surgery, 20 mg of HA (Hylartin V, Pfizer Animal Health, New York, NY) was injected into each stifle and doxycycline was given orally at 5 mg/kg b.i.d. for 10 weeks.

Clinical follow-up of HA/doxycycline-treated dogs

Follow-up visits were performed at 10 weeks and at least one year, except for one dog that died shortly before one year after surgery. At the long-term recheck each owner was asked to complete a specific outcome measure questionnaire based on the "Liverpool Osteoarthritis in Dogs" (LOAD) questionnaire [29]. In completing the LOAD questionnaire, owners were asked to score the function of the dog in the period immediately before surgery and then again in the period immediately before the long-term follow-up visit. The total possible score ranged from 0–52, with 0 being normal.

Force-plate analysis-of-gait was also performed at long-term follow-up. Peak vertical force (F_z) and vertical impulse (VI) normalized to body weight were obtained [30]. A biomechanical platform that measures 3-dimensional forces and impulses (OR6-6-1000 Biomechanics Platform with SGA6-4 Signal Conditioner/Amplifier, Advanced Mechanical Technologies Inc., Newton, MA) was used. The force plate was connected to a commercially available satellite data acquisition system (Sharon Software Inc., Dewitt, MI). The velocity of each trial was measured. At least 5 successful trials were obtained from each dog, other than one dog in which only 4 trials were obtained. A successful trial was defined by a thoracic limb hitting the plate followed by the ipsilateral pelvic limb within the predetermined velocity range of 1.1 to 1.8 m/s and an acceleration range of -0.5 m/s^2 to $+0.5$ m/s^2.

Collection of peripheral blood and joint tissue specimens from HA/doxycycline-treated dogs

A peripheral blood sample was collected into a vacutainer tube (BD Vacutainer^{TM} CPT^{TM}, Becton Dickinson, Franklin Lakes, NJ) during each visit. Peripheral blood mononuclear cells (PBMC) were subsequently isolated by centrifugation. During surgery, synovial membrane and synovial fluid specimens were collected bilaterally. Synovium was collected from the lateral suprapatellar region of the stifle at the site of the egress portal using aseptic technique [8]. Synovial fluid was also obtained bilaterally at both the 10 week and at long-term follow-up visits using aseptic technique and needle aspiration under sedation. Joint tissue specimens were then transported to a laboratory that was not used for routine bacteriological research. Specimens of synovium were divided in a laminar flow hood and portions of each biopsy were used for estimation of bacterial load and for histology. Synovial fluid cells were isolated by centrifugation. Synovial membrane, synovial fluid cells, and PBMC were stored at -80C until analyzed.

Determination of bacterial load by 16S rRNA real-time PCR in HA/doxycycline-treated dogs

DNA was isolated from synovium and synovial fluid and bacterial load was estimated in each sample using two broad-ranging standard primer sets optimized for detection of complementary genera of bacteria [24,31–33]. PCR reactions were carried out in a final volume of 25 μl using the TaqMan PCR core reagent kit (Applied Biosystems, Foster City, CA). The master mixture was filtered using a Centriprep YM-100 filter (Millipore, Billerica, MA), and then 1 μl of total DNA was added. All PCR reactions were performed in triplicate. To estimate bacterial copy number, the threshold cycle (C_t) of each sample was analyzed against a standard curve with serial 10-fold dilution of DNA from 10 ng to 10 fg, using DNA derived from a rapidly growing aerobic organism previously identified in canine joints (*Stenotrophomonas maltophilia* ATCC #13637, Manassas, VA) [24]. To prevent contamination, all work was performed within a laminar flow cabinet treated with UV light. PCR amplification was performed in a different room from DNA extraction. Aliquots from known negative samples were used as an extraction control in each PCR run, in addition to negative and positive controls. PCR runs were limited to no more than eight samples in order to minimize the risk of handling errors during the assay.

Quantitative reverse-transcriptase-polymerase chain reaction (qRT-PCR) of joint tissues from HA/doxycycline-treated dogs

cDNA was generated from 0.2–1 μg of total RNA isolated from synovium and synovial fluid as previously described [24]. qRT-PCR was performed using standard methods and SYBR green methodology using a Bio-Rad thermocycler (MyiQ and IQ-SYBR Green Supermix, Bio-Rad, Hercules, CA). Oligonucleotide primers for the following genes: variable region of the beta chain of the T lymphocyte antigen receptor (TCR Vβ), CD3ε, TRAP, interleukin-17 (IL-17), IL-10, IL-4, interferon-γ (IFN-γ), and tumor necrosis factor-α (TNF-α) (Table 1). The TCR complex consists of either a TCR α/β or γ/δ heterodimer co-expressed at the cell surface with invariant subunits (γ, δ, ε, η, ζ) of CD3 [34,35]. Primers were designed from known canine gene sequences or regions of homology between the specific genes of other higher mammals. The 18S rRNA gene was used as the housekeeping gene. All PCR reactions were carried out as described [24]. Assays were validated by the use of a no template control. In addition, we tested the CD3ε and TCR Vβ primers using an immortalized Madin Darby canine kidney cell line and found no expression, as would be expected with genes that are only expressed in T lymphocytes.

Synovial membrane histology in HA/doxycycline-treated dogs

After collection, a portion of each synovial membrane specimen was fixed in Zamboni's fixative for 1–2 days at 4°C [36]. Frozen sections 10 μm thick were prepared [24] and stained with hematoxylin and eosin. Sections were also stained histochemically for TRAP using naphthol AS-BI phosphate as a marker for activated macrophages [17]. For each batch of slides, a negative control was prepared by omission of the naphthol AS-BI phosphate. Synovial tissue sections were scored subjectively for severity of synovial inflammation (J.A.B.) and numbers of TRAP$^+$ synovial macrophages (P.M.) using a visual analog scale method [24].

Statistical Analysis

Gehan's generalized Wilcoxon test and the Kaplan-Meier Product-Limit estimate were used for multivariate survival analysis

Table 1. Canine oligonucleotide primers for quantitative real-time reverse-transcriptase polymerase chain reaction.

mRNA Targets	Primer Type	Olignonucleotides (5′ to 3′)	Amplicon Size (bp)	Sequence Reference
TCR-Vβ	Forward	ACAGTGACCCTGAGATGTTCCCTT	139	Laboratory of Dr. Muir
	Reverse	ATCTTGCCGGGATGTCTCCTTTGT		Dreitz et al. 1999 [65]
CD3â	Forward	CCAATTCCTTCCTACCCTTCAGAGGTAT	112	Laboratory of Dr. Muir
	Reverse	GAGCTGGAAAAACGGAAAGGT		Nash et al. 1991 [66]
TRAP	Forward	TGCTGGCCACGTACAAGGT	70	Laboratory of Dr. Muir
	Reverse	TCATCCTGAAGGTACTGCAGGTT		Partial canine sequence
IL-17	Forward	CACTCCTTCCGGCTAGAGAA	71	Maccoux et al. 2007 [54]
	Reverse	CACATGGCGAACAATAGGG		
IL-10	Forward	CGCTGTCACCGATTTCTTCC	78	Wang et al. 2007 [67]
	Reverse	CTGGAGCTTACTAAATGCGCTCT		
IL-4	Forward	CATCCTCACAGCGAGAAACG	83	Wang et al. 2007 [67]
	Reverse	CCTTATCGCTTGTGTTCTTTGGA		
IFN-γ	Forward	GCGCAAGGCGATAAATGAAC	82	Wang et al. 2007 [67]
	Reverse	CTGACTCCTTTTCCGCTTCCT		
TNF-α	Forward	GAGCCGACGTGCCAATG	79	Wang et al. 2007 [67]
	Reverse	CAACCCATCTGACGGCACTA		
18S rRNA	Forward	CGCCGCTAGAGGTGAAATTCT	100	Laboratory of Dr. Svaren
	Reverse	CGAACCTCCGACTTTCGTTCT		U. Wisconsin-Madison

Note: TCR-Vβ – variable region of the beta chain of the T lymphocyte antigen receptor; TRAP – tartrate-resistant acid phosphatase; IL – interleukin; IFN – interferon; TNF – tumor necrosis factor.

to determine whether there were significant differences in contralateral ligament survival between groups of dogs (Groups 1–3), as a baseline control. Similarly, effects of gender or breed on contralateral ligament survival were also examined. The ten most common breeds in the study were analyzed (in order of prevalence in the cohort, Labrador retriever, Golden retriever, Rottweiler, German shepherd, Cocker spaniel, Boxer, Pitbull terrier, Beagle, Newfoundland, Mastiff). Cox's proportional hazard model was also used to determine whether age, gender, bodyweight, or pre-operative TPA had significant effects on contralateral CrCL survival. Time-dependent analysis was performed for dog age. Gehan's generalized Wilcoxon test and the Chi-square test were also used to determine whether contralateral CrCL survival was influenced by treatment with our provisional disease-modifying therapy.

For analysis of long-term clinical follow-up data, the Kolmolgorov-Smironv test was used to determine whether data approximated a normal distribution. If a dog developed contralateral CrCLR during the study period, then this stifle was excluded from the short- or long-term follow-up data sets. Bacterial copy number was normalized to the DNA concentration and the result was expressed as #/μg of DNA. For analysis of gene expression data, the threshold cycle (C_t values) obtained from the exponential region of the PCR amplification plot from duplicate trials were averaged together. Relative expression for each of the genes-of-interest was then calculated using standard curves [37]. PBMC gene expression was used as an internal control and the 18S rRNA gene was used as the housekeeping gene. Dependent data from index and contralateral limbs were analyzed using the Student's t test for paired data, or the Friedman ANOVA and Wilcoxon matched-pairs tests, as appropriate. Within each group and time point, the single sample Student's t test with a hypothesized mean of zero was used to determine whether expression of TCR Vβ, CD3ε, TRAP, IL-17, IL-4, IL-10, IFN-γ

and TNF-α in synovial tissues and PBMC was different, after log-transformation of data. Results were considered significant at $p < 0.05$.

Correlations between the development of subsequent contralateral CrCLR and a priori clinical, radiographic, arthroscopic, and synovial tissue laboratory analyses were examined using the Pearson and Spearman Rank correlation tests. Where relevant, a Bonferroni correction for comparisons across three time points, such that values of $p < 0.025$ were considered significant.

Results

Contralateral Ligament Survival

In Group 1, median survival time for the contralateral ligament was 809 days. Subsequent contralateral rupture occurred in 67 of 125 dogs (54%). In Group 2, median survival time was 1227 days. Subsequent contralateral rupture occurred in 45 of 84 dogs (54%). In Group 3, median survival time was 836 days. Subsequent contralateral rupture occurred in 92 of 171 dogs (54%) (**Fig. 1**). There were no significant differences between groups in the clinical survival of the contralateral CrCL ($p = 0.57$). Overall, median survival time for the contralateral ligament was 947 days or 2.59 years; 204 of 380 dogs (54%) developed subsequent contralateral rupture within the study period.

In the combined cohort of 380 baseline dogs, dog age ($p < 0.05$), TPA ($p < 0.05$), and gender ($p < 0.05$) all significantly influenced contralateral CrCL survival. The effect of body weight ($p = 0.58$) and breed ($p = 0.62$) were not significant. Increasing age was associated with increased contralateral CrCL survival, whereas increasing TPA was associated with decreased contralateral CrCL survival (**Fig. 2**). Median survival time of the CrCL was longer in male (950 days) and female (923 days) dogs, and shorter in both castrated males (708 days) and ovariohysterectomized females (845 days).

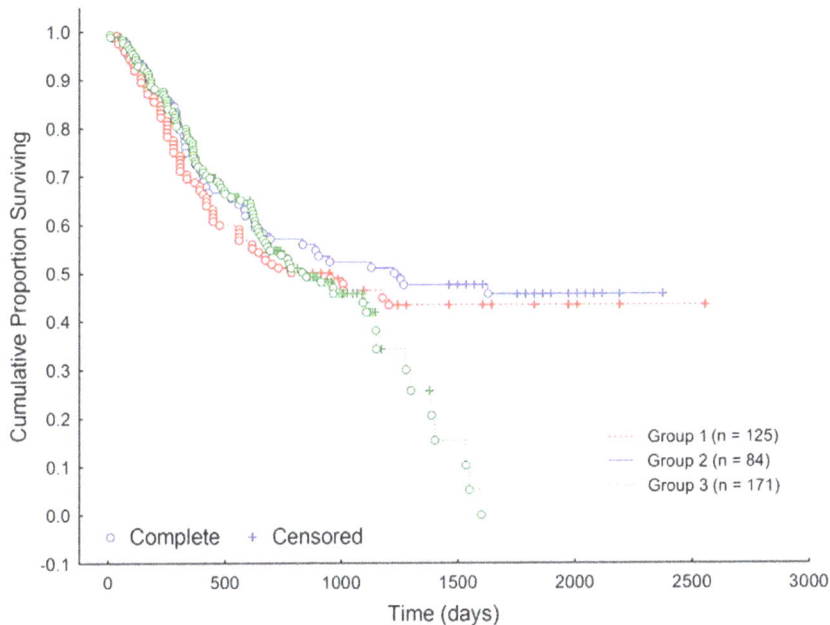

Figure 1. Contralateral cranial cruciate ligament (CrCL) survival. Kaplan-Meier plot for contralateral CrCL survival in three large populations of client-owned dogs. Overall median survival was 2.59 years. There was no significant difference in ligament survival between groups ($p = 0.57$). Complete – dogs that experienced contralateral CrCLR during the study period; Censored – dogs that did not experience contralateral CrCLR during the study period.

Clinical follow-up of HA/doxycycline-treated dogs

Of the cohort of 16 dogs, all dogs were re-examined at 10 weeks after surgery. Thirteen dogs were re-examined at long-term follow-up at least one year after surgery. Telephone follow-up with the owner was obtained for the remaining 3 dogs. The 16 client-owned dogs with stifle arthritis and CrCLR consisted of the following breeds: Golden retriever (n = 4), Labrador retriever (n = 3), and individual dogs of other breeds: American bulldog, Blood hound, Chesapeake Bay retriever, German shorthair pointer, Great Dane, Mastiff, Samoyed, Siberian Husky, Saint Bernard. In this group of dogs, age was 5.2 ± 2.5 years and body

weight was 40.7 ± 7.2 kg. Eight dogs were ovariohysterectomized females, 7 dogs were castrated males, and 1 dog was an intact male. Median duration of lameness was 19.5 weeks (range 1–156 weeks). None of the dogs had concurrent systemic disease, and all contralateral stifles were determined to be clinically stable by palpation under general anesthesia at diagnosis. At surgery, tearing of the medial meniscus was identified in the index stifle of 7 of 16 dogs (44%). No meniscal tears were found in the contralateral stable stifle.

All dogs were re-examined to evaluate clinical function and tibial osteotomy healing (10.2 ± 1.3 weeks after surgery). By this

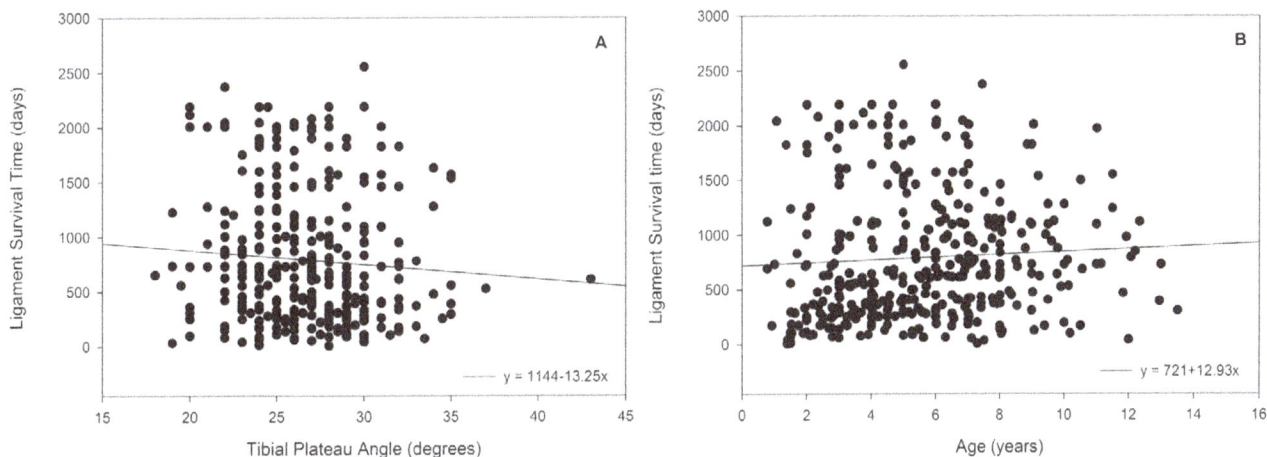

Figure 2. Tibial plateau angle (TPA) and age influence contralateral cranial cruciate ligament (CrCL) survival over time in dogs diagnosed with unilateral CrCL rupture. (A) Increasing TPA was associated with decreased contralateral CrCL survival, whereas increasing age at diagnosis was associated with increased contralateral CrCL survival (**B**). However, these effects appear minor, as the slope of the regression lines is small and data points are widely scattered.

time 1 of 16 dogs (6%) was diagnosed with contralateral CrCLR at 62 days after surgery. In the remaining 15 dogs, the contralateral stifle remained clinically stable. At long-term follow-up, an additional 4 dogs developed subsequent contralateral CrCLR, yielding a one-year incidence of 5 of 16 dogs (31%), which was not significantly different from the Group 3 dogs ($p = 0.12$). In two dogs with subsequent contralateral CrCLR, fraying of the CrCL was previously identified arthroscopically and estimated to involve 10% of the ligament, another dog was estimated to have a tear involving 30% of the ligament; in the two remaining dogs with subsequent contralateral CrCLR only minimal superficial fraying was observed.

One dog died during the study period shortly before the one-year long-term follow-up recheck examination was due. Doxycycline and intra-articular hyaluronic acid treatment after arthroscopic joint examination did not significantly influence contralateral CrCL survival time to rupture, when compared to the control population of 380 dogs that did not receive the provisional disease-modifying therapy ($p = 0.87$, **Fig. 3**).

Clinical metrology data were obtained from 11 of 13 dogs that were re-examined. Overall, load score showed a significant improvement in mobility at one-year after surgery, when compared with mobility at the time of initial diagnosis ($p < 0.05$). LOAD scores were 21 ± 11 and 10 ± 7 immediately before surgery and at long-term follow-up respectively.

Force-plate analysis-of-gait was performed in 10 of 15 dogs at long-term follow-up. In 8 dogs, the contralateral stifle was determined to be clinically stable at recheck, whereas in the remaining two dogs, contralateral CrCLR was diagnosed. In the dogs with stable contralateral stifles at recheck, no significance differences in Fz or VI were found between index and contralateral

stifles during force-plate analysis-of-gait ($p > 0.05$, **Table 2**); Fz was higher in the stable contralateral pelvic limb, with an index-contralateral difference in Fz of -4.6%. At follow-up, both of the dogs that developed subsequent contralateral CrCLR and underwent gait analysis exhibited reduced weight-bearing in the contralateral stifle (index-contralateral difference in Fz was 43.7%).

Stifle radiography in HA/doxycycline-treated dogs

Radiographic scores for overall change were significantly worse in the unstable index stifle, when compared to the stable contralateral stifle ($p < 0.05$, **Table 3**). In the stable contralateral stifle, effusion was identified in 12 of 16 stifles (75%) and all index stifles, and arthritis was identified in 15 of 16 stifles (94%), and all index stifles. Although the scores for overall change became higher over time, these changes were not significant in both the index and stable contralateral stifle ($p > 0.12$ and $p > 0.11$ respectively). Synovial effusion was also significantly worse in the index stifle at diagnosis, when compared with the stable contralateral stifle ($p < 0.01$), although this difference was not significant at the recheck visits. Scores for synovial effusion did not change significantly over time in both the index and stable contralateral stifle ($p > 0.78$ and $p > 0.14$ respectively).

Stress radiographic measurements supported the finding of clinical stability in the contralateral stifles at initial diagnosis. In the contralateral stifles that remained clinically stable over time, there were no significant differences in tibial translation ratio [median (range) at diagnosis of 0.025 (0.000–0.106), n = 11; 1 year follow-up ratio was 0.025 (0.00–0.048), n = 7]. However, in the 3 dogs that were determined to have experienced subsequent contralateral CrCLR at long-term follow-up visit, cranial tibial translation ratio was higher [0.075 (0.073–0.184)].

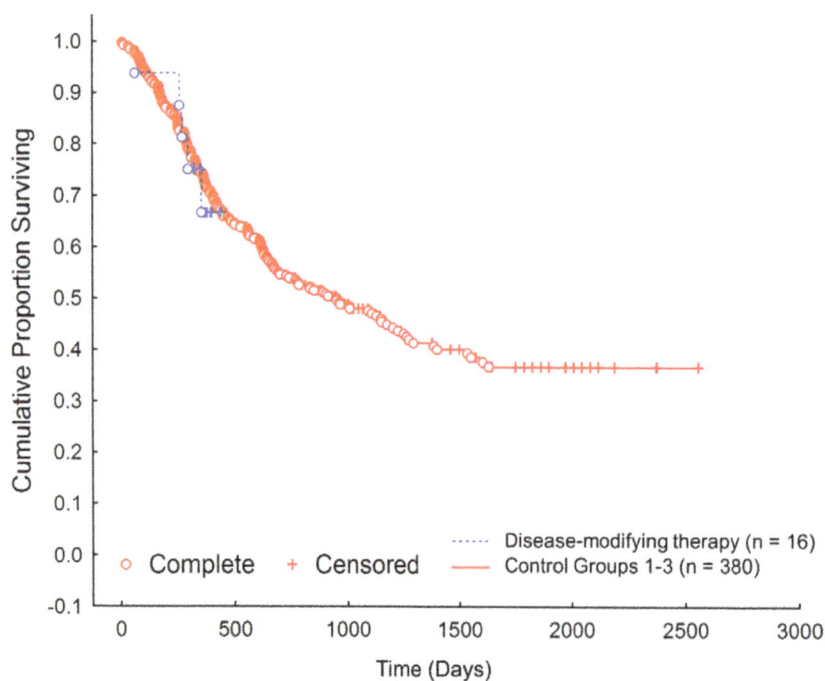

Figure 3. Contralateral cranial cruciate ligament (CrCL) survival after post-operative treatment with provisional disease-modifying therapy. Kaplan-Meier plot for contralateral CrCL survival in a population of client-owned dogs treatment with oral doxycycline after TPLO stabilization of unilateral CrCLR. Arthroscopic examination and associated lavage of the contralateral stable stifle, together with intra-articular hyaluronic acid and oral doxycycline did not significantly influence CrCL survival ($p = 0.87$). Complete – dogs that experienced contralateral CrCLR during the study period; Censored – dogs that did not experience contralateral CrCLR during the study period.

Table 2. Force-plate analysis-of-gait at long-term follow-up after surgical stabilization and hyaluronic acid/doxycycline treatment of stifle arthritis in dogs with unilateral cranial cruciate ligament rupture.

Parameter	Index stifle	Contralateral Stifle	Index-Contralateral difference (%)	Significance
Peak Vertical Force	46.4±8.9	48.5±11.9	−4.6	NS
Vertical Impulse	14.1±3.9	13.6±2.9	3.5	NS

Note: Data represent mean ± standard deviation. n = 8 dogs; NS – not significant ($p > 0.05$).

Histologic synovitis and bacterial load in HA/doxycycline-treated dogs

Both unstable index and stable contralateral stifles had macroscopic and histologic evidence of synovitis. Synovitis assessed arthroscopically was significantly increased in the index stifle, when compared with the contralateral stable stifle ($p < 0.001$, **Table 4**). Histologic synovitis was present in both stifles, with elevated severity scores in the unstable stifle; sub-intimal mononuclear inflammatory cells were often found (**Fig. 4**). Numbers of TRAP$^+$ mononuclear cells were increased in the unstable index stifle, when compared with the contralateral stable stifle. TRAP$^+$ mononuclear cells were identified in 11 of 14 unstable stifles, but only 2 of 10 stable stifles (**Fig. 4**).

No significant changes in bacterial load were identified using the Nadkarni 16S rRNA universal primer set. With the Yang 16S rRNA universal primer set, bacterial load within synovial fluid was increased in the contralateral stifle versus the unstable index stifle at diagnosis ($p < 0.05$, **Table 5**). At the 10-week recheck, bacterial load in synovial fluid in the unstable stifle was increased when compared to diagnosis ($p < 0.01$, **Table 5**). Bacterial load in synovial fluid in the contralateral stable stifle was also higher at the 10-week recheck ($p = 0.11$).

Synovial tissue gene expression in HA/doxycycline-treated dogs

Results are summarized in **Table 6**. Overall, expression of TCR Vβ and CD3ε were highly correlated ($S_R = 0.79$, $p < 0.0001$). At diagnosis, expression of TCR Vβ, CD3ε, IL-10, IFN-γ, and

TRAP in synovium was increased in the unstable index stifle, when compared with the stable contralateral stifle ($p < 0.05$). Expression of TNF-α was increased in synovial fluid in the unstable index stifle, when compared with the stable contralateral stifle ($p < 0.01$).

At the 10-week recheck, expression of IFN-γ ($p < 0.05$), TRAP ($p < 0.01$), and TNF-α ($p < 0.05$) in synovial fluid in the unstable index stifle was also higher, when compared with the stable contralateral stifle. Expression of IL-10 ($p < 0.01$) in synovial fluid from the unstable index stifle was also increased, when compared to diagnosis. No significant differences in gene expression were detected at the one-year recheck.

Correlative analyses in HA/doxycycline-treated dogs

Arthroscopic VAS synovitis severity score ($r^2 = 0.57$, $p = 0.005$) and the presence of TRAP$^+$ mononuclear cells in the stable stifle synovium ($S_R = 0.63$, $p = 0.05$) were significantly related to histologic synovitis score at diagnosis. No significant correlation was detected in the unstable index stifle. At diagnosis, bacterial load in synovium and synovial fluid was not significantly related to arthroscopic or histologic severity score, or numbers of TRAP$^+$ mononuclear cells in either stifle. Bacterial load was not significantly correlated with histologic inflammation or synovial gene expression at diagnosis, except that bacterial copy number estimated using the Nadkarni primers was correlated with expression of TNF-α in synovial fluid in the stable contralateral stifle ($S_R = 0.6$, $p < 0.05$). In the unstable stifle at diagnosis, histologic synovitis was inversely correlated with expression of IL-4 in synovium ($S_R = -0.77$, $p = 0.001$). Additionally, the presence of TRAP$^+$ mononuclear cells in synovium was significantly correlated with IL-10 expression in synovium ($S_R = 0.69$, $p < 0.01$). No significant correlations between the presence of a tear in the medial meniscus of the unstable index stifle and any marker of stifle joint inflammation were found.

Correlative analysis between a priori clinical variables and development of subsequent contralateral rupture revealed few significant results. Radiographic assessment of stifle arthritis and effusion, and arthroscopic assessment of synovial inflammation and CrCL fiber tearing were not significantly correlated with subsequent contralateral CrCLR. Pre-operative TPA was not significantly correlated with development of subsequent contralateral CrCLR.

At diagnosis, histologic inflammation in the unstable ($S_R = 0.39$, $p = 0.17$) and stable stifle ($S_R = 0.47$, $p = 0.13$) was not significantly related to subsequent contralateral rupture. Expression of CD3ε in synovium in the unstable stifle was significantly related to subsequent contralateral CrCLR ($S_R = 0.60$, $p = 0.01$), although this was not significant for the stable contralateral stifle. There was also a similar trend for expression of TCR Vβ and TRAP in unstable stifle synovium ($S_R = 0.54$, $p = 0.03$ and $S_R = 0.52$, $p = 0.05$ respectively). Expression of IL-17 in synovial fluid in the stable stifle was inversely correlated with development of

Table 3. Radiographic signs of stifle arthritis and synovial effusion in dogs with unilateral cranial cruciate ligament rupture after surgical stabilization and hyaluronic acid/doxycycline treatment.

Composite Score [28]	Index stifle	Contralateral Stifle	Significance
Diagnosis	6.5 (4–10)	4.5 (0–8)	$p < 0.005$
10 weeks after surgery	7 (4–8)	4 (2–7)	$p < 0.005$
1 year after surgery	8 (6–8)	6 (5–7)	$p < 0.05$
Synovial Effusion [28]			
Diagnosis	2 (1–2)	1 (0–2)	$p < 0.01$
10 weeks after surgery	2 (1–2)	2 (0–2)	NS
1 year after surgery	2 (1–2)	2 (1–2)	NS

Data represent median (range). Diagnosis, n = 16; 12 weeks after surgery, n = 15; 1 year after surgery, n = 8. NS – not significant ($p > 0.05$). Changes in composite score and synovial effusion were not significantly different over time. One dog was excluded from the analysis at the 10 week recheck, because of development of contralateral CCLR at 67 days after surgery, 5 dogs were excluded at long-term follow-up.

Table 4. Synovial inflammation in the unstable index and stable contralateral stifles of dogs with unilateral cranial cruciate ligament rupture.

	Unstable Index Stifle	Stable Contralateral Stifle	Significance
NRS Arthroscopic Synovitis (n = 16)	19 (11, 22)	12 (4, 20)	**p<0.001**
VAS Arthroscopic Synovitis (n = 16)	63±21	35±20	**p<0.001**
Histologic inflammation (n = 12–14)	33±23	20±20	**NS**
TRAP$^+$ mononuclear cells (n = 10–14)	19 (0, 42)	0 (0, 31)	**p<0.05**

Note: Synovitis was scored subjectively using arthroscopy using a compartmental numerical rating scale (NRS, score range 0–24) and a visual analogue scale (VAS). Histologic sections of synovium were also subjectively graded for inflammation and numbers of TRAP$^+$ mononuclear cells using a visual analogue scale; severity scores ranged from 0 (no inflammation) to 100 (could not be more severely inflamed). NS – not significant.

subsequent contralateral CrCLR (S_R = −0.65, p = 0.01). Correlations with IL-10, IL-4, IFN-γ, and TNF-α were not significant.

Discussion

It has been recognized for some time that dogs affected with CrCLR often ultimately develop bilateral ruptures. Bilateral rupture may be diagnosed at initial presentation, or by development of subsequent contralateral CrCLR, often within a relatively short period of time from diagnosis. Risk of subsequent contralateral CrCLR has typically been reported as a proportion at long-term follow-up, often around one year from diagnosis

[2,3,5–7]. This risk is in the range of 22–54% [2,3,5–7]. In the present study, this risk was 54% and was remarkably similar in the different cohorts within the study. Median survival time to subsequent contralateral CrCLR in our large baseline population of dogs treated surgically for unilateral rupture was 947 days overall. Interestingly, the Kaplan-Meier survival plot yielded an exponential shaped curve, particularly for Groups 1 and 2, which had the longest follow-up periods. The shape of the survival curve suggests that within the overall population, there are individual dogs that are protected from the trait, with a long contralateral CrCL survival time, as well as individual dogs that are susceptible to the trait and more rapidly experience subsequent contralateral

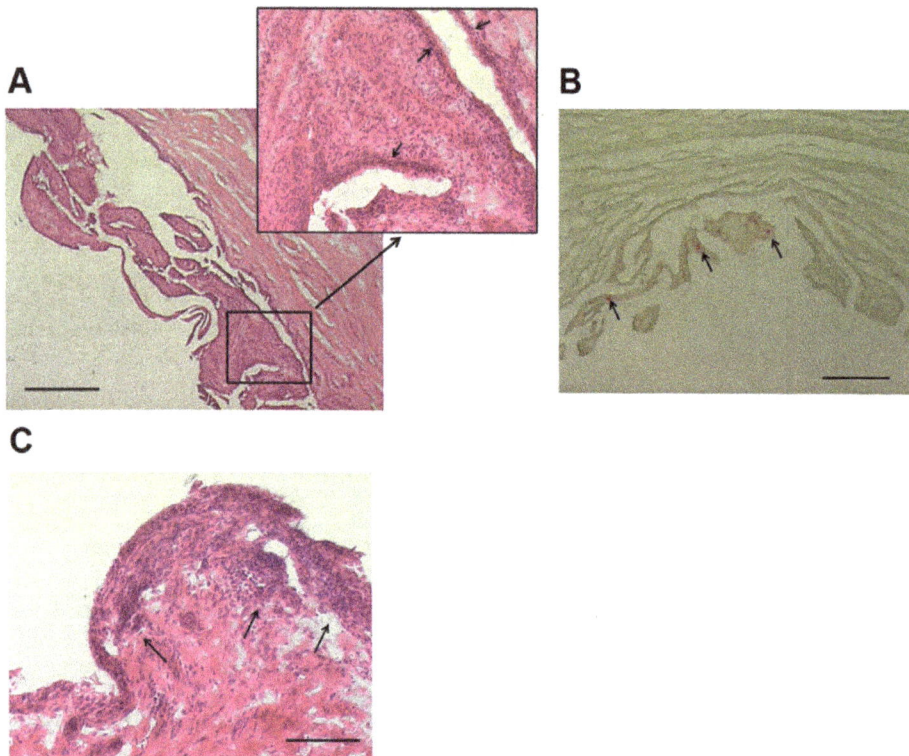

Figure 4. Photomicrographs of stifle synovium from dogs with unilateral cranial cruciate ligament rupture and a contralateral stable stifle. (**A**) Unstable stifle of a five-year-old neutered male Golden Retriever. Proliferation of the synovial intima with villus formation can be seen. Widening of intima (arrows) and infiltration of the intima and sub-intima with mononuclear inflammatory cells can also be seen. (**B**) Unstable stifle of a five-year-old Chesapeake Bay Retriever. TRAP$^+$ mononuclear cells (arrows) were identified in synovial villi in the intima and sub-intimal tissues. (**C**) Stable stifle from a six-year-old neutered male Golden Retriever. Proliferation of the synovial intima can also be seen, with accumulation of mononuclear inflammatory cells within the intima and the sub-intimal tissues (arrows). A,C – Hematoxylin and eosin stain; B – histochemical stain for tartrate-resistant acid phosphatase (TRAP). A – bar = 500 μm; B – bar = 200 μm; C – bar = 100 μm.

Table 5. Bacterial load in the unstable index and stable contralateral stifles of dogs with unilateral cranial cruciate ligament rupture.

16S rRNA Universal Primer Set	Unstable Index Stifle			Stable Contralateral Stifle		
	Diagnosis		10 Week Recheck	Diagnosis		10 Week Recheck
	Synovium	Synovial fluid	Synovial fluid	Synovium	Synovial fluid	Synovial fluid
Yang et al., (2002) [32]	53 (8, 1124)	41 (1, 514)	459## (7, 7931)	93 (10, 392)	212* (1, 2474)	1021 (86, 3882)
Nadkarni et al., (2002) [31]	40 (5, 442)	13 (3, 98)	15 (2, 64)	45 (2, 589)	17 (3, 89)	15 (2, 46)

Note: Data represent median (range). Bacterial load represents estimated 16S rRNA amplicon number using universal primers and real-time PCR.
*p<0.05 versus contralateral joint.
##p≤0.01 versus same tissue at diagnosis. (n = 13 to 16 dogs per group).

CrCLR. The factors that might influence this susceptibility are not fully understood. However, the presence of stifle synovitis histologically increases the risk of subsequent contralateral CrCLR [10], although there is no evidence of a MHC class II immunogenetic association [38]. Non-contact CrCLR is a complex trait, with multiple genes contributing to development of the phenotype [39]. Heritability is estimated to be 0.27 in Newfoundlands, suggesting that extrinsic factors also have a substantial effect on expression of the phenotype [40].

Both intrinsic and extrinsic factors are thought to contribute to the risk of developing CrCLR. Intrinsic factors include genetics, cruciate ligament matrix composition, stifle morphology, and body weight. Extrinsic factors include body condition, whether or not ovariohysterectomy or castration has been performed, and development of synovitis [4,10,39 45]. In the present study, we examined the effect of gender, breed, body weight, age, and TPA on risk of subsequent contralateral CrCLR in a large population of dogs. The effects of breed and body weight were not significant. However, we found that TPA significantly influenced the risk of contralateral CrCLR, suggesting that stifle morphology and functional loading of the CrCL during daily life is a risk factor for CrCLR, although this was not confirmed in our smaller cohort of dogs treated with HA/doxycycline. Although stifle morphological factors appear to confer some risk of CrCLR, stifle

Table 6. Relative expression of immune response genes in synovial fluid from unstable index and stable contralateral stifles of dogs with unilateral cranial cruciate ligament rupture.

Gene	Synovium	Synovial fluid		
	Unstable Index Stifle			
	Diagnosis		10 Week Recheck	1 Year Recheck
TCR Vβ	**0.03 (0.00, 3.33)	0.61 (0.01, 9.89)	0.64 (0.06, 13.8)	0.21 (0.05, 8.49)
CD3ε	*0.02 (0.00, 2.47)	**0.69** (0.01, 3.08)	**0.20** (0.03, 2.24)	**0.1** (0.01, 1.24)
IL-17	**2.59** (0.16, 337)	**3.84** (0.04, 451)	1.76 (0.08, 232)	
IL-10	** **7.98** (0.21, 184)	**14.2** (0.00, 331)	##**55.0** (0.13, 1686)	
IL-4	1.10 (0.00, 35.4)	**4.64** (0.27, 112)	1.17 (0.01, 785)	
IFN-γ	**1.38 (0.01, 10480)	12.4 (0.01, 3572)	*8.99 (0.51, 100)	
TRAP	**1.08 (0.01, 95.9)	**5.78** (0.48, 53.9)	**24.4 (0.06, 124)	
TNF-α	0.11 (0.00, 5.39)	**2.06 (0.00, 18.6)	*1.39 (0.32, 14.9)	2.75 (0.20, 16.8)
	Stable Contralateral Stifle			
TCR Vβ	**0.02** (0.00, 0.18)	**0.11** (0.01, 43.03)	0.21 (0.00, 1711)	0.40 (0.07, 1.16)
CD3ε	**0.02** (0.00, 0.08)	**0.15** (0.01, 22.3)	**0.04** (0.00, 1270)	0.17 (0.05, 1.00)
IL-17	2.71 (0.00, 122)	**4.58** (0.05, 23347)	1.87 (0.00, 84)	
IL-10	1.00 (0.02, 18.0)	**17.0** (0.04, 98.3)	**29.0** (0.18, 250)	
IL-4	0.80 (0.01, 15.8)	2.11 (0.00, 153)	**17.1** (0.80, 139407)	
IFN-γ	0.33 (0.00, 761)	0.63 (0.02, 126)	0.73 (0.00, 137)	
TRAP	**0.11** (0.01, 2.92)	**2.28** (0.26, 36.6)	1.87 (0.03, 92.0)	
TNF-α	**0.04** (0.00, 0.42)	**0.31** (0.00, 9.41)	0.38 (0.00, 5.50)	1.10 (0.46, 6.39)

Note: TCR Vβ - beta chain of the canine T cell receptor; TRAP – tartrate-resistant acid phosphatase; IL – interleukin; IFN – interferon; TNF – tumor necrosis factor. Data represent median (range). Median values in bold indicate that gene expression is significantly different from the peripheral blood mononuclear cell internal control (p<0.05).
*p<0.05,
**p<0.01 versus contralateral stifle.
##p<0.01 versus same tissue at diagnosis. n = 15–16 at diagnosis, n = 14–15 at 10 week recheck, n = 5–7 at 1 year recheck.

morphology alone and TPA, in particular, does not appear to be a primary causative factor [46]. The age range when CrCLR develops is typically between 2–10 years [43,44]. In the present study, we found that age significantly influenced CrCL survival, with increasing age being associated with increased contralateral CrCL survival, although this effect also appeared small in magnitude. This observation also fits with the concept that our overall study population consisted of dogs with a mixture of intrinsic (genetic) susceptibility to the CrCLR trait. Neutered dogs also had shortened contralateral CrCL survival, as previously described [43,44].

In a second experiment, we examined long-term CrCL survival in a small cohort of dogs with unilateral CrCLR that were treated with HA/doxycycline and surgical stabilization of the index stifle. We did not find a significant treatment effect with our provisional disease-modifying therapy. Correlative analysis revealed few significant associations between markers of stifle disease and subsequent development of contralateral CrCLR, although increased expression of T-cell associated genes in the unstable stifle at diagnosis was correlated with development of subsequent contralateral CrCLR. This observation fits with the concept that the presence of stifle synovitis is related to the risk of subsequent contralateral CrCLR [10], although the correlation between expression of IL-17 in synovial fluid in the stable stifle and development of subsequent contralateral CrCLR that we detected was an inverse one. Further work is needed studying association of the trait with MHC genotype, although current evidence suggests a strong class II association is unlikely [38]. Bacterial load was not significantly correlated with histologic synovitis, although increased copy number was detected in the unstable stifle, which increased over time. Although we have previously reported association and weak correlation between bacterial load and stifle synovitis/arthritis in CrCLR dogs [22–24], collectively these results suggest that bacterial load is not a key factor in development of stifle synovitis in affected dogs.

In this proof-of-principle study, we selected the test compounds used in the trial based on existing literature in the field of disease-modifying therapy, including both anti-inflammatory compounds, as well as compounds that may ameliorate connective tissue matrix degradation over time. Additionally, both of the treatments used are generic and inexpensive. Doxycycline has been widely studied as a potential therapeutic drug for arthritis. In-vitro, doxycycline can inhibit gelatinase-mediated degradation of type XI collagen, reduce activation of collagenase, and inhibit mRNA for inducible nitric oxide, a mediator of tissue catabolism [26,47,48]. In-vivo studies in dogs suggest that treatment can modify development of arthritis over time [27], using a treatment regimen of similar duration and dosage to that of the present study. Indirectly, this may suggest that disease-modifying therapy that targets synovial inflammation may be a more effective treatment strategy than therapy that targets ligament matrix degeneration, as the doxycycline regimen used in this study did not significantly influence CrCL survival. An additional point supporting this concept is the recent observation that synovitis is an early event in canine non-contact CrCL rupture, which precedes development of arthroscopically visible fraying of the cruciate ligament complex [8].

HA has also been widely studied as a disease-modifying treatment for arthritis both as a course of intra-articular injections, as well as using a single injection protocol [49,50]. Potential therapeutic effects on arthritic joints from intra-articular HA injection are complex and include reduction in both synovial inflammation, and connective tissue matrix degeneration through inhibition of MMP-13 expression, for example [51]. Pro-

inflammatory effects of HA fragmentation may occur through CD44 signaling [52]. However, treatment with intra-articular HA did not reduce CD44 expression in OA joints experimentally in an ovine meniscectomy model, but did reduce synovial vascularity and subintimal fibrosis [49]. In the present study, we also used arthroscopy to examine both the index and contralateral stifles at initial diagnosis [8]. The joint lavage associated with the arthroscopic procedure has the potential to exert a disease-modifying effect, by reducing synovial inflammation and production of pro-inflammatory cytokines, such as TNF-α [53].

In the dogs in this cohort, overall mobility was significantly improved at long-term follow-up, with equalization of weight-bearing between the index stifle treated with TPLO and the contralateral stifle, except for the dogs that developed subsequent contralateral CrCLR during the study period. Radiographic signs of arthritis were significantly worse in the unstable index stifle. There was also some evidence of worsening synovial effusion in the stable contralateral stifle over time, although no clinical or radiographically detectable changes in stability were identified. Synovial effusion was significantly worse in the index stifle at diagnosis, but not at the follow-up visits. Similarly, there was little change in expression of gene markers for T cells and macrophages over time. Increases in expression of the T-cell associated genes TCR Vβ, CD3ε, and IFN-γ that were identified in the unstable index stifle relative to the contralateral stable stifle were principally identified at diagnosis, although expression of IFN-γ remained increased in the unstable stifle at the 10 week recheck. Up-regulation of macrophage-associated genes (IL-10, TRAP, and TNF-α) was also identified in the unstable stifle at diagnosis and also at the 10-week recheck; there was no significant difference in TNF-α between index and contralateral stifles at the one-year recheck. These observations suggest that development of stifle synovitis may be mediated via T lymphocyte and macrophage signaling, which was not influenced by oral doxycycline treatment.

Interestingly, IL-10 was the only gene whose expression was increased in synovial fluid from the unstable stifle at the 10-week recheck. Relative expression was also higher in the contralateral stable stifle. IL-10 is a cytokine with anti-inflammatory properties that is typically up-regulated in arthritic joints [54,55]. Up-regulation of IL-10 in both stifles relative to internal control, with increased expression over time suggests that immune regulating cells, such as macrophages and regulatory T cells, are acting to inhibit effector T cells and activated macrophages, and suppress synovial inflammation in affected joints. In humans with rheumatoid arthritis, there is impairment of regulatory T cell function [56]. Polymorphisms in the promotor region of IL-10 are known to influence the risk of rheumatoid arthritis in human beings, by reducing IL-10 transcription and decreasing circulating IL-10 [57]. Similarly, IL-10 polymorphisms have been associated with immune-mediated disease in the dog [58]. Whether there is functional impairment of anti-inflammatory cytokine responses in dogs with stifle synovitis and non-contact CrCL rupture has not been determined. In the present study, the presence of TRAP+ mononuclear cells in synovium was significantly correlated with IL-10 expression in the unstable stifle at diagnosis, supporting the concept that IL-10 production by activated macrophages may be a functionally important anti-inflammatory factor within the joint environment, acting to ameliorate synovitis in this disease.

Although we did not identify an obvious treatment effect on CrCL survival, or significant progression of arthritis pathology over time, the lack of a treatment effect from arthroscopic lavage and associated medical therapy suggests that this in-vivo client-owned canine model of unilateral CrCLR (with contralateral incipient disease) may be valuable for future mechanistic and therapeutic studies, since pathogenesis of naturally occurring non-contact CrCLR in client-owned dogs is substantially different from traumatic CrCLR modeled by CrCL transection in the Pond-Nuki model [59], and has many similarities to the non-contact minimal trauma ACL rupture that is common in human beings, particularly women [60,61].

The lack of a significant treatment effect in this cohort, with a 31% contralateral rupture rate at one year, also suggests that our arthroscopic findings in the stable stifle at diagnosis are a valid reflection of incipient disease. Arthroscopic grading of synovitis has been widely performed in human beings with arthritic conditions [62], but not in dogs [8]. All client-owned dogs had medical treatment with non-steroidal anti-inflammatory drugs of variable duration before inclusion in this study [8], but this medical therapy did not prevent development of subsequent contralateral CrCLR in the cohort.

This study had several limitations. A potential concern with our ligament survival analysis was that limited phenotypic and clinical status data were available for each dog. It is common for CrCLR-affected dogs to be treated with a non-steroidal anti-inflammatory drug (NSAIDs). Whether NSAID medication has any effect on CrCL survival could not be determined from the present study. Given that stifle synovitis increases the risk of subsequent contralateral CrCLR in client-owned dogs [10], in future work it would be interesting to determine, in more detail, whether or not synovitis and the presence of specific T cell subsets in joint tissues or peripheral blood [63] have a significant effect on contralateral CrCL survival over time. Although difficult to obtain in a client-owned dog model, follow-up second-look arthroscopy and synovial biopsies may have also yielded additional data on synovitis status over time. Several dogs in the treatment cohort developed subsequent contralateral rupture during the study period. Collection and analysis of additional stifle joint tissue samples in these dogs at the time of contralateral stifle stabilization surgery may also have been informative. More detailed study of the phenotype of the inflammatory cells within the synovium of stable stifles [63] and analysis of other biomarkers of joint inflammation,

such as C-reactive protein [64], may also have yielded additional data on the relationship between synovitis and development of non-contact CrCLR. In addition, mobility questionnaire data were obtained retrospectively at long-term follow-up. Although efficacy of intra-articular HA has been described after use of a single injection [50], treatment is often given as a course of injections [49]. Efficacy of HA treatment may have been improved with a course of intra-articular injections, although risk of adverse effects may also be increased.

In conclusion, subsequent contralateral CrCLR is common in client-owned dogs, with a median ligament survival time of 947 days. Treatment with arthroscopic lavage, single intra-articular HA injection, and oral doxycycline does not significantly influence contralateral CrCL survival. In this client-owned model of stifle arthritis and non-contact minimal trauma CrCLR, development of cranial tibial translation is preceded by development of synovial inflammation, superficial fraying of the cruciate ligament complex, and rupture of ligament fibers, particularly within the caudolateral bundle of the CrCL [8]. The immunological mechanism that induces development of synovitis in stable stifles with incipient CrCLR should be the focus of future work on identification of targets for disease-modifying therapy. Here T cell-mediated synovitis appears important. More work is also needed on identification of a genetic marker or a clinically relevant biomarker that is a good predictor of progressive ligament rupture over time.

Acknowledgments

The laboratory of Dr. Christopher Olsen, University of Wisconsin-Madison, School of Veterinary Medicine kindly supplied the Madin Darby canine kidney cells. The assistance of Dr. Paul Manley is also gratefully acknowledged.

Author Contributions

Conceived and designed the experiments: PM. Performed the experiments: ZS SM AK JAB SLS GH ZH. Analyzed the data: ZH SM PM. Wrote the paper: PM. Contributed epidemiological data: SC NB.

References

1. Wilke VL, Robinson DA, Evans RB, Rothschild MF, Conzemius MG (2005) Estimate of the annual economic impact of treatment of cranial cruciate ligament injury in dogs in the United States. J Am Vet Med Assoc 227: 1604–1607.
2. Cabrera SY, Owen TJ, Mueller MG, Kass PH (2008) Comparison of tibial plateau angles in dogs with unilateral versus bilateral cranial cruciate ligament rupture: 150 cases (2000–2006). J Am Vet Med Assoc 232: 889–892.
3. Buote N, Fusco J, Radasch R (2009) Age, tibial plateau angle, sex, and weight as risk factors for contralateral rupture of the cranial cruciate ligament in Labradors. Vet Surg 38: 481–489.
4. Hayashi K, Manley PA, Muir P (2004) Cranial cruciate ligament pathophysiology in dogs with cruciate disease: a review. J Am Anim Hosp Assoc 40: 385–390.
5. de Bruin T, de Rooster H, Bosmans T, Duchateau L, van Bree H, et al. (2007) Radiographic assessment of the progression of osteoarthrosis in the contralateral stifle joint of dogs with a ruptured cranial cruciate ligament. Vet Rec 161: 745–750.
6. Doverspike M, Vasseur PB, Harb MF, Walls CM (1993) Contralateral cranial cruciate ligament rupture: incidence in 114 dogs. J Am Anim Hosp Assoc 29: 167–170.
7. Moore KW, Read RA (1995) Cranial cruciate ligament rupture in the dog – a retrospective study comparing surgical techniques. Aust Vet J 72: 281–285.
8. Bleedorn JA, Greuel EN, Manley PA, Schaefer SL, Markel MD, et al. (2011) Synovitis in dogs with stable stifle joints and incipient cranial cruciate ligament rupture: A cross-sectional study. Vet Surg 40: 531–543.
9. Sumner JP, Markel MD, Muir P (2010) Caudal cruciate ligament damage in dogs with cranial cruciate ligament rupture. Vet Surg 39: 936–941.
10. Erne JB, Goring RL, Kennedy FA, Schoenborn WC (2009) Prevalence of lymphoplasmacytic synovitis in dogs with naturally occurring cranial cruciate ligament rupture. J Am Vet Med Assoc 235: 386–390.
11. de Rooster H, de Bruin T, van Bree H (2006) Morphologic and functional features of the canine cruciate ligaments. Vet Surg 35: 769–780.

12. Kobayashi S, Baba J, Uchida K, Negoro K, Sato M, et al. (2006) Microvascular system of the anterior cruciate ligament in dogs. J Orthop Res 24: 1509–1520.
13. Goldberg VM, Burstein A, Dawson M (1982) The influence of an experimental immune synovitis on the failure mode and strength of the rabbit anterior cruciate ligament. J Bone Joint Surg 64A: 900–906.
14. Galloway RH, Lester SJ (1995) Histopathological evaluation of canine stifle joint synovial membrane collected at the time of repair of cranial cruciate ligament rupture. J Am Anim Hosp Assoc 31: 289–294.
15. Lemburg AK, Meyer-Lindenberg A, Hewicker-Trautwein M (2004) Immunohistochemical characterization of inflammatory cell populations and adhesion molecule expression in synovial membranes from dogs with spontaneous cranial cruciate ligament rupture. Vet Immunol Immunopathol 97: 231–240.
16. Klocke NW, Snyder PW, Widmer WR, Zhong W, McCabe GP, et al. (2005) Detection of synovial macrophages in the joint capsule of dogs with naturally occurring rupture of the cranial cruciate ligament. Am J Vet Res 66: 493–499.
17. Muir P, Schamberger GM, Manley PA, Hao Z (2005) Localization of cathepsin K and tartrate-resistant acid phosphatase in synovium and cranial cruciate ligament in dogs with cruciate disease. Vet Surg 34: 239–246.
18. Faldyna M, Zatloukal J, Leva L, Kohout P, Necas A, et al. (2004) Lymphocyte subsets in stifle joint synovial fluid of dogs with spontaneous rupture of the cranial cruciate ligament. Acta Vet Brno 73: 79–84.
19. de Rooster H, Cox E, van Bree H (2000) Prevalence and relevance of antibodies to type-I and -II collagen in synovial fluid of dogs with cranial cruciate ligament damage. Am J Vet Res 61: 1456–1461.
20. de Bruin T, de Rooster H, van Bree H, Cox E (2007) Evaluation of anticollagen type I antibody titers in synovial fluid of both stifle joints and the left shoulder joint of dogs with unilateral cranial cruciate disease. Am J Vet Res 68: 283–289.
21. de Bruin T, de Rooster H, van Bree H, Waelbers T, Cox E (2007) Lymphocyte proliferation to collagen type I in dogs. J Vet Med A Physiol Pathol Clin Med 54: 292–296.
22. Muir P, Oldenhoff WE, Hudson AP, Manley PA, Schaefer SL, et al. (2007) Detection of DNA from a range of bacterial species in the knee joints of dogs

with inflammatory knee arthritis and associated degenerative anterior cruciate ligament rupture. Microb Pathog 42: 47–55.

23. Muir P, Fox R, Wu Q, Baker TA, Zitzer NC, et al. (2010) Seasonal variation in detection of bacterial DNA in arthritic stifle joints of dogs with cranial cruciate ligament rupture using PCR amplification of the 16S rRNA gene. Vet Microbiol 141: 127–133.

24. Schwartz Z, Zitzer NC, Racette MA, Manley PA, Schaefer SL, et al. (2011) Are bacterial load and synovitis related in dogs with inflammatory stifle arthritis? Vet Microbiol 148: 308–316.

25. Brandt KD, Mazzuca SA, Katz BP, Lane KA, Buckwalter KA, et al. (2005) Effects of doxycycline on progression of osteoarthritis: results of a randomized, placebo-controlled, double-blind trial. Arthritis Rheum 52: 2015–2025.

26. Yu LP, Smith GN, Hasty KA, Brandt KD (1991) Doxycycline inhibits type XI collagenolytic activity of extracts from human osteoarthritic cartilage and of gelatinase. J Rheumatol 18: 1450–1452.

27. Yu LP, Jr., Smith GN, Jr., Brandt KD, Myers SL, O'Connor BL, et al. (1992) Reduction of the severity of canine osteoarthritis by prophylactic treatment with oral doxycycline. Arthritis Rheum 35: 1150–1159.

28. Innes JF, Costello M, Barr FJ, Rudorf H, Barr ARS (2004) Radiographic progression of osteoarthritis of the canine stifle joint: a prospective study. Vet Radiol Ultrasound 45: 143–148.

29. Hercock CA, Pinchbeck G, Giejda A, Clegg PD, Innes JF (2009) Validation of a client-based clinical metrology instrument for the evaluation of canine elbow osteoarthritis. J Small Anim Pract 50: 266–271.

30. Quinn MM, Keuler NS, Lu Y, Faria MLE, Muir P, et al. (2007) Evaluation of Agreement Between Numerical Rating Scales, Visual Analogue Scoring Scales, and Force Plate Gait Analysis in Dogs. Vet Surg 36: 360–367.

31. Nadkarni MA, Martin FE, Jacques NA, Hunter N (2002) Determination of bacterial load by real-time PCR using a broad-range (universal) probe and primers set. Microbiol 148: 257–266.

32. Yang S, Lin S, Kelen GD, Quinn TC, Dick JD, et al. (2002) Quantitative multiprobe PCR assay for simultaneous detection and identification to species level of bacterial pathogens. J Clin Microbiol 40: 3449–3454.

33. Horz HP, Vianna ME, Gomes BPFA, Conrads G (2005) Evaluation of universal probes and primer sets for assessing total bacterial load in clinical samples: General implications and practical use in endodontic microbial therapy. J Clin Microbiol 43: 5332–5337.

34. Samuelson LE, Harford JB, Klausner RD (1985) Identification of the components of the murine T cell antigen receptor complex. Cell 43: 223–231.

35. Baniyash M, Garcia-Morales P, Bonifacino JS, Samuelson LE, Klausner RD (1988) Disulfide linkage of the ζ and η chains of the T cell receptor. J Biol Chem 263: 9874–9878.

36. Stephanini M, De Martino C, Zamboni L (1967) Fixation of ejaculated spermatozoa for electron microscopy. Nature 216: 173–174.

37. Schefe JH, Lehmann KE, Buschmann IR, Unger T, Funke-Kaiser H (2006) Quantitative real-time RT-PCR data analysis: current concepts and the novel "gene expression's C_T difference" formula. J Mol Med 84: 901–910.

38. Clements DN, Kennedy LJ, Short AD, Barnes A, Ferguson J, et al. (2011) Risk of canine cranial cruciate ligament rupture is not associated with the major histocompatibility complex. Vet Comp Orthop Traumat 24: 262–265.

39. Wilke VL, Zhang S, Evans RB, Conzemius MG, Rothschild MF (2009) Identification of chromosomal regions associated with cranial cruciate ligament rupture in a population of Newfoundlands. Am J Vet Res 70: 1013–1017.

40. Wilke VL, Conzemius MG, Kinghorn BP, Macrossan PE, Cai W, et al. (2006) Inheritance of rupture of the cranial cruciate ligament in Newfoundlands. J Am Vet Med Assoc 228: 61–64.

41. Comerford EJ, Tarlton JF, Innes JF, Johnson KA, Amis AA, et al. (2005) Metabolism and composition of the canine anterior cruciate ligament relate to differences in knee joint mechanics and predisposition to ligament rupture. J Orthop Res 23: 61–66.

42. Guerrero TG, Geyer H, Hässig M, Montavon PM (2007) Effect of conformation of the distal portion of the femur and proximal portion of the tibia on the pathogenesis of cranial cruciate ligament disease in dogs. Am J Vet Res 68: 1332–1337.

43. Whitehair JG, Vasseur PB, Willits NH (1993) Epidemiology of cranial cruciate ligament rupture in dogs. J Am Vet Med Assoc 203: 1016–1019.

44. Witsberger TH, Villamil JA, Schultz LG, Hahn AW, Cook JL (2008) Prevalence of and risk factors for hip dysplasia and cranial cruciate ligament deficiency in dogs. J Am Vet Med Assoc 232: 1818–1824.

45. Doom M, de Bruin T, de Rooster H, van Bree H, Cox E (2008) Immunopathological mechanisms in dogs with rupture of the cranial cruciate ligament. Vet Immunol Immunopathol 125: 143–161.

46. Wilke VL, Conzemius MG, Besancon MF, Evans RB, Ritter M (2002) Comparison of tibial plateau angle between clinically normal greyhounds and Labrador retrievers with and without rupture of the cranial cruciate ligament. J Am Vet Med Assoc 221: 1426–1429.

47. Smith GN, Jr., Brandt KD, Hasty KA (1996) Activation of recombinant human neutrophil procollagenase in the presence of doxycycline results in fragmentation of the enzyme and loss of enzyme activity. Arthritis Rheum 39: 235–244.

48. Amin AR, Attur MG, Thakker GD, Patel PD, Vyas PR, et al. (1996) A novel mechanism of action of tetracyclines: effects on nitric oxide synthases. Proc Natl Acad Sci USA 93: 14014–14019.

49. Smith MM, Cake MA, Ghosh P, Schiavinato A, Read RA, et al. (2008) Significant synovial pathology in a meniscectomy model of osteoarthritis: modifications by intra-articular hyaluronan therapy. Rheumatology 47: 1172–1178.

50. Chevalier X, Jerosch J, Goupille P, van Dijk N, Luyten FP, et al. (2010) Single, intra-articular treatment with 6 ml hylan G-F 20 in patients with symptomatic primary osteoarthritis of the knee: a randomized, multicenter, double-blind, placebo controlled trial. Ann Rheum Dis 69: 113–119.

51. Hiraoka N, Takahashi KA, Arai Y, Sakao K, Mazda O, et al. (2011) Intra-articular injection of hyaluronan restores aberrant expression of matrix metalloproteinase-13 in osteoarthritic subchondral bone. J Orthop Res 29: 354–360.

52. Jiang D, Liang J, Noble PW (2011) Hyaluronan as an immune regulator in human diseases. Physiol Rev 91: 221–264.

53. Fu X, Lin L, Zhang J, Yu C (2009) Assessment of the efficacy of joint lavage in rabbits with osteoarthritis of the knee. J Orthop Res 27: 91–96.

54. Maccoux LJ, Salway F, Day PJR, Clements DN (2007) Expression profiling of select cytokines in canine osteoarthritis tissues. Vet Immunol Immunopathol 118: 59–67.

55. Fernandes JC, Martel-Pelletier J, Pelletier J-P (2002) The role of cytokines in osteoarthritis pathophysiology. Biorheology 39: 237–246.

56. Boissier M-C, Assier E, Biton J, Denys A, Falgarone G, et al. (2009) Regulatory T cells (Treg) in rheumatoid arthritis. Joint Bone Spine 76: 10–14.

57. Ying B, Shi Y, Pan X, Song X, Huang Z, et al. (2011) Association of polymorphisms in the human IL-10 and IL-18 genes with rheumatoid arthritis. Mol Biol Rep 38: 379–385.

58. Short AD, Catchpole B, Kennedy LJ, Barnes A, Lee AC, et al. (2009) T cell cytokine gene polymorphisms in canine diabetes mellitus. Vet Immunol Immunopathol 28: 137–146.

59. Pond MJ, Nuki G (1973) Experimentally-induced osteoarthritis in the dog. Ann Rheum Dis 32: 387–388.

60. Toth AP, Cordasco FA (2001) Anterior cruciate ligament injuries in the female athlete. J Gend Specif Med 4: 25–34.

61. Posthumus M, September AV, O'Cuinneagain D, van der Merwe W, Schwellnus MP, et al. (2009) The COL5A1 gene is associated with increased risk of anterior cruciate ligament rupture in female participants. Am J Sports Med 37: 2234–2240.

62. Ayral X, Mayoux-Benhamou A, Dougados M (1996) Proposed scoring system for assessing synovial membrane abnormalities at arthroscopy in knee osteoarthritis. Br J Rheumatol 35(suppl. 3): 14–17.

63. Muir P, Kelly JL, Marvel SJ, Heinrich DA, Schaefer SL, et al. (2011) Lymphocyte populations in joint tissues from dogs with inflammatory stifle arthritis and degenerative cranial cruciate ligament rupture. Vet Surg 40: 753–761.

64. Ohno K, Yokoyama Y, Nakashima K, Setoguchi A, Fujino Y, Tsujimoto H (2006) C-reactive protein concentration in canine idiopathic polyarthritis. J Vet Med Sci 68: 1275–1279.

65. Dreitz MJ, Ogilvie G, Sim GK (1999) Rearranged T lymphocyte antigen receptor genes as markers of malignant T cells. Vet Immunol Immunopathol 69: 113–119.

66. Nash RA, Scherf U, Storb R (1991) Molecular cloning of the CD3ε subunit of the T-cell receptor/CD3 complex in the dog. Immunogenetics 33: 396–398.

67. Wang YS, Chi KH, Chu RM (2007) Cytokine profiles of canine monocyte-derived dendritic cells as a function of lipopolysaccharide- or tumor necrosis factor-alpha-induced maturation. Vet Immunol Immunopathol 118: 186–198.

17

Two Major Medicinal Honeys Have Different Mechanisms of Bactericidal Activity

Paulus H. S. Kwakman[1], Anje A. te Velde[2], Leonie de Boer[1], Christina M. J. E. Vandenbroucke-Grauls[1,3], Sebastian A. J. Zaat[1]*

1 Department of Medical Microbiology, Center for Infection and Immunity Amsterdam (CINIMA), Academic Medical Center, University of Amsterdam, Amsterdam, The Netherlands, **2** Tytgat Institute for Liver and Intestinal Research, Academic Medical Center, University of Amsterdam, Amsterdam, The Netherlands, **3** Department of Medical Microbiology and Infectious Diseases, VU Medical Center, Amsterdam, The Netherlands

Abstract

Honey is increasingly valued for its antibacterial activity, but knowledge regarding the mechanism of action is still incomplete. We assessed the bactericidal activity and mechanism of action of Revamil® source (RS) honey and manuka honey, the sources of two major medical-grade honeys. RS honey killed *Bacillus subtilis*, *Escherichia coli* and *Pseudomonas aeruginosa* within 2 hours, whereas manuka honey had such rapid activity only against *B. subtilis*. After 24 hours of incubation, both honeys killed all tested bacteria, including methicillin-resistant *Staphylococcus aureus*, but manuka honey retained activity up to higher dilutions than RS honey. Bee defensin-1 and H_2O_2 were the major factors involved in rapid bactericidal activity of RS honey. These factors were absent in manuka honey, but this honey contained 44-fold higher concentrations of methylglyoxal than RS honey. Methylglyoxal was a major bactericidal factor in manuka honey, but after neutralization of this compound manuka honey retained bactericidal activity due to several unknown factors. RS and manuka honey have highly distinct compositions of bactericidal factors, resulting in large differences in bactericidal activity.

Editor: Pere-Joan Cardona, Fundació Institut Germans Trias i Pujol; Universitat Autònoma de Barcelona CibeRES, Spain

Funding: The authors have no support or funding to report.

Competing Interests: The authors have declared that no competing interests exist.

* E-mail: s.a.zaat@amc.uva.nl

Introduction

Antibiotic-resistant bacteria pose a very serious threat to public health. Resistance not only is a major problem in hospitals; resistant bacteria are now recognized among various groups in the community, such as pig-breeders, and in cattle [1–3]. Frequencies of bacterial resistance are increasing worldwide while very few new antibiotics are being developed [4,5]. Therefore alternative antimicrobial strategies are urgently needed.

For thousands of years honey has been used for treatment of wounds and as a gastrointestinal remedy [6,7]. Honey has broad-spectrum activity against pathogenic and food-spoiling bacteria [8–11]. The potent *in vitro* activity of honey against antibiotic-resistant bacteria [8] and its successful application in treatment of chronic wound infections not responding to antibiotic therapy [12] evoked interest in honey as antibacterial agent in modern medicine. Revamil® and manuka medical-grade honey have potent antibacterial activity [9,13] and are approved for application in wound management. RS honey, the source for Revamil®, is produced under standardized conditions in green-houses. The factors responsible for the bactericidal activity of this honey are the high sugar concentration, H_2O_2, the 1,2-dicarbonyl compound methylglyoxal (MGO), the cationic antimicrobial peptide bee defensin-1 and the low pH [14].

Manuka honey is produced from the manuka bush (*Leptospermum scoparium*) indigenous to New Zealand and Australia. Exceptionally high concentrations of the antibacterial compound MGO have been found in manuka honey [15,16], but the contribution this

and possible other compounds to the bactericidal activity of manuka honey is still unknown.

Incomplete knowledge of the antibacterial factors in honey and the contribution of these factors to the bactericidal activity hamper general applicability of honey. In the current study we determined the levels of all established honey antibacterial factors in RS and manuka honey and assessed the contribution of these factors to the bactericidal activity of both honeys against food-spoiling and pathogenic bacteria, including methicillin-resistant *Staphylococcus aureus*. We demonstrate that RS and manuka honey have highly distinct compositions of bactericidal factors, resulting in substantial differences in bactericidal activity. We show that in addition to MGO several other factors contribute substantially to the bactericidal activity of manuka honey. The implications of these findings for prudent application in medicine and for the potential use of honey in food preservation are discussed.

Methods

Honey

Unprocessed Revamil® source (RS) honey was kindly provided by Bfactory Health Products (Rhenen, The Netherlands). Non-sterilized UMF™ 16+ Active manuka honey was purchased from Nature's nectar Limited (Surrey, UK). To study the contribution of the sugars to the bactericidal activity of honey, a solution with a sugar composition similar to that of honey was prepared (333 g/kg glucose, 385 g/kg fructose, 73 g/kg sucrose and 62 g/kg maltose).

Microorganisms

Bactericidal activity of honey was assessed against *Bacillus subtilis* ATCC6633, Escherichia *coli* ML-35p [17], *Pseudomonas aeruginosa* PAO-1 (ATCC 15692) and against methicillin-resistant *S. aureus* (MRSA) strain AMC201 [14].

Quantification of H2O2 in honey

H_2O_2 concentrations that had accumulated in diluted honey were determined quantitatively as described previously [18]. In brief, 40 μl samples of honey were added to 135 μl reagent, consisting of 50 μg/ml o-dianisidine (Sigma-Aldrich, St. Louis, MI, USA) and 20 μg/ml horseradish peroxidase type IV (Sigma-Aldrich, St. Louis, MI, USA) in 10 mM phosphate buffer pH 6.5. After 5 min. of incubation at room temperature, reactions were stopped by addition of 120 μl 6 M H_2SO_4 and absorption at 540 nm was measured. H_2O_2 concentrations were calculated using a calibration curve of 2-fold serial dilutions of H_2O_2 ranging from 2200 to 2.1 μM.

Methylglyoxal (MGO) quantification and neutralization assay

Reduced glutathione (Sigma-Aldrich, St. Louis, MI, USA) was added to diluted honey to a final concentration of 15 mM, and conversion of MGO to S-D-lactoyl-glutathione (SLG) was initiated by addition of 0.5 U/ml glyoxalase I (Sigma-Aldrich, St. Louis, MI, USA). We previously determined that the bactericidal activity of a solution containing 20 mM MGO was completely neutralized by conversion to SLG [14]. The amount of MGO converted to SLG was determined using the extinction coefficient of SLG of 3.37 mM^{-1} at 240 nm [19]. As a control for complete conversion of MGO in honey, SLG formation was assessed for 40% honey solutions spiked with 10 mM of exogenous MGO.

Analysis of bee defensin-1 in honey

Bee defensin-1 was separated from other honey bactericidal factors and analysed as described previously [14]. In brief, 15 ml of 20% (v/v) honey was centrifuged in a 5 kDa molecular weight cut-off Amicon Ultra-15 tube (Millipore, Waters, Milford, MA, USA) at 4000×g for 45 min. at room temperature. The <5 kDa filtrate was collected, and the >5 kDa retentate, where bee defensin-1 would be retained, was subsequently washed three times in the filter tube with 15 ml of demineralized water and concentrated to 0.4 ml. Duplicate samples of retentate equivalent to 150 μl of undiluted honey were subjected to native acid-urea polyacrylamide gel electrophoresis (AU-PAGE). Bee defensin-1 was subsequently visualized by parallel Coomassie-staining and by a *B. subtilis* overlay assay.

Liquid bactericidal assay

Bactericidal activity of honey was quantified in 100 μl volume liquid tests, in polypropylene microtiterplates (Costar, Corning, NY, USA). For each experiment, a 50% (v/v) stock solution of honey was freshly prepared in incubation buffer containing 10 mM phosphate buffer pH 7.0 supplemented with 0.03% (w/v) trypticase soy broth (TSB; Difco, Detroit, MI, USA). Bacteria from logarithmic phase cultures in TSB were washed twice with incubation buffer and used at a final concentration of 1×10^6 CFU/ml, based on optical density. Plates were incubated at 37°C on a rotary shaker at 150 rpm. At indicated time points, duplicate 10 μl aliquots of undiluted and 10-fold serially diluted incubations of three independent incubations were plated on blood agar. Bacterial survival was quantified after overnight incubation at 37°C. The detection level of this assay is 100 CFU/ml. To assess the contribution of H_2O_2 and cationic compounds to the bactericidal activity of honey, 600 U/ml bovine liver catalase (Sigma-Aldrich, St. Louis, MI, USA) and 0.025% (w/v) sodium polyanetholesulfonate (SPS; Sigma-Aldrich, St. Louis, MI, USA), respectively, were added to incubations. Since bee defensin-1 is the only cationic bactericidal compound present in RS honey [14], addition of SPS to this honey specifically neutralizes bee defensin-1. The incubation buffer did not affect the pH of the concentrations of honey used in our experiments. A 1 M NaOH solution was used to titrate honey solutions to pH 7.0.

Ultrafiltration of honey components

Fifteen ml of 20% (v/v) honey was centrifuged in a 5 kDa molecular weight cut-off Amicon Ultra-15 tube (Millipore, Waters, Milford, MA, USA) at 4000×g for 45 min. at room temperature. The <5 kDa filtrate was collected, and the >5 kDa retentate was subsequently washed three times in the filter tube with 15 ml of demineralized water and concentrated to 0.4 ml.

Bacterial overlay assay

To visualize the antibacterial activity of bee defensin-1 from honey, a bacterial overlay assay was used. Amounts of >5 kDa honey retentate equivalent to 150 μl honey were separated by acid urea polyacrylamide gel electrophoresis (AU-PAGE) [20]. Gels were either stained with PAGE-Blue (Fermentas, Vilnius, Lithuania) or washed 3×8 min. in 10 mM phosphate buffer pH 7.0 for a bacterial overlay assay. After washing, the gel was incubated for 3 hours at 37°C on *B. subtilis*-inoculated nutrient-poor agarose to allow components to diffuse into the agarose. For this agarose, a *B. subtilis* inoculum suspension was prepared as described for the liquid bactericidal assay. Bacteria (10^7 CFU) were mixed with 20 ml nutrient-poor agar (0.03% (w/v) TSB in 10 mM sodium phosphate buffer, pH 7.0, with 1% low EEO agarose [Sigma-Aldrich, St. Louis, MI, USA]) of 45°C, and immediately poured into 10×10-cm culture plates. Subsequently, the gel was removed and the agarose was overlaid with 20 ml of double-strength nutrient agarose (6% TSB, 1% Bacto-agar, 45°C), and plates were incubated overnight at 37°C. Antibacterial activity resulting in zones devoid of bacterial growth is visualized as dark zones in a dark-field image.

Results

Bactericidal activity of RS and manuka honey

The bactericidal activity of RS and manuka honey was tested against the food-spoiling bacterium *Bacillus subtilis* and against the wound pathogens methicillin-resistant *Staphylococcus aureus* (MRSA), *Escherichia coli* and *Pseudomonas aeruginosa*. We determined the maximal dilution of honey which reduced bacterial survival 1000-fold after 2 and 24 hours of incubation, using 2-fold serial dilutions of 40% (v/v) honey. After 2 h up to 13.3±3.3-fold diluted RS honey killed *B. subtilis*, whereas manuka honey could only be 2.5-fold diluted (Fig. 1). After 24 hours, RS and manuka honey had potent activity against *B. subtilis*, up to 10- and 20-fold dilution, respectively. Neither RS nor manuka honey had bactericidal activity against MRSA after 2 hours. After 24 hours RS and manuka honey did kill MRSA, at dilutions of up to 10- and 80-fold, respectively (Fig. 1). *E. coli* and *P. aeruginosa* were killed by RS honey diluted 2.5-fold at 2 hours incubation, while manuka honey lacked rapid activity against these bacteria (Fig.1). After 24 hours RS honey had bactericidal activity against both bacteria up to 5-fold dilution, and manuka honey killed *E. coli* and *P. aeruginosa* up to dilution of 10- and 5-fold, respectively (Fig. 1). Overall, RS honey clearly had more potent bactericidal activity than manuka

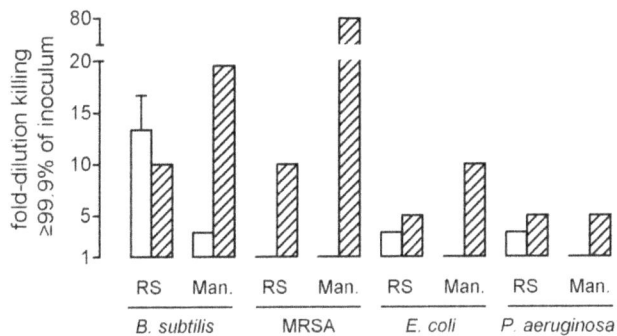

Figure 1. Bactericidal activity of RS and manuka honey. Indicated bacteria were incubated with serial dilutions of RS or manuka honey, starting at 40% honey. After 2 h (white bars) and 24 h (hatched bars) of incubation bacteria were quantitatively cultured. The bars represent the highest dilutions of honey causing a 1000-fold reduction in numbers of CFU relative to the initial inocula. The values are mean ± SEM of independent triplicate incubations.

after 2 hours of incubation, while manuka was the most potent honey after 24 hours.

Characterization of H2O2, MGO and bee defensin-1 in RS and manuka honey

We assessed the levels of the predominant bactericidal factors in RS and manuka honey, i.e. MGO, H_2O_2, and bee defensin-1. RS and manuka honey contained 0.25 ± 0.01 mM and 10.94 ± 1.70 mM MGO, respectively (Fig. 2A). Hydrogen peroxide is produced by the *Apis mellifera* (honey bee) glucose oxidase enzyme upon dilution of honey [18,21]. RS honey at a concentration of 40% (v/v) accumulated up to 3.47 ± 0.25 mM H_2O_2 in 24 hours, while no H_2O_2 was detected in diluted manuka honey (Fig. 2B).

Bee defensin-1 can be visualized by parallel Coomassie-staining and a *B. subtilis* overlay assay after separation of proteins of the >5 kDa fraction of honey by native acid-urea PAGE [14]. After gel electrophoresis, bee defensin-1 in the >5 kDa retentate of RS honey produced a clear zone of growth inhibition of *B. subtilis* in a gel overlay assay (Fig. 2C). In a similar amount of manuka honey retentate no bee defensin-1 was detected either by Coomassie-

staining or in a gel overlay assay (Fig. 2C). In a radial diffusion assay with *B. subtilis* an amount of RS honey retentate equivalent to 0.5 μl honey produced a zone of bacterial growth inhibition, while in an up to 20-fold larger amount of manuka retentate no antibacterial activity was observed (not shown).

Factors contributing to the bactericidal activity of manuka honey after 24 hours

We previously determined the contribution of H_2O_2, bee defensin-1, MGO and the low pH to the bactericidal activity of RS honey after 24 hours of incubation [14], which is summarized in Table 1. In manuka honey we did not detect H_2O_2 or bee defensin-1, but this honey contained an approximately 40-fold higher concentration of MGO compared to RS honey. To assess the contribution of MGO to the bactericidal activity of manuka honey after 24 hours, and to reveal potential other factors, we neutralized MGO by conversion to the non-bactericidal S-lactoylglutathione and assessed the remaining bactericidal activity. Neutralization of MGO reduced the activity against MRSA to a level identical to that of a honey-equivalent sugar solution (Fig. 3), indicating that MGO was responsible for the potent activity of manuka honey against MRSA. With MGO neutralized, 8- and 2-fold higher concentrations of manuka honey were required to kill *B. subtilis* and *P. aeruginosa*, respectively (Fig. 3). MGO-neutralized manuka honey still had more activity than a sugar solution against these species, and the activity of manuka honey against *E. coli* was not affected by neutralization of MGO (Fig. 3). This indicated the presence of other bactericidal factors beside MGO.

The polyanionic compound sodium polyanetholesulphonate (SPS) neutralizes cationic compounds. Addition of SPS to MGO-neutralized manuka honey abolished the residual activity against *P. aeruginosa* (Fig. 3) implying that this activity was due to cationic compound(s). As manuka honey does not contain detectable amounts of bee defensin-1, other cationic bactericidal component(s) must be present. Activity against *B. subtilis* and *E. coli* was also reduced but not abolished when SPS was added (Fig. 3), which indicates the contribution of both cationic and non-cationic factors to the non-MGO bactericidal activity of manuka honey.

When the pH of MGO- and cationic compound-neutralized manuka honey was adjusted from 3.9 to 7.0, all remaining activity against *E. coli* was abolished. Activity against *B. subtilis* was reduced,

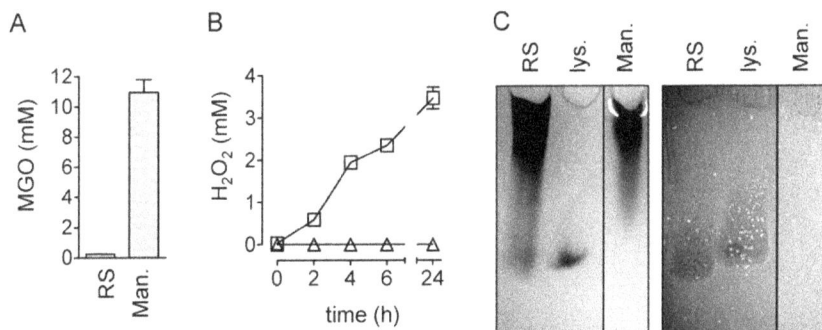

Figure 2. Comparison of levels of MGO, H_2O_2 and bee defensin-1 in RS and manuka honey. (A) Concentration of MGO in RS and manuka (Man.) honey, determined spectrophotometrically after its conversion to S-lactoylglutathione by glyoxalase I treatment. (B) H_2O_2 accumulation over time in 40% (v/v) RS (squares) and manuka honey (triangles). (C) Proteins were concentrated from honey by ultrafiltration with a 5 kDa molecular weight cut-off membrane. Amounts of >5 kDa retentate equivalent to 150 μl of undiluted honey, and 3 μg of lysozyme (lys.) as a reference, were run in duplicate on a single native acid-urea PAGE gel to separate cationic proteins. One half of the gel was Coomassie-stained (left), the other was used for a bacterial overlay assay with *B. subtilis* (right). Since a dark-field image was obtained, growth inhibition of the bacteria due to the presence of antibacterial proteins appears as a dark zone.

Table 1. Contribution of bactericidal factors to activity of RS and manuka honey.

	H₂O₂		bee defensin-1		MGO		pH		additional cationic		additional non-cationic	
	RS[a]	Man	RS	Man	RS	Man	RS	Man	RS	Man	RS	Man
B. subtilis	rapid[b]	-	rapid	-	slow	rapid	slow	rapid	-	rapid	-	rapid
MRSA	slow	-	slow	-	slow	slow	-	-	-	-	-	-
E. coli	rapid	-	slow	-	slow	slow	-	slow	-	slow	-	slow
P. aeruginosa	rapid	-	slow	-	slow	slow	slow	-	-	slow	-	-

[a]RS: RS honey, Man: manuka honey.
[b]Contribution is defined as ≥1 log reduction in numbers of CFU after 2 hours (rapid) or 24 hours (slow) of incubation.

but was still substantial (Fig. 3). So, the low pH was responsible for all non-cationic bactericidal activity of MGO-neutralized manuka honey against *E. coli*, while still other non-cationic bactericidal factor(s) were involved in activity against *B. subtilis*. As expected, addition of catalase – which neutralizes H_2O_2 – did not affect the bactericidal activity of manuka honey (not shown), since this honey did not contain detectable levels of H_2O_2 (Fig 2).

In summary, the high sugar concentration, MGO, low pH and as yet unidentified cationic factor(s) and non-cationic bactericidal factor(s) contributed to the bactericidal activity of manuka honey as recorded after 24 h.

Factors contributing to the rapid bactericidal activity of RS and manuka honey

In figure 1 we showed that RS honey had rapid activity (within 2 hours) against *B. subtilis*, *E. coli* and *P. aeruginosa* while manuka

honey exerted rapid activity only against *B. subtilis*. We subsequently assessed the contribution of individual factors to this rapid bactericidal activity. The entire *B. subtilis* inoculum was killed within 2 hours by 5% RS honey (Fig. 4A). When bee defensin-1 was neutralized by addition of SPS, 40% RS honey was required to kill *B. subtilis*. Subsequent neutralization of H_2O_2 reduced the activity of RS honey to that of a honey-equivalent sugar solution (Fig. 4A). So, bee defensin-1 and to a lesser extent H_2O_2, were the major factors involved in rapid activity of RS honey against *B. subtilis*.

Neutralization of bee defensin-1 did not affect the activity of RS honey against *E. coli* or *P. aeruginosa* (Fig. 4A). After neutralization of H_2O_2 the activity of RS honey against *E. coli* was reduced to that of a sugar solution and the activity of 40% RS honey against *P. aeruginosa* was reduced to a level at which the numbers of CFU were only about 1-log lower than after incubation in sugar (Fig. 4A). Titration of honey to pH 7

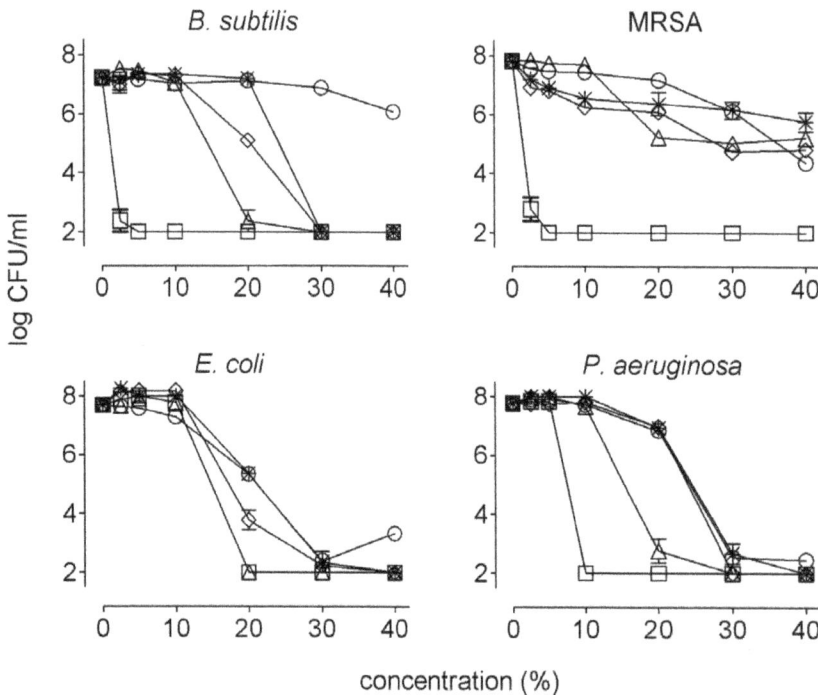

Figure 3. **Contribution of MGO to the bactericidal activity of manuka honey.** The indicated bacteria were incubated in various concentrations (v/v) of manuka honey in incubation buffer (squares), in manuka with addition of glyoxalase I (triangles) or glyoxalase I and SPS without (diamonds) or with adjustment of the pH to 7.0 (asterisks), or in a honey-equivalent sugar solution (circles). After 24 hours, numbers of surviving bacteria were determined.

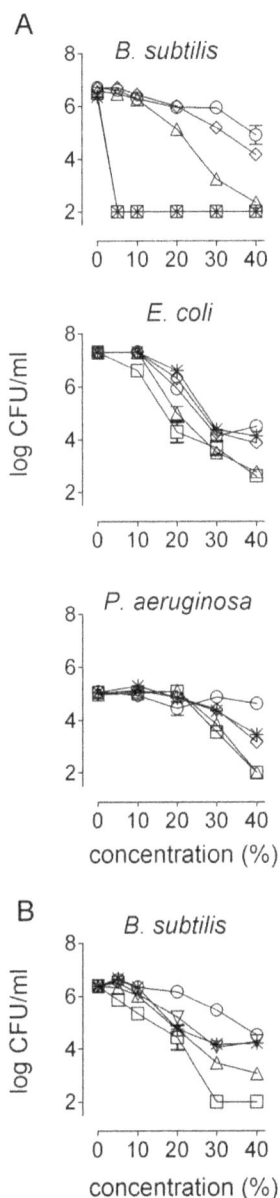

A *B. subtilis*, *E. coli*, *P. aeruginosa* (log CFU/ml vs concentration %)

B *B. subtilis* (log CFU/ml vs concentration %)

Figure 4. Factors contributing to rapid bactericidal activity of RS and manuka honey. (A) RS honey; bacteria were incubated for 2 hours in various concentrations (v/v) of RS honey in incubation buffer (squares), with either catalase (asterisks), SPS (triangles) or both (diamonds) added, or in sugar solution (circles). (B) Manuka honey; *B. subtilis* was incubated for 2 hours in various concentrations of manuka honey in incubation buffer (squares), with successive addition of glyoxalase I (triangles, top up), SPS (triangles, top down), and titration to pH 7.0 (asterisks), or in sugar solution (circles).

abolished all residual activity against *P. aeruginosa* (not shown). So, in different combinations, bee defensin, H_2O_2, sugars and the low pH contributed to the rapid activity of RS honey against specific bacterial species.

Concentrations of ≥30% manuka honey were required for rapid activity against *B. subtilis* (Fig. 4B). Neutralization of MGO in manuka honey reduced but did not abolish this rapid activity (Fig. 4B). The remaining activity was not affected by titration to pH 7 (Fig. 4B) or addition of catalase (not shown), but this activity was further reduced but not abolished by addition of SPS (Fig. 4B).

Both the cationic and non-cationic factor(s) involved in this rapid activity are unknown.

Discussion

General applicability of honey as antimicrobial agent requires safe preparations, knowledge of the composition of antibacterial factors and standardized antibacterial activity. Medical-grade honeys are gamma-irradiated to eradicate bacterial spores which may be present in raw honey. Revamil® and manuka medical-grade honey are approved as a medical product for wound care. Manuka honey obtained from manuka trees (*Leptospermum scoparium*) in New Zealand and Australia has large batch-to-batch variation in antibacterial activity [13]. Medical-grade manuka honey often carries a UMF™ (Unique Manuka Factor) value representing its antimicrobial activity. This value is based on activity against *S. aureus* in an agar diffusion assay. Standardization of RS honey, the source for Revamil®, is based on a controlled production process in greenhouses. We have previously shown that the bactericidal activity of Revamil® honey against *B. subtilis* varies by less than a factor two for eleven batches of honey [9], but the antibacterial activity of this honey is not routinely assessed.

In medicine, honey may be used either for treatment of infection or as antibacterial prophylaxis. Honey applied to wounds is diluted by wound exudate, so the active compounds need to be present in high concentrations. Treatment of infections particularly requires rapid bactericidal activity, whereas prophylactic application demands sustained and not necessarily very rapid bactericidal activity. We therefore assessed the rapid and slow bactericidal activity of RS and manuka honey, i.e. the activity after 2 and 24 hours of incubation, respectively. RS honey had much more potent rapid activity than manuka honey against *B. subtilis*, *E. coli* and *P. aeruginosa*. Both RS and manuka honey lacked rapid activity against MRSA. With respect to slow bactericidal activity, manuka honey was more potent than RS honey, most notably against MRSA and *B. subtilis*.

RS honey contains relatively high levels of bee defensin-1 and H_2O_2 and only a minor amount of MGO, whereas the opposite is true for manuka honey. The contribution of these compounds for rapid and slow bactericidal activity of RS and manuka honey is summarized in Table 1. The main conclusion is that these honeys exert bactericidal activity through entirely different sets of compounds, resulting in distinct bactericidal properties. MGO contributed substantially to the activity of manuka honey against *S. aureus* and *B. subtilis* but not against *E. coli* and *P. aeruginosa*. The activity against these latter bacteria involved compounds other than MGO including as yet unidentified cationic and non-cationic compounds. In earlier studies before the discovery of MGO, acidic [22] and phenolic compounds [23,24] were isolated from manuka honey. The contribution of these factors to the bactericidal activity was questioned at that time, since their concentrations in manuka honey were far too low to account for all observed activity [25]. It is possible that acidic and phenolic compounds are responsible for the non-MGO bactericidal activity of manuka honey. Bee defensin-1 and H_2O_2 were responsible for most of the rapid activity of RS honey and the absence of these compounds explains the limited rapid bactericidal activity of manuka honey.

Honeys show wide variation in their capacity to produce H_2O_2; some honeys – including the manuka honey used in our study - do not accumulate H_2O_2 at all [18,26]. Several causes for the absence of H_2O_2 in honey have been proposed. Factors known to affect H_2O_2 accumulation are the inactivation of glucose oxidase due to exposure to excess heat or light [27,28] degradation of H_2O_2 by catalase originating from nectar [29], and chemical scavenging

[30]. Another explanation for the variation in H_2O_2 accumulation in honeys could be differences in levels of glucose oxidase. To our knowledge no studies have been performed to assess the concentration of glucose oxidase in honey.

Bee defensin-1 is secreted in honey by the honey bee hypopharyngeal gland [14], but we did not detect bee defensin-1 in manuka honey. Secretions of the hypopharyngeal gland are used for production of royal jelly and honey [31,32]. The amount of bee defensin-1 in royal jellies (therein referred to as 'royalisin') obtained from different apiaries varies strongly [33], with some samples completely devoid of this peptide. This implies that bee defensin-1 expression in hypopharyngeal glands and/or the amount of gland secretions added may vary strongly. This could also explain the difference in bee defensin-1 levels in RS and manuka honey.

Recently, the 1,2-dicarbonyl compound MGO was identified as antibacterial compound present in exceptionally high levels in manuka honey [15,16]. In general, MGO can be formed from sugars during heat-treatment or prolonged storage of carbohydrate-containing foods and beverages [34]. MGO in manuka honey however is formed by conversion of dihydroxyacetone (DHA) present at exceptionally high concentrations in the nectar of manuka trees (*Leptospermum scoparium*) [35]. It is unknown how DHA is formed in nectar and why it is present in such large amounts in manuka trees. Concentrations of MGO in fermented milk products, wine, beer and roasted coffee have been reported to be in the range of 3 to 47 mg/kg, while up to 828 mg/kg (16.1 mM), has been found in manuka honey [15,16]. MGO is a reactive metabolite that can exert toxic effects [36]. Manuka honey has a long history of safe use, but nowadays batches of manuka honey with maximized levels of MGO are selected for medical and nutritional use. Concerns regarding potential toxicity of dietary MGO in honey and the effects on wound healing have been expressed by others [16,37] and this remains to be investigated.

The antibacterial properties of honey, or of individual honey components, could also be interesting for application in food technology, e.g. for food preservation or as functional food ingredients. It has for instance been reported that honey can inhibit opportunistic bacterial growth in milk [38]. We show that the food spoilage bacterium *B. subtilis* is highly susceptible to manuka honey, and also *Bacillus cereus* is effectively killed by this

honey (data not shown). Since manuka honey retains bactericidal activity against food-spoiling bacilli up to very high dilution, this honey has better potential than RS honey for food preservation.

Lack of standardization of antibacterial activity and incomplete knowledge of the active components are major limitations for the application of honey in medicine. The antibacterial activity of medical-grade manuka honey is commonly assessed by an agar diffusion assay with *S. aureus* [13]. This method has several major limitations. Firstly, antibacterial activity against a single bacterial species is not representative for activity against other species, since different species have varying susceptibility to honey and its antibacterial factors. We show for instance, that *E. coli* and *P. aeruginosa* are substantially less susceptible to manuka honey than *S. aureus* and *B. subtilis*. Secondly, in the agar diffusion assay the activity of honey is estimated by the size of the growth inhibition zone. Obviously, the size of such zones not only depends on the antimicrobial activity, but also on the rate of diffusion of antibacterial factors through the agar matrix. Honey with potent antibacterial activity due to compounds with relatively high molecular weight may thus erroneously be characterized as having low activity. Thirdly, the agar diffusion test does not discriminate between growth inhibiting and bactericidal activity and does not allow quantification of bactericidal activity or kinetics of killing.

To assess the potential of honey for treatment of infection it is important to discriminate between bacteriostatic and bactericidal activity, and to quantify the latter activity. This is also highly relevant for application of honey or honey-derived components in food preservation. In the current study, these limitations were overcome by the use of a quantitative liquid bactericidal assay with a panel of representative bacterial species.

Detailed analysis of antibacterial factors and bactericidal activity against a representative panel of bacteria is essential to characterize honeys. Such characterization will allow the production of standardized honeys with defined antibacterial activity, contributing to their applicability for medical, nutritional and food preservation purposes.

Author Contributions

Conceived and designed the experiments: PK AtV LdB SZ. Performed the experiments: PK LdB. Analyzed the data: PK AtV CV-G SZ. Wrote the paper: PK AtV CV-G SZ.

References

1. Khanna T, Friendship R, Dewey C, Weese JS (2008) Methicillin resistant Staphylococcus aureus colonization in pigs and pig farmers. Vet Microbiol 128: 298–303.
2. McEwen SA, Fedorka-Cray PJ (2002) Antimicrobial use and resistance in animals. Clin Infect Dis 34(Suppl 3): S93–S106.
3. Carattoli A (2008) Animal reservoirs for extended spectrum beta-lactamase producers. Clin Microbiol Infect 14(Suppl 1): 117–123.
4. Walsh C (2003) Antibiotics: Actions, Origins, Resistance. Washington DC: American Society for Microbiology (ASM) Press.
5. Fischbach MA, Walsh CT (2009) Antibiotics for Emerging Pathogens. Science 325: 1089–1093.
6. Majno G (1975) Man and wound in the ancient world. Massachusetts: Harvard University Press Cambridge.
7. Zumla A, Lulat A (1989) Honey–a remedy rediscovered. J R Soc Med 82: 384–385.
8. Cooper RA, Molan PC, Harding KG (2002) The sensitivity to honey of Gram-positive cocci of clinical significance isolated from wounds. J Appl Microbiol 93: 857–863.
9. Kwakman PHS, Van den Akker JPC, Guclu A, Aslami H, Binnekade JM, et al. (2008) Medical-grade honey kills antibiotic-resistant bacteria in vitro and eradicates skin colonization. Clin Infect Dis 46: 1677–1682.
10. Mundo MA, Padilla-Zakour OI, Worobo RW (2004) Growth inhibition of foodborne pathogens and food spoilage organisms by select raw honeys. International Journal of Food Microbiology 97: 1–8.
11. Taormina PJ, Niemira BA, Beuchat LR (2001) Inhibitory activity of honey against foodborne pathogens as influenced by the presence of hydrogen peroxide

and level of antioxidant power. International Journal of Food Microbiology 69: 217–225.
12. Efem SEE (1988) Clinical Observations on the Wound-Healing Properties of Honey. British Journal of Surgery 75: 679–681.
13. Allen KL, Molan PC, Reid GM (1991) A survey of the antibacterial activity of some New Zealand honeys. J Pharm Pharmacol 43: 817–822.
14. Kwakman PHS, Te Velde AA, de Boer L, Speijer D, Vandenbroucke-Grauls CMJE, et al. (2010) How honey kills bacteria. FASEB J 24: 2576–2582.
15. Adams CJ, Boult CH, Deadman BJ, Farr JM, Grainger MN, et al. (2008) Isolation by HPLC and characterisation of the bioactive fraction of New Zealand manuka (Leptospermum scoparium) honey. Carbohydr Res 343: 651–659.
16. Mavric E, Wittmann S, Barth G, Henle T (2008) Identification and quantification of methylglyoxal as the dominant antibacterial constituent of Manuka (Leptospermum scoparium) honeys from New Zealand. Mol Nutr Food Res 52: 483–489.
17. Lehrer RI, Barton A, Daher KA, Harwig SS, Ganz T, et al. (1989) Interaction of human defensins with Escherichia coli. Mechanism of bactericidal activity. J Clin Invest 84: 553–561.
18. White Jr. JW, Subers MH (1963) Studies on honey inhibine. 2. A chemical assay. Journal of Apicultural Research 2: 93–100.
19. Racker E (1951) The mechanism of action of glyoxalase. J Biol Chem 190: 685–696.
20. Harwig SS, Chen NP, Park AS, Lehrer RI (1993) Purification of cysteine-rich bioactive peptides from leukocytes by continuous acid-urea-polyacrylamide gel electrophoresis. Anal Biochem 208: 382–386.

21. Bang LM, Buntting C, Molan P (2003) The effect of dilution on the rate of hydrogen peroxide production in honey and its implications for wound healing. J Altern Complement Med 9: 267–273.
22. Bogdanov S (1997) Nature and origin of the antibacterial substances in honey. Food Science and Technology-Lebensmittel-Wissenschaft & Technologie 30: 748–753.
23. Weston RJ, Brocklebank LK, Lu YR (2000) Identification and quantitative levels of antibacterial components of some New Zealand honeys. Food Chemistry 70: 427–435.
24. Russell KM, Molan PC, Wilkins AL, Holland PT (1990) Identification of Some Antibacterial Constituents of New-Zealand Manuka Honey. Journal of Agricultural and Food Chemistry 38: 10–13.
25. Weston RJ, Mitchell KR, Allen KL (1999) Antibacterial phenolic components of New Zealand manuka honey. Food Chemistry 64: 295–301.
26. Molan PC (1992) The Antibacterial Activity of Honey. 2. Variation in the Potency of the Antibacterial Activity. Bee World 73: 59–76.
27. White JW Jr., Subers MH (1964) Studies on honey inhibine. 3. Effect of heat. Journal of Apicultural Research 3: 45–50.
28. White JW Jr., Subers MH (1964) Studies on honey inhibine. 4. Destruction of the peroxide accumulation system by light. J Food Sci 29: 819–828.
29. Schepartz AI (1966) Honey catalase: occurance and some kinetic properties. J Apic Res 5: 167–176.
30. White JW Jr., Subers MH, Schepartz AI (1963) The identification of inhibine, the antibacterial factor in honey, as hydrogen peroxide and its origin in a honey glucose oxidase system. Biochim Biophys Acta 73: 57–70.
31. Lensky Y, Rakover Y (1983) Separate Protein Body Compartments of the Worker Honeybee (Apis-Mellifera L). Comparative Biochemistry and Physiology B-Biochemistry & Molecular Biology 75: 607–615.
32. Knecht D, Kaatz HH (1990) Patterns of Larval Food-Production by Hypopharyngeal Glands in Adult Worker Honey-Bees. Apidologie 21: 457–468.
33. Bachanova K, Klaudiny J, Kopernicky J, Simuth J (2002) Identification of honeybee peptide active against Paenibacillus larvae larvae through bacterial growth-inhibition assay on polyacrylamide gel. Apidologie 33: 259–269.
34. Weigel KU, Opitz T, Henle T (2004) Studies on the occurrence and formation of 1,2-dicarbonyls in honey. European Food Research and Technology 218: 147–151.
35. Adams CJ, Manley-Harris M, Molan PC (2009) The origin of methylglyoxal in New Zealand manuka (Leptospermum scoparium) honey. Carbohydr Res 344: 1050–1053.
36. Kalapos MP (2008) The tandem of free radicals and methylglyoxal. Chem Biol Interact 171: 251–271.
37. Majtan J (2010) Methylglyoxal - a Potential Risk Factor of Manuka Honey in Healing of Diabetic Ulcers. eCAM: doi:10.1093/ecam/neq013.
38. Krushna NSA, Kowsalya A, Radha S, Narayanan RB (2007) Honey as a natural preservative of milk. Indian Journal of Experimental Biology 45: 459–464.

18

Reverse Zoonotic Disease Transmission (Zooanthroponosis): A Systematic Review of Seldom-Documented Human Biological Threats to Animals

Ali M. Messenger[1,2], Amber N. Barnes[1], Gregory C. Gray[1,2]*

1 College of Public Health and Health Professions, University of Florida, Gainesville, Florida, United States of America, 2 Emerging Pathogens Institute, University of Florida, Gainesville, Florida, United States of America

Abstract

Background: Research regarding zoonotic diseases often focuses on infectious diseases animals have given to humans. However, an increasing number of reports indicate that humans are transmitting pathogens to animals. Recent examples include methicillin-resistant *Staphylococcus aureus*, influenza A virus, *Cryptosporidium parvum*, and *Ascaris lumbricoides*. The aim of this review was to provide an overview of published literature regarding reverse zoonoses and highlight the need for future work in this area.

Methods: An initial broad literature review yielded 4763 titles, of which 4704 were excluded as not meeting inclusion criteria. After careful screening, 56 articles (from 56 countries over three decades) with documented human-to-animal disease transmission were included in this report.

Findings: In these publications, 21 (38%) pathogens studied were bacterial, 16 (29%) were viral, 12 (21%) were parasitic, and 7 (13%) were fungal, other, or involved multiple pathogens. Effected animals included wildlife (n = 28, 50%), livestock (n = 24, 43%), companion animals (n = 13, 23%), and various other animals or animals not explicitly mentioned (n = 2, 4%). Published reports of reverse zoonoses transmission occurred in every continent except Antarctica therefore indicating a worldwide disease threat.

Interpretation: As we see a global increase in industrial animal production, the rapid movement of humans and animals, and the habitats of humans and wild animals intertwining with great complexity, the future promises more opportunities for humans to cause reverse zoonoses. Scientific research must be conducted in this area to provide a richer understanding of emerging and reemerging disease threats. As a result, multidisciplinary approaches such as One Health will be needed to mitigate these problems.

Editor: Bradley S. Schneider, Metabiota, United States of America

Funding: This work was supported by the US Armed Forces Health Surveillance Center - Global Emerging Infections Surveillance Operations (multiple grants to GCG) and a supplement from the National Institute of Allergy and Infectious Diseases (R01 AI068803 to GCG). The funders had no role in study design, data collection and analysis, decision to publish, or preparation of the manuscript.

Competing Interests: The authors have declared that no competing interests exist.

* E-mail: gcgray@phhp.ufl.edu

Introduction

With today's rapid transport systems, modern public health problems are growing increasingly complex. A pathogen that emerges today in one country can easily be transported unnoticed in people, animals, plants, or food products to distant parts of the world in less than 24 hours [1]. This high level of mobility makes tracking and designing interventions against emerging pathogens exceedingly difficult, requiring close international and interdisciplinary collaborations. Fundamental to these efforts is an understanding of the ecology of emerging diseases. Published works often cite the large proportion of human emerging pathogens that originate in animals [2,3,4,5]. However, scientific reports seldom mention human contributions to the variety of emerging diseases that impact animals. The focus of this review is to examine and summarize the scientific literature regarding such zoonoses transmission. A comprehensive table of the results is included in this document.

Methods

For the purpose of this review several terms require definitions. Despite the fact that the term "zoonosis" usually refers to a disease that is transmitted from animals to humans (also called "anthropozoonosis") [6], in this paper, "zoonosis" was defined as any disease that is transmitted from animals to humans, or vice versa [6]. There are two related terms ("zooanthroponosis" and "reverse zoonosis") that refer to any pathogen normally reservoired in humans that can be transmitted to other vertebrates [6]. Acknowledging that the terms "reverse zoonosis" or "zooanthroponosis" are seldom used, and that the term "zoonosis" can have several meanings, search methods were designed to

```
┌─────────────────────────────────────────┐        ┌──────────────────────────────────────────┐
│ 4763 citations identified by literature  │◄───────┤ PubMed (n=1133)                            │
│ searchᵃ                                   │        │ Web of Knowledgeᵇ (n=2369)                 │
└─────────────────────────────────────────┘        │ ProQuestᶜ (n=1261)                         │
                                                    └──────────────────────────────────────────┘

                                                    ┌──────────────────────────────────────────┐
                                                    │ 2507 duplicates excluded by hand and using │
                                                    │ reference software                         │
                                                    └──────────────────────────────────────────┘

┌─────────────────────────────────────────┐
│ 2256 articles eligible for abstract      │
│ review                                    │
└─────────────────────────────────────────┘        ┌──────────────────────────────────────────┐
                                                    │ 2091 titles and abstracts excluded based on│
                                                    │ absence of evidence of direct human to     │
                                                    │ animal disease transmission                │
                                                    └──────────────────────────────────────────┘

┌─────────────────────────────────────────┐
│ 165 articles eligible for full text      │
│ review                                    │
└─────────────────────────────────────────┘        ┌──────────────────────────────────────────┐
                                                    │ 109 full text articles excluded based on:  │
                                                    │  • Full text in language other than English│
                                                    │  • No evidence of human-to-animal disease  │
                                                    │    transmission                            │
┌─────────────────────────────────────────┐        │  • Not accessible by any resources         │
│ 56 articles included in summary          │        │    available                               │
│  • 21 Bacterial Infection                │        └──────────────────────────────────────────┘
│  • 16 Viral Infection                    │
│  • 12 Parasitic Infection                │
│  • 4 Fungal Infection                    │
│  • 3 Other or Multiple Infections        │
└─────────────────────────────────────────┘
```

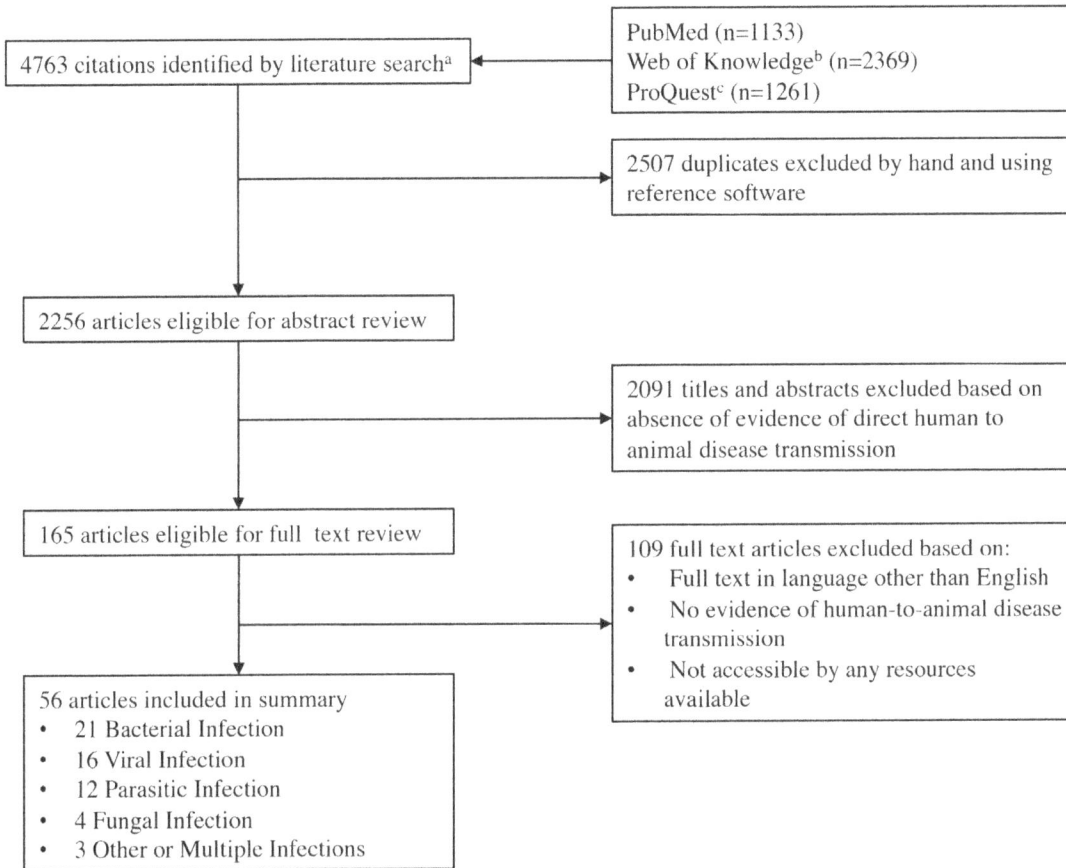

Figure 1. Flowchart demonstrating the identification and selection process for publications included in this review.

include all of these terms in an effort to capture the widest possible subset of publications with documented human-to-animal transmission.

Literature search

In June 2012, we searched PubMed in addition to several databases within Web of Knowledge and ProQuest to find articles documenting reverse zoonoses transmission. Search terms included: *reverse zoonosis, bidirectional zoonosis, anthroponosis, zooanthroponosis, anthropozoonosis,* and *human-to-animal disease transmission.* Articles were limited to clinical and observational type studies and were restricted to English only. Review articles were not included as they did not demonstrate a specific account of transmission. Letters to editors or similar correspondence were also excluded. Only publications with documented human-to-animal transmission were included. No time period was stipulated.

Four search strings were used for the PubMed database: ((bidirectional OR reverse) AND (zoono* or "disease transmission")) OR anthropono* OR "human-to-animal"), ((bidirectional OR reverse OR "human-to-animal") AND (zoono* or "disease transmission")) OR anthropono*), ("reverse zoonoses" OR " bidirectional zoonoses" OR "reverse zoonosis" OR " bidirectional zoonosis" OR "reverse zoonotic" OR " bidirectional zoonotic" OR anthropono* OR ("human-to-animal" AND disease* AND transmi*)), and (((bidirectional OR reverse OR "human-to-animal") AND (zoonoses[majr] OR "Disease Transmission, Infectious"[majr] OR zoonosis[tiab] OR zoonoses[tiab] OR zoonotic[tiab])) OR Anthroponos*[tiab] OR Zooanthroponos*[-

tiab] OR Anthropozoonos*[tiab]). In the ProQuest and Web of Knowledge databases, we only used one string: ((bidirectional OR reverse) AND (zoonosis OR zoonoses OR zoonotic)) OR anthropono* OR Zooanthropono* OR anthropozoono* OR "human-to-animal" OR "human to animal"). The lack of additional search strings for the latter databases was due to less comprehensive search capabilities. Duplicate articles were removed.

Literature analyses

Titles and abstracts were reviewed and articles were retained when there was evidence of disease transmission from humans to animals. During full text review, some citations proved straightforward in distinguishing transmission from humans to animals (e.g. via direct contact), while others were selected based on strong author suggestion or research implications toward reverse zoonotic transmission. In an effort to highlight trends in an otherwise diverse set of articles, citations were grouped by pathogen type and year of publication. To further clarify relationships, we also pictorially displayed the study locations and animal types discussed in the various articles.

Results

This comprehensive literature review yielded 4763 titles, 2507 of which were excluded as duplicates (Figure 1). During the review of abstracts, 2091 studies were excluded due to a lack of evidence of human-to-animal disease transmission. After consideration of the 165 eligible for full text review, 109 studies were excluded

Table 1. Descriptors of reports included in review with documented human-to-animal transmission.

Publications	Study Location	Specimen Source	Pathogen Name	Animal(s) Infected
Bacteria				
Cosivi et al (1995) [7]	Morocco	Assorted	*Mycobacterium tuberculosis, Mycobacterium bovis*[1]	Wildlife
Seguin et al (1999) [8]	United States	Veterinary hospital	Methicillin-resistant *Staphylococcus aureus* (MRSA)[1,2]	Livestock
Donnelly et al (2000) [9]	United States	4H project livestock	*Streptococcus pneumonia*[1]	Livestock
Nizeyi et al (2001) [10]	Uganda	National park	*Campylobacter* spp., *Salmonella* spp., *Shigella sonnei, Shigella boydii, Shigella flexneri*[1,3]	Wildlife
Michel et al (2003) [11]	South Africa	Zoo	*M. tuberculosis*[1,3]	Wildlife
Hackendahl et al (2004) [12]; also see Erwin et al (2004) [13]	United States	Veterinary hospital	*M. tuberculosis*[1,4]	Companion
Prasad et al (2005) [14]	India	Veterinary hospital	*M. tuberculosis*[3,4]	Livestock
Weese et al (2006) [15]	Canada, United States	Household; Veterinary hospital	MRSA[1]	Companion
Morris et al (2006) [16]	United States	Household; Veterinary hospital	MRSA[1]	Companion
Kwon et al (2006) [17]	Korea	Slaughterhouse	MRSA[1,3]	Companion; Livestock
Rwego et al (2008) [18]	Uganda	National park	*Escherichia coli*[1,3]	Livestock; Wildlife
Hsieh et al (2008) [19]	Taiwan	Livestock farm	Oxacillin-resistant *Staphylococcus aureus* (ORSA)	Livestock
Berg et al (2009) [20]	Ethiopia	Slaughterhouse	*M. tuberculosis*[3]	Livestock
Heller et al (2010) [21]	United Kingdom	Household; Veterinary hospital	MRSA[1,2]	Companion
Kottler et al (2010) [22]	United States	Household; Veterinary hospital	MRSA[1]	Companion
Ewers et al (2010) [23]	Germany, Italy, Netherlands, France, Spain, Denmark, Austria & Luxembourg	Veterinary hospital	*Escherichia coli*	Companion; Livestock
Every et al (2011) [24]	Australia	University zoology department	*Helicobacter pylori*[1]	Wildlife
Lin et al (2011) [25]	United States	Veterinary hospital	MRSA[1]	Companion; Livestock
Rubin et al (2011) [26]	Canada	Veterinary hospital; Human hospital	MRSA[1]	Companion
Price et al (2012) [27]	Austria, Belgium, Canada, Switzerland, China, Germany, Denmark, Spain, Finland, France, French Guiana, Hungary, Italy, the Netherlands, Peru, Poland, Portugal, Slovenia, and United States	Animal meat for sale	MRSA[1]	Livestock
Virus				
Meng et al (1998) [28]	United States	Veterinary laboratory; Human sample	Hepatitis E[5]	Wildlife
Willy et al (1999) [29]	United States	Veterinary laboratory	Measles[1,4]	Wildlife
Kaur et al (2008) [30]	Tanzania	National park	Human metapneumovirus (hMPV)[1,4]	Wildlife
Feagins et al (2008) [31]	United States	Commercially sold laboratory animals	Hepatitis E[5]	Livestock
Song et al (2010) [32]	South Korea	Livestock farm	Influenza A (2009 pandemic H1N1)[1]	Livestock
Swenson et al (2010) [33]	United States	Household; Veterinary hospital	Influenza A (2009 pandemic H1N1)[1,4]	Companion
Tischer et al (2010) [34]	Various; Unspecified	Unknown (previous reports cited)	Human herpesvirus 1, human herpesvirus 4[1,3,4]	Companion; Wildlife
Abe et al (2010) [35]	Japan	Wildlife	Rotavirus[1,3]	Wildlife
Berhane et al (2010) [36]	Canada, Chile	Livestock farm	Influenza A (2009 pandemic H1N1)[1,4,5]	Livestock
Poon et al (2010) [37]	Hong Kong	Slaughterhouse	Influenza A (2009 pandemic H1N1)	Livestock
Forgie et al (2011) [38]	Canada	Veterinary laboratory	Influenza A (2009 pandemic H1N1)	Livestock
Holyoake et al (2011) [39]	Australia	Livestock farm	Influenza A (2009 pandemic H1N1)[4]	Livestock

Table 1. Cont.

Publications	Study Location	Specimen Source	Pathogen Name	Animal(s) Infected
Scotch et al (2011) [40]	Mexico, United States, Canada, Australia, United Kingdom, France, Ireland, Argentina, Chile, Singapore, Norway, China, Italy, Thailand, South Korea, Indonesia, Germany, Japan, Russia, Finland, and Iceland	Unknown (previous reports cited)	Influenza A (2009 pandemic H1N1)	Companion; Livestock; Wildlife
Trevennec et al (2011) [41]	Vietnam	Livestock farm; Slaughterhouse	Influenza A (2009 pandemic H1N1)[1,2]	Livestock
Wevers et al (2011) [42]	Cameroon, Democratic Republic of the Congo, Gamiba, Côte d'Ivoire, Republic of Congo, Rwanda, Tanzania, Uganda, Germany (initial samples in Asia and South America)	Wildlife; Zoo	Human adenovirus A-F[1,3]	Wildlife
Crossley et al (2012) [43]	United States	Private zoo	Influenza A (2009 pandemic H1N1)[2,3]	Wildlife
Parasite				
Sleeman et al (2000) [44]	Rwanda	National park	*Chilomastix mesnili, Endolimax nana, Stronglyoides fuelleborni, Trichuris trichiura*[1,3]	Wildlife
Graczyk et al (2001) [45]	Uganda	National park	*Cryptosporidium parvum*	Wildlife
Graczyk et al (2002) [46]	Uganda	National park	*Encephalitozoon intestinalis*[1,3]	Wildlife
Graczyk et al (2002) [47]	Uganda	National park	*Giardia duodenalis*[1,3]	Wildlife
Guk et al (2004) [48]	Korea	Laboratory	*C. parvum*[5]	Livestock; Wildlife
Noël et al (2005) [49]	Singapore, Pakistan, Japan, Thailand, United States, France, Czech Republic	N/A	*Blastocystis* spp	Livestock; Wildlife
Coklin et al (2007) [50]	Canada	Livestock farm	*G. duodenalis, C. parvum*[1,3]	Livestock
Adejinmi et al (2008) [51]	Nigeria	Zoo	*Ascaris lumbricoides, T. trichiura*[1]	Wildlife
Teichroeb et al (2009) [52]	Ghana	Wildlife	*Isospora* spp., *Giardia duodenalis*[1,3]	Wildlife
Ash et al (2010) [53]	Zambia; Namibia; Australia	Wildlife; Zoo	*G. duodenalis*[1]	Wildlife
Johnston et al (2010) [54]	Uganda	National park	*G. duodenalis*[1,3]	Livestock; Wildlife
Dixon et al (2011) [55]	Canada	Livestock farm	*G. duodenalis, C. parvum*[1,3]	Livestock
Fungus				
Jacobs et al (1988) [56]	Unspecified	Assorted	*Microsporum* spp., *Trichophyton* spp.[1]	Assorted
Pal et al (1997) [57]	India	Household	*Trichophyton rubrum*[1]	Wildlife
Wrobel (2008) [58]	United States	Veterinary hospital	*Candida albicans*[3]	Companion; Livestock; Wildlife
Sharma et al (2009) [59]	India	Household; Veterinary hospital	*Microsporum gypseum*[1]	Wildlife
Other				
Epstein et al (2009) [60][+]	Assorted	Wildlife; Livestock farm; Zoo; Laboratory	Herpes simplex 1, influenza A, parasite spp, Measles, MRSA, *M. tuberculosis*[1,2,3,4,6]	Assorted
Guyader et al (2000) [61][&]	France	Shellfish-growing waters	Astrovirus, enterovirus, hepatitis A, Norwalk-like (norovirus), rotavirus[1,3]	Wildlife
Muehlenbein et al (2010) [62]^	Malaysia	Wildlife	Assorted illnesses[1,6]	Wildlife

Other assorted pathogen types:
[+]**virus; parasite/bacteria,**
[&]**virus/bacteria,**
^**assorted.**
Modes of transmission as indicated by authors:
[1]**direct contact,**
[2]**fomite,**
[3]**oral,**
[4]**aerosol,**
[5]**inoculation,**
[6]**other.**

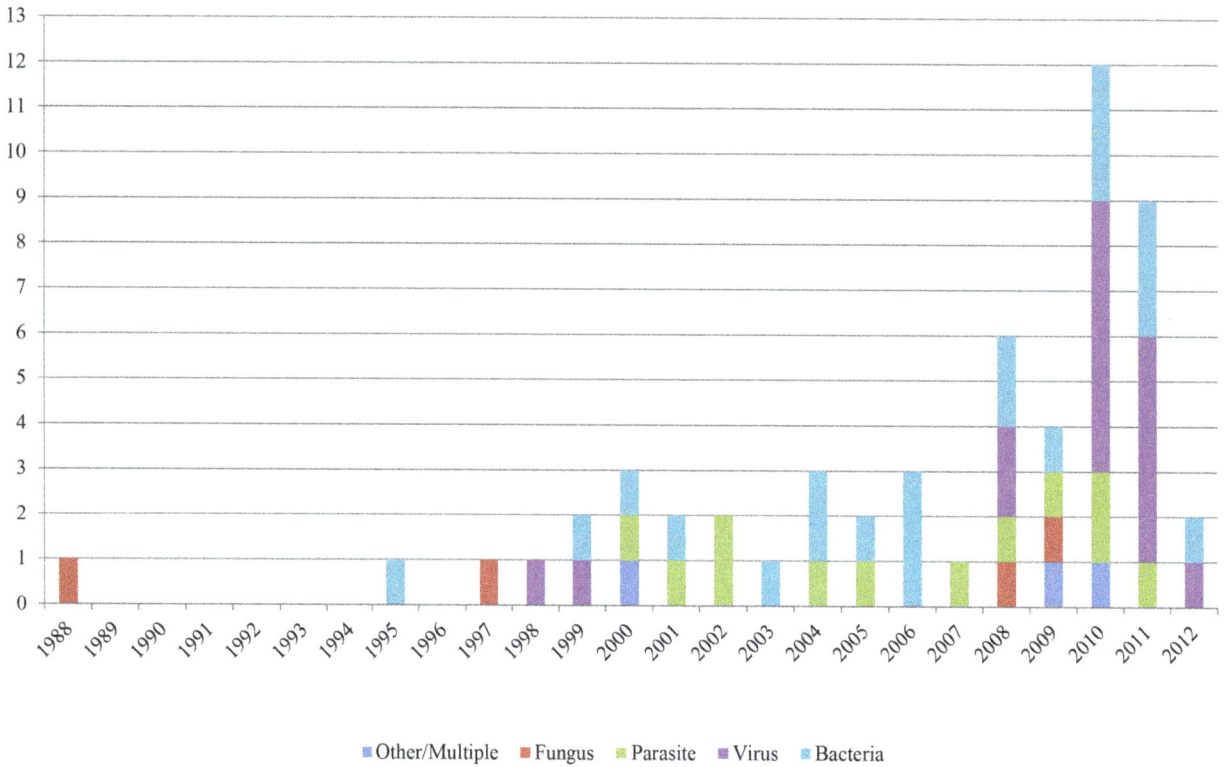

Figure 2. Timeline and frequency of reverse zoonoses publications included in this review shown by pathogen type.

based on full texts being written in a language other than English, absence of human-to-animal disease transmission, or full texts being unavailable. After all exclusions, 56 articles were considered for this review (Table 1).

Included reports were based in 56 different countries. Although the reports spanned three decades, there seems to be an increasing number of studies published in recent years (Figure 2). Twenty eight percent of the studies were conducted in the United States

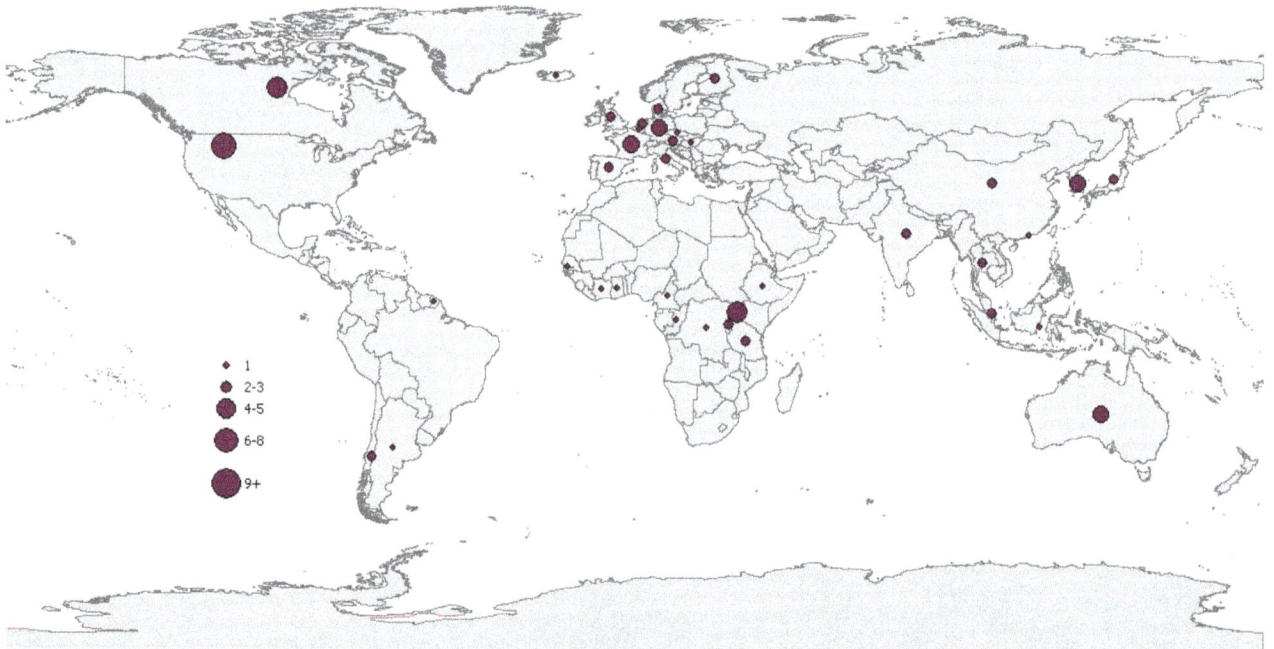

Figure 3. Proportion of reverse zoonoses scientific reports included in review as illustrated by study location. Note: Many reports identified several countries therefore each country in this figure does not necessarily represent a single corresponding publication.

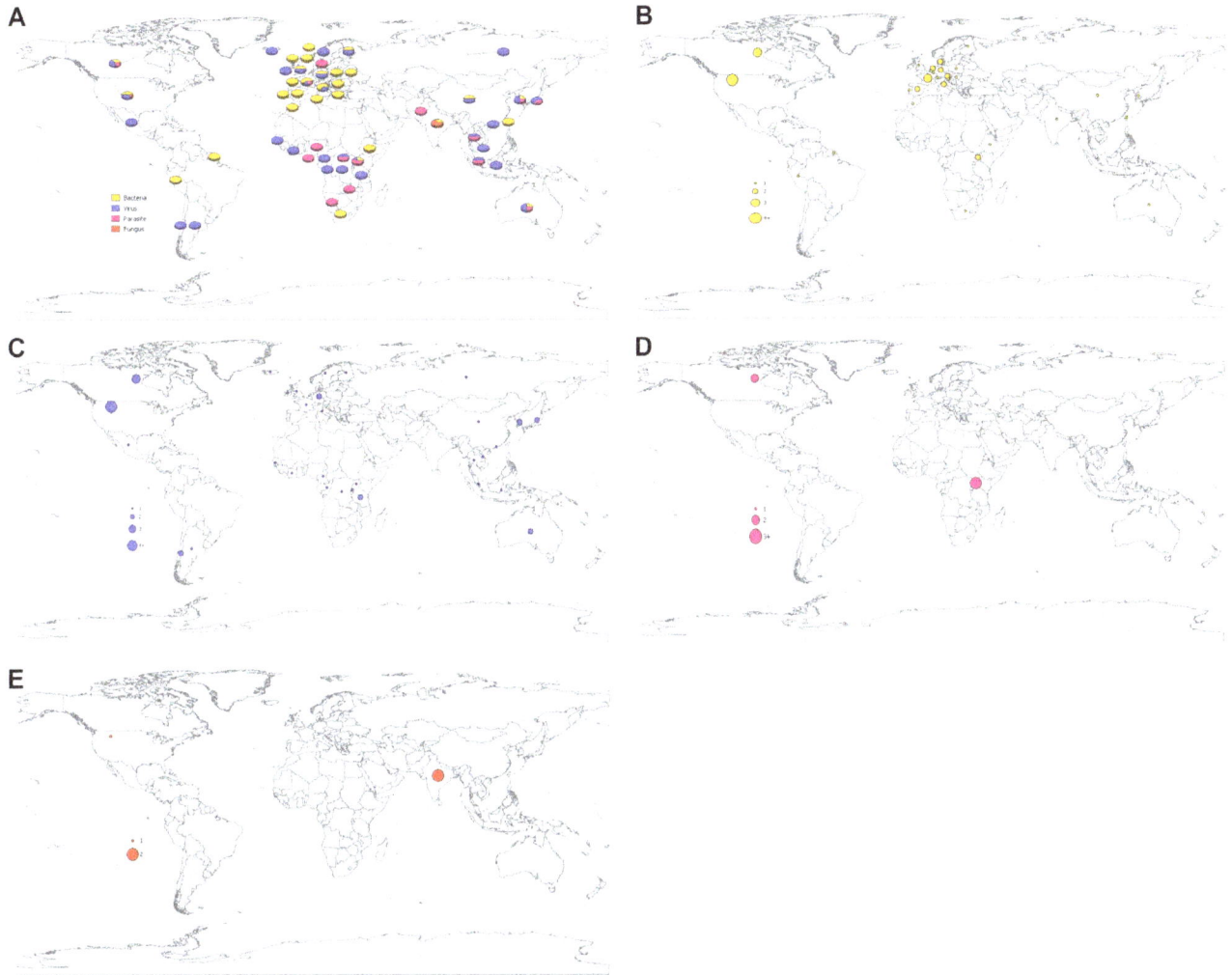

Figure 4. Study locations for literature included in review. A. Proportion of reverse zoonoses scientific reports as illustrated by study location and pathogen type; B. Proportion of reverse zoonoses scientific reports on bacterial pathogens as illustrated by study location; C. Proportion of reverse zoonoses scientific reports on viral pathogens as illustrated by study location; D. Proportion of reverse zoonoses scientific reports on parasitic pathogens as illustrated by study location; E. Proportion of reverse zoonoses scientific reports on fungal pathogens as illustrated by study location.

(n = 16), 14% in Canada (n = 8), and 13% in Uganda (n = 7) (Figure 3). Within the study results, 21 publications discussed human-to-animal transmission of bacterial pathogens (38%); 16 studies discussed viral pathogens (29%); 12 studies discussed human parasites (21%); and seven studies discussed transmission of fungi, other pathogens, or diseases of multiple etiologies (13%). Bacterial pathogen reports were centered in North America and Europe. Viral studies were well-distributed globally. Parasitic disease reports were conducted chiefly in Africa. Fungal studies were conducted almost exclusively in India (Figure 4).

Animals with reported infection or inoculation with human diseases included wildlife (n = 28, 50%), livestock (n = 24, 43%), companion animals (n = 13, 23%), and other animals or animals not explicitly mentioned (n = 2, 4%). The majority of companion and livestock animals were studied in North America and Europe, while wildlife studies were most prevalent in Africa (Table 1, Figure 5). Typically, diagnostic specimens were collected at veterinary hospitals (n = 15, 27%), national parks (n = 8, 14%) and livestock farms (n = 8, 14%). Direct contact was the suggested transmission route 71% of the time (n = 40). Other transmission routes included fomite, oral contact, aerosols, and inoculation.

As early as 1988, zoonoses research focusing on fungal pathogens was being conducted. Initial studies implied human transmission of *Microsporum* (n = 2) and *Trichophyton* (n = 2) to various animal species, with a later article centered on *Candida albicans* (n = 1) (Figure 2). These publications were set in India (n = 2) and the United States (n = 1).

Since 1988, research with implications of reverse zoonoses has been largely focused on infections of bacterial origin, beginning in 1995. The majority of articles in this review focused on methicillin-resistant *Staphylococcus aureus* (MRSA) (n = 9) and *Mycobacterium tuberculosis* (n = 5). Reports regarding these bacteria were primarily conducted in the United States (n = 8) among livestock (n = 10) or companion animals (n = 9).

Viruses were the second most common pathogen associated with human-to-animal transmission. Reverse zoonoses reports regarding viral pathogens began in 1998 and have since been focused primarily on influenza with great interest surrounding the 2009 H1N1 pandemic (n = 9). These studies were conducted largely in the United States (n = 6) in livestock (n = 8) and wildlife (n = 8).

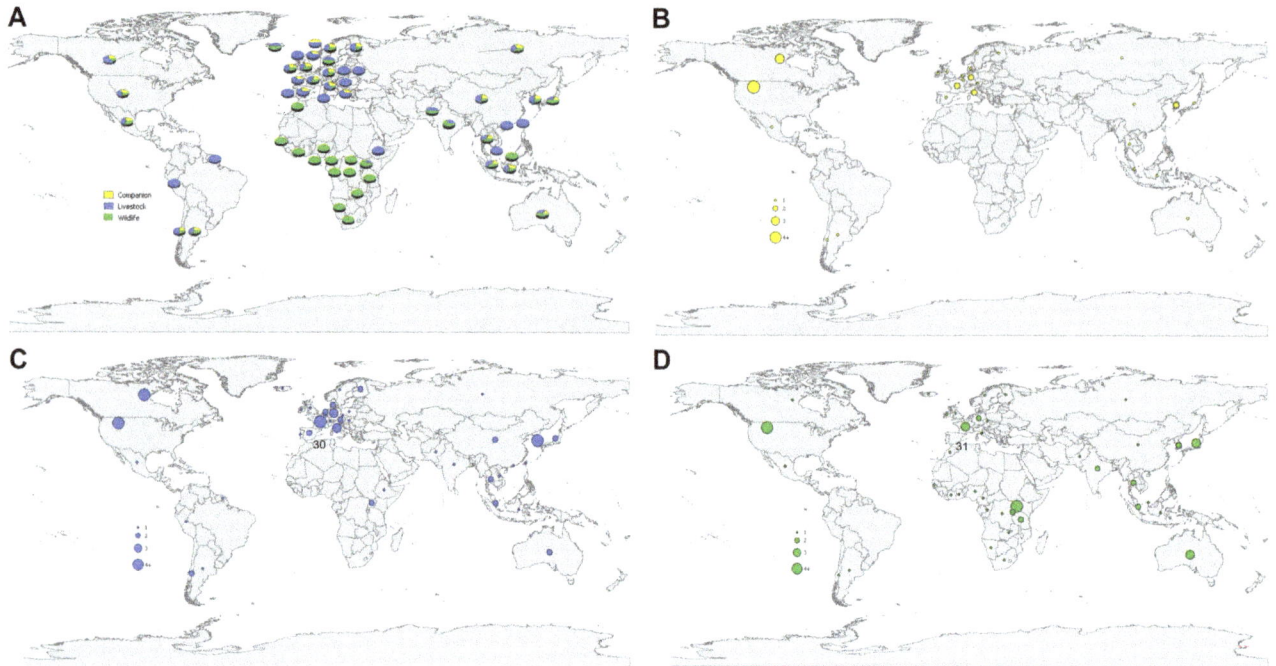

Figure 5. Animal type and study location included in review literature. A. Proportion of reverse zoonoses scientific reports as illustrated by study location and animal(s) infected; B. Proportion of reverse zoonoses scientific reports on companion animals as illustrated by study location; C. Proportion of reverse zoonoses scientific reports on livestock as illustrated by study location; D. Proportion of reverse zoonoses scientific reports on wildlife as illustrated by study location.

Studies suggestive of transmission of human parasites to animals were first published in 2000. The most commonly reported parasitic agents to be transmitted from humans to animals were *Giardia duodenalis* (n = 6) and *Cryptosporidium parvum* (n = 4). Parasitic research has been carried out most frequently in Uganda (n = 4) and Canada (n = 2). The authors investigated human parasitic infections chiefly in wildlife (n = 10) and livestock (n = 5).

Human-to-animal transmission is plausible for a large number of diseases because the pathogens concerned are known to infect multiple species [3]. For instance, 77.3% of the pathogens infecting livestock are considered "multiple species pathogens [3]." However, this review only found 24 reports which considered reverse zoonoses disease transmission as a potential threat to livestock, underscoring a need for further research in this area [3]. Similarly, in companion animals this review found even fewer studies (n = 13) that implied reverse zoonoses as a possible cause of infection, despite the fact that 90% of known pathogens for domestic carnivores are recognized as "multiple species pathogens [3]." The majority of publications in this reverse zoonoses review involved studies documenting human-to-wildlife transmission (n = 28). Unfortunately, they too were severely lacking in comparison to the research need. Each type of animal- livestock, companion, or wildlife, represents a unique set of risk factors for reverse zoonoses through their specific routes of human contact.

Discussion

Human and animal relationships are likely to continue to intensify worldwide over the next several decades due in part to animal husbandry practices, the growth of the companion animal market, climate change and ecosystem disruption, anthropogenic development of habitats, and global travel and commerce [2]. As the human-animal connection escalates, so does the threat for

pathogen spread [1,63]. This review notes a number of factors that influence the risk of disease transmission from humans to animals.

For instance, human population growth and expansion encourages different species to interact in ways and at rates previously not encountered, and to do so in novel geographical areas [4]. The term "pathogen pollution" refers to the process of bringing a foreign disease into a new locality due to human involvement [64]. In the case of the endangered African painted dog, wild dogs have been infected with human strains of *Giardia duodenalis*, leading researchers to believe that pathogen pollution occurred through open defecation in and around national parks by tourists and local residents [53]. Anthropogenic changes in the ecosystem increase the amount of shared habitats between humans and animals thus exposing both to new pathogens. Researchers discovered the human strain of pandemic *Escherichia coli* strain 025:H4-ST131 CTX-M-15 in many different species of animals indicating inter-species transmission from humans to pets and livestock [23]. This particular human strain found to be infecting animals was documented across Europe.

In addition to habitat change, growth, and/or destruction, there is the ever-increasing global movement of products and travelers that extends to both humans and animals. During the pandemic of 2009 H1N1 influenza, the novel virus was able to travel across the globe and from humans to swine in less than two months [32]. One driving force behind the movement of animals and animal products is the worldwide shipment of meat. This phenomenon is a relatively new event as developing countries adjust their diets to include more meat- and dairy-based products [4]. While food and animal safety guidelines attempt to keep up with the speed of global trade, international efforts appear to be outpaced by product demand. For example, it has been estimated that five tons of illegal bushmeat pass through Paris' main Roissy-Charles de Gaulle airport each week in personal luggage [65]. However, overt retail systems of animal and animal products can also contribute to the danger of zoonoses and reverse zoonoses transmission. Many animals are sold in markets which allow humans and a myriad of animal species to interact in conditions that are known to trigger emerging diseases [66]. Specifically, this is true for live animal markets and warehouses for exotic pets [4].

The pet industry is an enormous global business that now expands from domestic to exotic animals. A 2011–2012 national pet owners survey found that in the United States alone, 72.9 million homes or 62% of the population have a pet [67]. Of these pets, the majority of animals are dogs (78.2 million) or cats (86.4 million), but a large number of pets are birds (16.2 million), reptiles (13 million), or small animals (16 million) [67]. As pet ownership seems to be increasing worldwide and more exotic pets are being introduced to private homes, the potential for disease transmission between humans and animals will continue to increase. Veterinarians must more fervently protect animals under their care from human disease threats [68]. Adopting a One Health strategy for emerging disease surveillance and reporting will benefit both humans and animals and produce a more collaborative response plan.

Veterinarians, animal health workers, and public health professionals are not the only ones who should recognize the threat of reverse zoonoses. Increased awareness must also be communicated to the general public. Worldwide, there are 1,300 zoos and aquariums that sustain more than 700 million visitors each year [69]. The potential for pathogen spread to animals can come from a visitor with an illness, contamination of a shared environment or food, and the spread of disease through relocation of animals for captivity or educational purposes. In Tanzania, a fatal outbreak of human metapneumovirus in wild chimpanzees is believed to be the result of researchers and visitors viewing the animals in a national park that was once the great apes' territory [30]. Public education and awareness should be augmented to include the potential health threats inflicted on a susceptible animal by an unhealthy human.

This report has limitations. As demonstrated in this review paper, the trend for reporting pathogen spread of human-to-animal is increasing. However the route of human transmission to animal disease manifestation is often unknown in these reports and not well documented in this review. Also the report did not examine articles that did not document human-to-animal transmission. We acknowledge that many additional works that have recorded the existence of human pathogens in animals were not evaluated. However, this review was designed to summarize only the publications that document reverse zoonotic transmission.

Many common and dangerous pathogens have not, to the authors' knowledge, been researched as reverse zoonoses threats to animals representing a significant gap in the scientific literature. Future investigations of reverse zoonoses should take into account both transmission routes and disease prevalence. Prospective research should also include a wider variety of etiological agents and animal species. Scientific literature must document the presence and transmission of human diseases in animals such that the wealth of literature on this subject will become defined and accessible across multiple disciplines. A wider knowledge and understanding of reverse zoonoses should be sought for a successful One Health response. We recommend that future research be conducted on how human disease can, and does, affect the animals around us.

Acknowledgments

The authors especially thank Nancy Schaffer and Jennifer Lyon from the University of Florida Library Sciences for their research assistance.

Author Contributions

Analyzed the data: AM AB GG. Wrote the paper: AM AB GG.

References

1. Wilson ME (2003) The traveller and emerging infections: sentinel, courier, transmitter. J Appl Microbiol 94 Suppl: 1S–11S.
2. Worldbank (2010) People, pathogens and our planet: Volume 1: Towards a one health approach for controlling zoonotic diseases.
3. Cleaveland S, Laurenson MK, Taylor LH (2001) Diseases of humans and their domestic mammals: pathogen characteristics, host range and the risk of emergence. Philos Trans R Soc Lond B Biol Sci 356: 991–999.
4. Brown C (2004) Emerging zoonoses and pathogens of public health significance– an overview. Rev Sci Tech 23: 435–442.
5. World Health Organization (2010) The FAO-OIE-WHO Collaboration: Tripartite Concept Note: Sharing responsibilities and coordinating global activities to address health risks at the animal-human-ecosystems interfaces. Food and Agriculture Organization, World Organization for Animal Health, World Health Organization.
6. Hubalek Z (2003) Emerging human infectious diseases: anthroponoses, zoonoses, and sapronoses. Emerg Infect Dis 9: 403–404.
7. Cosivi O, Meslin FX, Daborn CJ, Grange JM (1995) Epidemiology of Mycobacterium bovis infection in animals and humans, with particular reference to Africa. Rev Sci Tech 14: 733–746.
8. Seguin JC, Walker RD, Caron JP, Kloos WE, George CG, et al. (1999) Methicillin-resistant Staphylococcus aureus outbreak in a veterinary teaching hospital: potential human-to-animal transmission. J Clin Microbiol 37: 1459–1463.
9. Donnelly TM, Behr MJ, Nims LJ (2000) What's your diagnosis? Septicemia in La Mancha goat kids - Apparent reverse zoonotic transmission of Streptococcus pneumoniae. Lab Animal 29: 23–25.
10. Nizeyi JB, Innocent RB, Erume J, Kalema G, Cranfield MR, et al. (2001) Campylobacteriosis, salmonellosis, and shigellosis in free-ranging human-habituated mountain gorillas of Uganda. J Wildl Dis 37: 239–244.
11. Michel AL, Venter L, Espie IW, Coetzee ML (2003) Mycobacterium tuberculosis infections in eight species at the National Zoological Gardens of South Africa, 1991–2001. J Zoo Wildl Med 34: 364–370.
12. Hackendahl NC, Mawby DI, Bemis DA, Beazley SL (2004) Putative transmission of Mycobacterium tuberculosis infection from a human to a dog. J Am Vet Med Assoc 225: 1573–1577.
13. Erwin PC, Bemis DA, Mawby DI, McCombs SB, Sheeler LL, et al. (2004) Mycobacterium tuberculosis transmission from human to canine. Emerg Infect Dis 10: 2258–2210.
14. Prasad HK, Singhal A, Mishra A, Shah NP, Katoch VM, et al. (2005) Bovine tuberculosis in India: potential basis for zoonosis. Tuberculosis (Edinb) 85: 421–428.
15. Weese JS, Dick H, Willey BM, McGeer A, Kreiswirth BN, et al. (2006) Suspected transmission of methicillin-resistant Staphylococcus aureus between domestic pets and humans in veterinary clinics and in the household. Vet Microbiol 115: 148–155.
16. Morris DO, Mauldin EA, O'Shea K, Shofer FS, Rankin SC (2006) Clinical, microbiological, and molecular characterization of methicillin-resistant Staphylococcus aureus infections of cats. Am J Vet Res 67: 1421–1425.
17. Kwon N, Park K, Jung W, Youn H, Lee Y, et al. (2006) Characteristics of methicillin resistant Staphylococcus aureus isolated from chicken meat and hospitalized dogs in Korea and their epidemiological relatedness. Vet Microbiol 117: 304–312.
18. Rwego IB, Isabirye-Basuta G, Gillespie TR, Goldberg TL (2008) Gastrointestinal bacterial transmission among humans, mountain gorillas, and livestock in Bwindi Impenetrable National Park, Uganda. Conserv Biol 22: 1600–1607.
19. Hsieh J, Chen R, Tsai T, Pan T, Chou C (2008) Phylogenetic analysis of livestock oxacillin-resistant Staphylococcus aureus. Vet Microbiol 126: 234–242.
20. Berg S, Firdessa R, Habtamu M, Gadisa E, Mengistu A, et al. (2009) The Burden of Mycobacterial Disease in Ethiopian Cattle: Implications for Public Health. PLoS One 4: e5068–e5068.
21. Heller J, Kelly L, Reid SWJ, Mellor DJ (2010) Qualitative Risk Assessment of the Acquisition of Methicillin-Resistant Staphylococcus aureus in Pet Dogs. Risk Anal 30: 458–472.

22. Kottler S, Middleton JR, Perry J, Weese JS, Cohn LA (2010) Prevalence of *Staphylococcus aureus* and Methicillin-Resistant *Staphylococcus aureus* Carriage in Three Populations. J Vet Intern Med 24: 132–139.

23. Ewers C, Grobbel M, Stamm I, Kopp PA, Diehl I, et al. (2010) Emergence of human pandemic O25:H4-ST131 CTX-M-15 extended-spectrum-beta-lactamase-producing *Escherichia coli* among companion animals. J Antimicrob Chemother 65: 651–660.

24. Every AL, Selwood L, Castano-Rodriguez N, Lu W, Windsor HM, et al. (2011) Did transmission of *Helicobacter pylori* from humans cause a disease outbreak in a colony of Stripe-faced Dunnarts (*Sminthopsis macroura*)? Vet Res 42: 26.

25. Lin Y, Barker E, Kislow J, Kaldhone P, Stemper ME, et al. (2011) Evidence of multiple virulence subtypes in nosocomial and community-associated MRSA genotypes in companion animals from the upper midwestern and northeastern United States. Clin Med Res 9: 7–16.

26. Rubin JEJ, Chirino-Trejo MM (2011) Antimicrobial susceptibility of canine and human *Staphylococcus aureus* collected in Saskatoon, Canada. Zoonoses Public Health 58: 454–462.

27. Price LB, Stegger M, Hasman H, Aziz M, Larsen J, et al. (2012) *Staphylococcus aureus* CC398: host adaptation and emergence of methicillin resistance in livestock. MBio 3.

28. Meng X, Halbur PG, Shapiro MS, Sugantha G, Bruna JD, et al. (1998) Genetic and experimental evidence for cross-species infection by swine hepatitis E virus. J Virol 72: 9714–9721.

29. Willy ME, Woodward RA, Thornton VB, Wolff AV, Flynn BM, et al. (1999) Management of a measles outbreak among Old World nonhuman primates. Lab Anim Sci 49: 42–48.

30. Kaur T, Singh J, Tong SX, Humphrey C, Clevenger D, et al. (2008) Descriptive epidemiology of fatal respiratory outbreaks and detection of a human-related metapneumovirus in wild chimpanzees (*Pan troglodytes*) at Mahale Mountains National Park, western Tanzania. Am J Primatol 70: 755–765.

31. Feagins AR, Opriessnig T, Huang YW, Halbur PG, Meng XJ (2008) Cross-species infection of specific-pathogen-free pigs by a genotype 4 strain of human hepatitis E virus. J Med Virol 80: 1379–1386.

32. Song M, Lee J, Pascua PNQ, Baek Y, Kwon H, et al. (2010) Evidence of human-to-swine transmission of the pandemic (H1N1) 2009 influenza virus in South Korea. J Clin Microbiol 48: 3204–3211.

33. Swenson SL, Koster LG, Jenkins-Moore M, Killian ML, DeBess EE, et al. (2010) Natural cases of 2009 pandemic H1N1 Influenza A virus in pet ferrets. J Vet Diagn Invest 22: 784–788.

34. Tischer BK, Osterrieder N (2010) Herpesviruses–a zoonotic threat? Vet Microbiol 140: 266–270.

35. Abe M, Yamasaki A, Ito N, Mizoguchi T, Asano M, et al. (2010) Molecular characterization of rotaviruses in a Japanese raccoon dog (*Nyctereutes procyonoides*) and a masked palm civet (*Paguma larvata*) in Japan. Vet Microbiol 146: 253–259.

36. Berhane Y, Ojkic D, Neufeld J, Leith M, Hisanaga T, et al. (2010) Molecular characterization of pandemic H1N1 influenza viruses isolated from turkeys and pathogenicity of a human pH1N1 isolate in turkeys. Avian Dis 54: 1275–1285.

37. Poon LL, Mak PW, Li OT, Chan KH, Cheung CL, et al. (2010) Rapid detection of reassortment of pandemic H1N1/2009 influenza virus. Clin Chem 56: 1340–1344.

38. Forgie SE, Keenliside J, Wilkinson C, Webby R, Lu P, et al. (2011) Swine outbreak of pandemic influenza A virus on a Canadian research farm supports human-to-swine transmission. Clin Infect Dis 52: 10–18.

39. Holyoake PK, Kirkland PD, Davis RJ, Arzey KE, Watson J, et al. (2011) The first identified case of pandemic H1N1 influenza in pigs in Australia. Aust Vet J 89: 427–431.

40. Scotch M, Brownstein JS, Vegso S, Galusha D, Rabinowitz P (2011) Human vs. animal outbreaks of the 2009 swine-origin H1N1 influenza A epidemic. Ecohealth 8: 376–380.

41. Trevennec K, Leger L, Lyazrhi F, Baudon E, Cheung CY, et al. (2011) Transmission of pandemic influenza H1N1 (2009) in Vietnamese swine in 2009–2010. Influenza Other Respi Viruses.

42. Wevers D, Metzger S, Babweteera F, Bieberbach M, Boesch C, et al. (2011) Novel adenoviruses in wild primates: a high level of genetic diversity and evidence of zoonotic transmissions. J Virol 85: 10774–10784.

43. Crossley B, Hietala S, Hunt T, Benjamin G, Martinez M, et al. (2012) Pandemic (H1N1) 2009 in captive cheetah. Emerg Infect Dis 18: 315–317.

44. Sleeman JM, Meader LL, Mudakikwa AB, Foster JW, Patton S (2000) Gastrointestinal parasites of mountain gorillas (*Gorilla gorilla beringei*) in the Parc National des Volcans, Rwanda. J Zoo Wildl Med 31: 322–328.

45. Graczyk TK, DaSilva AJ, Cranfield MR, Nizeyi JB, Kalema G, et al. (2001) *Cryptosporidium parvum* Genotype 2 infections in free-ranging mountain gorillas (*Gorilla gorilla beringei*) of the Bwindi Impenetrable National Park, Uganda. Parasitol Res 87: 368–370.

46. Graczyk TK, Bosco-Nizeyi J, da Silva AJ, Moura IN, Pieniazek NJ, et al. (2002) A single genotype of *Encephalitozoon intestinalis* infects free-ranging gorillas and people sharing their habitats in Uganda. Parasitol Res 88: 926–931.

47. Graczyk TK, Bosco-Nizeyi J, Ssebide B, Thompson RCA, Read C, et al. (2002) Anthropozoonotic *Giardia duodenalis* genotype (assemblage) a infections in habitats of free-ranging human-habituated gorillas, Uganda. J Parasitol 88: 905–909.

48. Guk S, Yong T, Park S, Park J, Chai J (2004) Genotype and animal infectivity of a human isolate of *Cryptosporidium parvum* in the Republic of Korea. Korean J Parasitol 42: 85–89.

49. Noel C, Dufernez F, Gerbod D, Edgcomb VP, Delgado-Viscogliosi P, et al. (2005) Molecular phylogenies of Blastocystis isolates from different hosts: implications for genetic diversity, identification of species, and zoonosis. J Clin Microbiol 43: 348–355.

50. Coklin T, Farber J, Parrington L, Dixon B (2007) Prevalence and molecular characterization of *Giardia duodenalis* and *Cryptosporidium* spp. in dairy cattle in Ontario, Canada. Vet Parasitol 150: 297–305.

51. Adejinmi OJ, Ayinmode AB (2008) Preliminary investigation of zooanthroponosis in a Nigerian Zoological Garden. Vet Res (Pakistan) 2: 38–41.

52. Teichroeb JA, Kutz SJ, Parkar U, Thompson RCA, Sicotte P (2009) Ecology of the Gastrointestinal Parasites of *Colobus vellerosus* at Boabeng-Fiema, Ghana: Possible Anthropozoonotic Transmission. Am J Phys Anthropol 140: 498–507.

53. Ash A, Lymbery A, Lemon J, Vitali S, Thompson RCA (2010) Molecular epidemiology of *Giardia duodenalis* in an endangered carnivore - The African painted dog. Vet Parasitol 174: 206–212.

54. Johnston AR, Gillespie TR, Rwego IB, McLachlan TL, Kent AD, et al. (2010) Molecular epidemiology of cross-species *Giardia duodenalis* transmission in western Uganda. PLoS Negl Trop Dis 4: e683.

55. Dixon B, Parrington L, Cook A, Pintar K, Pollari F, et al. (2011) The potential for zoonotic transmission of *Giardia duodenalis* and *Cryptosporidium* spp. from beef and dairy cattle in Ontario, Canada. Vet Parasitol 175: 20–26.

56. Jacobs PHP (1988) Dermatophytes that infect animals and humans. Cutis; cutaneous medicine for the practitioner 42: 330–331.

57. Pal M, Matsusaka N, Chauhan P (1997) Zooanthroponotic significance of *Trichophyton rubrum* in a rhesus monkey (*Macaca mulatta*). Verh. ber. Erkrg. Zootiere 38: 355–358.

58. Wrobel L, Whittington JK, Pujol C, Oh S-H, Ruiz MO, et al. (2008) Molecular Phylogenetic Analysis of a Geographically and Temporally Matched Set of *Candida albicans* Isolates from Humans and Nonmigratory Wildlife in Central Illinois. Eukaryot Cell 7: 1475–1486.

59. Sharma DK, Gurudutt J, Singathia R, Lakhotia RL (2009) Zooanthroponosis of *Microsporum gypseum* infection. Haryana Veterinarian 48: 108–109.

60. Epstein JH, Price JT (2009) The significant but understudied impact of pathogen transmission from humans to animals. Mt Sinai J Med 76: 448–455.

61. Guyader Fl, Haugarreau L, Miossec L, Dubois E, Pommepuy M (2000) Three-year study to assess human enteric viruses in shellfish. Appl Environ Microbiol 66: 3241–3248.

62. Muehlenbein MP, Martinez LA, Lemke AA, Ambu L, Nathan S, et al. (2010) Unhealthy travelers present challenges to sustainable primate ecotourism. Travel Med Infect Dis 8: 169–175.

63. DeHart RL (2003) Health issues of air travel. Annu Rev Public Health 24: 133–151.

64. Daszak P, Cunningham AA, Hyatt AD (2000) Emerging infectious diseases of wildlife–threats to biodiversity and human health. Science 287: 443–449.

65. Chaber A-L, Allebone-Webb S, Lignereux Y, Cunningham AA, Marcus Rowcliffe J (2010) The scale of illegal meat importation from Africa to Europe via Paris. Conservation Letters 3: 317–321.

66. Fournie G, Pfeiffer DU (2013) Monitoring and controlling disease spread through live animal market networks. Vet J 195: 8–9.

67. American Pet Products Association Pet Industry Market Size & Ownership Statistics.

68. Leighton FA (2004) Veterinary medicine and the lifeboat test: a perspective on the social relevance of the veterinary profession in the 21st century. Can Vet J 45: 259–263.

69. World Association of Zoos and Aquariums (2013) Zoos and Aquariums of the World.

19

Prevalence of Disorders Recorded in Dogs Attending Primary-Care Veterinary Practices in England

Dan G. O'Neill[1]*, **David B. Church**[2], **Paul D. McGreevy**[3], **Peter C. Thomson**[3], **Dave C. Brodbelt**[1]

1 Veterinary Epidemiology, Economics and Public Health, Royal Veterinary College, London, United Kingdom, 2 Small Animal Medicine and Surgery Group, Royal Veterinary College, London, United Kingdom, 3 Faculty of Veterinary Science, University of Sydney, Sydney, New South Wales, Australia

Abstract

Purebred dog health is thought to be compromised by an increasing occurence of inherited diseases but inadequate prevalence data on common disorders have hampered efforts to prioritise health reforms. Analysis of primary veterinary practice clinical data has been proposed for reliable estimation of disorder prevalence in dogs. Electronic patient record (EPR) data were collected on 148,741 dogs attending 93 clinics across central and south-eastern England. Analysis in detail of a random sample of EPRs relating to 3,884 dogs from 89 clinics identified the most frequently recorded disorders as otitis externa (prevalence 10.2%, 95% CI: 9.1–11.3), periodontal disease (9.3%, 95% CI: 8.3–10.3) and anal sac impaction (7.1%, 95% CI: 6.1–8.1). Using syndromic classification, the most prevalent body location affected was the head-and-neck (32.8%, 95% CI: 30.7–34.9), the most prevalent organ system affected was the integument (36.3%, 95% CI: 33.9–38.6) and the most prevalent pathophysiologic process diagnosed was inflammation (32.1%, 95% CI: 29.8–34.3). Among the twenty most-frequently recorded disorders, purebred dogs had a significantly higher prevalence compared with crossbreds for three: otitis externa (P = 0.001), obesity (P = 0.006) and skin mass lesion (P = 0.033), and popular breeds differed significantly from each other in their prevalence for five: periodontal disease (P = 0.002), overgrown nails (P = 0.004), degenerative joint disease (P = 0.005), obesity (P = 0.001) and lipoma (P = 0.003). These results fill a crucial data gap in disorder prevalence information and assist with disorder prioritisation. The results suggest that, for maximal impact, breeding reforms should target commonly-diagnosed complex disorders that are amenable to genetic improvement and should place special focus on at-risk breeds. Future studies evaluating disorder severity and duration will augment the usefulness of the disorder prevalence information reported herein.

Editor: Cheryl S. Rosenfeld, University of Missouri, United States of America

Funding: This study was part of a Ph.D. study that was financially supported by the RSPCA (http://www.rspca.org.uk/sciencegroup/companionanimals). The funders had no role in study design, data collection and analysis, decision to publish, or preparation of the manuscript.

Competing Interests: The authors have declared that no competing interests exist.

* E-mail: doneill@rvc.ac.uk

Introduction

The domestic dog (*Canis lupus familiaris*) has become integral to modern human family life, with the UK dog population estimated to be 8–10 million [1,2,3] and 24–31% of UK households estimated to own at least one dog [1,2]. Although humans benefit from dog ownership both physically [4,5] and mentally [6,7], it is increasingly questioned whether modern breeding practices have allowed dog health and welfare to derive comparable benefits [8,9]. Although the dog is now the most phenotypically diverse mammal at a species level [10], genetic diversity has been greatly reduced within modern breeds [11] because of breeding practices that include closed stud books [12], structured inbreeding [11] and reproductive dominance of popular sires [13]. Additionally, selection pressure within breeds towards phenotypic exaggeration driven by breed standards [8], have increased the potential for conformation-associated disease [14]. Each of the 50 most popular breeds in the UK has at least one reported conformational predisposition to disease [15] and almost 400 non-conformational inherited disorders have been identified [16]. Conversely, implicit acceptance of the statement that purebred dogs are plagued with many inherited diseases [17] has contributed to a widespread belief that crossbred dogs are substantially healthier than purebreds [18].

Following claims in the BBC documentary *Pedigree Dogs Exposed* that purebred dog health was deteriorating because of inbreeding and ill-advised breed standards [19], three major reports concurred that pedigree breeding practices did impose welfare costs on dogs but, more crucially, concluded that a critical data gap on disorder prevalence information in UK dogs constrained effective reforms [20,21,22]. Prevalence data have been published on only 1% of inherited disorders affecting popular UK dog breeds [23]. Effective welfare reform of pedigree dog-breeding must be underpinned by scientifically valid prioritisation of disorders based on reliable and comparable prevalence data [12,24]. However, differing case definitions, study populations, geographical locations, data quality and data collection periods between published studies, combined with substantial data gaps, have constrained efforts to prioritise disorders in domestic dogs [9]. Application of health data collected via a single national surveillance system has been proposed for effective disorder prioritisation, with the critical first step being the generation of reliable disorder prevalence values [12].

Systematised collection, mergence and analysis of electronic patient record (EPR) data from primary-care veterinary practices has been proposed for generation of reliable prevalence data relating to the overall dog population [12,20]. Contemporaneous recording of clinical information by veterinary health professionals during episodes of care for every patient treated minimises selection and recall biases in primary-care practice EPR data [20]. By contrast, referral caseloads may show selection bias towards more complicated disorders [25], questionnaire surveys may incur selection, recall and misclassification biases [26], and pet insurance data are limited by selection bias emerging from age restrictions, financial excesses and owner attributes [27].

This study aimed to use a database of merged primary-care practice EPRs to estimate the prevalence of the most frequently recorded disorders and syndromes in dogs attending primary-care veterinary practices in England. The study further aimed to evaluate associations between the occurrence of common disorders with purebred/crossbred status and with popular breeds. It was hypothesised that purebred dogs have a higher prevalence of common disorders compared with crossbred dogs.

Materials and Methods

Ethics statement: Ethics approval was granted by the RVC Ethics and Welfare Committee (reference number 2010 1076).

The VetCompass Animal Surveillance project collates de-identified EPR data from primary-care veterinary practices in the UK for epidemiological research [28]. The current study included data collected from all clinics within the Medivet Veterinary Group, a large network of integrated veterinary practices covering central and south-eastern England [29]. Practitioners recorded summary diagnosis terms from an embedded standard nomenclature, the VeNom codes [30], at episodes of clinical care. EPR data were extracted from practice management systems (PMSs) using integrated clinical queries [31] and uploaded to a secure structured query language (SQL) database. Information collected included patient demographic (animal identification number, species, breed, date of birth, sex, neuter status, insurance status, microchip number and weight) and clinical information (free-form text clinical notes, VeNom summary diagnosis terms and treatment, with relevant dates) data fields.

The study sampling frame included all dogs that had at least one EPR (clinical note, weight recording or treatment dispensed) recorded within the VetCompass Animal Surveillance database from September 1, 2009 to March 31, 2013. Sample size calculations estimated that, from a study population of 140,000 dogs, a sample of 3,648 animals was required to represent a disorder with 2.5% expected frequency with a precision of 0.5% at a 95% confidence level [32].

A random sample of dogs was selected from the overall sampling frame using an online random number generator (www.random.org). Clinical notes and VeNom summary diagnosis terms recorded during the study period were reviewed in detail, and the most definitive diagnostic term recorded for each disorder diagnosed within individual dogs was manually coded using the most appropriate VeNom term. Elective (e.g. neutering) or prophylactic (e.g. vaccination) clinical events were not included. Multiple counting of disorder events for ongoing cases was avoided by including recurring diagnoses of ongoing conditions only once (e.g. repeated events of otitis externa) and by including only the final diagnosis term recorded in cases with diagnosis revision over time (e.g. following clinical work-up or trial therapy), based on the assumption that diagnostic accuracy increased over time [33]. The parent term was used for disorders that encompassed multiple child terms [34] (e.g. a parent term *road traffic accident* (RTA) may have multiple child terms such as *laceration*, *fracture* and *hypovolaemic*

shock). Disorder events that were aetiologically independent despite sharing the same disorder term name (e.g. novel traumatic events) were included separately. No distinction was made between pre-existing and incident disorder presentations. Disorders described within the clinical notes using presenting sign terms (e.g. 'vomiting and diarrhoea'), but without a formal clinical diagnostic term being recorded, were included using the first sign listed (e.g. vomiting). Dental disorders were included only if surgical or medical intervention were recommended.

Recognisable single breeds [35] were grouped as 'purebred' while all other dogs were grouped as 'crossbred'. Purebreds were further categorised by Kennel Club (KC) breed-recognition (recognised/not recognised) and KC breed group (gundog, hound, pastoral, terrier, toy, utility, working) [36]. Neuter status was defined by the final EPR neuter value and was combined with sex to create four categories: female entire, female neutered, male entire and male neutered. Insurance and microchip values characterized the existence of a positive status at any time during the study period. The maximum bodyweight (kg) recorded for dogs aged over one year was categorised into seven groups (<10.0, 10.0–19.9, 20.0–29.9, 30.0–39.9, 40.0–49.9, ≥50.0, and 'no recorded weight'). The age (years) at the final EPR was categorised into five groups (<1.0, 1.0–2.9, 3.0–5.9, 6.0–9.9, ≥10.0). Time contributed to the study for each dog was calculated as the period from the date of the earliest EPR to the date of the latest EPR. The date and manner (euthanasia or non-assisted) [37] of deaths recorded during the study were identified.

VeNom diagnostic terms for all recorded disorders were extracted and mapped to three systems of terms for analysis: diagnosis-level precision, mid-level precision and syndromic classification. Diagnosis-level terms were one-to-one descriptors of the original extracted terms at the maximal diagnostic precision recorded within the clinical notes (e.g. *inflammatory bowel disease* would remain as *inflammatory bowel disease*). Mid-level precision terms were one-to-one descriptors of original diagnosis terms defined at a general level of diagnostic precision (e.g. *inflammatory bowel disease* would map to *enteropathy*). Syndromic classification used three taxonomic groupings: body location, organ system and pathophysiologic process. The number of syndromic terms that could be mapped from each original diagnostic term was not limited.

Study data were exported from the VetCompass database to a spreadsheet (Microsoft Office Excel 2007, Microsoft Corp.) for checking and cleaning before further export to Stata Version 11.2 (Stata Corporation) for statistical analyses. Demographic variables were described statistically for the overall study population and the sample group. Prevalence values with 95% confidence intervals (CI) were tabulated for the twenty most prevalent diagnosis-level and mid-level disorders and for all syndromic terms, and were reported across all sampled dogs, purebreds only and crossbreds only. Prevalence values for purebred and crossbred dogs were compared statistically using the chi-squared test with Holm-adjusted P-values to account for multiple testing effects [38]. Statistical significance was set at the 5% level. The CI estimates were derived from standard errors based on approximation to the normal distribution for disorders with ten or more events recorded [39], but the Wilson approximation method was used for disorders with fewer than ten events recorded [40]. Prevalence (95% CI) values for the twenty most prevalent diagnosis-level and mid-level disorders and for all syndromic terms were similarly derived, reported and compared for popular breeds and crossbreds (popular breeds had ≥100 dogs in the sample group).

Results

The overall population comprised 148,741 dogs attending 93 clinics across central and south-eastern England. Demographic examination of dogs with information available indicated that 117,179 (78.9%) were purebred, 71,002 (48.0%) were female, 61,120 (41.1%) were neutered, 43,435 (29.2%) were insured and 41,071 (27.6%) were microchipped. The median weight was 18.2 kg (interquartile range (IQR): 9.4–29.0, range: 0.68–105.0) and the median age was 4.5 years (IQR: 1.6–8.7, range: 0.0–27.4) (Table 1).

The study sample comprised 3,884 dogs attending 89 clinics. Of dogs with information available, 3,079 (79.4%) were purebred, 1,817 (47.0%) were female, 1,735 (44.7%) were neutered, 1,226 (31.6%) were insured and 1,151 (29.6%) were microchipped. The median weight was 17.3 kg (IQR: 9.1–28.4, range: 1.3–100.6) and the median age was 4.8 years (IQR: 1.8–9.1, range: 0.0–21.24). The most popular seven breeds accounted for 1,431 (36.8%) of the study sample dogs (Table 1). Of the sampled dogs, 378 (9.7%) died during the study period, with a median (IQR, range) age at death of 12.3 years (9.2–14.4, 0.0–21.0) and 336 (88.9%) deaths involving euthanasia. Overall, 2,945 (75.8%) dogs had at least one disorder diagnosed, with the remainder having no disorders diagnosed during the study period. The median (IQR, range) number of disorders diagnosed per dog was 1.0 (1.0–3.0, 0.0–21.0). The median (IQR, range) time contributed to the study per dog was 0.7 years (0.0–3.5, 0.0–1.9). The sample and study populations were similar across all measures assessed.

Among the sampled dogs, 8,025 unique disorder events were recorded encompassing 430 distinct diagnosis-level disorder terms. The most prevalent diagnosis-level disorders recorded were otitis externa (number of events: 396, prevalence: 10.2%, 95% CI: 9.1–11.3), periodontal disease (361, 9.3%, 95% CI: 8.3–10.3), anal sac impaction (277, 7.1%, 95% CI: 6.1–8.1) and overgrown nails (276, 7.1%, 95% CI: 6.1–8.2). Purebred dogs had a significantly higher prevalence compared with crossbreds for three of the twenty most-prevalent diagnosis-level disorders: otitis externa (P = 0.001), obesity (P = 0.006) and skin mass lesion (P = 0.033) (Table 2). The prevalence of five of the twenty most-prevalent diagnosis-level disorders differed statistically significantly between popular breeds: periodontal disease (P = 0.002), overgrown nails (P = 0.004), degenerative joint disease (P = 0.005), obesity (P = 0.001) and lipoma (P = 0.003) (Table 3).

Within 54 mid-level diagnosis terms, the most prevalent disorders were enteropathic (n = 692, prevalence: 17.8%, 95% CI: 16.0–19.6), dermatological (602, 15.5%, 95% CI: 13.9–17.1), musculoskeletal (457, 11.8%, 95% CI: 10.6–12.9) and aural (426, 11.0%, 95% CI: 9.8–12.2). Purebred dogs showed a significantly higher prevalence than crossbreds for four of the twenty most-prevalent mid-level disorders: dermatological (P = 0.004), aural (P = 0.001), ophthalmological (P = 0.032) and obesity (P = 0.009) (Table 4). Statistically significant differences in prevalence values were shown between the most popular breeds in eight of the twenty most-frequent mid-level disorders: musculoskeletal (P = 0.002), claw/nail (P = 0.008), dental (P = 0.007), neoplastic (P = 0.001), anal sac (P = 0.006), obesity (P = 0.004), cardiac (P = 0.005) and brain (P = 0.003) (Table 5).

Syndromic classification analysis indicated that the most prevalent body locations affected in dogs were the head-and-neck (n = 1,273, prevalence = 32.8%, 95% CI: 30.7–34.9), abdomen (993, 25.6%, 95% CI: 23.6–27.5) and limb (679, 17.5%, 95% C: 15.9–19.1). Purebreds had significantly higher prevalence values compared with crossbreds for two of the eight body locations: head-and-neck (P = 0.003) and tail (P = 0.038) disorders. The most

prevalent organ systems affected were the integument (1,408, 36.3%, 95% CI: 33.9–38.6), digestive (1,144, 29.5%, 95% CI: 27.5–31.5) and musculoskeletal (573, 14.8%, 95% CI: 13.8–16.0) (Table 6). Purebreds had significantly higher prevalence values than crossbreds for two of fifteen organ systems, namely integument (P = 0.001) and auditory (P = 0.002) (Table 6). The most prevalent pathophysiologic processes recorded were inflammation (1,246, 32.1%, 95% CI: 29.8–34.3), mass/swelling (625, 16.1%, 95% CI: 14.6–17.6) and traumatic (557, 14.3%, 95% CI: 12.8–15.9). Purebreds had significantly higher prevalence values than crossbreds for two of twenty-one pathophysiological processes: inflammatory (P = 0.006) and nutritional (P = 0.0014) disorders (Table 7). Statistically significant differences in prevalence values between the most popular breeds were shown for 5/8 body location terms, 5/15 organ system terms and 5/21 pathophysiologic processes (Tables 8, 9 &10).

Discussion

This study reported the most prevalent disorders recorded in dogs attending primary-care veterinary practices in England as otitis externa, periodontal disease and anal sac impaction, while the most prevalent disorder groups were enteropathic, dermatological and musculoskeletal. The head-and-neck was the most prevalent body location affected, the integument was the most prevalent organ system affected, and inflammation was the most prevalent pathophysiologic process. Some evidence was shown to support higher disorder prevalence in purebred dogs compared with crossbred dogs and for important differences in disorder prevalence between breeds.

The current study was designed to fill a critical data gap relating to disorder prevalence information that has been identified as a constraint to improving dog welfare by effective reform of purebred dog-breeding [20,21,22]. Unacceptably high occurrence of inherited disorders in purebred dogs has been discussed since over half a century ago [41,42,43,44], leading to implementation of disease control measures such as defined health schemes [45,46,47,48] and revised KC recommendations and rules for registration and showing [44,49]. However, the current state and predicted trajectory of purebred dog health remain contentious despite these and other ongoing health measures, suggesting that these earlier breeding reforms that were developed without access to prioritisation information on the overall disorder burden may at best have been sub-optimal, and potentially even counter-productive [50].

Primary-care veterinary clinical data have been proposed as a superior data resource for clinical research in dogs [12,20]. Although useful, alternative data sources including referral practice data [51,52,53], pet insurance databases [27], official health schemes [54,55,56] and large scale questionnaire surveys [26,57,58,59] are reported to suffer many limitations for the generation of prevalence values that can be generalised to the wider dog population. Analyses based on primary-care veterinary EPR data benefit from open-ended data collection allowing generation of stronger evidence from cohort compared with cross-sectional study designs [60,61,62]. Selection bias is reduced by merging data collected from a miscellany of practices [63] and recall and misclassification biases are reduced by collection of clinical notes recorded contemporaneously by veterinary clinicians during episodes of care [64]. Veterinary primary-care denominator populations are well-characterised demographically within PMSs and include all practice-attending animals, whether presenting healthy or sick, linked with comprehensive clinical documentation that facilitates internal validation [27]. Registra-

Table 1. Demographic information for sampled (n = 3,884) and overall study population (n = 148,741) dogs attending primary veterinary practices in England.

Variable	Category	Sample: No. (%)	Population: No. (%)
Sex/neuter	Female entire	981 (25.4)	40,514 (27.4)
	Female neutered	836 (21.6)	30,488 (20.6)
	Male entire	1,152 (29.8)	46,459 (31.4)
	Male neutered	899 (23.2)	30,635 (20.7)
Microchip	Not microchipped	2,733 (70.4)	107,670 (72.4)
	Microchipped	1,151 (29.6)	41,071 (27.6)
Purebred status	Crossbred	797 (20.6)	31,354 (21.1)
	Purebred	3,079 (79.4)	117,179 (78.9)
Popular breeds	Crossbreed	797 (20.5)	31,354 (21.1)
	Labrador Retriever	339 (8.7)	13,328 (9.0)
	Staffordshire Bull Terrier	334 (8.6)	12,212 (8.2)
	Jack Russell Terrier	262 (6.8)	10,006 (6.7)
	Cocker Spaniel	133 (3.4)	5,579 (3.8)
	German Shepherd Dog	132 (3.4)	5,314 (3.6)
	Yorkshire Terrier	127 (3.3)	4,880 (3.3)
	Border Collie	104 (2.7)	3,997 (2.7)
	Other named breeds	1,656 (42.6)	62,071 (41.7)
KC[a]- breed[b]	Not KC-recognised	306 (9.9)	11,717 (10.0)
	KC-recognised	2,773 (90.1)	105,462 (90.0)
KC[a] group[c]	Gundog	737 (26.6)	28,832 (27.3)
	Hound	178 (6.4)	6,505 (6.2)
	Pastoral	284 (10.2)	11,530 (10.9)
	Terrier	561 (20.2)	21,481 (20.4)
	Toy	474 (17.1)	17,215 (16.3)
	Utility	330 (11.9)	11,573 (11.0)
	Working	209 (7.5)	8,326 (7.9)
Weight (kg)	No recorded weight	1,260 (32.4)	52,308 (35.2)
	<10.0	769 (19.8)	26,786 (18.0)
	10.0–19.9	695 (17.9)	25,278 (17.0)
	20.0–20.99	579 (14.9)	21,869 (14.7)
	30.0–30.9	390 (10.0)	15,255 (10.3)
	40.0–40.9	130 (3.4)	5,118 (3.4)
	≥50.0	61 (1.6)	2,127 (1.4)
Age (years)	<1.0	588 (15.2)	24,915 (16.8)
	1.0–2.9	791 (20.4)	30,747 (20.7)
	3.0–5.9	877 (22.6)	33,500 (22.5)
	6.0–9.9	811 (20.9)	30,811 (20.7)
	≥10.0	814 (21.0)	28,664 (19.3)
Insurance	Non-insured	2,658 (68.4)	105,306 (70.8)
	Insured	1,226 (31.6)	43,435 (29.2)

[a]KC The Kennel Club.
[b]Percentage values based on purebred only.
[c]Percentage values based on KC-recognised dogs only.

tion databases from primary-care practices are more representative of the national dog population than other databases available for research purposes; 77% of UK dogs are registered with a veterinary practice compared with just 42% of UK dogs that are insured and 31% of UK dogs that are registered with the KC [2].

Previous large-scale studies using primary-care practice clinical data have been variably successful and have encountered problems with sustainability. A cross-sectional study of paper-based clinical records for 7,146 dogs from eight UK practices described demographic and morbidity results but concluded that direct electronic extraction of clinical data and implementation of

Table 2. Prevalence results for the most frequent disorders recorded in dogs, purebreds only and crossbreds only that attended primary veterinary practices in England.

Disorder	Overall			Purebred		Crossbred		
	No.	Prev[a]%	95% CI[b]	Prev[a]%	95% CI[b]	Prev[a]%	95% CI[b]	P-value
Otitis externa	396	10.2	9.1–11.3	11.2	10.0–12.4	6.5	4.7–8.3	**0.001**
Periodontal disease	361	9.3	8.3–10.3	9.4	8.2–10.5	9.2	7.4–11.0	1.000
Anal sac impaction	277	7.1	6.1–8.1	7.1	6.0–8.1	7.5	5.7–9.4	1.000
Overgrown nails	276	7.1	6.1–8.2	6.9	5.8–8.0	8.0	6.1–9.9	1.000
Degenerative joint disease	256	6.6	5.7–7.5	6.4	5.3–7.4	7.5	5.7–9.4	1.000
Diarrhoea	249	6.4	5.5–7.4	6.8	5.6–8.0	4.9	3.4–6.4	0.255
Obesity	238	6.1	5.2–7.1	6.7	5.6–7.9	3.9	2.3–5.5	**0.006**
Traumatic injury	214	5.5	4.7–6.4	5.5	4.4–6.5	5.7	3.6–7.7	1.000
Conjunctivitis	192	4.9	4.1–5.8	5.2	4.2–6.2	4.1	2.8–5.5	1.000
Vomiting	159	4.1	3.3–4.9	4.0	3.1–4.9	4.5	3.0–6.0	1.000
Heart murmur	153	3.9	3.3–4.5	4.1	3.5–4.7	3.4	2.1–4.7	1.000
Lipoma	137	3.5	2.8–4.2	3.5	2.7–4.2	3.8	2.7–4.9	1.000
Dermatitis	134	3.5	2.8–4.1	3.5	2.8–4.3	3.1	1.9–4.4	1.000
Skin hypersensitivity	113	2.9	2.3–3.5	3.2	2.5–3.9	1.8	0.9–2.6	0.116
Skin mass	110	2.8	2.3–3.4	3.2	2.6–3.8	1.5	0.6–2.4	**0.033**
Claw injury	103	2.7	2.1–3.2	2.6	2.0–3.2	2.6	1.5–3.8	1.000
Behavioural	99	2.6	2.1–3.0	2.6	2.1–3.1	2.4	1.4–3.4	1.000
Gastroenteritis	99	2.6	2.0–3.1	2.4	1.9–2.9	3.1	2.0–4.3	1.000
Dog bite injury	97	2.5	1.9–3.1	2.4	1.7–3.1	2.9	1.8–4.0	1.000
Laceration	92	2.4	1.8–2.9	2.5	1.8–3.1	2.0	1.1–2.9	0.446

P-values (Holm-adjusted) represent comparison between purebreds and crossbreds.
[a]Prev prevalence.
[b]95% CI 95% confidence interval.

standardised coding for breeds and disorders were required to sustain long-term data collection [65]. In the US, the National Companion Animal Study (NCAS) reported overall disorder prevalence values using electronic records from 86,772 dogs attending 63 private practices. However, prevalence estimation was based only on the 36% of animals that had at least one coded disorder term recorded and the full clinical notes were not accessible for case-finding and internal validation exercises [66]. The National Companion Animal Surveillance System (NCASP) was established using EPR data from over 500 Banfield Pet Hospitals, but this system focused on the threat of emerging infection, terrorist attack or natural disaster rather than disorder prevalence [67] and has since been discontinued [68].

A standardised veterinary lexicon is critical for large-scale epidemiological application of secondary clinical data [52,65,69,70]. The VeNom codes [30] offers an open-access veterinary nomenclature that has been developed collaboratively between university and primary-care practice groups and facilitates both direct coding by attending clinicians at the point of clinical care and also retrospective coding by researchers during analysis. The VeNom coding ontology that is made available for point-of-care coding defines multiple clinical fields including species (45 terms), dog breeds (767), cat breeds (101), presenting complaints (201), diagnostic tests (39), diagnoses (2,291) and procedures (780).

The current study indicated that otitis externa (10.2%), periodontal disease (9.3%), anal sac impaction (7.1%) and overgrown nails (7.1%) were the most prevalent disorders recorded

in dogs attending veterinary practices in England. A US primary-care study similarly identified dental calculus (20.5%), gingivitis (19.5) and otitis externa (13.0%) as the most prevalent diagnoses in dogs, but reported the prevalence of anal sac disease at only 2.5%, and did not even include nail disorders within the common disorders diagnosed [70]. An under-developed coding system, inconsistent case definitions and selection bias from inclusion of only the one-third of animals that had at least one coded diagnosis term within the US study may explain these differing prevalence trends and underscores the importance of standardised coding systems for reliable comparisons between studies. The high frequency of dental disease reported in the US study may have resulted from inclusion of animals with any recorded dental abnormality, regardless of severity. By contract, the current study aimed to report the occurrence of dental disorders that currently warranted treatment in the opinion of the attending clinician. Study-inclusion of dental abnormalities of any nature provides information on the summative effects from both current and potential future clinically-significant dental disease whereas including just current clinically-significant cases provides evidence on the current welfare implications of dental disease. Both approaches have merit and add to our understanding of the substantial clinical relevance of dental disorders to the health and welfare of dogs. A UK primary-care study using paper-based clinical records identified the most prevalent disorders of dogs as overgrown nails (2.7%), ascarid worm problems (2.3%), anal sac impaction (2.1%), dental calculus (1.8%), fleas (1.8%), bacterial otitis externa (1.7%), waxy otitis externa (1.2%), diarrhoea/

Table 3. Prevalence results for frequent disorders recorded in popular breeds (number of dogs) from 3,884 randomly sampled dogs attending primary veterinary practices in England.

Disorder	Prevalence percentage (95% confidence interval)								P-Value
	Crossbred (797)	Labrador Retriever (339)	Staffordshire Bull Terrier (334)	Jack Russell Terrier (262)	Cocker Spaniel (133)	German Shepherd Dog (132)	Yorkshire Terrier (127)	Border Collie (104)	
Otitis externa	6.5 (4.7–8.3)	11.8 (8.8–15.7)	9.9 (7.1–13.6)	6.9 (4.4–10.6)	8.3 (4.7–14.2)	11.4 (7.0–17.9)	7.9 (4.3–13.9)	1.9 (0.5–6.7)	0.084
Periodontal disease	9.2 (7.4–11.0)	3.2 (1.8–5.7)	2.4 (1.2–4.7)	9.5 (6.6–13.7)	12.8 (8.1–19.5)	4.5 (2.1–9.6)	25.2 (18.6–33.4)	6.7 (3.3–13.3)	**0.002**
Anal sac impaction	7.5 (5.7–9.4)	4.7 (2.9–7.5)	3.3 (1.9–5.8)	6.9 (4.4–10.6)	12.0 (7.5–18.6)	6.1 (3.1–11.5)	6.3 (3.2–11.9)	2.9 (1.0–8.1)	0.066
Overgrown nails	8.0 (6.1–9.9)	6.5 (4.3–9.6)	3.9 (2.3–6.5)	13.7 (10.1–18.4)	2.3 (0.8–6.4)	1.5 (0.4–5.4)	15.0 (9.8–22.2)	1.0 (0.2–5.3)	**0.004**
Degenerative joint disease	7.5 (5.9–9.6)	11.5 (8.5–15.3)	5.4 (3.4–8.4)	4.2 (2.4–7.4)	1.5 (0.4–5.3)	6.8 (3.6–12.5)	1.6 (0.4–5.6)	11.5 (6.7–19.1)	**0.005**
Diarrhoea	4.9 (3.4–6.4)	8.3 (5.8–11.7)	4.8 (3.0–7.6)	4.6 (2.6–7.8)	9.8 (5.8–16.0)	8.3 (4.7–14.3)	5.5 (2.7–10.9)	7.7 (4.0–14.5)	1.000
Obesity	3.9 (2.3–5.5)	13.0 (9.8–17.0)	6.0 (3.9–9.1)	5.3 (3.2–8.8)	8.3 (4.7–14.2)	2.3 (0.8–6.5)	0.8 (0.1–4.3)	6.7 (3.3–13.3)	**0.001**
Traumatic injury	5.7 (3.6–7.7)	5.3 (3.4–8.2)	4.5 (2.7–7.3)	6.1 (3.8–9.7)	5.3 (2.6–10.5)	4.6 (2.1–9.6)	3.2 (1.2–7.8)	4.8 (2.1–10.8)	1.000
Conjunctivitis	4.1 (2.8–5.5)	4.1 (2.5–6.8)	5.1 (3.2–8.0)	4.2 (2.4–7.4)	6.8 (3.6–12.4)	0.0 (0.0–2.8)	7.1 (3.8–12.9)	4.8 (2.1–10.8)	1.000
Vomiting	4.5 (3.0–6.0)	3.8 (2.3–6.5)	3.9 (2.3–6.5)	5.7 (3.5–9.2)	2.3 (0.8–6.4)	4.6 (2.1–9.6)	3.2 (1.2–7.8)	1.9 (0.5–6.7)	1.000
Heart murmur	3.4 (2.1–4.7)	1.5 (0.6–3.4)	2.7 (1.4–5.0)	3.8 (2.1–6.9)	3.8 (1.6–8.5)	1.5 (0.4–5.4)	7.1 (3.8–12.9)	4.8 (2.1–10.8)	0.837
Lipoma	3.8 (2.7–4.9)	9.1 (6.5–12.7)	2.1 (1.0–4.3)	2.7 (1.3–5.4)	6.0 (3.1–11.4)	1.5 (0.4–5.4)	2.1 (0.0–2.9)	5.8 (2.7–12.0)	**0.003**
Dermatitis	3.1 (1.9–4.4)	1.5 (0.6–3.4)	3.6 (2.1–6.2)	3.4 (1.8–6.4)	3.0 (1.2–7.5)	3.0 (1.2–7.5)	4.7 (2.2–9.9)	6.7 (3.3–13.3)	1.000
Skin hypersensitivity	1.8 (0.9–2.6)	3.8 (2.3–6.5)	5.1 (3.2–8.0)	3.1 (1.6–5.9)	1.5 (0.4–5.3)	3.0 (1.2–7.5)	3.2 (1.2–7.8)	2.9 (1.0–8.1)	1.000
Skin mass	1.5 (0.6–2.4)	3.2 (1.8–5.7)	3.9 (2.3–6.5)	2.3 (1.1–4.9)	3.8 (1.6–8.5)	3.0 (1.2–7.5)	2.4 (0.8–6.7)	3.0 (1.0–8.1)	1.000
Claw injury	2.6 (1.5–3.8)	3.8 (2.3–6.5)	3.6 (2.1–6.2)	2.7 (1.3–5.4)	2.3 (0.8–6.4)	3.0 (1.2–7.5)	3.9 (1.7–8.9)	2.9 (1.0–8.1)	1.000
Undesirable behaviour	2.4 (1.4–3.4)	3.0 (1.6–5.3)	2.7 (1.4–5.0)	1.5 (0.6–3.9)	3.0 (1.2–7.5)	7.6 (4.2–13.4)	2.4 (0.8–6.7)	5.8 (2.7–12.0)	0.208
Gastro-enteritis	3.1 (2.0–4.3)	4.4 (2.7–7.3)	1.5 (0.6–3.5)	1.9 (0.8–4.4)	3.0 (1.2–7.5)	0.8 (0.1–4.2)	3.9 (1.7–8.9)	3.9 (1.5–9.5)	1.000
Dog bite injury	2.9 (1.8–4.0)	1.5 (0.6–3.4)	3.0 (1.6–5.4)	3.8 (2.1–6.9)	3.8 (1.6–8.5)	1.5 (0.4–5.4)	0.0 (0.0–2.9)	1.0 (0.2–5.3)	1.000
Laceration	2.0 (1.2–3.2)	3.5 (2.0–6.1)	2.4 (1.2–4.7)	2.7 (1.3–5.4)	3.0 (1.2–7.5)	0.8 (0.1–4.2)	1.6 (0.4–5.6)	2.9 (1.0–8.1)	1.000

P-values (Holm-adjusted) represent comparison between breeds.

Table 4. Prevalence results for the most frequent mid-level disorders recorded in dogs, purebreds only and crossbreds only that attended primary veterinary practices in England.

Mid-level disorder	Overall			Purebred		Crossbred		
	No.	Prev[a]%	95% CI[b]	Prev[a]%	95% CI[b]	Prev[a]%	95% CI[b]	P-value
Enteropathic	692	17.8	16.0–19.6	17.7	15.8–19.7	18.3	15.4–21.2	1.000
Dermatological	602	15.5	13.9–17.1	16.5	14.6–18.4	11.9	10.0–13.9	**0.004**
Musculoskeletal	457	11.8	10.6–12.9	11.2	9.8–12.6	14.1	11.8–16.3	0.130
Aural	426	11.0	9.8–12.2	12.0	10.7–13.3	7.2	5.3–9.0	**0.001**
Ophthalmological	406	10.5	9.1–11.8	11.1	9.7–12.6	7.9	6.1–9.7	**0.032**
Claw/nail	400	10.3	9.1–11.5	10.1	8.8–11.5	10.9	9.0–12.9	1.000
Dental	386	9.9	8.8–11.1	10.0	8.8–11.2	9.8	7.9–11.7	1.000
Neoplastic	367	9.5	8.2–10.7	9.6	8.2–10.9	9.2	7.2–11.1	1.000
Traumatic injury (not incl. bites)	351	9.0	8.0–10.1	9.1	7.8–10.3	8.9	6.6–11.2	1.000
Anal sac	337	8.7	7.5–9.8	8.6	7.3–9.9	9.0	7.1–11.0	1.000
Obesity	238	6.1	5.2–7.1	6.7	5.6–7.9	3.9	2.3–5.5	**0.009**
Mass lesion	235	6.1	5.2–6.9	6.4	5.3–7.4	4.9	3.4–6.4	0.726
Behavioural	233	6.0	5.3–6.85	5.8	4.9–6.7	6.9	5.1–8.7	1.000
Upper respiratory tract	223	5.7	4.9–6.5	5.6	4.6–6.6	6.4	4.6–8.2	1.000
Cardiac	219	5.6	4.8–6.5	5.9	5.0–6.7	4.9	3.1–6.7	1.000
Parasitic	172	4.4	3.8–5.1	4.2	3.5–5.0	5.3	3.7–6.8	1.000
Congenital	171	4.4	3.7–5.1	4.6	3.7–5.4	3.9	2.6–5.2	1.000
Bite injury	148	3.8	3.0–4.6	3.7	2.9–4.6	4.1	2.8–5.5	1.000
Urinary	126	3.2	2.7–3.8	3.4	2.7–4.1	2.8	1.6–3.9	1.000
Brain	122	3.1	2.5–3.7	3.2	2.6–3.8	3.1	1.9–4.4	1.000

P-values (Holm-adjusted) represent comparison between purebreds and crossbreds.
[a]Prev prevalence.
[b]95% CI 95% confidence interval.

vomiting (1.0%) and *Otodectes* otitis externa (0.9%) [65]. Although the predominance of aural, nail, anal sac and dental disorders identified was consistent with the current study, the older study reported *prevalence per consultation* values, leading to apparently lower prevalence values than the current study that reported *period prevalence per dog*. The substantially lower prevalence of parasitic disorders reported in the current study may also reflect increasing adoption and effectiveness of prophylactic parasiticides in the intervening fifteen years since the previous study [71,72].

Although diagnosis-level disorder terms are useful to describe disorders at their precision of clinical diagnosis, sole reliance on these terms for research may mask important underlying disorder concepts because of fragmentation into multiple terms along diagnostic pathways. The current study grouped clinically-related diagnosis-level terms (430 unique terms) into appropriate, composite mid-level disorder terms (54 unique terms) for further analysis. Selection of cut-off points for amalgamation along diagnostic precision pathways aimed to optimise interpretability whilst still retaining adequate precision [73]. The predominant mid-level disorders (enteropathic, dermatological, musculoskeletal and aural) differed from the predominant diagnosis-level disorders (otitis externa, periodontal disease, anal sac impaction, overgrown nails), suggesting that such hierarchical analysis can offer useful insights that may otherwise be missed.

Syndromic surveillance is based on clinical features that are discernible even from early presentation and are not dependent on complete or even correct diagnosis for elucidation of diagnostic patterns [74]. Although veterinary clinical diagnostic accuracy

may have improved over recent years, diagnostic discrepancies have been identified in 15% of cases undergoing necropsy [75]. Syndromic surveillance has been applied within human bioterrorism surveillance [76] and for analysis of canine insurance data [77,78]. The three syndromic classification systems used in the current study (body location, organ system and pathophysiology) were selected for their potential welfare importance via breed conformation and genetic effects [15]. The syndromic coding system used in the current study was adapted from VeNom codes and other published veterinary lexicons in line with the disorder types recorded within the study [25,79]. Progression towards a standardised syndromic terminology would facilitate future inter-study comparisons and meta-analyses [80].

The results from syndromic analyses in the current study identified the most prevalent body locations affected by disorders in dogs as the head-and-neck (32.8%), abdomen (25.6%) and limb (17.5%). Morphologic diversity between breeds resulting from artificial selection towards the extremes of breed standard morphometrics [81] has been associated with conformational predisposition for disorders [15,20]. The predominance of disorders identified affecting the head-and-neck reaffirm the importance of this body area to dog health [82].

The most affected organ systems identified by the current study were the integument (36.3%), digestive (29.5%) and musculoskeletal (14.8%). Swedish insurance data analysis similarly identified the most prevalently affected organs systems as the integument (3.2%), gastrointestinal (2.7%) and genital (2.5%) [83]. A consistently high prevalence reported by these studies for disorders

Table 5. Prevalence results for frequent mid-level disorders recorded in popular breeds (number of dogs) attending primary veterinary practices in England.

Mid-level disorder	Prevalence percentage (95% confidence interval)								P-value
	Crossbred (797)	Labrador Retriever (339)	Staffordshire Bull Terrier (334)	Jack Russell Terrier (262)	Cocker Spaniel (133)	German Shepherd Dog (132)	Yorkshire Terrier (127)	Border Collie (104)	
Enteropathic	18.3 (15.4–21.2)	22.7 (18.6–27.5)	13.2 (10.0–17.2)	15.3 (11.4–20.1)	18.8 (13.1–26.3)	20.5 (14.5–28.1)	16.5 (11.1–24.0)	17.3 (11.2–25.7)	1.000
Dermatological	11.9 (10.0–13.9)	16.8 (13.2–21.2)	14.7 (11.38–18.9)	13.0 (9.4–17.6)	9.8 (5.8–16.0)	18.9 (13.2–26.5)	18.1 (12.4–25.7)	18.3 (12.0–26.8)	0.715
Musculoskeletal	14.1 (11.8–16.3)	16.2 (12.7–20.5)	8.4 (5.9–11.9)	7.3 (4.7–11.1)	3.0 (1.2–7.5)	16.7 (11.3–24.0)	6.3 (3.2–11.9)	16.4 (10.5–24.6)	**0.002**
Aural	7.2 (5.3–9.0)	12.1 (9.0–16.0)	11.1 (8.1–14.9)	7.6 (5.0–11.5)	9.0 (5.2–15.1)	11.4 (7.0–17.9)	7.9 (4.3–13.9)	4.8 (2.1–10.8)	0.828
Ophthalmo-logical	7.9 (6.1–9.7)	6.8 (4.6–10.0)	8.1 (5.6–11.5)	8.0 (5.3–11.9)	12.0 (7.5–18.7)	2.3 (0.8–6.5)	12.6 (7.9–19.5)	12.5 (7.5–20.2)	0.261
Claw/nail	10.9 (9.0–12.9)	10.9 (8.0–14.7)	7.5 (5.1–10.8)	14.9 (11.1–19.7)	5.3 (2.6–10.5)	5.3 (2.6–10.5)	19.7 (13.7–27.5)	5.8 (2.7–12.0)	**0.008**
Dental	9.8 (7.9–11.7)	3.8 (2.3–6.5)	3.0 (1.6–5.4)	11.5 (8.1–15.9)	12.8 (8.1–19.5)	5.3 (2.6–10.5)	25.2 (18.5–33.4)	7.7 (4.0–14.5)	**0.007**
Neoplastic	9.2 (7.2–11.1)	14.8 (11.4–18.9)	6.6 (4.4–9.8)	4.6 (2.6–7.8)	13.5 (8.7–20.4)	4.6 (2.1–9.6)	6.3 (3.2–11.9)	8.7 (4.6–15.6)	**0.001**
Traumatic injury (not bites or claw)	8.9 (6.6–11.2)	11.2 (8.3–15.0)	7.88 (5.4–11.2)	9.2 (6.2–13.3)	10.5 (6.4–16.9)	6.1 (3.1–11.5)	3.9 (1.7–8.9)	9.6 (5.3–16.8)	1.000
Anal sac	9.0 (7.1–11.0)	5.9 (3.9–8.9)	3.6 (2.1–6.2)	9.9 (6.9–14.1)	13.5 (8.7–20.4)	6.8 (3.6–12.5)	6.3 (3.2–11.9)	2.9 (1.0–8.1)	**0.006**
Obesity	3.9 (2.3–5.5)	12.98 (9.81–16.98)	6.0 (3.9–9.1)	5.3 (3.2–8.8)	8.3 (4.7–14.2)	2.3 (0.8–6.5)	0.8 (0.1–4.3)	6.7 (3.3–13.3)	**0.004**
Mass lesion	4.9 (3.4–6.4)	8.26 (5.78–11.68)	6.6 (4.4–9.8)	5.0 (2.9–8.3)	6.8 (3.6–12.4)	6.1 (3.1–11.5)	7.9 (4.3–13.9)	8.7 (4.6–15.6)	1.000
Behavioural	6.9 (5.1–8.7)	4.7 (2.9–7.5)	5.1 (3.2–8.0)	7.6 (5.0–11.5)	6.8 (3.6–12.4)	12.9 (8.2–19.7)	3.9 (1.7–8.9)	8.7 (4.6–15.6)	0.460
Upper respiratory tract	6.4 (4.6–8.2)	6.2 (4.1–9.3)	6.3 (4.2–9.4)	5.7 (3.5–9.2)	2.3 (0.8–6.4)	3.0 (1.2–7.5)	7.1 (3.8–12.9)	2.9 (1.0–8.1)	1.000
Cardiac disorder	4.9 (3.1–6.7)	1.5 (0.6–3.4)	3.0 (1.6–5.4)	6.5 (4.1–10.1)	4.5 (2.1–9.5)	1.5 (0.4–5.4)	10.2 (6.1–16.7)	5.8 (2.7–12.0)	**0.005**
Parasitic	5.3 (3.7–6.8)	3.5 (2.0–6.1)	4.8 (3.0–7.6)	3.4 (1.8–6.4)	8.3 (4.7–14.2)	2.3 (0.8–6.5)	4.7 (2.2–9.9)	1.9 (0.5–6.7)	1.000
Congenital	3.9 (2.6–5.2)	2.4 (1.2–4.6)	2.1 (1.0–4.3)	3.8 (2.2–6.9)	3.8 (1.6–8.5)	0.8 (0.1–4.2)	6.3 (3.2–11.9)	1.9 (0.5–6.7)	1.000
Bite injury	4.1 (2.8–5.5)	3.8 (2.3–6.5)	4.29 (2.5–6.9)	5.0 (2.9–8.3)	4.5 (2.1–9.5)	2.3 (0.8–6.5)	1.6 (0.4–5.6)	1.9 (0.5–6.7)	1.000
Urinary	2.8 (1.6–3.9)	4.7 (2.9–7.5)	2.4 (1.2–4.6)	1.9 (0.8–4.4)	3.0 (1.2–7.5)	3.0 (1.2–7.5)	2.4 (0.8–6.7)	3.9 (1.5–9.5)	1.000
Brain	3.1 (1.9–4.4)	3.2 (1.8–5.7)	0.6 (0.2–2.2)	2.3 (1.1–4.9)	3.0 (1.2–7.5)	4.6 (2.1–9.6)	1.6 (0.4–5.6)	9.6 (5.3–16.8)	**0.003**

P-values (Holm–adjusted) represent comparison between breeds. (n = 3,884).

Table 6. Prevalence of syndromic disorders affecting body location and organ system recorded in overall dogs, purebreds only and crossbreds only that attended primary veterinary practices in England.

	Overall		Purebred		Crossbred		
	No.	Prev[a]%	95% CI[b]	Prev[a]%	95% CI[b]	Prev[a]%	95% CI[b]	P–value
Body Location								
Head/neck	1,273	32.8	30.7–34.9	34.0	31.7–36.2	28.5	24.9–32.0	**0.003**
Abdomen	993	25.6	23.6–27.5	25.9	23.7–28.0	24.6	21.5–27.7	1.000
Limb	679	17.5	15.9–19.1	17.3	15.5–19.1	18.3	15.7–20.9	1.000
Anus/perineum	359	9.2	8.1–10.4	9.1	7.8–10.5	9.8	7.6–12.0	1.000
Thorax	353	9.1	8.1–10.1	9.2	8.1–10.4	8.7	6.5–10.8	1.000
Vertebral column	78	2.0	1.5–2.5	2.0	1.5–2.6	2.0	1.0–3.0	1.000
Pelvis	33	0.9	0.6–1.2	0.9	0.7–1.4	0.5	0.2–1.3	0.684
Tail	21	0.5	0.4–0.8	0.7	0.5–1.0	0.0	0.0–0.5	**0.038**
Organ system								
Integument	1,408	36.3	33.9–38.6	37.6	35.0–40.2	31.4	28.0–34.7	**0.001**
Digestive	1,144	29.5	27.5–31.5	29.4	27.2–31.6	30.0	26.6–33.3	1.000
Musculoskeletal	573	14.8	13.5–16.0	14.1	12.6–15.6	17.3	14.8–19.8	0.110
Connective/Soft tissue	503	13.0	11.6–14.3	13.2	11.6–14.7	12.3	10.2–14.4	1.000
Ocular	447	11.5	10.2–12.8	12.2	10.6–13.7	9.2	7.2–11.1	0.057
Auditory	437	11.3	10.0–12.5	12.3	11.0–13.6	7.4	5.5–9.3	**0.002**
Nervous	301	7.8	6.8–8.7	7.7	6.7–8.7	7.9	6.2–9.6	1.000
Respiratory	273	7.0	6.2–7.9	7.0	6.0–8.1	7.2	5.2–9.1	1.000
Cardiovascular	241	6.2	5.3–7.1	6.5	5.5–7.4	5.3	3.5–7.1	1.000
Urinary	227	5.8	5.1–6.6	5.9	4.9–6.8	5.8	4.1–7.5	1.000
Reproductive	184	4.7	4.1–5.4	4.7	4.0–5.5	4.9	3.5–6.3	1.000
Endocrine	72	1.9	1.5–2.3	1.8	1.3–2.3	2.1	1.2–3.1	1.000
Haematopoietic	53	1.4	1.0–1.7	1.4	1.0–1.8	1.3	0.5–2.1	1.000
Hepatobiliary	29	0.8	0.5–1.1	0.9	0.6–1.3	0.1	0.0–0.7	0.088
Lymphatic	26	0.7	0.5–1.0	0.6	0.4–1.0	0.9	0.4–1.8	1.000

P–values (Holm–adjusted) represent comparison between purebreds and crossbreds.
[a]Prev prevalence.
[b]95% CI 95% confidence interval.

Table 7. Prevalence of syndromic disorders related to pathophysiologic processes recorded in overall dogs, purebreds only and crossbreds only that attended primary veterinary practices in England.

Pathophysiologic process	Overall			Purebred		Crossbred		
	No.	Prev[a]%	95% CI[b]	Prev[a]%	95% CI[b]	Prev[a]%	95% CI[b]	P–value
Inflammation	1,246	32.1	29.8–34.3	33.2	30.7–35.7	28.1	25.1–31.2	**0.006**
Mass/swelling	625	16.1	14.6–17.6	16.7	15.0–18.4	14.1	11.8–16.3	0.222
Traumatic	557	14.3	12.8–15.9	14.3	12.7–16.0	14.3	11.6–17.0	1.000
Degenerative	411	10.6	9.4–11.8	10.4	9.0–11.7	11.4	9.1–13.8	1.000
Infectious	388	10.0	9.0–11.0	10.3	9.1–11.4	9.0	6.9–11.2	1.000
Neoplastic	336	8.7	7.6–9.8	8.6	7.3–9.8	9.0	7.2–10.9	1.000
Congenital/developmental	332	8.6	7.4–9.7	8.9	7.6–10.2	7.3	5.6–9.2	0.870
Nutritional	320	8.2	7.1–9.4	8.9	7.5–10.2	5.9	4.3–7.5	**0.014**
Behavioural	262	6.8	5.9–7.6	6.5	5.5–7.4	7.9	6.0–9.8	1.000
Hereditary	232	6.0	5.1–6.9	6.2	5.1–7.3	5.3	3.5–7.0	1.000
Parasitic	221	5.7	5.0–6.4	5.5	4.6–6.3	6.7	5.0–8.4	1.000
Iatrogenic	150	3.9	3.3–4.5	3.7	3.1–4.4	4.4	2.9–5.9	1.000
Foreign body	109	2.8	2.3–3.3	2.8	2.3–3.4	2.8	1.6–3.9	1.000
Death	65	1.7	1.2–2.2	1.6	1.1–2.1	2.1	1.2–3.1	1.000
Intoxicative	49	1.3	1.0–1.7	1.3	1.0–1.8	1.1	0.6–2.1	1.000
Haemostatic	38	1.0	0.7–1.3	1.1	0.8–1.5	0.5	0.2–1.3	0.496
Immune–mediated	38	1.0	0.7–1.3	1.1	0.8–1.5	0.5	0.2–1.3	0.620
Allergic	35	0.9	0.7–1.3	0.9	0.6–1.3	0.9	0.4–1.8	1.000
Thermoregulatory	17	0.4	0.3–0.7	0.4	0.2–0.7	0.6	0.3–1.5	1.000
Metabolic	8	0.2	0.1–0.4	0.2	0.1–0.4	0.3	0.1–0.9	1.000
Effusion	1	0.0	0.0–0.2	0.0	0.0–0.2	0.0	0.0–0.5	1.000

P–values (Holm-adjusted) represent comparison between purebreds and crossbreds.
[a]Prev prevalence.
[b]95% CI 95% confidence interval.

affecting the integument and digestive systems suggests the importance of clinical emphasis on maintaining the health of these systems.

The current study identified inflammation (32.1%), mass/swelling (16.1%) and trauma (14.3%) as the most prevalent pathophysiologic processes affecting dogs. Similarly, a Swedish insurance study identified inflammation (5.4%), symptomatic (3.0%), trauma (2.7%) and neoplasia (2.1%) as the pathological processes with the highest risk of morbidity [83]. Although an essential adaptive response to injury, inflammation can behave both physiologically (restoring homeostasis) and pathologically (contributing to ongoing disease) [84]. The preponderance of inflammatory disorders affecting dogs identified by the current study suggests welfare gains from increased awareness by owners of judicious use of anti-inflammatory medications and also the value from ongoing research to better harness the healing aspects of inflammation while limiting detrimental effects [85].

The current study hypothesised that purebred dogs have higher prevalence of common disorders compared with crossbreds. This hypothesis was founded on reports and studies that concluded substantial detriment to purebred dog welfare from increasing inherited health problems induced by inbreeding and selection for extreme morphologies [15,16,20,21,22]. The study hypothesis was tested by comparing prevalence values between purebreds and crossbreds for each of the twenty most prevalent diagnosis-level and mid-level disorders and for all syndromic presentations. Purebreds showed significantly higher prevalence values for 13 of

the 84 (15.5%) disorders and syndromes evaluated. No instances were identified in which prevalence values were significantly higher in crossbred than in purebred dogs. These results provided moderate evidence for higher disorder prevalence in purebreds compared with crossbreds. However, additional analyses of severity and duration data for these disorders would enable a more comprehensive understanding of health disparities between the groups [23].

Failure to show overwhelming evidence for disorder disparity between purebred and crossbred dogs appears initially at odds with the large body of literature apparently to the contrary [20,21,22,86,87]. There are a number of possibilities for this dissonance. Breed-specific conformational disorders within purebreds may be under-reported or under-recognised by both veterinarians and owners because 'normal for breed' may have become confused with 'normal' [88]. A study of dogs clinically diagnosed with brachycephalic obstructive airway syndrome (BOAS) identified that 58% of owners reported these dogs not to have 'breathing problems' [82]. Purebred and crossbred dog categories comprise heterogeneous mosaics of size, shape and genetics. Merging this variation into single categories may have masked important effects related to specific conformational, physiological or behavioural features. Analyses of purebred or crossbred subgroups based on breed, behaviour or body attributes may better elucidate important health hazards, benefits and associations.

Table 8. Prevalence of syndromic diagnoses affecting body location recorded in crossbred dogs and popular breeds (number of dogs) from 3,884 randomly sampled dogs attending primary veterinary practices in England.

Body Location	Prevalence percentage (95% confidence interval)								P-Value
	Crossbred (797)	Labrador Retriever (339)	Staffordshire Bull Terrier (334)	Jack Russell Terrier (262)	Cocker Spaniel (133)	German Shepherd Dog (132)	Yorkshire Terrier (127)	Border Collie (104)	
Head/neck	28.5 (24.9-32.0)	28.6 (24.1-33.6)	24.0 (19.7-28.8)	30.5 (25.3-36.4)	33.1 (25.7-41.5)	22.7 (16.4-30.6)	43.3 (35.0-52.0)	35.6 (27.0-45.1)	0.006
Abdomen	24.6 (21.5-27.7)	32.4 (27.7-37.6)	21.0 (16.9-25.6)	21.0 (16.5-26.3)	27.1 (20.2-35.2)	25.8 (19.1-33.8)	20.5 (14.4-28.3)	30.8 (22.7-40.2)	0.045
Limb	18.3 (15.7-20.9)	20.4 (16.4-25.0)	14.1 (10.7-18.2)	20.2 (15.8-25.5)	7.5 (4.1-13.3)	13.6 (8.8-20.5)	22.0 (15.7-30.0)	16.3 (10.5-24.6)	0.036
Anus/perineum	9.8 (7.6-12.0)	6.2 (4.1-9.3)	3.9 (2.3-6.5)	9.9 (6.9-14.1)	15.0 (10.0-22.1)	9.1 (5.3-15.2)	7.1 (3.8-12.9)	3.8 (1.5-9.5)	0.001
Thorax	8.7 (6.5-10.8)	6.5 (4.3-9.6)	6.0 (3.9-9.1)	8.8 (5.9-12.8)	6.0 (3.1-11.4)	3.0 (1.2-7.5)	13.4 (8.5-20.4)	6.7 (3.3-13.2)	0.294
Vertebral column	2.0 (1.0-3.0)	1.5 (0.6-3.4)	0.3 (0.1-1.7)	1.1 (0.4-3.3)	3.8 (1.6-8.5)	1.5 (0.4-5.4)	0.8 (0.1-4.3)	2.9 (1.0-8.1)	1.000
Pelvis	0.5 (0.2-1.3)	0.6 (0.2-2.1)	0.6 (0.2-2.2)	0.0 (0.0-1.4)	0.0 (0.0-2.8)	0.0 (0.0-2.8)	1.6 (0.4-5.6)	1.0 (0.2-5.2)	1.000
Tail	0.0 (0.0-0.5)	2.4 (1.2-4.6)	0.3 (0.1-1.7)	0.0 (0.0-1.4)	1.5 (0.4-5.3)	0.0 (0.0-2.8)	0.0 (0.0-2.9)	1.0 (0.2-5.2)	0.002

P-values (Holm-adjusted) represent comparison between breeds.

Purebred dogs comprise 75-80% of the overall UK dog population [3,28], suggesting that a high proportion of crossbreds are likely to be first or second filial offspring from purebred progenitors and could be reasonably expected to show conformational and polygenic disorder occurrence at the midpoint between the values for their parent breeds, with any additional health benefits in crossbreds resulting from hybrid vigour effects [89]. From this perspective, the less-than-overwhelming evidence provided by the current study for substantially lower prevalence values in crossbred compared with purebred dogs does not refute claims in the literature of rising prevalence values for inherited disorders within purebred dogs. Instead, this suggests that the overall disorder burden within crossbred dogs may reflect the overall disorder burden in purebreds at any point in time. For optimal understanding, disorder prevalence in purebreds should be quantified by analysing cohort health data to identify trends over time.

The most prevalent disorders identified in dogs within the current study were complex disorders that have multiple interacting environmental and genetic casual factors [90]: otitis externa [91], periodontal disease [92], anal sac disorders [93], nail disorders [94,95], degenerative joint disease [96], diarrhoea [97,98], obesity [99], traumatic injury [100], conjunctivitis [101], vomiting [101,102] and heart murmur [103,104]. It may be useful for canine health research to move away from viewing individual disorders as necessarily either inherited or non-inherited [105] and towards an acknowledgement of relevant roles for both genetic and environmental components in the majority of canine disorders [106,107,108]. This acceptance will improve decision-making on effective disease-control and breeding programs [109]. Application of estimated breeding values (EBVs) developed from summative health information derived from a range of sources, including health schemes and veterinary primary-care data, could contribute integrally to novel disorder-control programs [14,110,111].

A large body of literature supports the existence of disorder predispositions affecting most dog breeds [15,16,112]. Despite inclusion of just seven breeds in the current analysis, breed associations were identified for 33.3% (28/84) of the disorders and syndromes evaluated (diagnosis-level disorders 20% (5/20), mid-level disorders 40% (8/20) and syndromic terms 34% (15/44)). The high-risk breeds differed considerably between the disorders in the current study, suggesting that rational health control measures should focus on highly-predisposed disorders within at-risk breeds. Future breed-specific studies are recommended to report more precise prevalence estimates and for a wider range of breeds. Early studies could focus on the fourteen high-profile breeds identified by the KC as having higher health risks, mainly due to conformational problems [113].

There were some limitations to the current study. The practices participating in the study formed a single veterinary group that extended across central and south-east England and may not be representative of the overall veterinary practice structure in England. Case definitions and diagnosis recording relied heavily on the clinical acumen and note-making of attending practitioners. The researchers made no attempts to second-guess underlying disorders in cases with presenting signs (e.g. vomiting) recorded *in lieu* of formal diagnoses. Inclusion of umbrella terms such as *road traffic accident* without additional inclusion of the individual specific injuries sustained within the primary event may have reduced the apparent prevalence of fractures and lacerations but avoided multiple counting of disorder events along axes of diagnostic precision. The analyses based on popular breeds were exploratory in nature and should be validated within larger confirmatory

Table 9. Prevalence of syndromic diagnoses affecting organ system recorded in crossbred dogs and popular breeds (number of dogs) from 3,884 randomly sampled dogs attending primary veterinary practices in England.

Organ system	Prevalence percentage (95% confidence interval)								P-Value
	Crossbred (797)	Labrador Retriever (339)	Staffordshire Bull Terrier (334)	Jack Russell Terrier (262)	Cocker Spaniel (133)	German Shepherd Dog (132)	Yorkshire Terrier (127)	Border Collie (104)	
Integument	31.4 (28.0–34.7)	39.2 (34.2–44.5)	36.2 (31.3–41.5)	34.0 (28.5–39.9)	33.8 (26.3–42.2)	34.8 (27.3–43.3)	42.5 (34.3–51.2)	29.8 (21.9–39.2)	0.816
Digestive	30.0 (26.6–33.3)	29.8 (25.2–34.9)	19.2 (15.3–23.7)	28.6 (23.5–34.4)	36.1 (28.4–44.5)	27.3 (20.4–35.4)	44.1 (35.8–52.8)	26.9 (19.3–36.2)	**0.002**
Musculoskeletal	17.3 (14.8–19.8)	19.2 (15.3–23.7)	9.6 (6.9–13.2)	9.5 (6.5–13.7)	6.8 (3.6–12.4)	18.9 (13.2–26.5)	8.7 (4.9–14.8)	22.1 (15.2–31.0)	**0.005**
Connective/ Soft tissue	12.3 (10.2–14.4)	16.2 (12.7–20.5)	9.9 (7.1–13.6)	9.5 (6.5–13.7)	14.3 (9.3–21.2)	5.3 (2.6–10.5)	9.4 (5.5–15.8)	17.3 (11.2–25.7)	0.060
Ocular	9.2 (7.2–11.1)	9.1 (6.5–12.7)	8.7 (6.1–12.2)	8.8 (5.9–12.8)	12.8 (8.1–19.5)	2.3 (0.8–6.5)	13.4 (8.5–20.4)	14.4 (8.9–22.4)	0.203
Auditory	7.4 (5.5–9.3)	12.4 (9.3–16.3)	11.1 (8.1–14.9)	8.4 (5.6–12.4)	10.5 (6.4–16.9)	11.4 (7.0–17.9)	7.9 (4.3–13.9)	5.8 (2.7–12.0)	1.000
Nervous	7.9 (6.2–9.6)	8.3 (5.8–11.7)	3.0 (1.6–5.4)	5.7 (3.5–9.2)	9.0 (5.2–15.1)	12.9 (8.2–19.7)	3.1 (1.2–7.8)	15.4 (9.7–23.5)	**0.003**
Respiratory	7.2 (5.2–9.1)	8.0 (5.5–11.3)	6.9 (4.6–10.1)	7.3 (4.7–11.0)	3.0 (1.2–7.5)	3.8 (1.6–8.6)	8.7 (4.9–14.8)	3.8 (1.5–9.5)	1.000
Cardiovascular	5.3 (3.5–7.1)	1.5 (0.6–3.4)	3.3 (1.8–5.8)	7.6 (5.0–11.5)	5.3 (2.6–10.5)	1.5 (0.4–5.4)	11.0 (6.7–17.7)	6.7 (3.3–13.2)	**0.001**
Urinary	5.8 (4.1–7.5)	5.3 (3.4–8.2)	3.6 (2.1–6.2)	4.6 (2.6–7.8)	6.8 (3.6–12.4)	4.5 (2.1–9.6)	6.3 (3.2–11.9)	6.7 (3.3–13.2)	1.000
Reproductive	4.9 (3.5–6.3)	2.7 (1.4–5.0)	6.0 (3.9–9.1)	5.0 (2.9–8.3)	5.3 (2.6–10.5)	2.3 (0.8–6.5)	3.9 (1.7–8.9)	1.0 (0.2–5.2)	1.000
Endocrine	2.1 (1.2–3.1)	1.5 (0.6–3.4)	1.2 (0.5–3.0)	2.3 (1.1–4.9)	0.0 (0.0–2.8)	0.8 (0.1–4.2)	2.4 (0.8–6.7)	1.9 (0.5–6.7)	1.000
Haematopoietic	1.3 (0.7–2.3)	2.1 (1.0–4.2)	1.2 (0.5–3.0)	0.4 (0.1–2.1)	1.5 (0.4–5.3)	1.5 (0.4–5.4)	0.0 (0.0–2.9)	0.0 (0.0–3.6)	1.000
Hepatobiliary	0.1 (0.0–0.7)	1.8 (0.8–3.8)	0.0 (0.0–1.1)	0.4 (0.1–2.1)	0.0 (0.0–2.8)	0.0 (0.0–2.8)	0.0 (0.0–2.9)	3.8 (1.5–9.5)	**0.004**
Lymphatic	0.9 (0.4–1.8)	0.6 (0.2–2.1)	0.6 (0.2–2.2)	0.4 (0.1–2.1)	0.8 (0.1–4.1)	0.0 (0.0–2.8)	0.0 (0.0–2.9)	1.0 (0.2–5.2)	1.000

P-values (Holm–adjusted) represent comparison between breeds.

Table 10. Prevalence of syndromic diagnoses relating to pathophysiologic processes recorded in crossbred and popular breeds (number of dogs) attending primary veterinary practices in England.

Pathophysiologic process	Prevalence percentage (95% confidence interval)								P-Value
	Crossbred (797)	Labrador Retriever (339)	Staffordshire Bull Terrier (334)	Jack Russell Terrier (262)	Cocker Spaniel (133)	German Shepherd Dog (132)	Yorkshire Terrier (127)	Border Collie (104)	
Inflammation	28.1 (25.1–31.2)	37.8 (32.8–43.0)	29.6 (25.0–34.7)	25.2 (20.3–30.8)	27.8 (20.9–36.0)	32.6 (25.2–41.0)	35.4 (27.7–44.1)	27.9 (20.2–37.2)	0.120
Mass/swelling	14.1 (11.8–16.3)	23.3 (19.1–28.1)	14.1 (10.7–18.2)	11.1 (7.8–15.4)	20.3 (14.3–27.9)	12.1 (7.6–18.8)	14.2 (9.2–21.3)	24.0 (16.8–33.1)	**0.004**
Traumatic	14.3 (11.6–17.0)	18.3 (14.5–22.8)	14.1 (10.7–18.2)	14.5 (10.8–19.3)	16.5 (11.2–23.8)	11.4 (7.0–17.9)	7.1 (3.8–12.9)	15.4 (9.7–23.5)	1.000
Degenerative	11.4 (9.1–13.8)	15.6 (12.2–19.9)	7.5 (5.1–10.8)	7.6 (5.0–11.5)	4.5 (2.1–9.5)	9.8 (5.8–16.1)	6.3 (3.2–11.9)	18.3 (12.0–26.8)	**0.001**
Infectious	9.0 (6.9–11.2)	13.9 (10.6–17.9)	7.8 (5.4–11.2)	8.0 (5.3–11.9)	9.0 (5.2–15.1)	10.6 (6.4–17.0)	7.9 (4.3–13.9)	13.5 (8.2–21.3)	0.990
Neoplastic	9.0 (7.2–10.9)	15.3 (11.9–19.6)	6.3 (4.1–9.4)	4.6 (2.6–7.8)	12.8 (8.1–19.5)	2.3 (0.8–6.5)	3.9 (1.7–8.9)	9.6 (5.3–16.8)	**0.003**
Congenital	7.3 (5.6–9.2)	5.0 (3.2–7.9)	4.8 (3.0–7.6)	6.5 (4.1–10.1)	7.5 (4.1–13.3)	6.1 (3.1–11.5)	11.0 (6.7–17.7)	5.8 (2.7–12)	1.000
Nutritional	5.9 (4.3–7.5)	16.5 (12.9–20.8)	7.5 (5.1–10.8)	6.9 (4.4–10.6)	9.8 (5.8–16.0)	3.8 (1.6–8.6)	2.4 (0.8–6.7)	9.6 (5.3–16.8)	**0.002**
Behavioural	7.9 (6.0–9.8)	5.0 (3.2–7.9)	6.6 (4.4–9.8)	8.8 (5.9–12.8)	6.8 (3.6–12.4)	13.6 (8.8–20.5)	3.9 (1.7–8.9)	8.7 (4.6–15.6)	0.400
Hereditary	5.3 (3.5–7.0)	4.4 (2.7–7.2)	3.3 (1.8–5.8)	3.4 (1.8–6.4)	3.0 (1.2–7.5)	7.6 (4.2–13.4)	11.8 (7.3–18.6)	2.9 (1.0–8.1)	**0.025**
Parasitic	6.7 (5.0–8.4)	6.2 (4.1–9.3)	5.7 (3.7–8.7)	5.0 (2.9–8.3)	9.8 (5.8–16.0)	3.0 (1.2–7.5)	5.5 (2.7–10.9)	2.9 (1.0–8.1)	1.000
Iatrogenic	4.4 (2.9–5.9)	4.4 (2.7–7.2)	3.0 (1.6–5.4)	4.2 (2.4–7.4)	3.8 (1.6–8.5)	4.5 (2.1–9.6)	4.7 (2.2–9.9)	4.8 (2.1–10.8)	1.000
Foreign body	2.8 (1.6–3.9)	3.2 (1.8–5.7)	1.2 (0.5–3.0)	2.7 (1.3–5.4)	2.3 (0.8–6.4)	2.3 (0.8–6.5)	0.0 (0.0–2.9)	3.8 (1.5–9.5)	1.000
Death	2.1 (1.2–3.1)	1.8 (0.8–3.8)	1.5 (0.6–3.5)	0.8 (0.2–2.7)	0.8 (0.1–4.1)	2.3 (0.8–6.5)	3.1 (1.2–7.8)	4.8 (2.1–10.8)	1.000
Intoxicative	1.1 (0.6–2.1)	1.5 (0.6–3.4)	0.9 (0.3–2.6)	1.5 (0.6–3.9)	0.8 (0.1–4.1)	0.0 (0.0–2.8)	1.6 (0.4–5.6)	1.0 (0.2–5.2)	1.000
Haemostatic	0.5 (0.2–1.3)	1.5 (0.6–3.4)	1.8 (0.8–3.9)	1.1 (0.4–3.3)	0.0 (0.0–2.8)	0.8 (0.1–4.2)	0.0 (0.0–2.9)	2.9 (1.0–8.1)	1.000
Immune–mediated	0.5 (0.2–1.3)	0.0 (0.0–1.1)	0.3 (0.1–1.7)	0.8 (0.2–2.7)	2.3 (0.8–6.4)	0.0 (0.0–2.8)	2.4 (0.8–6.7)	1.0 (0.2–5.2)	0.189
Allergic	0.9 (0.4–1.8)	2.1 (1.0–4.2)	0.6 (0.2–2.2)	0.8 (0.2–2.7)	0.8 (0.1–4.1)	0.8 (0.1–4.2)	1.6 (0.4–5.6)	0.0 (0.0–3.6)	1.000
Thermoregulatory	0.6 (0.3–1.5)	0.0 (0.0–1.1)	0.6 (0.2–2.2)	0.8 (0.2–2.7)	0.8 (0.1–4.1)	0.0 (0.0–2.8)	1.6 (0.4–5.6)	1.0 (0.2–5.2)	1.000
Metabolic	0.3 (0.1–0.9)	0.0 (0.0–1.1)	0.0 (0.0–1.1)	0.0 (0.0–1.4)	0.8 (0.1–4.1)	0.0 (0.0–2.8)	0.0 (0.0–2.9)	0.0 (0.0–3.6)	1.000
Effusion	0.0 (0.0–0.5)	0.0 (0.0–1.1)	0.0 (0.0–1.1)	0.0 (0.0–1.4)	0.0 (0.0–2.8)	0.0 (0.0–2.8)	0.0 (0.0–2.9)	0.0 (0.0–3.6)	1.000

P-values (Holm–adjusted) represent comparison between breeds.

studies [114,115]. Holm adjustments to P-values were used to constrain the number of false-positive findings resulting from interpretation of multiple comparisons [38,115,116]. The current study reported prevalence values but effective welfare prioritisation would additionally benefit from the generation of accurate data on disorder severity and duration [117].

Conclusion

This study describes the most frequently recorded disorders in dogs in England and provides a prevalence baseline against which to measure progress in canine health. The most prevalent disorders recorded in dogs attending primary-care veterinary practices in England were otitis externa, periodontal disease and anal sac impaction, and the most prevalent disorder groups were enteropathic, dermatological and musculoskeletal. The head-and-neck was the body location most frequently affected by the disorders recorded, the integument was the most prevalent organ system affected and inflammation was the most prevalent pathophysiologic process. The study identified some evidence that purebred dogs had higher disorder prevalence compared with crossbred dogs. Substantial variation was shown across breeds in

their prevalence of common disorders. These results suggest that breeding reforms should target commonly diagnosed complex disorders that are amenable to genetic improvement on a breed-by-breed basis for the greatest population impact. The prevalence information provided by this study fills a crucial data gap. Future studies of disorder severity and duration would augment the current results and contribute to increasingly effective strategies to improve dog welfare based on disorder prioritisation.

Acknowledgments

We thank Peter Dron (RVC) for VetCompass database development and Noel Kennedy (RVC) for software and programming development. We are especially grateful to the Medivet Veterinary Partnership and the other UK practices and clients who are participating in VetCompass.

Author Contributions

Conceived and designed the experiments: DON DBC PDM PCT DCB. Performed the experiments: DON DBC PDM PCT DCB. Analyzed the data: DON DBC PDM PCT DCB. Contributed reagents/materials/analysis tools: DON DBC PDM PCT DCB. Wrote the paper: DON DBC PDM PCT DCB.

References

1. Murray JK, Browne WJ, Roberts MA, Whitmarsh A, Gruffydd-Jones TJ (2010) Number and ownership profiles of cats and dogs in the UK. Veterinary Record 166: 163–168.

2. Asher L, Buckland E, Phylactopoulos CL, Whiting M, Abeyesinghe S, et al. (2011) Estimation of the number and demographics of companion dogs in the UK. BMC Veterinary Research 7: 74.

3. PFMA (2012) The Pet Food Manufacturers' Association 'Statistics'. In: Association TPFM, editor: The Pet Food Manufacturers' Association.

4. Ownby DR, Johnson C, Peterson EL (2002) Exposure to dogs and cats in the first year of life and risk of allergic sensitization at 6 to 7 years of age. Journal of the American Medical Association 288: 963–972.

5. Friedmann E, Son H (2009) The human–companion animal bond: how humans benefit. Veterinary Clinics of North America: Small Animal Practice 39: 293–326.

6. Virués-Ortega J, Buela-Casal G (2006) Psychophysiological effects of human-animal interaction: theoretical issues and long-term interaction effects. Journal of Nervous and Mental Disease 194: 52–57.

7. Walsh F (2009) Human-animal bonds I: the relational significance of companion animals. Family Process 48: 462–480.

8. McGreevy PD, Nicholas FW (1999) Some practical solutions to welfare problems in dog breeding. Animal Welfare 8: 329–341.

9. Rooney NJ (2009) The welfare of pedigree dogs: cause for concern. Journal of Veterinary Behavior: Clinical Applications and Research 4: 180–186.

10. Wayne RK, Leonard JA, Vila C (2006) Genetic analysis of dog domestication. In: Zeder MA, editor. Documenting domestication: new genetic and archaeological paradigms. Berkeley, California: University of California Press. pp. 279–293.

11. Leroy G (2011) Genetic diversity, inbreeding and breeding practices in dogs: results from pedigree analyses. The Veterinary Journal 189: 177–182.

12. McGreevy PD (2007) Breeding for quality of life. Animal Welfare 16: 125–128.

13. Calboli FC, Sampson J, Fretwell N, Balding DJ (2008) Population structure and inbreeding from pedigree analysis of purebred dogs. Genetics 179: 593–601.

14. Lewis TW (2010) Optimisation of breeding strategies to reduce the prevalence of inherited disease in pedigree dogs. Animal Welfare 19: 93–98.

15. Asher L, Diesel G, Summers JF, McGreevy PD, Collins LM (2009) Inherited defects in pedigree dogs. Part 1: disorders related to breed standards. The Veterinary Journal 182: 402–411.

16. Summers JF, Diesel G, Asher L, McGreevy PD, Collins LM (2010) Inherited defects in pedigree dogs. Part 2: Disorders that are not related to breed standards. The Veterinary Journal 183: 39–45.

17. Mellersh CS, Ostrander EA (1997) The canine genome. In: Dodds WJ, James EW, editors. Advances in Veterinary Medicine: Academic Press. pp. 191–216.

18. Starkey MP, Scase TJ, Mellersh CS, Murphy S (2005) Dogs really are man's best friend: canine genomics has applications in veterinary and human medicine! Briefings in Functional Genomics & Proteomics 4: 112–128.

19. BBC (2008) Pedigree Dogs Exposed.

20. Bateson P (2010) Independent inquiry into dog breeding. Cambridge: University of Cambridge.

21. Rooney N, Sargan D (2008) Pedigree dog breeding in the UK: a major welfare concern? Horsham, West Sussex: RSPCA.

22. APGAW (2009) A healthier future for pedigree dogs. London: The Associate Parliamentary Group for Animal Welfare.

23. Collins LM, Asher L, Summers J, McGreevy P (2011) Getting priorities straight: risk assessment and decision-making in the improvement of inherited disorders in pedigree dogs. The Veterinary Journal 189: 147–154.

24. Collins LM, Asher L, Summers JF, Diesel G, McGreevy PD (2010) Welfare epidemiology as a tool to assess the welfare impact of inherited defects on the pedigree dog population. Animal Welfare 19: 67–75.

25. Fleming JM, Creevy KE, Promislow DEL (2011) Mortality in North American dogs from 1984 to 2004: an investigation into age-, size-, and breed-related causes of death. Journal of Veterinary Internal Medicine 25: 187–198.

26. Adams VJ, Evans KM, Sampson J, Wood JLN (2010) Methods and mortality results of a health survey of purebred dogs in the UK. Journal of Small Animal Practice 51: 512–524.

27. Egenvall A, Nødtvedt A, Penell J, Gunnarsson L, Bonnett BN (2009) Insurance data for research in companion animals: benefits and limitations. Acta Veterinaria Scandinavica 51: 42.

28. VetCompass (2013) VetCompass: Health surveillance for UK companion animals. http://wwwrvcacuk/VetCompass. London: RVC Electronic Media Unit.

29. Medivet (2014) Medivet: the veterinary partnership. Medivet Partnership LLP.

30. The VeNom Coding Group (2013) VeNom Veterinary Nomenclature. In: Group TVC, editor. http://wwwvenomcodingorg: VeNom Coding Group.

31. Kearsley-Fleet L, O'Neill DG, Volk HA, Church DB, Brodbelt DC (2013) Prevalence and risk factors for canine epilepsy of unknown origin in the UK. Veterinary Record 172: 338.

32. Epi Info 7 CDC (2012) Centers for Disease Control and Prevention (US): Introducing Epi Info 7. http://wwwncdcgov/epiinfo/7. Atlanta, Georgia: CDC.

33. Willard MD, Tvedten H (2004) Small animal clinical diagnosis by laboratory methods. St. Louis, Miss.: Saunders.

34. Sleator DD, Endre Tarjan R (1983) A data structure for dynamic trees. Journal of Computer and System Sciences 26: 362–391.

35. Irion DN, Schaffer AL, Famula TR, Eggleston ML, Hughes SS, et al. (2003) Analysis of genetic variation in 28 dog breed populations with 100 microsatellite markers. Journal of Heredity 94: 81–87.

36. The Kennel Club (2012) Kennel Club's Breed Information Centre. In: Club TK, editor. http://wwwthe-kennel-cluborguk/services/public/breed/Defaultaspx. London: The Kennel Club.

37. McMillan FD (2001) Rethinking euthanasia: death as an unintentional outcome. Journal of the American Veterinary Medical Association 219: 1204–1206.

38. Aickin M, Gensler H (1996) Adjusting for multiple testing when reporting research results: the Bonferroni vs Holm methods. American Journal of Public Health 86: 726–728.

39. Kirkwood BR, Sterne JAC (2003) Essential Medical Statistics. Oxford: Blackwell Science.

40. Agresti A, Coull BA (1998) Approximate is better than "exact" for interval estimation of binomial proportions. The American Statistician 52: 119–126.

41. Hein HE (1963) Abnormalities and defects in pedigree dogs-II. Hereditary aspects of hip dysplasia. Journal of Small Animal Practice 4: 457–462.

42. Hodgman SFJ (1963) Abnormalities and defects in pedigree dogs-I. An investigation into the existence of abnormalities in pedigree dogs in the British Isles. Journal of Small Animal Practice 4: 447–456.

43. Knight GC (1963) Abnormalities and defects in pedigree dogs—III. Tibio-femoral joint deformity and patella luxation. Journal of Small Animal Practice 4: 463-464.

44. Willis MB (1963) Abnormalities and defects in pedigree dogs—V. Cryptorchidism. Journal of Small Animal Practice 4: 469-474.

45. BVA/KC (2013) Hip Dysplasia Scheme. In: British Veterinary Association/Kennel Club, editor. London: British Veterinary Association,.

46. BVA/KC (2013) Chiari Malformation/Syringomyelia Scheme (CM/SM Scheme). In: Club BVAK, editor. London: British Veterinary Association.

47. BVA/KC (2013) Elbow Scheme. London: British Veterinary Association.

48. BVA/KC/ISS (2013) Eye Scheme. In: Society BVAKCIS, editor. Loondon: British Veterinary Association,.

49. KC (2013) DNA Screening Schemes and Results. In: The Kennel Club, editor. London: The Kennel Club,.

50. Indrebo A (2007) Animal welfare in modern dog breeding. Acta Veterinaria Scandinavica 50 Supplement S6.

51. Froom P, Froom J (1992) Selection bias in using data from one population to another: common pitfalls in the interpretation of medical literature. Theoretical Medicine 13: 255-259.

52. Bartlett PC, Van Buren JW, Neterer M, Zhou C (2010) Disease surveillance and referral bias in the veterinary medical database. Preventive Veterinary Medicine 94: 264-271.

53. Soll-Johanning H, Hannerz H, Tüchsen F (2004) Referral bias in hospital register studies of geographical and industrial differences in health. Danish Medical Bulletin 51: 207-210.

54. KC (2013) The Kennel Club. London: The Kennel Club,.

55. Platt S, Freeman J, di Stefani A, Wieczorek L, Henley W (2006) Prevalence of unilateral and bilateral deafness in Border Collies and association with phenotype. Journal of Veterinary Internal Medicine 20: 1355-1362.

56. Powers MY, Karbe GT, Gregor TP, McKelvie P, Culp WTN, et al. (2010) Evaluation of the relationship between Orthopedic Foundation for Animals' hip joint scores and PennHIP distraction index values in dogs. Journal of the American Veterinary Medical Association 237: 532-541.

57. Slater MR, Scarlet JM, Donoghue S, Erb HN (1992) The repeatability and validity of a telephone questionnaire on diet and exercise in dogs. Preventive Veterinary Medicine 13: 77-91.

58. Pearce N, Checkoway H, Kriebel D (2007) Bias in occupational epidemiology studies. Occupational and Environmental Medicine 64: 562-568.

59. Gobar GM (1998) Program for surveillance of causes of death of dogs, using the Internet to survey small animal veterinarians. Journal of the American Veterinary Medical Association 213: 251-256.

60. Hudson JI, Pope HG, Glynn RJ (2005) The cross-sectional cohort study: an underutilized design. Epidemiology (Cambridge, Mass) 16: 355-359.

61. Dohoo I, Martin W, Stryhn H (2009) Veterinary Epidemiologic Research. Charlottetown, Canada: VER Inc.

62. Aragon CL, Budsberg SC (2005) Applications of evidence-based medicine: cranial cruciate ligament injury repair in the dog. Veterinary Surgery 34: 93-98.

63. John U, Rumpf H-J, Hapke U (1999) Estimating prevalence of alcohol abuse and dependence in one general hospital: an approach to reduce sample selection bias. Alcohol and Alcoholism 34: 786-794.

64. Chodick G, Freedman MD, Kwok RK, Fears TR, Linet MS, et al. (2007) Agreement between contemporaneously recorded and subsequently recorded time spent outdoors: implications for environmental exposure studies. Annals of Epidemiology 17: 106-111.

65. Edney ATB (1997) An observational study of presentation patterns in companion animal veterinary practices in England. London: University of London. 290 p.

66. Lund EM (1997) Development and evaluation of a model for diagnostic surveillance in companion animal practice. St Paul: University of Minnesota.

67. Glickman L, Glickman N (2012) The National Companion Animal Surveillance System NCASP. Purdue University.

68. Brady S, Norris JM, Kelman M, Ward MP (2012) Canine parvovirus in Australia: the role of socio-economic factors in disease clusters. The Veterinary Journal 193: 522-528.

69. Egenvall A, Bonnett BN, Olson P, Hedhammar Å (1998) Validation of computerized Swedish dog and cat insurance data against veterinary practice records. Preventive Veterinary Medicine 36: 51-65.

70. Lund EM, Armstrong PJ, Kirk CA, Kolar LM, Klausner JS (1999) Health status and population characteristics of dogs and cats examined at private veterinary practices in the United States. Journal of the American Veterinary Medical Association 214: 1336-1341.

71. Rust MK (2005) Advances in the control of Ctenocephalides felis (cat flea) on cats and dogs. Trends in Parasitology 21: 232-236.

72. NOAH (2013) Facts and Figures About the UK Animal Medicines Industry. In: National Office of Animal Health, editor: NOAH,.

73. Royston P, Altman DG, Sauerbrei W (2006) Dichotomizing continuous predictors in multiple regression: a bad idea. Statistics in Medicine 25: 127-141.

74. Mandl KD, Overhage JM, Wagner MM, Lober WB, Sebastiani P, et al. (2004) Implementing syndromic surveillance: a practical guide informed by the early experience. Journal of the American Medical Informatics Association 11: 141-150.

75. Dank G, Segev G, Moshe D, Kent MS (2012) Follow-up study comparing necropsy rates and discrepancies between clinical and pathologic diagnoses at a veterinary teaching hospital: 2009 versus 1989 and 1999. Journal of Small Animal Practice 53: 679-683.

76. Lober WB, Thomas Karras B, Wagner MM, Marc Overhage J, Davidson AJ, et al. (2002) Roundtable on bioterrorism detection: information system-based surveillance. Journal of the American Medical Informatics Association 9: 105-115.

77. Egenvall A, Hedhammar A, Bonnett BN, Olson P (2000) Gender, age and breed pattern of diagnoses for veterinary care in insured dogs in Sweden during 1996. Veterinary Record 146: 551-557.

78. Vilson Å, Bonnett B, Hansson-Hamlin H, Hedhammar Å (2013) Disease patterns in 32,486 insured German Shepherd Dogs in Sweden: 1995-2006. Veterinary Record 173: 116.

79. Bonnett BN, Egenvall A, Hedhammar Å, Olson P (2005) Mortality in over 350,000 insured Swedish dogs from 1995-2000: I. breed-, gender-, age- and cause-specific rates. Acta Veterinaria Scandinavica 46: 105-120.

80. Stone AB, Hautala JA (2008) Meeting Report: Panel on the potential utility and strategies for design and implementation of a National Companion Animal Infectious Disease Surveillance System. Zoonoses and Public Health 55: 378-384.

81. Neff MW, Rine J (2006) A fetching model organism. Cell 124: 229-231.

82. Packer RMA, Hendricks A, Burn CC (2012) Do dog owners perceive the clinical signs related to conformational inherited disorders as 'normal' for the breed? A potential constraint to improving canine welfare. Animal Welfare 21: 81-93.

83. Egenvall A, Bonnett BN, Olson P, Hedhammar Å (2000) Gender, age, breed and distribution of morbidity and mortality in insured dogs in Sweden during 1995 and 1996. Veterinary Record 146: 519-525.

84. Medzhitov R (2010) Inflammation 2010: new adventures of an old flame. Cell 140: 771-776.

85. Mountziaris PM, Spicer PP, Kasper FK, Mikos AG (2011) Harnessing and modulating inflammation in strategies for bone regeneration. Tissue Engineering Part B, Reviews 17: 393-402.

86. Rooney NJ, Sargan DR (2010) Welfare concerns associated with pedigree dog breeding in the UK. Animal Welfare 19: 133-140.

87. Crispin S (2011) Tackling the welfare issues of dog breeding. Veterinary Record 168: 53.

88. Anon (2009) Balancing pedigree dog breed standards and animal welfare - is it possible? Veterinary Record 164: 481-482.

89. Bell J. The clinical truths about pure breeds, mixed breeds, and designer breeds; 2012 Feb 19-23; Las Vegas. 22-23.

90. Page GP, George V, Go RC, Page PZ, Allison DB (2003) "Are we there yet?": Deciding when one has demonstrated specific genetic causation in complex diseases and quantitative traits. The American Journal of Human Genetics 73: 711-719.

91. Marsella R, Girolomoni G (2009) Canine models of atopic dermatitis: a useful tool with untapped potential. The Journal of Investigative Dermatology 129: 2351-2357.

92. Albuquerque C, Morinha F, Requicha J, Martins T, Dias I, et al. (2012) Canine periodontitis: the dog as an important model for periodontal studies. The Veterinary Journal 191: 299-305.

93. Scott DW, Miller WH, Griffin CE, Muller GH (2001) Muller & Kirk's Small Animal Dermatology. Philadelphia: Saunders.

94. Neuber A (2009) Nail diseases in dogs. Companion Animal 14: 56-62.

95. Smith FJD (2003) The molecular genetics of keratin disorders. American Journal of Clinical Dermatology 4: 347-364.

96. Lewis T, Blott S, Woolliams J (2013) Comparative analyses of genetic trends and prospects for selection against hip and elbow dysplasia in 15 UK dog breeds. BMC Genetics 14: 16.

97. German AJ, Hall EJ, Day MJ (2003) Chronic intestinal inflammation and intestinal disease in dogs. Journal of Veterinary Internal Medicine 17: 8-20.

98. Kathrani A, Werling D, Allenspach K (2011) Canine breeds at high risk of developing inflammatory bowel disease in the south-eastern UK. Veterinary Record 169: 635.

99. German AJ (2006) The growing problem of obesity in dogs and cats. The Journal of Nutrition 136: 1940S-1946S.

100. Houlton JE (2008) A survey of gundog lameness and injuries in Great Britain in the shooting seasons 2005/2006 and 2006/2007. Veterinary and comparative Orthopaedics and Traumatology 21: 231-237.

101. Lourenço-Martins AM, Delgado E, Neto I, Peleteiro MC, Morais-Almeida M, et al. (2011) Allergic conjunctivitis and conjunctival provocation tests in atopic dogs. Veterinary Ophthalmology 14: 248-256.

102. Batt RM, Hall EJ (1989) Chronic enteropathies in the dog. Journal of Small Animal Practice 30: 3-12.

103. Pedersen HD, Häggström J (2000) Mitral valve prolapse in the dog: a model of mitral valve prolapse in man. Cardiovascular Research 47: 234-243.

104. Lewis T (2011) Heritability of premature mitral valve disease in Cavalier King Charles Spaniels. The Veterinary Journal 188: 73.

105. Bellumori TP, Famula TR, Bannasch DL, Belanger JM, Oberbauer AM (2013) Prevalence of inherited disorders among mixed-breed and purebred dogs: 27,254 cases (1995-2010). Journal of the American Veterinary Medical Association 242: 1549-1555.

106. Rand JS, Fleeman LM, Farrow HA, Appleton DJ, Lederer R (2004) Canine and feline diabetes mellitus: nature or nurture? The Journal of Nutrition 134: 2072S–2080S.

107. Wood JLN (2002) Heritability and epidemiology of canine hip-dysplasia score and its components in Labrador retrievers in the United Kingdom. Preventive Veterinary Medicine 55: 95–108.

108. Hillier A, Griffin CE (2001) The ACVD task force on canine atopic dermatitis (I): incidence and prevalence. Veterinary Immunology and Immunopathology 81: 147–151.

109. Mellersh C (2012) DNA testing and domestic dogs. Mammalian Genome 23: 109–123.

110. Lewis TW (2010) Genetic evaluation of hip score in UK Labrador Retrievers. PLoS One 5.

111. Wilson B, Nicholas FW, Thomson PC (2011) Selection against canine hip dysplasia: success or failure? The Veterinary Journal 189: 160–168.

112. Gough A, Thomas A (2010) Breed Predispositions to Disease in Dogs and Cats. Chicester, West Sussex: Wiley-Blackwell.

113. Anon. (2013) High profile best of breed winners pass vet checks at Crufts. Veterinary Record 172: 277.

114. Bender R, Lange S (2001) Adjusting for multiple testing - when and how? Journal of Clinical Epidemiology 54: 343–349.

115. Greenland S (2008) Multiple comparisons and association selection in general epidemiology. International Journal of Epidemiology 37: 430–434.

116. Feise R (2002) Do multiple outcome measures require p-value adjustment? BMC Medical Research Methodology 2: 8.

117. CAWC (2006) Breeding and welfare in companion animals: welfare aspects of modifications, through selective breeding or biotechnological methods, to the form, function, or behaviour of companion animals. Sidmouth, Devon: Companion Animal Welfare Council.

20

Student Attainment of Proficiency in a Clinical Skill: The Assessment of Individual Learning Curves

Robert D. Campbell[1¤], Kent G. Hecker[2], David J. Biau[3], Daniel S. J. Pang[2,4]*

1 Calgary Animal Referral and Emergency Centre, Calgary, Alberta and the Faculty of Veterinary Medicine, University of Calgary, Calgary, Alberta, Canada, **2** Veterinary Clinical and Diagnostic Sciences, Faculty of Veterinary Medicine, University of Calgary, Calgary, Alberta, Canada, **3** Département de Biostatistique et Informatique Médicale, Hôpital Saint-Louis, AP-HP Paris, France, **4** Hotchkiss Brain Institute, University of Calgary, Calgary, Alberta, Canada

Abstract

The aims of this study were to determine if the learning curve cumulative summation test (LC-CUSUM) can differentiate proficiency in placing intravenous catheters by novice learners, and identify the cause of failure when it occurred. In a prospective, observational study design 6 undergraduate students with no previous experience of placing intravenous catheters received standardized training by a board certified veterinary anesthesiologist in intravenous catheter placement technique. Immediately following training, each student attempted 60 intravenous catheterizations in a dog mannequin thoracic limb model. Results were scored as a success or failure based upon completion of four specific criteria, and where catheter placement failure occurred, the cause was recorded according to pre-defined criteria. Initial acceptable and unacceptable failure rates were set by the study team and the LC-CUSUM was used to generate a learning curve for each student. Using 10% and 25% acceptable and unacceptable failure rates, 3 out of 6 students attained proficiency, requiring between 26 to 48 attempts. Applying 25% and 50% acceptable and unacceptable failure rates, 5 of 6 students obtained proficiency, requiring between 18 and 55 attempts. Wide inter-individual variability was observed and the majority of failed catheterisation attempts were limited to two of the four pre-defined criteria. These data indicate that the LC-CUSUM can be used to generate individual learning curves, inter-individual variability in catheter placement ability is wide, and that specific steps in catheter placement are responsible for the majority of failures. These findings may have profound implications for how we teach and assess technical skills.

Editor: Pascal Launois, World Health Organization, Switzerland

Funding: Funding for this study was provided by the Veterinary Education Research Fund of the Faculty of Veterinary Medicine, University of Calgary. The funders had no role in study design, data collection and analysis, decision to publish, or preparation of the manuscript.

Competing Interests: The authors have declared that no competing interests exist.

* E-mail: dsjpang@ucalgary.ca

¤ Current address: Cornell University Hospital for Animals, Ithaca, New York, United States of America

Introduction

Attainment of proficiency in a technical skill, such as intravenous (IV) catheterization, is often based on an arbitrary distinction such as experience, or instructor observation of one or more successful attempts. Evidence suggests there is wide variation between individual attainment of proficiency in a technical skill. [1,2] The concept of quantitatively assessing proficiency in clinical skills for individual students is relatively new to the health professions and has garnered recent prominence in human medicine as a result infamous cases such as increased mortality rates following cardiac surgery [3–5].

Statistical process control charts, originally designed for use in the manufacturing industry to assess production processes have recently been adapted to quantitatively assess attainment and maintenance of proficiency in medicine, particularly in surgery and anesthesia. [1,6,7] The cumulative summation (CUSUM) method tests the hypothesis that a process (e.g. surgical performance in cardiac surgery) is deviating from a target of adequate performance (process is out of control), or that a process remains within an acceptable limit (process is in control). [8] If a process is deemed to be 'out of control', an intervention takes place, such as a period of re-training. The limitation of this technique during an

initial period of learning is that the learner will be frequently assessed as out of control due to poor performance, triggering an unacceptable failure rate. Biau and Porcher modified the CUSUM test to provide monitoring and assessment of when a process reaches an in control state, creating the LC-CUSUM (the cumulative summation test for learning curve). This approach considers that a process is out of control initially (as a result of initial trainee performance), and indicates when the process is in control (adequate trainee performance achieved). [9].

Training and assessing veterinary students to an acceptable level of proficiency in clinical skills, such as venous catheterization, and decisions regarding exposure to practical classes (with mannequins, simulators or live animals) should be based on evidence. This is particularly important as the use of in vivo models for teaching purposes must be defensible, in keeping with the principles of the 3 Rs (replacement, reduction, refinement) of animal use. [10,11] Furthering our understanding of the learning curve would allow an optimal use of training resources, thereby reducing associated costs. To use IV catheterization as an example, the choice of training tool (live animal versus model) could be guided by the principle of the right tool at the right time: a low fidelity model may be adequate for understanding the basic steps of IV catheter placement while a high fidelity simulator or live animals may only be necessary when attempting to create a clinical scenario.

For the first time in veterinary medicine the LC-CUSUM test was applied to evaluate whether proficiency in placing intravenous (IV) catheters could be achieved by subjects with no previous experience with this skill.

Materials and Methods

This research project received ethics approval from the University of Calgary Conjoint Health Research Ethics Board (E-24326). All participants provided informed signed consent.

Six undergraduate students (from the Bachelor of Health Sciences program at the University of Calgary) participated in the study. Exclusion criteria included previous experience observing or performing IV catheter placement in any species. Students were required to perform 60 IV catheter attempts in a dog forelimb mannequin (K9 IV Trainer, Rescue Critters, Van Nuys, CA, USA). The artificial veins were filled with artificial blood maintained at a pressure of approximately 100 mmHg. This was achieved by placing the fluid bag in an inflatable pressure sac. All students used the same model of IV catheter (PROTECTIV ® 20G 1.25″, Smiths Medical, Markham, ON, Canada). Prior to proceeding with the experiment students were instructed individually by a board- certified anesthesiologist (DP) using a standardized series of instructions. Testing was video-recorded to allow for retrospective analysis and ensure uniformity of grading between examiners. Students were assigned a binary score for each attempt (0 = failure, 1 = success), which were used to generate a learning curve. The scorers did not provide students with any feedback during the simulations.

To be deemed successful each student was required to (Figure 1):

1. Pierce the skin with the catheter and stylet at a 20–40 degree angle (relative to long axis of mannequin limb)
2. Advance the catheter and stylet into the vein (confirmed by observation of a "flash" of blood in the catheter hub).
3. Reduce the angle of the catheter and stylet and advance them 1–2 mm further to ensure placement in the vein before advancing the catheter in to the vein while holding the stylet in place.
4. Observe blood flow from the catheter hub

Participants who did not complete all of these components were scored as a failure. An additional sub-score was recorded reflecting at which point of the 4 steps failed catheterization attempts occurred. Students were not provided a time limit for the simulation, but were required to take a 1-minute break after every 3 attempts.

The LC-CUSUM sequentially tests, after each procedure, the null hypothesis that performance is inadequate. A score is computed from successive procedures with successes yielding an increase in the score and failures yielding a decrease. [9] Once the score reaches a predefined value (h, the in-control limit), the null hypothesis is rejected and performance is considered adequate. The in-control limit, which defines when proficiency is achieved, is based on numerical simulations of the probability of early detection of proficiency (see Marshall et al. and Biau and Porcher for statistical review). [9,12] Graphically, the LC-CUSUM score is displayed on the y-axis and procedure number on the x-axis. Performance of the trainee is considered to be unacceptable as long as the score remains below the in-control limit, h. The trainee is considered proficient when the in-control limit line is reached. A

holding barrier at y = 0 ensures that a student's learning curve will not suffer unduly (become negative) for poor previous performance, thereby allowing the test to remain responsive to present performance.

Defining adequate and inadequate performance should be based on expert consensus or existing specialty college guidelines; such guidelines do not exist in veterinary medicine. Because these parameters control the weighting allocated to failure or success at a task, adequate and inadequate performance should be set according to context i.e. the level of experience/training of the population being studied. In this study the acceptable and unacceptable failure rates were initially assigned after consultation with a board certified anesthesiologist (DP) with experience of training undergraduate and postgraduate trainees.

For the present study, the adequate performance level was initially set at 10% failure, inadequate performance at 25% failure, and the acceptable deviation from adequate performance was 5%. An in-control limit, h = 0.95, was chosen to give a true discovery rate (probability of declaring competency if the trainee's true performance is adequate; true alarm, akin to power) of 87% and a false discovery rate (probability of declaring competency if the trainee's false performance is inadequate; false alarm, akin to type I error) of 14% over 60 procedures. Adequate and inadequate performance, and acceptable deviation criteria were then adjusted to be more lenient (25%, 50%, and 10% respectively) to assess when (or if) more students achieved proficiency. In this case, a limit h = 1.15 was chosen to give a true discovery rate of 94% and a false discovery rate of 10% over 60 procedures.

Results

Figure 2 presents the results comparing student proficiency based upon the two sets of acceptable and unacceptable failure rates. With acceptable and unacceptable failure rates of 10 and 25% (Figure 2A) respectively, 3 out of 6 students achieved proficiency. The number of attempts required to achieve proficiency (reach the in-control limit line) were 26, 32 and 48. Three students did not achieve proficiency within 60 attempts. Lowering the standard for acceptable and unacceptable failure rates to 25 and 50% respectively resulted in 5 of 6 students attaining proficiency (Figure 2B). Considerable inter-individual variability was reflected in the number of attempts required to attain proficiency, varying from 18 to 55 (Figure 2B).

Examination of the point of failure for individual students (Table 1), reveals that the overwhelming majority (95.7%) of failed catheterizations occurred during steps 2 and 3 of the 4-step procedure. Of these, 57 (39.8%) were accounted for by step 2, and 80 (55.9%) accounted for by step 3.

Discussion

Clinical proficiency has historically been determined by utilizing subjective criteria; for example, after an arbitrary number of procedural attempts, or after a certain amount of time has passed with assumed proficiency (Rush et al, 2011). [13] Assuming proficiency based on generalized criteria does not take into account inter-individual variability in learning, nor does it provide for continued assessment of maintained proficiency over time. Recent research in human anesthesia has shown that achieving clinical proficiency varies widely from individual to individual (de Oliveira Filho, 2002; Naik et al, 2003; Konrad et al, 1999). [1,2,14] de Oliveira Filho (2002) reported successful endotracheal intubation ranges from 9 to 88 (43±33.49, mean ± SD) attempts in novice anesthesia residents. [1] Another study reported wide individual variation in first year anesthesia residents achieving

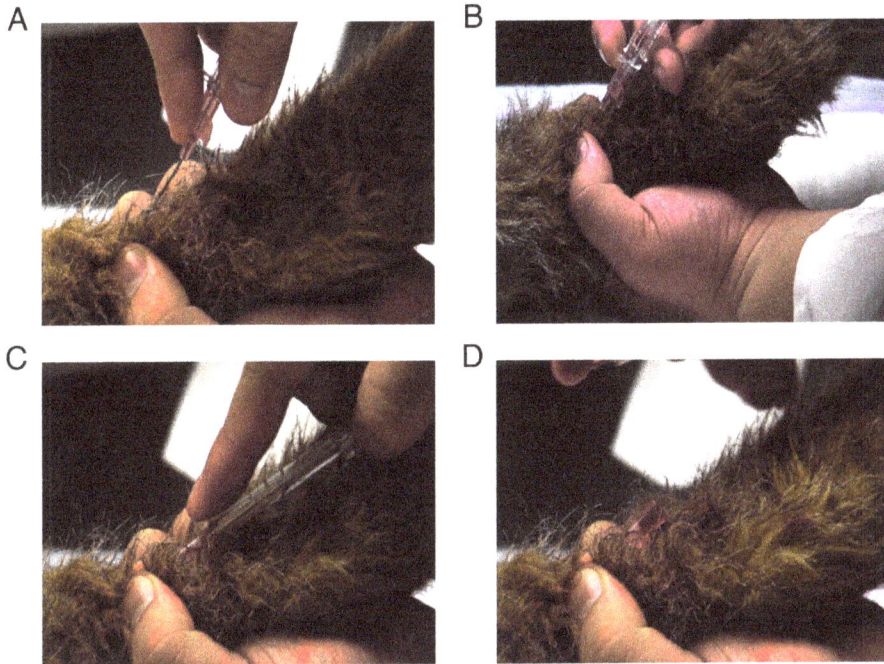

Figure 1. Video stills showing key steps in the successful catheter placement being implemented in the canine IV training model. A: Piercing the skin with the catheter and stylet at a 20–40 degree angle (relative to long axis of mannequin limb) B: Advancing the catheter and stylet into the vein (confirmed by observation of a "flash" of blood in the catheter hub). C: Reducing the angle of the catheter and stylet and advancing them 1–2 mm further to ensure placement in the vein before advancing the catheter in to the vein while holding the stylet in place. D: Observing blood flow from the catheter hub.

clinical proficiency in epidural anesthesia (ranging from 1 to 85 attempts, with one resident failing to achieve proficiency after 75 attempts). [2] We have identified large inter-individual variation in achieving proficiency in IV catheter placement, demonstrating the need for increased scrutiny in candidate performance in veterinary medicine, and reform of current training paradigms.

The LC-CUSUM has been previously employed successfully to evaluate achievement of clinical proficiency in human medicine. [15,16] Definition of acceptable and unacceptable failure rates are crucial to successful utilization of LC-CUSUM, and are typically set by experts in a given field (for example; board certified anesthesiologists for anesthesia procedures). Despite the use of expert consensus there is potential for bias when setting these values, and if criteria are set too strictly achievement of proficiency may be delayed (or in some cases, never achieved by an individual), hence the importance of establishing success and failure rates appropriate to the candidates' level of training. Ideally bias is decreased by setting acceptable and unacceptable failure rates according to empirical data rather than opinion; empirical training data does not currently exist in veterinary medicine. In this study, when stricter acceptable and unacceptable failure rates were set (10% and 25% respectively, and acceptable deviation from adequate performance of 5%) 3 out of the 6 students failed to achieve proficiency over 60 attempts, and of those who did achieve proficiency it took between 26 and 48 attempts. Changing the threshold for proficiency (changing the acceptable and unacceptable failure rates to 25% and 50% respectively, and acceptable deviation to 10%) affects the number of students attaining proficiency as expected, however wide inter-individual variability remained. These data indicate that traditional methods for assessing proficiency, typically after an arbitrary number of

attempts, or time in training, may not adequately cater for individual variation in learning.

These data provide two important pieces of information, the steps associated with impeding the learning curve in a group of naïve students, and the benefit of tracking performance at an individual level.

Examination of the causes of failed catheter placements (Figures 1 and 2), there are multiple sources: 1. Each step of catheter placement must be completed successfully to allow progression to the next step. For example, completion of step 3 is necessary to advance to step 4. There were no failures occurring at step 4 (Table 1), indicating that the critical steps occur earlier in the sequence. Furthermore this indicates that while evaluation of step 4 alone would reflect successful catheter placement, it will not allow identification of the source of failed attempts. In this study, failed attempts occurred primarily at steps 2 and 3. 2. There were a low number (6) of attempts failing at step 1, indicating that this is not a critical step though it is possible that the orientation of the catheter with respect to the long axis of the vein contributed to failures at step 2. Catheter orientation was not evaluated in this study. 3. Additional factors potentially contributing to failure at step 2 include the speed of catheter and stylet advancement and the ability of candidates to identify penetration of the vein from the sensation of advancing the catheter. 4. Successful completion of step 3 requires three distinct steps (reducing the angle of insertion, advancing the catheter and stylet a 1–2 mm further, and threading the catheter in to the vein) which may explain the greater failure rate. 5. Achievement of proficiency (attaining the in-control limit line) is reflected not simply by having a lesser number of total failure rates, but also the number of successive failures. Taking the student represented by the solid black line as an example (Figure 2A), the student approaches the in-control limit following

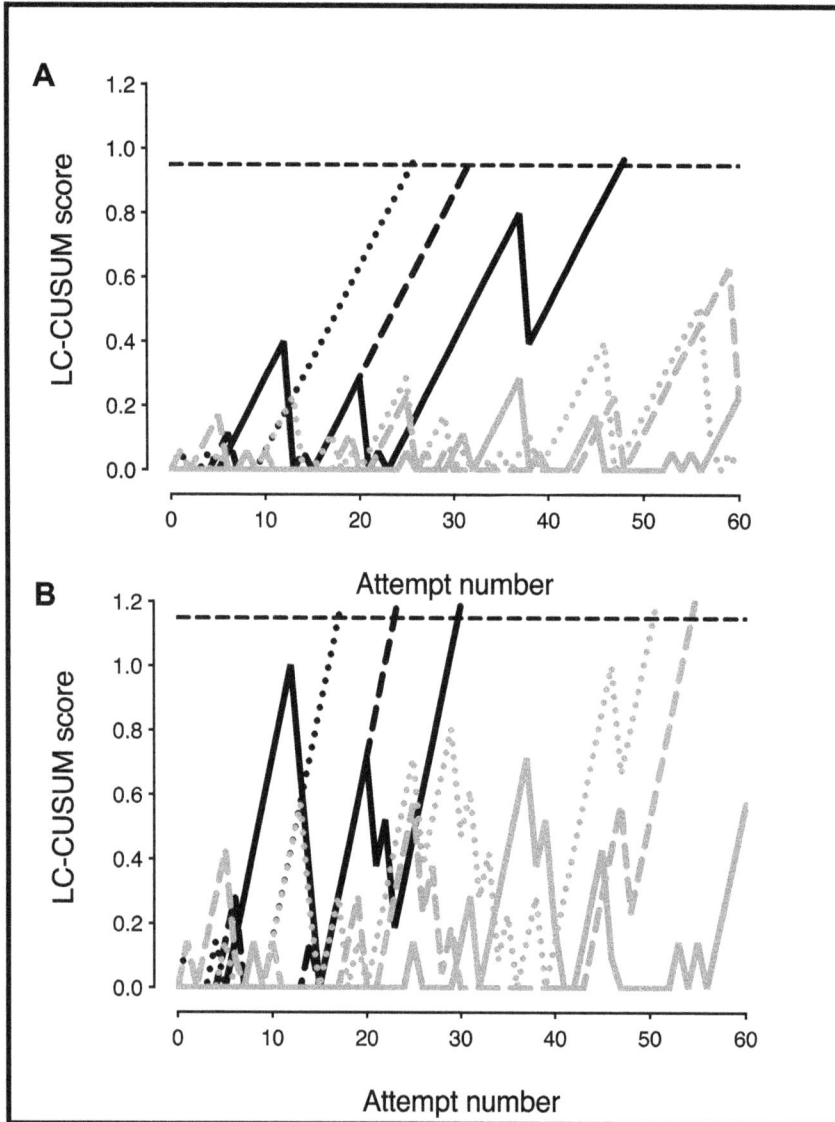

Figure 2. A, LC-CUSUM plot. Horizontal dashed line represents the in-control limit, the threshold for achieving proficiency. Lines represent individual student learning curves. Three students achieved proficiency within 60 attempts as depicted by transection of the in-control limit. Two students did not. Acceptable and unacceptable failure rates were set at 10% and 25%, respectively. N = 6 students. B, Same raw data as in 2A, but acceptable and unacceptable failure rates were set at 25% and 50%, respectively. This change in performance levels results in students attaining proficiency sooner, and two additional students attain proficiency. The in-control limit (horizontal dashed line) changes with a change in performance levels in order to control Type 1 and II errors. Student 1 (—), student 2 (---), student 3 (---), student 4 (....), student 5 (—), student 6 (....).

Table 1. Total number of unsuccessful catheter placement attempts per student, categorised according to observable criteria.

Criteria	Student 1	Student 2	Student 3	Student 4	Student 5	Student 6
Pierce skin with catheter at 20–40°	0	0	0	1	5	0
Advance catheter and stylet – observe flash of blood	0	6	3	17	24	7
Thread catheter off stylet	10	15	29	4	12	10
Observe blood flow	0	0	0	0	0	0

See text for full description of criteria.

a run of successful catheter placements. However, one failed attempt results in a descent of the learning curve towards zero, requiring a further run of 10 consecutive successes to achieve proficiency.

The performance tracking of individual students allows identification of areas needing further training or practice, or both. For example, student 4 (Table 1) is relatively successful in step 3, with only 4 unsuccessful attempts as a result of failure to thread the catheter in to the vein, but recorded the second highest failure rate at step 2. This contrasts with student 3, where the opposite is apparent, with the second lowest incidence of failures at step 2, but the highest number of failures at step 3. This information could be used to supported targeted training, allowing students and trainers to focus on key areas.

Our results indicate that LC-CUSUM can be used to generate individual learning curves for a technical skill in veterinary medicine and the technique is simple to implement, providing an individualized approach to learning. The results provide further evidence of performance variation by student within task reinforcing the need for learner specific feedback in order to achieve proficiency. In other words, the LC-CUSUM provides instructors and learners specific information which can be used to complement more traditional evaluations of skill performance, such as number of times skill has been performed and duration of time on task. Once students are deemed proficient, CUSUM can

be applied to analyze the maintenance of proficiency over time. By increasing the number of students in the experiment, we hope to generate individualized learning curves that can be trended and extrapolated to populations of students to better design teaching methodologies. LC-CUSUM provides data (rather then speculation) that may facilitate guidelines on acceptable levels of proficiency for students at different levels of training and application of the LC-CUSUM derived data may allow for evaluation of teaching techniques (computer simulated learning vs. lectures vs. mannequin models vs live models etc.) in terms of their educational merit in contributing to skilled practitioners.

Acknowledgments

Thank you to Dr. Gemai Chen for useful discussions, Dr. Valerie Madden for assistance with data collection, Michelle Hasiuk for assistance with video analysis, and to the six volunteer students from the BHSc programme. Intravenous catheters (PROTECTIV ® 20G 1.25″) kindly donated by Anna Rae of Smiths Medical.

Author Contributions

Conceived and designed the experiments: DSP KGH DJB. Performed the experiments: RDC DSP KGH. Analyzed the data: DJB DSP. Contributed reagents/materials/analysis tools: DSP KGH DJB. Wrote the paper: DSP KGH DJB RDC.

References

1. de Oliveira Filho GR (2002) The construction of learning curves for basic skills in anesthetic procedures: an application for the cumulative sum method. Anesth Analg 95: 411–416.
2. Naik VN, Devito I, Halpern SH (2003) Cusum analysis is a useful tool to assess resident proficiency at insertion of labour epidurals. Can J Anaesth 50: 694–698.
3. de Leval MR, Francois K, Bull C, Brawn W, Spiegelhalter D (1994) Analysis of a cluster of surgical failures. Application to a series of neonatal arterial switch operations. J Thorac Cardiovasc Surg 107: 914–923.
4. Kennedy I The Bristol Royal Infirmary Inquiry. Available: http://www.official-documents.gov.uk/document/cm53/5363/5363.asp. Accessed: 9 October 2013.
5. Spiegelhalter D, Grigg O, Kinsman R, Treasure T (2003) Risk-adjusted sequential probability ratio tests: applications to Bristol, Shipman and adult cardiac surgery. Int J Qual Health Care 15: 7–13.
6. Biau DJ, Williams SM, Schlup MM, Nizard RS, Porcher R (2008) Quantitative and individualized assessment of the learning curve using LC-CUSUM. Br J Surg 95: 925–929.
7. Dagash H, Chowdhury M, Pierro A (2003) When can I be proficient in laparoscopic surgery? A systematic review of the evidence. J Pediatr Surg 38: 720–724.
8. Page ES (1954) Continuous inspection schemes. Biometrika 41: 100–115.
9. Biau DJ, Porcher R (2010) A method for monitoring a process from an out of control to an in control state: Application to the learning curve. Stat Med 29: 1900–1909.
10. Anon. CCAC Three Rs Microsite. Available: http://threers.ccac.ca/en/alternatives/ Accessed: 9 October 2013.
11. Anon. NC3Rs-National Centre for the Replacement, Refinement and Reduction of Animals in Research. Available: http://www.nc3rs.org.uk/ Accessed: 9 October 2013.
12. Marshall M, Best N, Bottle A, Aylin P (2004) Statistical issues in the prospective monitoring of health outcomes across multiple units. J R Statist Soc A 167: 541–559.
13. Rush BR, Biller DS, Davis EG, Higginbotham ML, Klocke E et al. (2011) Web-based documentation of clinical skills to assess the competency of veterinary students. J Vet Med Educ 38: 242–250.
14. Konrad C, Schupfer G, Wietlisbach M, Gerber H (1998) Learning manual skills in anesthesiology: Is there a recommended number of cases for anesthetic procedures? Anesth Analg 86: 635–639.
15. Dessolle L, Freour T, Barriere P, Jean M, Ravel C et al. (2010) How soon can I be proficient in embryo transfer? Lessons from the cumulative summation test for learning curve (LC-CUSUM). Hum Reprod 25: 380–386.
16. Papanna R, Biau DJ, Mann LK, Johnson A, Moise KJJ (2011) Use of the Learning Curve-Cumulative Summation test for quantitative and individualized assessment of competency of a surgical procedure in obstetrics and gynecology: fetoscopic laser ablation as a model. Am J Obstet Gynecol 204: 218.e1–218.e9.

21

Detection of *Mycobacterium bovis* in Bovine and Bubaline Tissues Using Nested-PCR for TbD1

Cristina P. Araújo[1], Ana Luiza A. R. Osório[1], Kláudia S. G. Jorge[1], Carlos Alberto N. Ramos[2], Antonio Francisco S. Filho[1], Carlos Eugênio S. Vidal[3], Eliana Roxo[4], Christiane Nishibe[5], Nalvo F. Almeida[5], Antônio A. F. Júnior[6], Marcio R. Silva[7], José Diomedes B. Neto[8], Valíria D. Cerqueira[8], Martín J. Zumárraga[9], Flábio R. Araújo[10]*

1 Programa de Pós-graduação em Ciência Animal FAMEZ, UFMS, Campo Grande, MS, Brazil, 2 Bolsista DTI, CNPq, Campo Grande, MS, Brazil, 3 PPGMV, UFSM, Santa Maria, RS, Brazil, 4 Instituto Biológico de São Paulo, São Paulo, SP, Brazil, 5 Faculdade de Computação, UFMS, Campo Grande, MS, Brazil, 6 Laboratório Nacional Agropecuário, Pedro Leopoldo, MG, Brazil, 7 Embrapa Gado de Leite, Juiz de Fora, MG, Brazil, 8 UFPA, Castanhal, PA, Brazil, 9 Instituto de Biotecnología, Instituto Nacional de Tecnología Agropecuaria, Buenos Aires, Argentina, 10 Embrapa Gado de Corte, Campo Grande, MS, Brazil

Abstract

In the present study, a nested-PCR system, targeting the TbD1 region, involving the performance of conventional PCR followed by real-time PCR, was developed to detect *Mycobacterium bovis* in bovine/bubaline tissue homogenates. The sensitivity and specificity of the reactions were assessed with DNA samples extracted from tuberculous and non-tuberculous mycobacteria, as well as other actinomycetales species and DNA samples extracted directly from bovine and bubaline tissue homogenates. In terms of analytical sensitivity, the DNA of *M. bovis* AN5 was detected up to 1.56 ng with conventional PCR, 97.6 pg with real-time PCR, and 1.53 pg with nested-PCR in the reaction mixture. The nested-PCR exhibited 100% analytical specificity for *M. bovis* when tested with the DNA of reference strains of environmental mycobacteria and closely-related Actinomycetales. A clinical sensitivity value of 76.0% was detected with tissue samples from animals that exhibited positive results in the comparative intradermal tuberculin test (CITT), as well as from those with lesions compatible with tuberculosis (LCT) that rendered positive cultures. A clinical specificity value of 100% was detected with tissue samples from animals with CITT- results, with no visible lesions (NVL) and negative cultures. No significant differences were found between the nested-PCR and culture in terms of detecting CITT+ animals with LCT or with NVL. No significant differences were recorded in the detection of CITT- animals with NVL. However, nested-PCR detected a significantly higher number of positive animals than the culture in the group of animals exhibiting LCT with no previous records of CITT. The use of the nested-PCR assay to detect *M. bovis* in tissue homogenates provided a rapid diagnosis of bovine and bubaline tuberculosis.

Editor: Joao Inacio, National Institute for Agriculture and Veterinary Research, IP (INIAV, I.P.), Portugal

Funding: CNPq (grants 578278/2008, 479394/2011-3, 305857/2013-4 and 310165/2010-5), FUNDECT (grants 23/200.152/2009, 23/200.582/2012 and TO-0096/2012), Embrapa (grants 03.11.22.003.00.00) and CAPES (PhD fellowship). The funders had no role in study design, data collection and analysis, decision to publish, or preparation of the manuscript.

Competing Interests: The authors have declared that no competing interests exist.

* E-mail: flabio.araujo@embrapa.br

Introduction

Tuberculosis is a chronic infectious disease caused by members of the *Mycobacterium tuberculosis* complex (MTC), including *M. tuberculosis*, *M. bovis*, *M. microti* [1], *M. africanum* [2], *M. canettii* [3], *M. caprae* [4], *M. pinnipedii* [5], *M. mungi* [6] and *M. orygis* [7]. In cattle, *M. bovis* is the species most frequently involved in tuberculosis cases. However other species of the MTC have been detected [7,8,9].

Bovine/bubaline tuberculosis causes financial losses in many countries and it is a zoonotic risk [10]. In Brazil, the control of bovine/bubaline tuberculosis is regulated by the Brazilian National Program for the Control and Eradication of Animal Brucellosis and Tuberculosis (PNCEBT). These regulations involve the slaughter of cattle with positive reactions to the intradermal tuberculin test (*ante-mortem* diagnosis) and the inspection of carcasses for gross lesions in abattoirs (*post-mortem* diagnosis) [11]. However, there is an increasing pressure from beef markets for a definitive diagnosis of tuberculosis in cattle exhibiting lesions compatible with tuberculosis (LCT). Since 2012, the Brazilian Ministry of Agriculture, Livestock and Food Supply (MAPA) determined that farms with cases of bovine/bubaline tuberculosis cannot export beef to the Customs Union of Belarus, Kazakhstan, and Russia. All lots of animals from a farm with suspicious animals are sequestered and the LCT are submitted to an official laboratory for etiological diagnosis [12].

The culture is considered to be the "gold standard" and definitive test for the confirmation of bovine tuberculosis. However, the microbiological diagnosis of *M. bovis* is an extremely slow procedure which may take as long as 2 to 3 months. Additional 2 to 3 weeks are required for the biochemical identification of isolates [13]. Therefore, the need for more rapid diagnostic systems is evident. Molecular diagnostic systems, particularly those based on real-time PCR technology, are faster [14].

The aim of the present study was to describe the development and assessment of a nested-PCR system, which involved a conventional reaction followed by real-time PCR, in terms of detecting *M. bovis* in bovine tissue homogenates.

Materials and Methods

Biological samples

Table 1 displays the reference bacterial strains used for the analytical sensitivity (*M. kansasii*, *M. smegmatis*, and *R. equi*) or specificity testing, as well as optimization of the nested-PCR. These include members of the MTC (*M. bovis* and *M. tuberculosis*), *Mycobacterium avium* complex (*M. avium*), atypical non-tuberculosis mycobacteria (*Mycobacterium abscessus*, *Mycobacterium fortuitum*, *Mycobacterium gordonae*, *Mycobacterium kansasii* and *Mycobacterium smegmatis*), and non-*Mycobacterium* Actinomycetales (*Corynebacterium pseudotuberculosis*, *Rhodococcus equi*).

The following materials were also used: a) 92 DNA samples obtained from cultures of lesions from cattle that had been naturally-infected with *M. bovis*. These samples were obtained from commercial cattle showing LCT during routine sanitary inspection in abattoirs, and lesions were submitted for etiological diagnosis at the Ministry of Agriculture – LANAGRO, MG, Brazil (n = 50) and *Instituto Biológico*, São Paulo, Brazil (n = 42), according to the regulation of the PNCEBT [11]; b) DNA from culture samples (n = 3) of *M. avium* from LANAGRO-MG. *M. bovis* and *M. avium* strains were identified using standard biochemical methods (samples from LANAGRO-MG) or PCR with the primers JB21 and JB22 for MTC [15]. Reference AN5 strain of *M. bovis* was cultured in Stonebrink medium, while the other *Mycobacterium* spp. reference strains were cultured in Löwenstein Jensen and Middlebrook media. Non-mycobacterium strains were not cultured and the DNA was purified directly from lyophilized bacterial suspension.

Bacterial strains DNA isolation

DNA of reference bacteria was purified with DNEasy Blood & Tissue kit (Qiagen), following the manufacturer's instructions. The quality and concentration of the DNA samples were assessed by spectrophotometry (NanoDrop ND-1000, Thermo Scientific) and electrophoresis in 0.8% agarose gel, stained with SYBR Gold (Invitrogen).

Primers and probes

Based on the DNA sequences of MTC members available at GenBank-NCBI (http://www.ncbi.nlm.nih.gov) and BLAST (http://blast.ncbi.nlm.nih.gov) searchers, specific targets were selected for DNA amplification of *M. bovis*. The primers and probe for nested-PCR were designed using Primer Express v2.0 software (Applied Biosystems).

The selected target for amplification was TbD1, a region that comprises the *mmpS6* gene (ID: 1092456) and the 5′ region of *mmpL6*. TbD1 is present in *M. bovis* (including BCG strains), *M. africanum*, *M. canettii*, and East-African Indian ancestral isolates of *M. tuberculosis*. In modern strains of *M. tuberculosis*, *mmpS6* is absent and *mmpL6* is truncated [03, 16, 17].

Two sets of primers were designed: outer primers, for conventional PCR amplification; internal primers and probe, for *TaqMan* MGB real-time PCR amplification. The first reaction was included to enrich *M. bovis* DNA, since the higher relative concentration of the host DNA isolated from cattle tissues may interfere with the amplification of the target gene. Sequences of the primers and probe are shown in Table 2.

Nested-PCR standardization

Conventional PCR (first step) was carried out in a volume of 25 µl, containing 10 mM of Tris-HCl (pH 8.3); 50 µM of KCl; 1.5 mM of $MgCl_2$, 0.2 mM of each dNTP, 7.5 pmol of each primer, 1.25 U of *Taq* DNA polymerase (Sigma), and 400 ηg of DNA.

Table 2. Primers and probes used for first conventional PCR and second real-time PCR for *Mycobacterium bovis* TbD1.

Target region	DNA sequences (5′→3′)
TbD1	Forward outer: GTGGCGGTCGCGGGATTCAGCGTCTAT
	Forward internal: GCGGTCTTCGCCAATGTT
	Probe: 6FAM TCGCGCAAGGCGA MGBNFQ
	Reverse internal: GCAGCCGATGGAATTGCT
	Reverse outer: TTATGGCGGCCACACCCACCCAAAACAG

Table 1. Bacterial standard strains used for evaluation of analytical specificity or analytical sensitivity of the nested-PCR.

Bacterial strains	Strain/origin
Corynebacterium pseudotuberculosis	LGCM/FIOCRUZ*
Mycobacterium abscessus	ATCC 19977/FIOCRUZ
Mycobacterium avium	ATCC 25291/FIOCRUZ
Mycobacterium bovis	AN5 strain, Agricultural Ministry – LANAGRO-MG
Mycobacterium fortuitum	ATCC 6841/FIOCRUZ
Mycobacterium gordonae	ATCC 14470/FIOCRUZ
Mycobacterium kansasii	ATCC 12478/FIOCRUZ
Mycobacterium tuberculosis	H37Rv/FIOCRUZ
Mycobacterium smegmatis	ATCC 700044/FIOCRUZ
Rhodococcus equi	ATCC 6939/FIOCRUZ

*Fundação Oswaldo Cruz, Instituto Nacional de Controle de Qualidade em Saúde.

Real-time PCR reactions (second step) for MTC were carried out in a volume of 12.5 μl, containing 6.25 μl of TaqMan Master Mix (ref 4352042, Applied Biosystems), 600 nM of each primer, 100 nM of the probe and 3 μl of the first step PCR reaction.

First step amplifications were carried out in an MJ Mini Biorad thermocycler. Initial denaturation was carried out at 95°C for 4 minutes, followed by 35 cycles of denaturation at 95°C for 90 seconds, annealing at 65°C for 30 seconds, and extension at 72°C for 45 seconds. A single 72°C final extension step was carried out for 3 minutes. Real-time PCR amplifications were carried out in a StepOne Plus thermocycler (Applied Biosystems, USA). Initial denaturation was carried out at 95°C for 10 minutes, followed by 35 cycles of denaturation at 95°C for 15 seconds and annealing/extension at 62°C for 30 seconds.

For all of the nested-PCR reactions, a positive control with DNA of M. bovis AN5, a blank control with no DNA and a negative control with DNA of H37Rv were included.

The primers/probe for M. bovis were tested for analytical specificity with 50 ηg of DNA of C. pseudotuberculosis, M. abscessus, M. avium, M. fortuitum, M. gordonae, M. kansasii, M. smegmatis and R. equi. Since TbD1 is absent in modern strains of M. tuberculosis, the strain H37Rv was also tested for PCR analytical specificity.

To test for PCR inhibitors, aliquots of DNA from the above species, used to assess specificity, were spiked with DNA of M. bovis AN5 and tested by nested-PCR. The amplification conditions were the same as those for the specific target.

The primers and probe were tested for analytical sensitivity with serial dilutions of DNA from reference strains of M. bovis AN5, in triplicate, but with one reaction mix for each replicate. The DNA samples were tested by real-time PCR singly, conventional PCR singly, and nested-PCR (both conventional and real-time reactions), and sensitivity was expressed as the minimum amount of DNA detected in the reaction mixture. In the case of nested-PCR, the volume of the first reaction (25 μl) was considered.

The primers and probe were also tested for analytical sensitivity with DNA extracted from 92 tissue cultures from naturally-infected cattle, provided by LANAGRO and the Instituto Biológico.

Direct detection of M. bovis in bovine and water buffalo tissues

Direct detection of M. bovis in tissue homogenates was carried out with 172 bovines and 62 water buffaloes (Bubalus bubalis) from commercial herds. No animals were slaughtered specifically for research. Tissue samples were collected during sanitary inspection in abattoirs from states of Amapá, Espírito Santo, Mato Grosso do Sul, Minas Gerais, Pará, Pernambuco, Rio Grande do Sul and São Paulo, Brazil, as follows:

a)   127 comparative intradermal tuberculin test (CITT) positive animals, including 80 with lesions compatible with tuberculosis (LCT) and 47 with no visible lesions (NVL). These animals, from different age groups and zootechnical categories (dairy and beef cattle and water buffaloes), were culled following the recommendations of the PNCEBT [11].

b)   51 CITT negative animals with NVL. These animals came from a mixed commercial farm (dairy and beef cattle and water buffaloes), with a previous history of tuberculosis.

c)   51 animals with no records of CITT (dairy and beef cattle and water buffaloes) with LCT, detected during routine inspections in abattoirs.

Comparative intradermal tuberculin tests were conducted according to the regulations of PNCEBT [11]. A positive CITT reaction was defined as a relative increase in skin thickness at the injection site for bovine PPD of at least 4 mm greater than the increase in skin thickness at the injection site for avian PPD [11].

LCT were obtained for the present study from hepatic, iliac, mandibular, mediastinal, mesenteric, pre-scapular, retropharyngeal and tracheobronchial lymph nodes or the lungs, tonsils, liver or diaphragm. When cattle exhibited NVL, the hepatic, mediastinal, mesenteric, retropharyngeal and tracheobronchial lymph nodes were collected. The organs were kept on ice until they reached the laboratory, where they were kept at −30°C until processing. The organs were thawed and divided into two samples, one for culturing and the other for DNA isolation.

For DNA isolation, the samples were cut into pieces of 100 mg, corresponding to the transition between gross lesions and apparently healthy areas. These pieces were completely homogenized with 1 ml of phosphate buffered saline (PBS). From these tissue suspensions, 200 μl was used for DNA isolation with the DNEasy Blood & Tissue kit (Qiagen), following the manufacturer's instructions. Nested-PCR reactions were carried out as described above.

For culturing, the samples were thawed and homogenized with an equivalent amount of sterile sand and saline. The tissue suspensions were filtered through sterile gauze and centrifuged at 1200 g for 15 minutes. The sediments were suspended with 2 ml of sterile saline, decontaminated using Petroff's method [18], and cultured on the Stonebrink medium. The cultures were incubated at 37°C and searched for bacterial colonies for at least 90 days, with weekly observations. The smears from the isolated colonies were stained using the Ziehl-Neelsen method (ZN) for acid-fast bacilli (AFB). All the AFB cultures were analyzed by PCR, with primers JB21 and JB22, for MTC [15].

Cattle were considered positive for tuberculosis when at least a single tissue sample exhibited amplification in the nested-PCR or exhibited AFB cultures confirmed by the PCR with primers JB21 and JB22. Cattle were considered negative for tuberculosis when the cultures exhibited no AFB, when AFB cultures were negative for MTC in the PCR with primers JB21 and JB22, and when the tissues were negative in the nested-PCR.

Statistical analysis

The agreement between the nested-PCR and the culture was assessed by the Kappa index [19]. Paired comparisons were performed using McNemar's test, with the level of significance set at 0.05. The chi-square test and Fisher's exact test were carried out to assess associations between the categorical variables, with the level of significance set at 0.05. The chi-square for linear trend was also used and, whenever possible, univariate logistic regression was performed to assess whether there was a dose-response relationship between the levels of presumptive evidence for bovine TB. Based on a combination of both diagnoses (CITT and LCT) and the result of the nested-PCR for each level of "exposure," an odds ratio was calculated to compare the proportion of positive results with the baseline level or level 0 (no visible lesions and negative CITT) [20].

Results

In silico analysis of the DNA primer and probe sequences exhibited complete identity with TbD1 sequences of M. bovis AF2122/97, different M. bovis BCG strains, M. africanum and M. canettii, available in the NCBI. Complete identity was also found for 7 strains of M. bovis from Argentina (including 04-303, accession number AVSW00000000), 10 strains of M. bovis from Brazil, and AN5 strain (accession number AWPL00000000), the genomes of which were sequenced by our group in other study. Regarding *M. tuberculosis*, the primers and probe exhibited complete identity with an ancestral strain (accession number AJ426486) [03], but no homology was detected with modern strains of *M. tuberculosis* available at GenBank.

No amplification was recorded in the following cases: DNA from the H37Rv strain or from clinical isolates of *M. tuberculosis*; DNA from reference strains of the non-tuberculous mycobacteria *M. abscessus*, *M. avium*, *M. fortuitum*, *M. gordonae*, *M. kansasii* and *M. smegmatis*; DNA from closely-related Actinomycetales *C. pseudotuberculosis*; *R. equi*. DNA aliquots of non-target microorganisms spiked with the DNA of *M. bovis* AN5 were positive in the nested-PCR.

With regards to analytical sensitivity, DNA of *M. bovis* AN5 was detected in the reaction mixture up to 1.56 ηg with conventional PCR, 97.6 pg with real-time PCR, and 1.53 pg with nested-PCR. Of the 50 DNA samples isolated from cultures from lesions of cattle that had been naturally-infected with *M. bovis* from the Ministry of Agriculture – LANAGRO, 49 (98.0%) were positive in the nested-PCR for *M. bovis*. All of the 42 (100%) DNA samples isolated from cultures of *M. bovis* from the *Instituto Biológico*, were positive in the nested-PCR for *M. bovis*.

Tissue samples from 229 bovines/bubalines were tested directly by nested-PCR for *M. bovis*. The nested-PCR and culture results are shown in Table 3. Aliquots of all the samples that showed negative results in the nested-PCR were spiked with DNA of *M. bovis* AN5 strain and re-tested in the nested-PCR, showing positive results. Of the 51 animals with CITT- results and NVL, 50 exhibited negative cultures. These 50 animals were included for the calculation of clinical specificity, which was 100%. Of the 50 animals with CITT+ results and LCT that rendered positive cultures, 38 were also positive in the nested-PCR, corresponding to a clinical sensitivity of 76.0%.

With regards to the agreement between the nested-PCR and the culture, there were 51 nested-PCR+/culture+ animal (22.27%), 120 nested-PCR-/culture- animals (52.40%), 36 nested-PCR+/culture- animals (15.72%) and 22 nested-PCR-/culture+ animals (9.61%). The agreement assessed by the Kappa index was 0.445, with a standard error of 0.061 and a 95% confidence interval from 0.325 to 0.565. The strength of the agreement is considered to be moderate [19].

Results from the nested-PCR and cultures revealed no significant differences in terms of detecting CITT+ animals with LCT or with NVL. No significant differences were found in the

detection of CITT- animals with NVL. However, the nested-PCR detected a significantly higher number of positive animals than the culture in the group of animals with no records of CITT, but exhibiting LCT (p<0.05).

There was a linear trend between increasing presumptive evidence of bovine tuberculosis and the chance of positive results in the culture (p<0.001) or in the nested-PCR (p<0.001). The presumptive results of LCT or positive CITT produced 13.75 and 15.27 times more chance of a positive result in the culture, and 59.10 and 72.61 times more chance of a positive result in the nested-PCR, respectively, when compared with the group with no presumptive results. In the group with the two presumptive positive results, LCT and CITT produced 83.33 and 161.86 times more chance of a positive result in the culture and in the nested-PCR, when compared with the group with no presumptive results, respectively (Table 3).

Discussion

One of the most essential systems applied to the eradication of bovine tuberculosis by *M. bovis* is the epidemiological surveillance of animals slaughtered in abattoirs. This surveillance is conducted by means of inspection and taking samples of LCT, confirming the existence of the disease through the culture and molecular detection, which takes weeks before a result can be obtained [21].

The aim of the present study was to develop a *post-mortem* diagnostic system for bovine and bubaline tuberculosis, applicable directly to bovine clinical samples, that could substantially reduce the time between the detection of CITT+ animals and/or LCT and the etiological diagnosis, when compared to the traditional method of culturing, which takes up to 90 days.

A nested-PCR system targeting the TbD1 was developed. This region comprises the *mmpS6* gene and the 5′ region of *mmpL6*, which are present in the genomes of *M. bovis*, *M. africanum*, *M. canettii* and in ancestral strains of *M. tuberculosis* [03, 22]. As expected, BLASTn analysis of the sequences of the primers and probe for TbD1 exhibited complete identity with the above MTC species. However, there is little genomic information about field strains of *M. bovis* to assess the conservation of the target sequences of the nested-PCR. Our research group sequenced the genomes of 7 strains of *M. bovis* from Argentina and 11 strains from Brazil, and target sequences were conserved in all 18 strains.

The analytical specificity of the nested-PCR was analyzed *in vitro*. No amplification was detected when the primers/probe for

Table 3. Nested-PCR for *Mycobacterium bovis* TbD1 and culture results of 229 bovine and bubaline tissue homogenates.

Status		Total Number	Test			Odds ratio**	
Ante-mortem	Post-mortem		Culture* (%)	Nested-PCR (%)	P-value	Culture	Nested-PCR
CITT-	NVL	51	1 (1.96)a	0 (0.00)a	1.0	1.0A	1.0A
No CITT	LCT	51	11 (21.57)a	21 (41.18)b	0.0329	13.75B	72.61B
CITT+	NVL	47	11 (23.40)a	17 (36.17)a	0.176	15.27B	59.10B
CITT+	LCT	80	50 (62.50)a	49 (61.25)a	0.8707	83.33C	161.86C
	Total	229	73 (31.88)	87 (37.99)	0.17	-	-

CITT = Comparative intradermal tuberculin test.
LCT = Lesions compatible with tuberculosis.
NVL = No visible lesions.
*Confirmed by PCR with primers JB21 and JB22 [15].
**p-value for chi-square of linear trend <0.001.
Different lowercase letters in rows indicate significant differences (p<0.05) within the paired comparisons between culture and nested-PCR.
Different capital letters in the columns indicate proportions significantly different (p<0.05).

TbD1 were used with DNA of *M. tuberculosis* H37Rv or from cultures of clinical isolates of *M. tuberculosis*. However, only H37Rv was tested in the present study and this is a modern genotype of *M. tuberculosis* [23].

There are reports of *M. tuberculosis* infecting cattle worldwide [24,25,26,27]. In Brazil, more than 2000 culture samples from cattle with presumptive lesions of tuberculosis were tested for *M. tuberculosis* at LANAGRO-MG (Brazilian Ministry of Agriculture) and no positive results were found (A. A. Fonseca Júnior, 2013, personal communication).

In humans, modern genotype strains (TbD1 deleted) of *M. tuberculosis* are most commonly found in Morocco, Cameroon, Ethiopia, Pakistan, Myanmar [17,28,29,30,31]. However, in Bangladesh, 65% of the *M. tuberculosis* isolates were ancestral (TbD1+) [32]. In India, modern genotypes are predominant in the south of the country, whereas ancestral genotypes are more common in central and northern areas of the country [33].

No amplification was detected with the primers/probe for TbD1, DNA of the environmental mycobacteria *M. abcessus*, *M. avium*, *M. fortuitum*, *M. gordonae*, *M. kansasii* and *M. smegmatis*, or with the DNA of the closely-related bacteria tested. This is particularly significant since environmental mycobacteria present in lymph nodes submitted for diagnostic testing can confound assays that lack sufficient specificity [34]. Furthermore, closely-related Actinomycetales, such as *R. equi* and *C. pseudotuberculosis*, may cause lesions to be mistakenly diagnosed as tuberculosis [35,36].

Nested-PCR for TbD1 was not tested with the DNA of *M. africanum* or *M. canettii*, which are TbD1 positive. However, both species are essentially human pathogens [03, 37] and have not been described in Brazil. A number of reports of *M. africanum* in cattle have been described in Europe and Asia [08, 38, 39]. The epidemiological importance of this pathogen in cattle must be clarified, especially in new world countries.

Traditionally, clinical sensitivity and specificity for PCR reactions to tuberculosis are assessed with tissue samples that are positive or negative, respectively, in the culture for *Mycobacterium* sp., since the culture is considered to be the gold-standard diagnostic test for tuberculosis [21]. In this sense, nested-PCR exhibited a moderate clinical sensitivity and a high clinical specificity. Nevertheless, in terms of the use of an additional diagnostic tool as part of a control/eradication program of bovine tuberculosis, this information is limited. Depending on the stage of the infection or even the condition of the biological sample, PCR may detect more animals than the culture [21], or vice-versa [40,41]. Feasibility is another important factor, since carcasses with LCT in abattoirs require rapid diagnostic results.

In the present study, nested-PCR detected 36 nested-PCR+/culture- animals, which corresponded to 15.72% of the number of samples tested. Additional suggestions that these animals were really infected include the presence of other presumptive evidence of tuberculosis in all animals (positive CITT: 26 animals; LCT: 21 animals; CITT and LCT: 11 animals). On the other hand, there were 22 culture+/nested-PCR- animals (9.61%). Since different methods of DNA purification from tissue may influence the presence of PCR inhibitors in the sample being tested [42], DNA aliquots from tissues of these 22 culture+/nested-PCR- animals were spiked with DNA from *M. bovis* AN5 strain and were re-tested by nested-PCR, showing positive results.

In Brazil, skin tuberculinization is the official *ante-mortem* test for bovine/bubaline tuberculosis. CITT+ animals are considered positive for tuberculosis and must be slaughtered in a maximum of 30 days [11], preferably in an official abattoir in which tissue samples are to be taken for microbiological diagnosis. Nested-PCR for TbD1 and the culture detected similar numbers of CITT+ animals (P = 0.5304). No statistically significant differences were found between nested-PCR and the culture in the numbers of CITT- animals detected.

During meat inspection at abattoir level, the main concerns are animals exhibiting LCT, which are considered inappropriate for consumption. However, in the bovine/bubaline samples of the present study, 37% of the CITT+ animals exhibited NVL, of which 14.9% were positive both in the culture and in the nested-PCR. This raises concerns that zoonotic transmission, such as that of *M. bovis*, can survive the cooking process [43]. For this reason, sanitary policies involving PCR testing of CITT+/NVL animals should be considered.

In Brazil, carcasses that exhibit LCT during routine sanitary inspections are condemned for consumption. Some countries that import meat from Brazil are imposing the requirement of an etiological diagnosis of such lesions. The nested-PCR was more sensitive than the culture when detecting *M. bovis* in animals that were not tested by CITT, but exhibited LCT during sanitary inspections at abattoirs. One of the possible reasons for this result is that this group included 23 water buffaloes from the Amazon region (State of Amapá), whose tissues were transported for a long period in high temperatures. Despite being stored in ice, the samples started to deteriorate, resulting in negative cultures, although the nested-PCR reactions were positive.

Several methodologies have previously been used to increase the sensitivity of real-time PCR when detecting *Mycobacterium* sp. directly from tissue homogenates. Parra et al. [21] used a capture probe to isolate mycobacterial DNA from tissue homogenates, achieving a lower sensitivity (65.6%) than that found in the present study. Taylor et al. [40] also reported a sensitivity of 70% when performing PCR directly on tissue homogenates, although the sensitivity increased to 91% when PCR was only performed on DNA isolated from lesions excised from the tissues rather than whole tissue homogenates. The limitation of this method is that the assay can only be performed on tissues that have LCT, thus excluding samples without readily apparent lesions. Thacker et al. [34] used a strategy that was similar to the present study, with conventional PCR followed by a real-time reaction, but targeting IS*6110*, and found a sensitivity of 66.7% in detecting positive culture samples.

One of the concerns about nested-PCR, particularly in relation to real-time reactions, is the possibility of cross-contamination. Throughout the DNA extraction procedure, gloves were changed frequently. DNA purification was carried out at biosafety level 3, with the PCR set-up on a laminar flow PCR cabinet with UV light. Separate sets of micropipettes were used for DNA purification and PCR set-up. Filter tips were used routinely. Surfaces and equipment in contact with sample tubes were cleaned before each assay. Blank and negative controls were always used.

Nested-PCR allowed the identification of *M. bovis* in tissues with a performance that was similar or superior to the culture. Individual results from the nested-PCR were obtained in a short period of time (2 days), in contrast with the culture, which took up to 90 days. This suggests that nested-PCR can be used for *post-mortem* etiological diagnoses of bovine/bubaline tuberculosis during routine inspections at abattoirs. However, a large-scale study and an inter-laboratory validation of the method are required to determine whether the method is adequate for the PNCEBT.

Finally, there was a linear positive trend, confirming a dose–response relationship between the increase of presumptive results, both in terms of the negative level (CITT – and NVL) and the positive level (CITT + and LCT), as well as the odds ratio for positive results in the culture and the nested-PCR. Dose-response and trend analysis are commonly employed in epidemiology and public health. In the present study, the dose-response was shown to be useful in terms of demonstrating the logic of laboratory results with the clinical data of the animals and assisting the decision-making process in diagnostic tests related to animal health surveillance and food inspection.

Supporting Information

Table S1 Identification of isolates of Mycobacterium bovis by origin and abattoir, and results of culture and nested-PCR.

Author Contributions

Conceived and designed the experiments: ALARO FRA. Performed the experiments: CPA ALARO CANR AFSF CESV ER CN NFA AAFJ MRS JDBN VDC MJZ FRA KSGJ. Analyzed the data: NFA MRS FRA CANR. Contributed reagents/materials/analysis tools: FRA ALARO. Wrote the paper: MRS FRA CANR.

References

1. Wells AQ (1937) Tuberculosis in wild voles, Lancet 1, 1221.
2. Castets M, Sarrat H (1969) Experimental study of the virulence of *Mycobacterium africanum* (preliminary note). Bull Soc Med Afr Noire Lang Fr 14: 693–696.
3. Brosch R, Gordon SV, Marmiesse M, Brodin P, Buchrieser C, et al. (2002) A new evolutionary scenario for the *Mycobacterium tuberculosis* complex. Proc Natl Acad Sci EUA 99: 3684–3689.
4. Aranaz A, Cousins D, Mateos A, Domínguez L (2003) Elevation of Mycobacterium tuberculosis subsp. caprae Aranaz, et al. 1999 to species rank as Mycobacterium caprae comb. nov., sp. nov. Int J Syst Evol Microbiol 53: 785–1789.
5. Cousins DV, Bastida R, Cataldi A, Quse V, Redrobe S, et al. (2003) Tuberculosis in seals caused by a novel member of the *Mycobacterium tuberculosis* complex: *Mycobacterium pinnipedii* sp. nov. Int J Syst Evol Microbiol 53: 1305–1334.
6. Alexander KA, Laver PN, Michel AL, Williams M, van Helden PD, et al. (2010) Novel *Mycobacterium tuberculosis* complex pathogen, *M. mungi*. Emerg Infect Dis 16: 1296–1299.
7. Van Ingen J, Rahim Z, Mulder A, Boeree MJ, Simeone R, et al. (2012) Characterization of *Mycobacterium orygis* as *M. tuberculosis* complex subspecies. Emerg Infect Dis 18: 653–655.
8. Alfredsen S, Saxegaard F (1992) An outbreak of tuberculosis in pigs and cattle caused by *Mycobacterium africanum*. Vet Rec 131: 51–53.
9. Johansen IS, Thomsen VO, Forsgren A, Hansen BF, Lundgren B (2004) Detection of *Mycobacterium tuberculosis* complex in formalin-fixed, paraffin-embedded tissue specimens with necrotizing granulomatous inflammation by strand displacement amplification. J Mol Diagn 6: 231–236.
10. Müller B, Dürr S, Alonso S, Hattendorf J, Laisse CJ, et al. (2013) Zoonotic *Mycobacterium bovis*-induced tuberculosis in humans. Emerg Infect Dis 19: 899–908.
11. Brasil (2006) Programa Nacional de Controle e Erradicação da Brucelose e Tuberculose – PNCEBT. Manual Técnico, Ministério da Agricultura, Pecuária e Abastecimento, Brasília.
12. Brasil (2012) Norma Interna DAS n°02/2012. Ministério da Agricultura, Pecuária e Abastecimento. Secretaria de Defesa Agropecuária.
13. Duffield BJ, Norton JH, Hoffmann D (1989) An analysis of recent isolations of *Mycobacterium bovis* and saprophytic *mycobacteria* from cattle in northern Queensland. Aust J Vet 66: 307–308.
14. Soini H, Musser JM (2001) Molecular diagnosis of mycobacteria. Clin Chem 47: 809–814.
15. Rodriguez JG, Mejia GA, Del Portillo P, Patarroyo ME, Murillo LA (1995) Species-specific identification of *Mycobacterium bovis* by PCR. Microbiology 141: 2131–2138.
16. Mostowy S, Inwald J, Gordon S, Martin C, Warren R, et al. (2005) Revisiting the evolution of *Mycobacterium bovis*. J Bacteriol 187: 6386–6395.
17. Lahlou O, Millet J, Chaoui I, Sabouni R, Filali-Maltouf A, et al. (2012) The genotypic population structure of *Mycobacterium tuberculosis* complex from Moroccan patients reveals a predominance of Euro-American lineages. PLos One 7: 47113.
18. Petroff SA (1915) A new and rapid method for the isolation and cultivation of tubercle bacilli directly from the sputum and feces. J Exp Med 21: 38–42.
19. Ansari-Lari M (2005) Comparison between two tests results, kappa statistic instead of simple overall agreement. Veterinary Parasitol 133: 369–370.
20. Schlesselman JJ (1982) Case-Control Studies, Oxford Univ. Press, NY, p. 205.
21. Parra A, García N, García A, Lacombe A, Moreno F, et al. (2008) Development of a molecular diagnostic test applied to experimental abattoir surveillance on bovine tuberculosis. Vet Microbiol 127: 315–324.
22. Garnier T, Eiglmeier K, Camus JC, Medina N, Mansoor H, et al. (2003) The complete genome sequence of *Mycobacterium bovis*. Proc Natl Acad Sci U S A 100: 7877–7882.
23. Cole ST, Brosch R, Parkhill J, Garnier T, Churcher C, et al. (1998) Deciphering the biology of *Mycobacterium tuberculosis* from the complete genome sequence. Nature 393: 537–544.
24. Ameni G, Vordermeier M, Firdessa R, Aseffa A, Hewinson G, et al. (2011) *Mycobacterium tuberculosis* infection in grazing cattle in central Ethiopia. Vet J 188: 359–361.
25. Romero B, Rodríguez S, Bezos J, Diaz R, Copano MF, et al. (2011) Humans as source of *Mycobacterium tuberculosis* infection in cattle, Spain. Emerg Infect Dis 17: 2393–2395.
26. Mbugi EV, Katale BZ, Kendall S, Good L, Kibiki GS, et al. (2012) Tuberculosis cross-species transmission in Tanzania: Towards a One-Health concept, Onderstepoort. J Vet Res 79:1–6.
27. Thakur A, Sharma M, Katoch VC, Dhar P, Katoch RC (2012) Detection of *Mycobacterium bovis* and *Mycobacterium tuberculosis* from Cattle: Possible Public Health Relevance. Indian J Microbiol 52: 289–291.
28. Niobe-Eyangoh SN, Kuaban C, Sorlin P, Thonnon J, Vincent V, et al. (2004) Molecular characteristics of strains of the cameroon family, the major group of *Mycobacterium tuberculosis* in a country with a high prevalence of tuberculosis. J Clin Microbiol 42: 5029–5035.
29. Stavrum R, Valvatne H, Bo TH, Jonassen I, Hinds J, et al. (2008) Genomic diversity among Beijing and non-Beijing *Mycobacterium tuberculosis* isolates from Myanmar. PLoS One 3: 1973.
30. Tanveer M, Hasan Z, Siddiqui AR, Ali A, Kanji A, et al. (2008) Genotyping and drug resistance patterns of *M. tuberculosis* strains in Pakistan. BMC Infect Dis 8: 171.
31. Beyene D, Bergval I, Hailu E, Ashenafi S, Yamuah L, et al. (2009) Identification and genotyping of the etiological agent of tuberculous lymphadenitis in Ethiopia. J Infect Dev Ctries 3: 412–419.
32. Banu S, Uddin MK, Islam MR, Zaman K, Ahmed T, et al. (2012) Molecular epidemiology of tuberculosis in rural Matlab. Bangladesh. Int J Tuberc Lung Dis 16: 319–326.
33. Thomas SK, Iravatham CC, Moni BH, Kumar A, Archana BV, et al. (2011) Modern and ancestral genotypes of *Mycobacterium tuberculosis* from Andhra Pradesh, India. Plos One 6: 27584.
34. Thacker TC, Harris B, Palmer MV, Waters WR (2011) Improved specificity for detection of *Mycobacterium bovis* in fresh tissues using IS6110 real-time PCR. BMC Vet Res 7: 50.
35. Flynn O, Quigley F, Costello E, O'Grady D, Gogarty A, et al. (2001) Virulence-associated protein characterization of *Rhodococcus equi* isolated from bovine lymph nodes. Vet Microbiol 78: 221–228
36. Sahraoui N, Müller B, Guetarni D, Boulahbal F, Yala D, et al. (2009) Molecular characterization of *Mycobacterium bovis* strains isolated from cattle slaughtered at two abattoirs in Algeria. BMC Vet Res 5: 4.
37. Niemann S, Richter E, Rüsch-Gerdes S (2000) Differentiation among members of the *Mycobacterium tuberculosis* complex by molecular and biochemical features: evidence for two pyrazinamide-susceptible subtypes of *M. bovis*. J Clin Microbiol 38: 152–157.
38. Weber A, Reischl U, Naumann L (1998) Demonstration of *Mycobacterium africanum* in a bull from North Bavaria. Berl Munch Tierarztl Wochenschr 111: 6–8.
39. Rahim Z, Möllers M, te Koppele-Vije A, de Beer J, Zaman K, et al. (2007) Characterization of *Mycobacterium africanum* subtype I among cows in a dairy farm in Bangladesh using spoligotyping. Southeast Asian J Trop Med Public Health 38: 706–713.
40. Taylor GM, Worth DR, Palmer S, Jahans K, Hewinson RG (2007) Rapid detection of *Mycobacterium bovis* DNA in cattle lymph nodes with visible lesions using PCR. BMC Vet Res 3:12.
41. Costa P, Ferreira AS, Amaro A, Albuquerque T, Botelho A, et al. (2013). Enhanced detection of tuberculous mycobacteria in animal tissues using a semi-nested probe-based real-time PCR. PLoS One 8: e81337.
42. Barandiaran S, Garbaccio SG, Kiernicki MC, Martinez Vivot, M, Zumarraga MJ (2013) Evaluación de distintas metodologias de extracción de ADN para la detección de *Mycobacterium bovis* en tejidos. Rev Argent Microbiol 45: 91.
43. Van der Merwe M, Bekker JL, van der Merwe P, Michel AL (2009) Cooking and drying as effective mechanisms in limiting the zoonotic effect of *Mycobacterium bovis* in beef. J S Afr Vet Assoc 80: 142–145.

22

Evaluation of Change in Canine Diagnosis Protocol Adopted by the Visceral Leishmaniasis Control Program in Brazil and a New Proposal for Diagnosis

Wendel Coura-Vital[1,2,7], **Henrique Gama Ker**[1,3], **Bruno Mendes Roatt**[1,3], **Rodrigo Dian Oliveira Aguiar-Soares**[1,3], **Gleisiane Gomes de Almeida Leal**[1,3], **Nádia das Dores Moreira**[1,3], **Laser Antônio Machado Oliveira**[1], **Evandro Marques de Menezes Machado**[3], **Maria Helena Franco Morais**[4], **Rodrigo Corrêa-Oliveira**[5,7], **Mariângela Carneiro**[2,6], **Alexandre Barbosa Reis**[1,3,7]*

1 Laboratório de Pesquisas Clínicas, Ciências Farmacêuticas, Escola de Farmácia, Universidade Federal de Ouro Preto, Morro do Cruzeiro, Ouro Preto, Minas Gerais, Brazil, **2** Infectologia e Medicina Tropical, Faculdade de Medicina, Universidade Federal de Minas Gerais, Minas Gerais, Brazil, **3** Laboratório de Imunopatologia, Núcleo de Pesquisas em Ciências Biológicas, Instituto de Ciências Exatas e Biológicas, Universidade Federal de Ouro Preto, Morro do Cruzeiro, Ouro Preto, Minas Gerais, Brazil, **4** Secretaria Municipal de Saúde, Prefeitura de Belo Horizonte, Belo Horizonte, Minas Gerais, Brazil, **5** Laboratório de Imunologia Celular e Molecular, Centro de Pesquisas René Rachou, Fundação Oswaldo Cruz, Belo Horizonte, Minas Gerais, Brazil, **6** Laboratório de Epidemiologia de Doenças Infecciosas e Parasitárias, Departamento de Parasitologia, Instituto de Ciências Biológicas, Universidade Federal de Minas Gerais, Belo Horizonte, Minas Gerais, Brazil, **7** Instituto Nacional de Ciência e Tecnologia em Doenças Tropicais (INCTDT), Salvador, Bahia, Brazil

Abstract

The techniques used for diagnosis of canine visceral leishmaniasis (CVL) in Brazil ELISA and IFAT have been extensively questioned because of the accuracy of these tests. A recent change in the diagnosis protocol excluded IFAT and included the Dual-Path Platform (DPP). We evaluated the prevalence and incidence rates of *Leishmania* spp. before and after the change in the protocol. In addition, based on our results, we propose a new alternative that is less expensive for the screening and confirmation of CVL. Plasma samples were obtained from a serobank from dogs evaluated in a cross-sectional study (1,226 dogs) and in a cohort study of susceptible animals (n = 447), followed for 26 months. Serology testing was performed using ELISA, IFAT, and DPP. The incidence and prevalence of CVL were determined by using the protocol of the Visceral Leishmaniasis Control and Surveillance Program until 2012 (ELISA and IFAT using filter paper) and the protocol used after 2012 (DPP and ELISA using plasma). The prevalence was 6.2% and the incidence was 2.8 per 1,000 dog-months for the protocol used until 2012. For the new diagnosis protocol for CVL resulted in an incidence of 5.4 per 1,000 dog-months and a prevalence of 8.1%. Our results showed that the prevalence and incidence of infection were far greater than suggested by the previously used protocol and that the magnitude of infection in endemic areas has been underestimated. As tests are performed sequentially and euthanasia of dogs is carried out when the serological results are positive in both tests, the sequence does not affect the number of animals to be eliminated by the Control Program. Then we suggest to municipalities with a large demand of exams to use ELISA for screening and DPP for confirmation, since this allows easier performance and reduced cost.

Editor: Dario S. Zamboni, University of São Paulo, Brazil

Funding: This study was supported by the following grants: Federal University of Ouro Preto; Brazilian Ministry of Health; DECIT/MS/CNPq/BR/grant: 576062/2008-1; FAPEMIG/BR/grant: CBB-APQ-3073-4.01/07, CNPq/BR/grant: 472554/2007-7; PPSUS/MS/CNPq/FAPEMIG/SES-MG/grant CBB-APQ-00356-10; FAPEMIG/PPM and PNPD/Institutional/2011. The funders had no role in the study design, the data collection and analysis, the decision to publish the manuscript, or the preparation of the manuscript. ABR, MC, and RCO are grateful for CNPq fellowships. WCV is supported by a PNPD/CAPES postdoctoral fellowship.

Competing Interests: The authors have declared that no competing interests exist.

* E-mail: alexreis@nupeb.ufop.br

Introduction

In recent decades visceral leishmaniasis (VL) has become a major public health problem in Brazil, affecting approximately 3,379 individuals per year, with an annual incidence rate of 1.9 cases per 100,000 [1]. Zoonotic VL is a potentially fatal disease that is transmitted by the Phlebotominae sandfly species and is caused by the intracellular protozoan parasite *Leishmania infantum* (*Leishmania chagasi*), which is endemic in South America, Central America, the Mediterranean basin, and parts of Asia [2].

Dogs are highly susceptible to leishmaniasis infection and represent the major source of infection because of intense skin parasitism, independent of their clinical presentation [3–5]. The domestic dog has been identified as the main urban reservoir for *L. infantum*, and canine VL (CVL) is considered to be an emerging and re-emerging disease, as indicated by an increase in the number of seropositive dogs and by the geographical expansion of the disease [6–10].

To control the spread of disease, the Brazilian Ministry of Health through the Visceral Leishmaniasis Control and Surveillance Program (VLCSP) has instituted various measures including

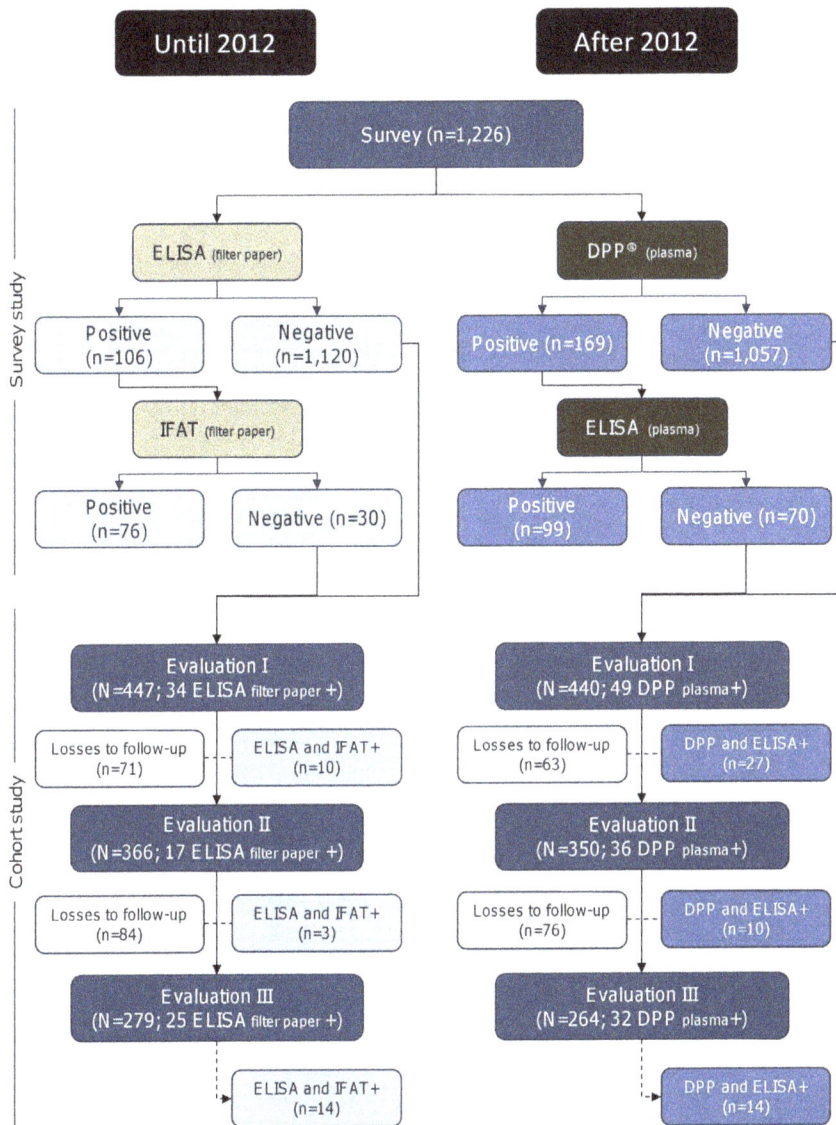

Figure 1. Diagnostic protocols used for canine visceral leishmaniasis in Brazil until 2012 and after 2012.

early diagnosis and treatment of human cases, identification and culling of seropositive infected dogs, control of insect vectors, and health education [1]. The VLCSP mainly relies on the euthanasia of seropositive dogs to control VL; however, this measure is controversial and some reports suggest that it has little impact on the reduction of human and canine cases [11–13]. This failure has been attributed to delays in detecting and eliminating infected dogs, the tendency to replace infected dogs with susceptible puppies, and the low sensitivity of the serological methods used [14–19]. Some studies have estimated that the sensitivity of the immunofluorescent antibody test (IFAT) ranges from 68% to 100% and that the specificity ranges from 52% to 100%, whereas the sensitivity of enzyme-linked immunosorbent assay (ELISA) ranges from 91% to 97% and the specificity of ELISA ranges from 83% to 98% [16,20–23].

Until 2012, CVL had been diagnosed using IFAT, a method recommended for confirming positive cases detected by ELISA. These serological tests were performed using serum or blood samples collected on filter paper [1,19]. Recently, to improve

accuracy in the diagnosis of CVL, the VLCSP has recommended using an immunochromatographic rapid test comprising rK26 and rK39 recombinant antigens, the Dual-Path Platform (DPP; Bio-Manguinhos/Fiocruz, Rio de Janeiro, Brazil), for the screening of infected dogs and ELISA to confirm the positive results [24–25]. Moreover, changing the eluate from dried blood collected on filter paper to serum or plasma samples has been recommended [24]. However, this measure has not yet been widely adopted by all health departments of the municipalities located in many endemic areas around the country because of some operational difficulties.

Herein, we report the results of a baseline canine survey followed by a cohort study using the conventional serological methods used by the VLCSP until 2012 (ELISA and IFAT with filter paper) and after 2012 (DPP and ELISA with plasma) to evaluate the prevalence and incidence of *Leishmania* spp. infection in a large canine population in an endemic area of Brazil. In addition, based on our results, we propose a new alternative that is less expensive for the screening and confirmation of CVL.

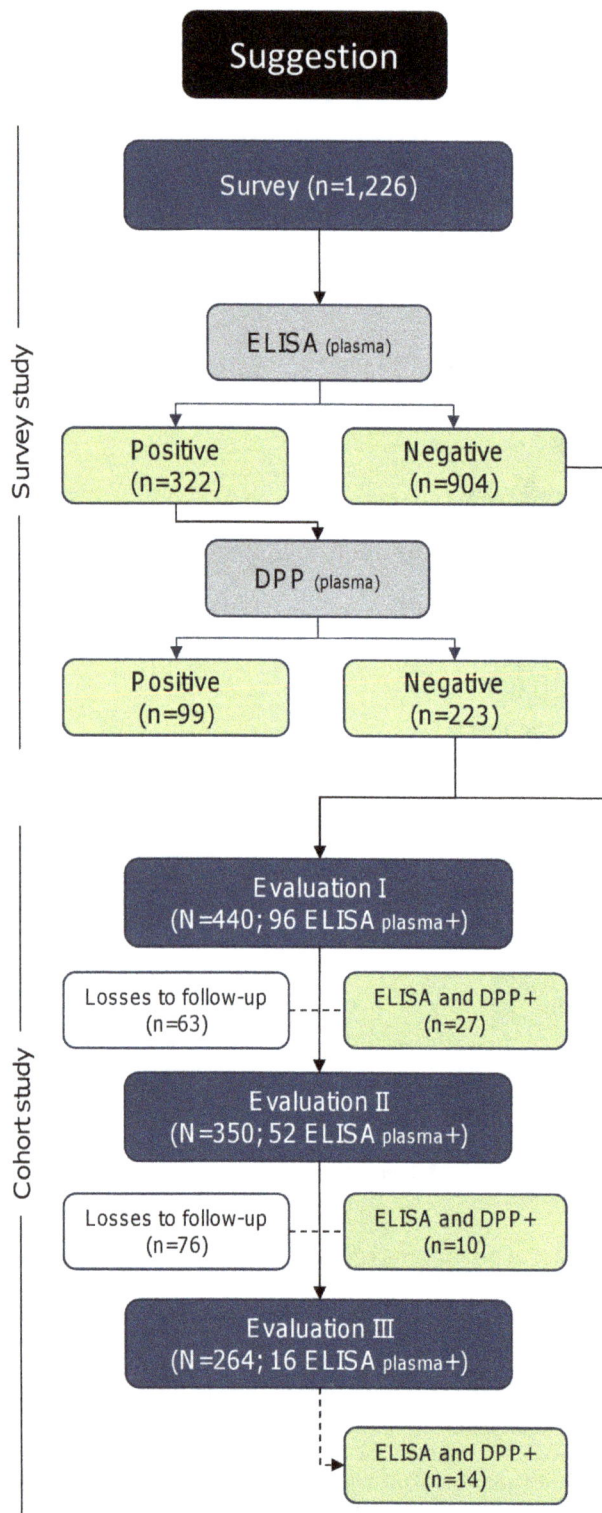

Figure 2. Study design using a new proposed method for screening and confirmation of canine visceral leishmaniasis.

Methods

Ethical Statement

The study was approved by the Committees of Ethics in Animal Experimentation of the Universidade Federal de Ouro Preto (protocol no. 083/2007), of the Universidade Federal de Minas Gerais (protocol no. 020/2007), and of the City Council of Belo Horizonte (protocol no. 001/2008). All procedures in this study were according to the guidelines set by the Brazilian Animal Experimental Collage (COBEA), Federal Law number 11794. Owners of the dogs participating in the project were informed of the research objectives and were required to sign the Informed Consent Form before sample collection.

Study Design: Initial Survey and Follow-up

Plasma samples were provided by the serobank of the Clinical Research Laboratory of the School of Pharmacy at the Federal University of Ouro Preto and were selected from a baseline survey and prospective cohort study performed from June 2008 to August 2010 in Belo Horizonte, Minas Gerais State, Brazil [7,10]. Briefly, a cross-sectional study was performed in the northwest sanitary district (36,874 km^2) of Belo Horizonte. According to zoonosis control management, the canine population comprised 20,883 dogs. With an expected positive rate of 5% to 10% for CVL in the study area 95% confidence interval (CI) and an estimated precision rate of 1.5%, the appropriate sample size for the study was 1,226 dogs. The field work was performed in close collaboration with the Municipal Health Service, and the data were collected during the canine survey census conducted by health agents as a routine procedure of the VLCSP.

The follow-up study was initiated 10 months after the baseline (evaluation I) with 447 dogs and blood samples were collected by venipuncture. Evaluations II and III were conducted 16 and 26 months after the baseline, respectively. All dogs included in evaluations II and III underwent the same procedures as used in evaluation I.

During the follow-up, losses occurred due to seropositivity in sequential tests, death, change of address, household closed, refusal, and dog escape (Fig. 1 and 2). The number of losses during follow-up in each evaluation changed according to the protocol employed in the diagnosis.

Collection of Blood Samples

A sample of peripheral blood (5 mL) was collected by puncture of the brachiocephalic vein, and an aliquot was transferred to a glass vial containing sufficient anticoagulant (ethylenediaminetet-raacetic acid) to achieve a final concentration of 1 mg/mL. Then the blood sample was transferred from the syringe to filter paper and maintained at room temperature until dry out. The filter paper sample was then sent to the Laboratory of Zoonosis of the Municipality of Belo Horizonte and analyzed. The blood sample was centrifuged (1,500–1,800 g, 20 min), and the plasma was collected and stored at −70°C from 3 to 5 years until it was assayed for the serological tests (DPP and ELISA) in the Laboratory of Immunopathology of the Federal University of Ouro Preto. Serological tests conducted in the Laboratory of Immunopathology were performed blind.

Serological Tests (ELISA, IFAT, and DPP)

Each sample was tested using two protocols established by the Brazilian Ministry of Health and a third protocol proposed by our group. In all protocols the tests were performed sequentially. The first used ELISA (Canine Leishmaniasis EIE Kit; Bio-Manguinhos/Fiocruz) for screening and IFAT (Canine Leishmaniasis IFI

Table 1. Estimated prevalence of canine visceral leishmaniasis using two strategies of serological sequential testing.

Diagnostics Methods	Prevalence (95% CI)
ELISA and IFAT (filter paper)	6.2 (4.9–7.7)
DPP and ELISA (plasma)	8.1 (6.6–9.8)

CI, confidence interval; DPP, Dual-Path Platform; ELISA, enzyme-linked immunosorbent assay; IFAT, immunofluorescent antibody test.

Kit; Bio-Manguinhos/Fiocruz) as a confirmatory test. This protocol used blood collected on filter paper (eluate) to perform the serological tests. The second protocol used the DPP CVL rapid test (Bio-Manguinhos/Fiocruz) for screening and ELISA (Canine Leishmaniasis EIE Kit) as a confirmatory test. This protocol used plasma for the serological tests. Both protocols followed the manufacturer's instructions. As an alternative, the third protocol used ELISA (Canine Leishmaniasis EIE Kit) for screening and DPP CVL rapid test for confirmation. The cut-off of the EIE Kit was defined based on the manufacturer's instructions and by considering the mean of the optical density of the negative controls multiplied by two. IFAT to detect anti-*Leishmania* IgG antibodies was performed as described by Camargo [26] using the Canine Leishmaniasis IFI Kit. Dogs with antibody titrations equal or higher than 1:40 were considered to be positive for disease.

Statistical Analysis

Statistical analysis was performed using Stata software (version 11.0; Stata Corp, College Station, TX). The prevalence and incidence rates indicated by ELISA, IFAT, and DPP were estimated using 95% CI.

Results

Serological Baseline Survey

Among the 1,226 dogs, 106, 169, and 322 dogs had seropositive results according to ELISA using filter paper (ELISA-FP), DPP, and ELISA using plasma (ELISA-PL), with estimated prevalence rates of 8.6% (95% CI, 7.1–10.4), 13.8% (95% CI, 11.8–16.0), and 26.3% (95% CI, 23.8–28.8), respectively. Among the ELISA-FP–positive results (106), 76 (71.7%) were confirmed by IFAT. Independent of the protocol of diagnostic test used in screening or confirmatory phase (DPP or ELISA-PL), the same number of dogs (99) was found positive for infection in both tests (Figs. 1 and 2).

After the confirmatory tests (sequential), the prevalence rates were 6.2% (95% CI, 4.9–7.7) for the first protocol (ELISA-FP and IFAT), 8.1% (95% CI, 6.6–9.8) for the second protocol (DPP and ELISA-PL), and 8.1% (95% CI, 6.6–9.8) for the third protocol (ELISA-PL and DPP) (Table 1).

Incidence of Seroconversion using Sequential Testing

According to ELISA-FP and IFAT, 27 seroconversions were observed in both tests within the study cohort, with an overall incidence rate of 2.8 per 1,000 dog-months (95% CI, 1.9–4.1). However, for DPP and ELISA-PL 51 seroconversions were observed, with an incidence rate of 5.4 per 1,000 dog-months (95% CI, 4.1–7.1) (Table 2).

Discussion

In the present study we compared, for the first time, the change of the protocols for the diagnosis of CVL in Brazil. We performed a baseline survey using 1,226 dogs, followed by a cohort study using 447 dogs. Our results showed that the protocol using the DPP and ELISA detected a higher prevalence (8.1%) and incidence (5.4/1,000 dog-months) of infected dogs than did the protocol using ELISA and IFAT (prevalence, 6.2%; incidence, 2.8/1,000 dog-months). Previous studies showed that DPP had good performance, with sensibility ranging from 93% to 100% and specificity ranging from 92% to 100% [25,27–29]. However, Grimaldi et al. [25] observed that the sensitivity depended on the clinical status, which was higher in symptomatic than in asymptomatic dogs. In the present study, the majority of dogs evaluated were classified as asymptomatic [7,10]; however, DPP and ELISA still showed better performance. It is important to note that the sensitivity of a diagnostic test changes during the clinical course of infection [30–31]. Quinnell et al. [33] evaluated the diagnostic performance of immunochromatographic dipstick

Table 2. Dog-months of follow-up, seroconversion in sequential testing, and incidence rates in Brazil.

Follow-up	Diagnostic Methods				
	ELISA and IFAT (Filter Paper)		DPP and ELISA (Plasma)		
	Seroconversion	Incidence Rate[d] (95% CI)	Seroconversion	Incidence Rate[d] (95% CI)	
Evaluation I[a]	10	1.9 (1.0–3.5)	27	5.1 (3.5–7.4)	
Evaluation II[b]	3	1.4 (0.5–4.5)	10	5.0 (2.7–9.3)	
Evaluation III[c]	14	6.2 (3.6–10.4)	14	6.4 (3.8–10.8)	
Total	27	2.8 (1.9–4.1)	51	5.4 (4.1–7.1)	

[a]At 10 months after baseline.
[b]At 16 months after baseline.
[c]At 26 months after baseline.
[d]Incidence rate per 1,000 dog-months. CI, confidence interval; DPP, Dual-Path Platform; ELISA, enzyme-linked immunosorbent assay; IFAT, immunofluorescent antibody test.

RDTs using rK39 antigen for CVL and showed that antibody responses to rK39 in natural infection develop slower than do responses to crude antigen. However, as observed in the present study, the combination of recombinant antigens rK39 and rK26, as in DPP, can improve this performance.

IFAT is the most widespread diagnostic method. For many years, IFAT was considered the serological reference test for CVL. However, this technique presented limitations such as low reproducibility, especially when filter paper was used, higher false-positive results because of cross-reactivity with *Trypanosoma cruzi*, *Trypanosoma caninum*, *Leishmania braziliensis*, and *Ehrlichia canis*, and false-negative results attributable to other factors [19–20,29]. Moreover, IFAT may be impractical for use in rural areas because of the lack of laboratory equipment and qualified technicians to interpret the results. Although ELISA also presented cross-reactivity, its sensitivity, specificity, and reproducibility were better than that of IFAT [20,28]. Furthermore, ELISA is an automated technique that enables the testing of a large number of samples simultaneously and is less subjective than IFAT. During the evaluation of serological cross-reactivity between CVL and *T. caninum*, Alves et al. [29] observed that a large percentage of dogs were erroneously diagnosed with CVL even after screening by ELISA and confirmation by IFAT. When evaluating the DPP test, this authors observed minor cross-reactivity [29]. Use of recombinant proteins, such as rK39 and rK26, has led to excellent results in the detection of human VL and CVL, independent of the diagnostic method used [28,31–34]. Additionally to the aspects mentioned above, the best results obtained with the new protocol are also associated to the quality of the samples analyzed; considering the higher sensitivity in plasma than when filter paper is used [15,35].

An improvement in the accuracy of the tests used for the diagnosis of CVL is critical for the VLCSP [18]. Considering the new protocol for CVL diagnosis and the results obtained in the present study, we believe it is important to discuss the factors related to the viability of using DPP in accordance with the logistics of the VLCSP.

The DPP has advantages such as easy storage, rapidity as a diagnostic method, ease of use, and flexibility in the type of biological samples used (blood, serum, or plasma) [24–25]. However, although the test can be used in the field with a simple visual assessment of positivity, the use of an optical reader increases the credibility of the results, as previously recommended by Grimaldi et al. [25]. Furthermore, the use of DPP in the field, in municipalities with a large number of cases, leads to a reduction in the number of dogs monitored daily by health agents, because it is necessary to collect samples, perform the assay in the home, and subsequently performs new blood collection in seropositive dogs for confirmation by ELISA. Another option is to perform the sample collection in seropositive dogs later; however, returning home with dogs that are declared seropositive by DPP results in a great loss of time and a loss of dogs, making this option impracticable in large municipalities or in large-scale surveys. With the first option, it is necessary to establish a daily routine of sending the blood samples to the laboratory for storage and processing. Because the logistics and structure of sending and processing are the same for large or small numbers of samples, collecting samples from all dogs and using diagnostic tests in the laboratory are better options. In this context, in many Brazilian states the recommendation is that blood collection in the field is carried out in all animals and sent to the Zoonosis Control Centers for DPP testing. Next, the positive samples are sent to the Central

Public Health Laboratories (LACENS). This eliminates the need to maintain a structured laboratory for performing ELISA in small municipalities. By using this methodology the Brazilian Ministry of Health reduces the demand for tests performed (ELISA) in the LACENS.

However, based on the current guidelines of the Ministry of Health and the data obtained in this study, we suggest to municipalities with a large demand of exams to use ELISA for automated screening and DPP as confirmatory test. This strategy would allow diagnosis in a laboratory where quality control can be easily implemented, thus facilitating the performance of large-scale screening tests. In addition, the cost of the ELISA reaction is lower (US $1.63) than the cost of the DPP test (US $2.72), when performed on large scale. Moreover, these values are related to the price of the tests only and do not include the transportation of inputs, acquisition and maintenance of equipment or training of specialized technicians.

All these methods need to be significantly improved because the results determine whether seropositive dogs in endemic areas will be euthanized. In addition to the direct consequence experienced by the dogs (euthanization), there are also consequences for the dog owners, such as emotional trauma. Furthermore, false-negative results are unacceptable because they may lead to the perpetuation of infection. A possible way to improve canine diagnosis is the use of ELISA with recombinant antigen, such as rK39 and rK26, since they exhibit excellent performance [15,34,36].

Important features of this study must be highlighted. The analysis assays were carried out with samples obtained in the epidemiological studies (i.e., cross-sectional and concurrent cohort) to evaluate prevalence and incidence in a large number of dogs evaluated in an urban endemic area.

To avoid diagnosis bias, the assays were performed in blind (DPP and ELISA). Also, we took care not to identify sample results according to previous exams of ELISA and IFAT carried out in filter paper.

In conclusion, the new protocol for diagnosis of CVL (DPP and ELISA) shows that the prevalence and incidence of infection are far greater than suggested by the previous protocol (ELISA and IFAT), indicating that the magnitude of infection in endemic areas has been underestimated. As tests are performed sequentially and euthanasia of the dog is carried out when the serological results are positive in both tests, the sequence does not affect the number of animals to be eliminated by the Control Program. Then, we suggest to municipalities with a large demand of exams to use ELISA for screening and DPP for confirmation because of its easy use and reduced costs.

Acknowledgments

The authors thank Bio-Manguinhos/Fiocruz, Rio de Janeiro, for providing the DPP, EIE Kit, and IFI Kit. The authors also thank the staff of the Secretaria Municipal de Saúde de Belo Horizonte, Minas Gerais, for their cooperation, logistical support, and special dedication to this work.

Author Contributions

Conceived and designed the experiments: WCV MC ABR. Performed the experiments: WCV HGK BMR RDOAS GGdAL NdDM LAMO EMdMM MHFM. Analyzed the data: WCV MC ABR. Contributed reagents/materials/analysis tools: MC ABR RCO. Wrote the paper: WCV MC ABR RCO HGK MHFM.

References

1. Ministério da Saúde (2006) Manual de vigilância e controle da leishmaniose visceral, 1st ed. Secretaria de Vigilância em Saúde, Brasília. Available: http://portal.saude.gov.br/portal/arquivos/pdf/manual_leish_visceral2006.pdf Accessed 8 December.

2. WHO (2010) Working to overcome the global impact of neglected tropical diseases: First WHO report on neglected tropical diseases. In: WHO, editor. Geneva. 184.

3. Molina R, Amela C, Nieto J, San-Andres M, Gonzalez F, et al. (1994) Infectivity of dogs naturally infected with *Leishmania infantum* to colonized *Phlebotomus perniciosus*. Trans R Soc Trop Med Hyg 88: 491–493.

4. Michalsky EM, Rocha MF, da Rocha Lima AC, Franca-Silva JC, Pires MQ, et al. (2007) Infectivity of seropositive dogs, showing different clinical forms of leishmaniasis, to *Lutzomyia longipalpis* phlebotomine sand flies. Vet Parasitol 147: 67–76.

5. Giunchetti RC, Mayrink W, Genaro O, Carneiro CM, Correa-Oliveira R, et al. (2006) Relationship between canine visceral leishmaniosis and the *Leishmania (Leishmania) chagasi* burden in dermal inflammatory foci. J Comp Pathol 135: 100–107.

6. Fraga DB, Solca MS, Silva VM, Borja LS, Nascimento EG, et al. (2012) Temporal distribution of positive results of tests for detecting *Leishmania* infection in stray dogs of an endemic area of visceral leishmaniasis in the Brazilian tropics: A 13 years survey and association with human disease. Vet Parasitol 190: 591–594.

7. Coura-Vital W, Marques MJ, Veloso VM, Roatt BM, Aguiar-Soares RD, et al. (2011) Prevalence and factors associated with *Leishmania infantum* infection of dogs from an urban area of Brazil as identified by molecular methods. PLoS Negl Trop Dis 5: e1291.

8. Barata RA, Peixoto JC, Tanure A, Gomes ME, Apolinario EC, et al. (2013) Epidemiology of visceral leishmaniasis in a reemerging focus of intense transmission in minas gerais state, Brazil. Biomed Res Int 2013: 405083.

9. Malaquias LC, do Carmo Romualdo R, do Anjos JB, Jr., Giunchetti RC, Correa-Oliveira R, et al. (2007) Serological screening confirms the re-emergence of canine leishmaniosis in urban and rural areas in Governador Valadares, Vale do Rio Doce, Minas Gerais, Brazil. Parasitol Res 100: 233–239.

10. Coura-Vital W, Reis AB, Fausto MA, Leal GGdA, Marques MJ, et al. (2013) Risk Factors for Seroconversion by *Leishmania infantum* in a Cohort of Dogs from an Endemic Area of Brazil. PLoS One 8: e71833.

11. Courtenay O, Quinnell RJ, Garcez LM, Shaw JJ, Dye C (2002) Infectiousness in a cohort of brazilian dogs: why culling fails to control visceral leishmaniasis in areas of high transmission. J Infect Dis 186: 1314–1320.

12. Costa CH (2011) How effective is dog culling in controlling zoonotic visceral leishmaniasis? A critical evaluation of the science, politics and ethics behind this public health policy. Rev Soc Bras Med Trop 44: 232–242.

13. Grimaldi G, Jr., Teva A, Santos CB, Ferreira AL, Falqueto A (2012) The effect of removing potentially infectious dogs on the numbers of canine *Leishmania infantum* infections in an endemic area with high transmission rates. Am J Trop Med Hyg 86: 966–971.

14. Nunes CM, Lima VM, Paula HB, Perri SH, Andrade AM, et al. (2008) Dog culling and replacement in an area endemic for visceral leishmaniasis in Brazil. Vet Parasitol 153: 19–23.

15. Rosario EY, Genaro O, Franca-Silva JC, da Costa RT, Mayrink W, et al. (2005) Evaluation of enzyme-linked immunosorbent assay using crude *Leishmania* and recombinant antigens as a diagnostic marker for canine visceral leishmaniasis. Mem Inst Oswaldo Cruz 100: 197–203.

16. Lira RA, Cavalcanti MP, Nakazawa M, Ferreira AG, Silva ED, et al. (2006) Canine visceral leishmaniosis: a comparative analysis of the EIE-leishmaniose-visceral-canina-Bio-Manguinhos and the IFI-leishmaniose-visceral-canina-Bio-Manguinhos kits. Vet Parasitol 137: 11–16.

17. Falqueto A, Ferreira AL, dos Santos CB, Porrozzi R, da Costa MV, et al. (2009) Cross-sectional and longitudinal epidemiologic surveys of human and canine Leishmania infantum visceral infections in an endemic rural area of southeast Brazil (Pancas, Espirito Santo). Am J Trop Med Hyg 80: 559–565.

18. Romero GA, Boelaert M (2010) Control of visceral leishmaniasis in Latin America a systematic review. PLoS Negl Trop Dis 4: e584.

19. Silva DA, Madeira MF, Teixeira AC, de Souza CM, Figueiredo FB (2011) Laboratory tests performed on *Leishmania* seroreactive dogs euthanized by the leishmaniasis control program. Vet Parasitol 179: 257–261.

20. Ferreira EC, de Lana M, Carneiro M, Reis AB, Paes DV, et al. (2007) Comparison of serological assays for the diagnosis of canine visceral leishmaniasis in animals presenting different clinical manifestations. Vet Parasitol 146: 235–241.

21. da Silva ES, van der Meide WF, Schoone GJ, Gontijo CM, Schallig HD, et al. (2006) Diagnosis of canine leishmaniasis in the endemic area of Belo Horizonte, Minas Gerais, Brazil by parasite, antibody and DNA detection assays. Vet Res Commun 30: 637–643.

22. Scalone A, De Luna R, Oliva G, Baldi L, Satta G, et al. (2002) Evaluation of the Leishmania recombinant K39 antigen as a diagnostic marker for canine leishmaniasis and validation of a standardized enzyme-linked immunosorbent assay. Vet Parasitol 104: 275–285.

23. de Arruda MM, Figueiredo FB, Cardoso FA, Hiamamoto RM, Brazuna JC, et al. (2013) Validity and reliability of enzyme immunoassays using Leishmania major or L. infantum antigens for the diagnosis of canine visceral leishmaniasis in Brazil. PLoS One 8: e69988.

24. Ministério da Saúde (2011) Esclarecimento sobre substituição do protocolo diagnóstico da leihsmaniose visceral canina; Nota técnica conjunta n° 01/2011 - CGDT-CGLAB/DEVIT/SVS/MS.

25. Grimaldi G, Jr., Teva A, Ferreira AL, dos Santos CB, Pinto IS, et al. (2012) Evaluation of a novel chromatographic immunoassay based on Dual-Path Platform technology (DPP(R) CVL rapid test) for the serodiagnosis of canine visceral leishmaniasis. Trans R Soc Trop Med Hyg 106: 54–59.

26. Camargo ME (1966) Fluorescent antibody test for the serodiagnosis of American trypanosomiasis. Technical modification employing preserved culture forms of Trypanosoma cruzi in a slide test. Rev Inst Med Trop Sao Paulo 8: 227–235.

27. Marcondes M, de Lima VM, de Araujo MD, Hiramoto RM, Tolezano JE, et al. (2013) Longitudinal analysis of serological tests officially adopted by the Brazilian Ministry of Health for the diagnosis of canine visceral leishmaniasis in dogs vaccinated with Leishmune. Vet Parasitol 197: 649–652.

28. Silva DA, Madeira Mde F, Abrantes TR, Filho CJ, Figueiredo FB (2013) Assessment of serological tests for the diagnosis of canine visceral leishmaniasis. Vet J 195: 252–253.

29. Alves AS, Mouta-Confort E, Figueiredo FB, Oliveira RV, Schubach AO, et al. (2012) Evaluation of serological cross-reactivity between canine visceral leishmaniasis and natural infection by Trypanosoma caninum. Res Vet Sci 93: 1329–1333.

30. Quinnell RJ, Courtenay O, Davidson S, Garcez L, Lambson B, et al. (2001) Detection of *Leishmania infantum* by PCR, serology and cellular immune response in a cohort study of Brazilian dogs. Parasitology 122: 253–261.

31. Quinnell RJ, Carson C, Reithinger R, Garcez LM, Courtenay O (2013) Evaluation of rK39 rapid diagnostic tests for canine visceral leishmaniasis: longitudinal study and meta-analysis. PLoS Negl Trop Dis 7: e1992.

32. da Costa RT, Franca JC, Mayrink W, Nascimento E, Genaro O, et al. (2003) Standardization of a rapid immunochromatographic test with the recombinant antigens K39 and K26 for the diagnosis of canine visceral leishmaniasis. Trans R Soc Trop Med Hyg 97: 678–682.

33. Romero HD, Silva Lde A, Silva-Vergara ML, Rodrigues V, Costa RT, et al. (2009) Comparative study of serologic tests for the diagnosis of asymptomatic visceral leishmaniasis in an endemic area. Am J Trop Med Hyg 81: 27–33.

34. Maia Z, Lirio M, Mistro S, Mendes CM, Mehta SR, et al. (2012) Comparative study of rK39 Leishmania antigen for serodiagnosis of visceral leishmaniasis: systematic review with meta-analysis. PLoS Negl Trop Dis 6: e1484.

35. Figueiredo FB, Madeira MF, Nascimento LD, Abrantes TR, Mouta-Confort E, et al. (2010) Canine visceral leishmaniasis: study of methods for the detection of IgG in serum and eluate samples. Rev Inst Med Trop Sao Paulo 52: 193–196.

36. Porrozzi R, Santos da Costa MV, Teva A, Falqueto A, Ferreira AL, et al. (2007) Comparative evaluation of enzyme-linked immunosorbent assays based on crude and recombinant leishmanial antigens for serodiagnosis of symptomatic and asymptomatic Leishmania infantum visceral infections in dogs. Clin Vaccine Immunol 14: 544–548.

23

Increased Mortality in Groups of Cattle Administered the β-Adrenergic Agonists Ractopamine Hydrochloride and Zilpaterol Hydrochloride

Guy H. Loneragan[1]*, Daniel U. Thomson[2], H. Morgan Scott[3]

1 International Center for Food Industry Excellence, Department of Animal and Food Sciences, College of Agriculture and Natural Resources, Texas Tech University, Lubbock, Texas, United States of America, 2 Department of Clinical Sciences, College of Veterinary Medicine, Kansas State University, Manhattan, Kansas, United States of America, 3 Department of Diagnostic Medicine/Pathobiology, College of Veterinary Medicine, Kansas State University, Manhattan, Kansas, United States of America

Abstract

The United States Food and Drug Administration (FDA) approved two β-adrenergic agonists (βAA) for in-feed administration to cattle fed in confinement for human consumption. Anecdotal reports have generated concern that administration of βAA might be associated with an increased incidence of cattle deaths. Our objectives, therefore, were to a) quantify the association between βAA administration and mortality in feedlot cattle, and b) explore those variables that may confound or modify this association. Three datasets were acquired for analysis: one included information from randomized and controlled clinical trials of the βAA ractopamine hydrochloride, while the other two were observational data on zilpaterol hydrochloride administration to large numbers of cattle housed, fed, and cared for using routine commercial production practices in the U.S. Various population and time at-risk models were developed to explore potential βAA relationships with mortality, as well as the extent of confounding and effect modification. Measures of effect were relatively consistent across datasets and models in that the cumulative risk and incidence rate of death was 75 to 90% greater in animals administered the βAA compared to contemporaneous controls. During the exposure period, 40 to 50% of deaths among groups administered the βAA were attributed to administration of the drug. None of the available covariates meaningfully confounded the relationship between βAA and increased mortality. Only month of slaughter, presumably a proxy for climate, consistently modified the effect in that the biological association was generally greatest during the warmer months of the year. While death is a rare event in feedlot cattle, the data reported herein provide compelling evidence that mortality is nevertheless increased in response to administration of FDA-approved βAA and represents a heretofore unquantified adverse drug event.

Editor: William Barendse, CSIRO, Australia

Funding: Initial funding for the evaluation of an association of ractopamine hydrochloride with death loss was provided by Elanco Animal Health, Greenfield, IN. In preparation for manuscript development, further analyses of ractopamine hydrochloride data and all analyses of zilpaterol hydrochloride data were performed solely in the service of the first author's employment at Texas Tech University. The funders had no role in study design, data collection and analysis, decision to publish, or preparation of the manuscript.

Competing Interests: I have read the journal's policy and have the following conflicts: GHL has accepted consulting fees for service on scientific advisory boards for Elanco Animal Health, and Intervet/Schering Plough (now known as Merck Animal Health) an dZoetis. In addition, GHL has received honoraria and paid travel expenses from Elanco Animal Health and Zoetis, and has served as a co-author with, and graduate advisor of, Elanco Animal Health personnel. DUT reports that Elanco Animal Health provided funds in support of the Beef Cattle Institute at Kansas State University of which DUT is the director. HMS reports no conflicts of interest related to either drug sponsor. The authors have no other competing interests such as employment, patents, products in development or marketed products.

* E-mail: Guy.Loneragan@TTU.edu

Introduction

The United States Food and Drug Administration (FDA) approved two β-adrenergic agonists (βAA) for in-feed administration to cattle that are fed in confinement (i.e., typically feedlot operations) for human consumption [1,2]. When administered according to label directions, βAA result in well-characterized and predictable improvements in the rate and efficiency of weight gain, as well as increased leanness and yield of edible products derived from beef carcasses [3–7]. Ractopamine hydrochloride (RH) was the first βAA approved in cattle; further, RH may be used in a variety of dosages and has also been approved for administration to swine and turkeys. Ractopamine hydrochloride is included in cattle feed during the final 28 to 42 days of the fattening period. Zilpaterol hydrochloride (ZH), the second βAA approved by the

FDA, may only be used at a single rate of inclusion in cattle feeds. It is included in cattle feed for 20 to 40 days prior to slaughter; however, in contrast to RH, a 3-day period during which ZH may not be administered must be observed prior to shipment to the abattoir (i.e., slaughter withholding).

In addition to their production uses in food-animal production, β-adrenergic agonists are routinely used in human clinical medicine for various conditions such as acute therapeutic intervention and maintenance care of asthma and chronic obstructive pulmonary disease (i.e., COPD). In human clinical medicine, these drugs are not innocuous in that side effects (or adverse unintended consequences) of approved medical uses of βAA have been observed and include an increased risk of asthma exacerbations and hospitalizations, arrhythmias, myocardial infarction, and death [8–12]. Unintended consequences have also been observed with βAA use in several animal species. For example, observations both in non-ruminant and ruminant species indicate that administration of βAA is associated, albeit somewhat inconsistently, with elevated heart rates, body temperature, physical activity, lameness or foot lesions, and aggression [13–18]. Given the widespread distribution of β-adrenoreceptors in the body, some of these unintended consequences, such as elevated heart rate, might (or ought to) be expected with βAA administration.

With some similarity to observations of increased risk of mortality associated with use of certain βAA in human clinical medicine [9,19], unpublished reports from some end-users of RH and ZH indicated the potential for an increase in mortality in cattle associated with FDA-approved administration of βAA. Mortality in feedlot cattle represents a clear and meaningful economic loss to producers. Death loss also raises broader societal concerns about the welfare of animals fed βAA in that progression from a healthy status to death may include in pain and suffering in affected animals. If a relationship between βAA administration and increased risk of mortality exists, it ought to stimulate discussion of the pros and cons of the use of drugs approved purely to improve the efficiencies of production yet offering no offsetting health benefits to the animals. As an example, some antibiotics are believed to improve production efficiency, at least in part, by controlling or preventing subclinical disease. To our knowledge, no beneficial 'side-effect' favoring improved health or welfare, or control or prevention of disease in response to FDA-approved βAA administration in cattle is believed to exist. Our objectives, therefore, were to: a) quantify the association between βAA administration and mortality in feedlot cattle, and b) explore those variables that may confound or modify this association.

Methods

Three confidential datasets were received either through solicitation by the first author in the case of RH or following requests for analytical support from the owners of the data (i.e., feedlot operators) in the case of ZH. The authors adhere to all the PLOS ONE policies on sharing data and materials. Different models were constructed and where possible and appropriate, a number of covariates (as potential and plausible confounders and effect modifiers) were evaluated. Datasets analyzed included both experimental trials (i.e., clinical trials involving randomized treatment allocation) and observational studies (i.e., treatment allocation was determined by factors other than a random process).

Description of Datasets

The first dataset (hereafter *4-company RH dataset*) included information concerning administration of RH. A convenience sample of cattle-feeding companies was contacted to evaluate whether or not they had performed field-based experiments of RH administration and, if so, to ascertain their willingness to provide their data for further analysis. Inclusion criteria included: a) experimental observations of RH administered to cattle pens according to label directions so as to provide a target dose of 200 mg/animal/day for the 28 to 42 days immediately prior to shipment to the abattoir, b) inclusion of appropriate contemporaneous control pens, and c) randomization performed either at the group level, or at the individual level. Groups were then classified as either unexposed in that all animals within the group were fed the usual fattening diet, or else as exposed in that all

animals within the group were fed the usual fattening diet with RH incorporated to provide the target dose.

This first aggregated dataset included information from four companies and collectively included 12 separate randomized experiments. All experiments used a randomized block design in that there were at least 2 groups per block, i.e., one administered RH and the other not. These data included information suitable for analysis on a total of 79,171 cattle. These animals were aggregated into 509 groups that averaged 155.5 (standard deviation [SD] = 70.9, minimum [MIN] = 42, maximum [MAX] = 381) animals per group. The number of studies and groups varied by company in that company A provided data on 1,510 animals that were enrolled in 1 study and housed in 24 groups, company B provided data on 5,696 animals across 3 studies and housed in 52 groups, company C provided data on 62,379 animals across 3 studies and housed in 329 groups, and company D provided data on 9,586 animals across 5 studies and housed in a total of 104 groups. The combined 6 studies conducted by companies B and C were conducted in 6 different feedlots whereas the 5 studies of company D were all conducted in the same feedlot. The vast majority of cattle were steers (i.e., castrated males; n = 72,868 in 441 groups) with the balance being females (i.e., heifers; n = 6,303 in 68 groups). Heifers were exclusively enrolled as the study population in 3 of the 5 experiments of company D.

The second dataset (*multi-feedlot ZH dataset*) concerned administration of ZH and included observational data from nine feedlots. Data on 722,704 animals were provided and the cattle were housed in 3,110 groups of an average size of 232.4 animals per group (SD = 91.3, MIN = 32, MAX = 943). Out of these animals, 79.3% (n = 573,076) were steers and 20.7% (n = 149,628) were heifers. The at-risk period of interest for exposed animals included both the period during which ZH was administered as well as the slaughter-withholding period. This slaughter-withholding period must be a minimum of 3 days but may be longer depending on various marketing strategies used by the feedlots. For the unexposed population in the multi-feedlot ZH dataset, the at-risk period was calculated by including the typical number of days ZH was administered to the exposed cohort and the typical slaughter-withholding period. Based on the observed and calculated at-risk periods for the exposed and unexposed cohorts, respectively, the mean at-risk periods consisted of the final 29.4 and 29.2 days prior to shipment, respectively. The data were unbalanced in that there were 2,775 groups comprised of 637,339 animals administered ZH (i.e., exposed cohort) and 335 groups comprised of 85,365 animals that served as comparative controls (i.e., unexposed cohort). The mean group sizes were 229.7 (SD = 90.7, MIN = 32, MAX = 943) and 254 (SD = 94.0, MIN = 55, MAX = 610), respectively. The number of animals per feedlot for which data were provided varied from 61,059 to 123,679. Heifers were represented in the data from 8 of the 9 feedlots.

The third dataset (*single-feedlot ZH dataset*) included observational data on 149,636 animals that were housed in 835 groups in a single feedlot. Of the population at risk, 88.7% (n = 132,725) were steers and 11.3% (n = 16,911) were heifers. The data were more balanced than the multi-feedlot ZH dataset in that 56.1% of the cattle (n = 83,865 in 470 groups) were administered ZH (i.e., exposed cohort) whereas 43.9% of the cattle (n = 65,711 in 365 groups) served as the contemporaneous control cohort. The mean group sizes were 178.4 (SD = 76.3, MIN = 30, MAX = 352) and 180.2 (SD = 63.9, MIN = 54, MAX = 382), respectively. The feedlot was managed in such a way that ZH was administered 21 days prior to shipment and a 3-day withdrawal period was observed. This 24-day period was considered the at-risk period.

Consequently, the final 24 days prior to shipment were considered the comparative at-risk period for those animals not administered ZH.

Data Analyses

The primary outcome variable of interest across all datasets was the number of animals that died in each group during the at-risk period (consequently, the group may be considered the experimental unit of interest). This outcome variable, therefore, represents a count response and the approaches described herein to model count data within groups in which the outcome may be clustered have been described [20–23]. Two offset variables were used as denominators in the various statistical models. The first was the natural logarithm of the population within a group (i.e., the at-risk population) at the start of the exposure period; the use of this offset allows calculation of model-adjusted estimates of the proportion the population at risk that died within each cohort [20]. Where the at-risk period varied across groups, i.e., in the 4-company RH and multi-feedlot ZH datasets, the natural logarithm of time at-risk was used (in other words, the total number of cattle-days within a group during the period of interest); the use of this offset allows calculation of model-adjusted estimates of the incidence of death (i.e., deaths per unit time) within each cohort [20]. Because information on the day during the at-risk period that individual animals died was only available for Company C in the RH dataset, a uniform approach to estimating time at risk (expressed as cattle-days) was used for the 4-company RH and multi-feedlot ZH datasets. Time at risk was estimated as a function of the at-risk period (days) multiplied by the population at risk. To account for withdrawals due to death, half of the total possible days at-risk was subtracted from the group's time at risk for each animal that died within the group.

Consistent across all datasets, therefore, were deaths within a group, whether they were administered a βAA or not, and population at risk. In addition, for the 4-company RH and multi-feedlot ZH datasets, time at risk was calculated using a common approach. Generalized linear mixed models were constructed using commercially available statistical analysis software (SAS System for Windows release 9.3, SAS Institute, Cary, NC) and parameterized similarly across datasets to account for the hierarchical nature of the data. A Poisson distribution was used with a log-link function. In all models, a group-level term was forced into the model to account for potential over-dispersion of the data (i.e., extra-Poisson variation). In the model of the 4-company RH dataset, random intercept terms were included for company, study within company, and block within study. In the multi-feedlot ZH dataset, a random intercept term was included to account for potential clustering of the outcome within feedlots. To explore potential modification of βAA effect on death loss across companies in the 4-company RH dataset and across feedlots in the multi-feedlot ZH dataset, the highest-level random-intercept term was changed from a random effect to a fixed effect to explore the interaction with exposure. Because of model convergence issues due to sparsely populated cells in the former dataset, when evaluating the interaction of feedlot and RH administration, data from company A was dropped from the model (i.e., n = 1,510 animals in 24 groups where no deaths were reported in either cohort).

Covariates were variably recorded across the three datasets. For example, within the 4-company RH dataset, the number of deaths within a group prior to exposure was relatively consistently recorded whereas month of shipment was only recorded for Company C. Further, in the multi-feedlot ZH dataset, a variety of covariates were consistently recorded and included: sex of the animals within a group, percentage of a group that died prior to the at-risk period, percentage of a group that were treated prior to the at-risk period, percentage of cattle within a group that had a predominantly black hide, mean carcass weight of the surviving animals that were shipped to slaughter, and month in which the at-risk period ended (i.e., animals were shipped to an abattoir for slaughter). However, in the single-feedlot ZH dataset only sex of the animal and the month in which the animals were shipped to an abattoir for slaughter were available for analysis. For each dataset, therefore, covariates that could potentially confound or modify the association between βAA use and death loss were evaluated in univariate models to test their association with mortality. Model structures were similar to those described above. Covariates with P values less than or equal to 0.20 were included as fixed effects in multivariable models that included main effects (i.e., potential confounders) and terms for the interaction of each of these main effects with exposure to βAA (i.e., effect-measure modifiers). While maintaining hierarchy within variables, terms were removed from the model in a backward, stepwise manner using $\alpha = 0.10$ level of significance for retention. For all models, measures of burden (proportion of population at risk and incidence of mortality per time at risk) and measures of effect (cumulative relative risk [RR] and incidence rate ratio [IRR], respectively) were computed from the model estimates and presented with their 95% confidence limits (CL) and P values where appropriate.

In addition to the primary outcome of mortality, secondary outcomes were available for both the multi-feedlot ZH and single-feedlot ZH datasets. Secondary count-based outcomes included number of animals treated for illness during the at-risk period and the number of carcasses that were classified as *dark, firm and dry* (which is colloquially referred to as *dark cutter* in the beef cattle industry). In addition, the proportion of cattle that could not be shipped to slaughter because they were within a slaughter-withholding period at the time the rest of the group was shipped was available in the single-feedlot dataset. This so-called *medicine hold* results from administration of a therapeutic drug, such as an injectable antimicrobial drug to treat bacterial bronchopneumonia; most such FDA-approved antimicrobial drugs have slaughter-withholding periods and these must be observed prior to shipment to slaughter for human consumption.

To explore the extent of unexplained model variation attributable to the levels of company and study within company, a multilevel, hierarchical model was constructed for the 4-company RH dataset using commercially available software (MLwiN 2.26, Centre for Multilevel Modelling, University of Bristol, Bristol, UK). Four levels of organization were included in the model: company, study within company, block within study, and group within block; generalized linear mixed models within a Poisson distribution were constructed. The dependent and offset variables were those described above and RH administration was the independent variable of interest. After accounting for RH administration as a fixed effect in the model, unexplained variation was partitioned to the highest 3 level terms (i.e., level 1 variance was not calculated given the assumptions of the Poisson model) [22]. Model estimation was performed using reweighted iterative generalized least squares and 2nd-order penalized quasi-likelihood approximation, while allowing for over-dispersion of the data [24].

Multivariable semi-parametric survival analysis was performed on the data provided by Company C owing to the rich level of detail available (Stata version 12.1, Stata Corp., College Station, TX). The multivariable model accounted for fixed effects of study, month of shipment to slaughter, prior mortality events experienced within the cohort, and exposure to RH. In addition, the model accounted for the shared frailty experience of animals within each group. Backwards elimination was employed to yield the final model (accounting for potential confounding variables and effect modifiers) and the importance of the shared group frailty was determined using the parameter Theta.

Results

4-company RH Dataset

Overall, 0.27% (n = 211) of the 79,171 cattle died during the at-risk period (Table 1). After accounting for various levels of clustering, the estimates of cumulative risk and the incidence rate of death were 0.26% (95% confidence limits [CL] = 0.16, 0.40) and 0.86 (95% CL = 0.58, 1.30) deaths per 10,000 cattle days, respectively. Model-adjusted estimates of risk and incidence of death for cattle administered RH were 0.34% (95% CL = 0.25, 0.45) and 1.12 (95% CL = 0.85, 1.45) deaths per 10,000 cattle days at risk, respectively. For cattle not administered RH, risk and incidence of death were 0.18% (95% CL = 0.13, 0.25) and 0.59 (95% CL = 0.43, 0.83) deaths per 10,000 cattle days, respectively.

After controlling for clustering within company, study, block and group, cattle administered RH were 91% more likely to die than control animals during the at-risk period (RR = 1.90 [95% CL = 1.38, 2.60]; $P<0.01$). A very similar measure of effect was observed for the incidence rate ratio (IRR = 1.90 [95% CL = 1.38, 2.61]; $P<0.01$). The only potential covariate collected across multiple studies was the number of animals that died in each group prior to the at-risk period. This variable neither modified the effect of exposure on mortality ($P=0.77$) nor did it confound the association between βAA and increased death loss ($P=0.63$). There was no evidence that the association between RH administration and increased death loss varied across the 3 companies that supplied data in which at least one death was observed ($P=0.66$; Figure 1). Moreover, in the multilevel hierarchical model that included all 4 companies, there was no unexplained variation attributed to unmeasured factors across companies (model variance = 0.00 [SE = 0.00]). At lower levels of organization, the unexplained model variation was 4-fold greater among blocks within studies (model variance = 0.169 [SE = 0.120]) than among studies within companies (model variance = 0.048 [SE = 0.072]).

Company C provided information on 167 deaths across 1,983,564 animal-days and within this company, the incidence of death was 83% greater among those animals administered RH compared to controls (IRR = 1.83; 95% CL = 1.32, 2.56; $P<0.01$). A graphical representation of the unadjusted Kaplan-Meier non-parametric survival experiences for each set of treatment cohorts is presented in Figure 2. The smoothed instantaneous force of mortality for each cohort set (i.e., the hazard function [h(t)]) is presented in Figure 3 and suggests that the constant hazard assumption was met for approximately the first 25–28 days of the at risk period. Moreover, the proportional hazards assumption was met throughout the entire at-risk period. In addition, the pen-level mortality rate prior to exposure was evaluated as a covariate but was neither associated with the incidence of death during exposure ($P=0.61$), nor did this variable confound the relation between exposure to RH and survivor function. Importantly, the multi-variable adjusted treatment hazard ratio (HR) of 2.00 (95% CL = 1.36, 2.96; $P<0.01$) was greater than that observed when the other significant covariates (i.e., fixed effects of feedlot and month of slaughter) and the shared frailties of group were ignored. Because the force of mortality (hazard) was relatively constant over time, the HR is comparable to IRR; the observed IRR was 1.83 and was included within the 95% confidence interval of the HR.

Multi-feedlot ZH Dataset

Of the 722,704 cattle at risk, 0.51% (n = 3,657) of animals died during the exposure period (Table 1). After accounting for feedlot- and group-level clustering, the estimates of risk and incidence of death were 0.50% (95% CL = 0.44, 0.57) and 1.68 (95% CL = 1.51, 1.86) deaths per 10,000 animal-days, respectively. Model-adjusted estimates of the risk and incidence of death for cattle administered ZH were 0.53% (95% CL = 0.47, 0.59) and 1.77 (95% CL = 1.62, 1.92) deaths per 10,000 animal-days, respectively. Model-adjusted estimates among the unexposed cohort were 0.30 (95% CL = 0.25, 0.36) and 1.01 (95% CL = 0.85, 1.19) deaths per 10,000 animal-days, respectively. After adjusting for the various levels of clustering, administration of ZH was associated with a significant increase in the likelihood of death (RR = 1.76 [95% CL = 1.50, 2.05]; $P<0.01$). When time at risk during the exposure period was used as the offset variable instead of population at risk, the measure of effect was similar in that the IRR was 1.75 (95% CL = 1.50, 2.05; $P<0.01$).

Covariates included in the multivariable model as main effects (i.e., potential confounders) along with terms representing their interactions with exposure to ZH (i.e., effect modifiers) included (Table 2):

- Sex of the animals within a group,
- Percentage of a group that died prior to the at-risk period,
- Percentage of a group that were treated prior to the at-risk period,
- Percentage of cattle within a group that had a predominantly black hide,
- Mean carcass weight of the surviving animals that were shipped to slaughter, and
- Month in which the at-risk period ended (i.e., animals were shipped to an abattoir for slaughter).

Of the main effect terms, only percentage of a group that died prior to the at-risk period and mean carcass weight of animals shipped to slaughter were removed from the final model. The only effect modifier (i.e., interaction term) that was retained was month in which the animals were shipped to the abattoir ($P=0.07$). While controlling for the other covariates, RR estimates were 1.17 (95% CL = 0.64, 2.14; $P=0.60$; Figure 4); 1.56 (95% CL = 0.86, 2.82; $P=0.15$); 1.23 (95% CL = 0.87, 1.73; $P=0.24$); 2.69 (95% CL = 1.86, 3.90; $P<0.01$); 1.80 (95% CL = 1.28, 2.53; $P<0.01$); 1.86 (95% CL = 1.42, 2.43; $P<0.01$) and 1.71 (95% CL = 1.18, 2.49; $P=0.01$) for March, April, May, June, July, August, and September, respectively.

Averaged across the means of all other terms in the model, treatment remained significantly associated with mortality (RR = 1.66 [95% CL = 1.40, 1.96]; $P<0.01$). Thus, its effect did not appear to be confounded to any meaningful extent by other variables (those listed in bullet form above) in that the measure of effect from the multivariable model was similar to the reduced model in which only exposure was included as a fixed effect.

The same set of covariates listed above were associated with the incidence rate of death in univariate models; that is, the models in which when time at risk was included as the offset variable. These variables were subsequently included as covariates (main effects and effect modifiers) in the multivariable model of the incidence of death. While the same main effects were retained in the final model as those for the population at-risk model, no effect modifiers were retained in the final model (i.e., $P>0.14$ for all interaction terms). Controlling for the covariates that remained in the model (i.e., sex, month shipped to slaughter, percent of the group with a

Table 1. Summary statistics for death loss (counts, and crude and model-adjusted estimates) by dataset for all cattle, the exposed cohort (i.e., groups of cattle administered either ractopamine hydrochloride [RH] or zilpaterol hydrochloride [ZH]), and the unexposed cohort.

Dataset	Cohort	Statistic						
		Population at risk (n)	Deaths (n)	Crude estimate of cumulative risk (%)	Model-adjusted cumulative risk (%)	95% confidence limits	Model-adjusted incidence (deaths/10,000 animal days)	95% confidence limits
4-company RH dataset	All cattle	79,171	211	0.27	0.26	0.16, 0.40	0.86	0.58, 1.30
	Exposed	39,890	139	0.35	0.34	0.25, 0.41	1.12	0.85, 1.45
	Unexposed	39,281	72	0.18	0.18	0.13, 0.25	0.59	0.43, 0.83
Multi-feedlot ZH dataset	All cattle	722,704	3,657	0.51	0.50	0.44, 0.57	1.68	1.51, 1.86
	Exposed	637,339	3,405	0.53	0.53	0.44, 0.59	1.77	1.62, 1.92
	Unexposed	85,365	252	0.30	0.30	0.25, 0.36	1.01	0.85, 1.19
Single-feedlot ZH dataset	All cattle	149,636	571	0.38	0.38	0.35, 0.42	*	*
	Exposed	83,865	401	0.48	0.48	0.43, 0.43	*	*
	Unexposed	65,771	170	0.26	0.26	0.22, 0.31	*	*

* Not calculated as both cohorts had the same exposure period of 24 days.

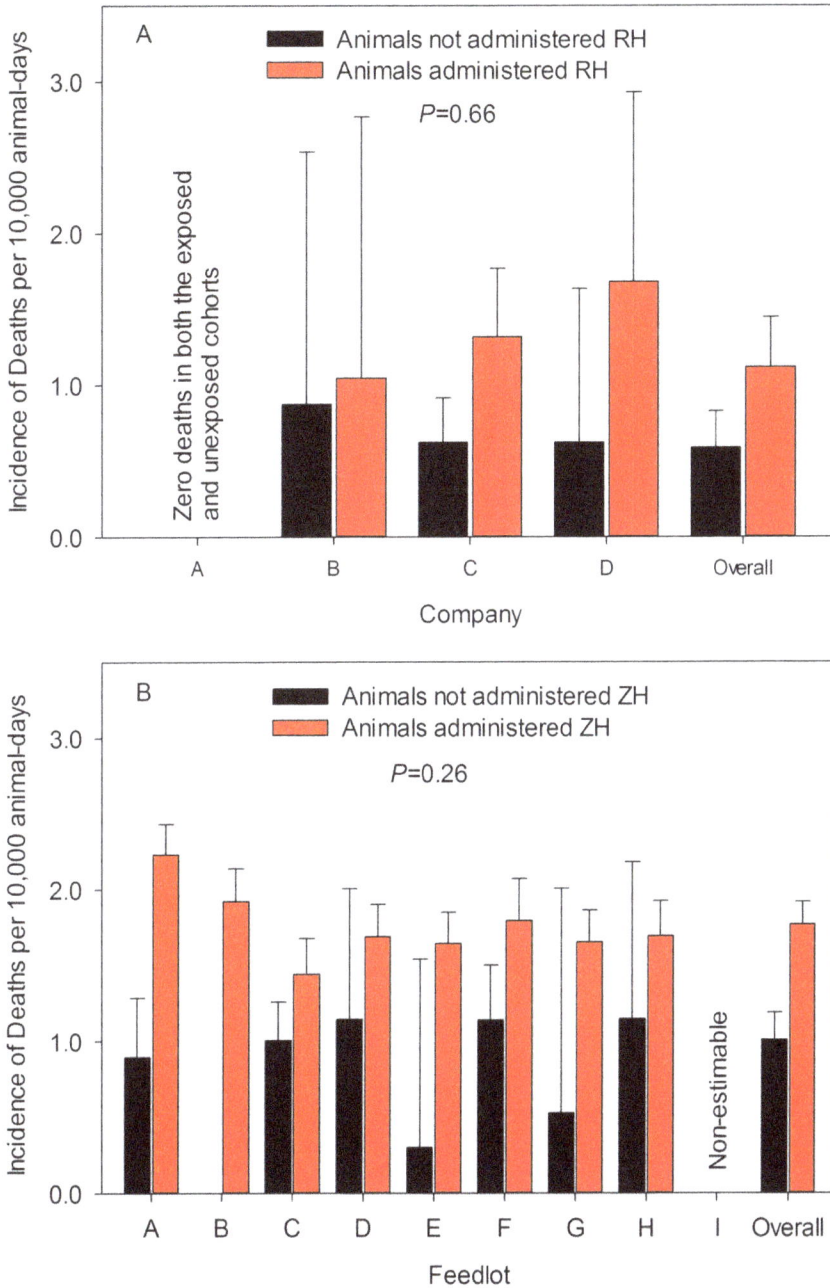

Figure 1. Association between β-adrenergic agonist administration and mortality. Model-adjusted estimates of incidence of death per 10,000 animal-days for cattle administered either ractopamine hydrochloride (RH – graph A) or zilpaterol hydrochloride (ZH – graph B) compared to a diet without a beta agonist. No deaths were reported for Company A (graph A) and rates for Feedlot I (graph B) were non-estimable. P values are those associated with interaction term for exposure by company (graph A) or feedlot (graph B). Bars represent upper 95% confidence limit.

black hide, and percent of pen treated prior to the at-risk period), the incidence of death was 80% greater in animals administered ZH than the comparative control cohort (IRR = 1.80 [95% CL = 1.55, 2.10]; P<0.01). The association between incidence rate of death and administration of βAA, therefore, did not appear to be confounded by the covariates available for analysis.

There was little evidence of feedlot-to-feedlot variation in the association between ZH and increased risk of death. In the population at-risk model, for example, the covariance parameter was much greater at the group-level (1.14 [SE = 0.03]) than that observed at the feedlot-level (0.04 [SE = 0.02]). In the alternative

model that treated feedlot and its interaction with exposure as ZH fixed effects, there was no evidence that the association between administration of ZH and increased mortality was modified by which feedlot the animals were housed in either the population at risk (P = 0.16) or time at risk models (P = 0.26; Figure 1).

Two secondary outcomes were available for analysis (Table 3). Cattle administered ZH were 33% more likely (RR = 1.33 [95% CL = 1.18, 1.50]; P<0.01) to require treatment for illness during the at-risk period than animals not administered ZH. In addition, an association between ZH administration and an increased likelihood of the animal's beef being classified as *dark, firm and dry*

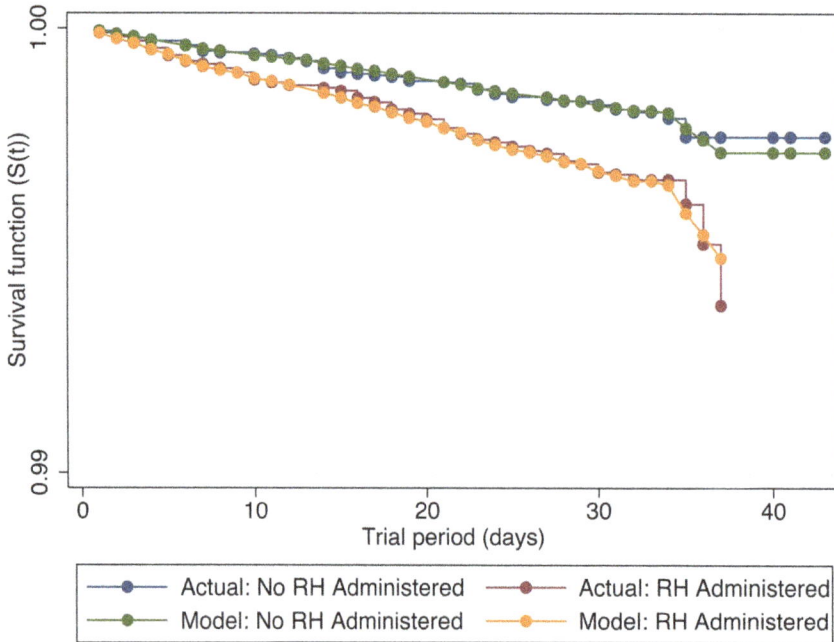

Figure 2. Survival analysis for cattle administered a β-adrenergic agonist. Kaplan-Meier non-parametric (actual) and Cox proportional hazards (predicted) survivor functions (S(t)) for cattle administered a diet containing ractopamine hydrochloride (RH) compared to a diet without RH in Company C.

was detected (Table 4); however, this latter association was modified by the sex of the animal ($P = 0.01$). The carcasses derived from steers administered ZH were 2.31 times more likely to be classified as *dark, firm and dry* compared to carcasses of steers not administered ZH (RR = 2.31 [95% CL = 1.77, 3.02]; $P<0.01$). Of the steer carcasses, 1.87 and 0.81%, of those administered ZH and

the unexposed cohort, respectively, were classified as *dark, firm and dry*. No such association was observed with treatment among the carcasses derived from heifers ($P = 0.36$); of the heifer carcasses, 1.30 and 1.07%, of those administered ZH and the unexposed cohort, respectively, were classified as *dark, firm and dry*.

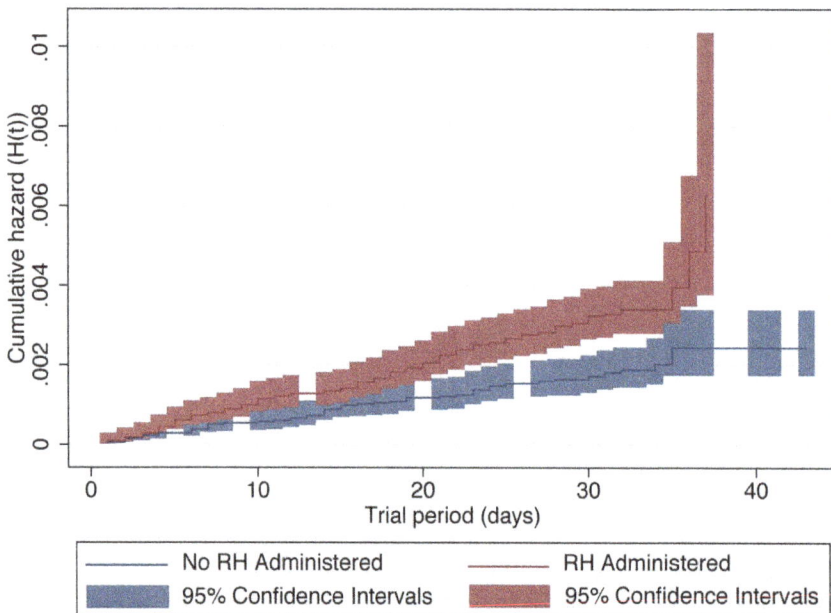

Figure 3. Force of mortality among cattle administered a β-adrenergic agonist. Empirical cumulative hazard function (H(t)) and 95% confidence intervals (during those time periods where mortalities occurred) for cattle administered a diet containing ractopamine hydrochloride (RH) compared to a diet without RH in Company C.

Table 2. Covariates evaluated for an association with mortality in groups of cattle either administered zilpaterol hydrochloride (ZH) or not in the multi-feedlot ZH dataset in univariate and multivariable models.

Measure of mortality in groups of cattle	Covariate	Univariate model		Multivariable model			
		P value	Included in multivariate model	Main effect P value*	Retained in final model	P value* of interaction term**	Retained in final model
Cumulative risk (%)	Sex of the animals within a group	<0.01	Yes	<0.01	Yes	0.46	No
	Percentage of a group that died prior to the at-risk period	0.13	Yes	0.31	No	0.39	No
	Percentage of a group that were treated prior to the at-risk period	<0.01	Yes	<0.01	Yes	0.41	No
	Percentage of cattle within a group that had a predominantly black hide	<0.01	Yes	<0.01	Yes	0.66	No
	Mean carcass weight of the surviving animals that were shipped to slaughter	<0.01	Yes	0.77	No	0.73	No
	Month in which the at-risk period ended	<0.01	Yes	<0.01	Yes	0.07	Yes
	Days at the feedlot prior to exposure	0.23	No	–	–	–	–
Incidence (deaths/10,000 animal-days)	Sex of the animals within a group	<0.01	Yes	<0.01	Yes	0.42	No
	Percentage of a group that died prior to the at-risk period	0.05	Yes	0.70	No	0.49	No
	Percentage of a group that were treated prior to the at-risk period	<0.01	Yes	<0.01	Yes	0.50	No
	Percentage of cattle within a group that had a predominantly black hide	<0.01	Yes	<0.01	Yes	0.85	No
	Mean carcass weight of the surviving animals that were shipped to slaughter	<0.01	Yes	0.50	No	0.95	No
	Month in which the at-risk period ended	<0.01	Yes	<0.01	Yes	0.14	No
	Days at the feedlot prior to exposure	0.91	No	–	–	–	–

Administration of ZH was associated with mortality ($P < 0.01$) in all multivariable models.
*P value indicated was that observed at the time of removal from the multivariable model if > 0.10, or if retained, i.e., ≤ 0.10, its value in the final multivariable model.
** Interaction term of the covariate with administration of ZH, i.e., evaluation of potential modification of the association between death loss and administration.

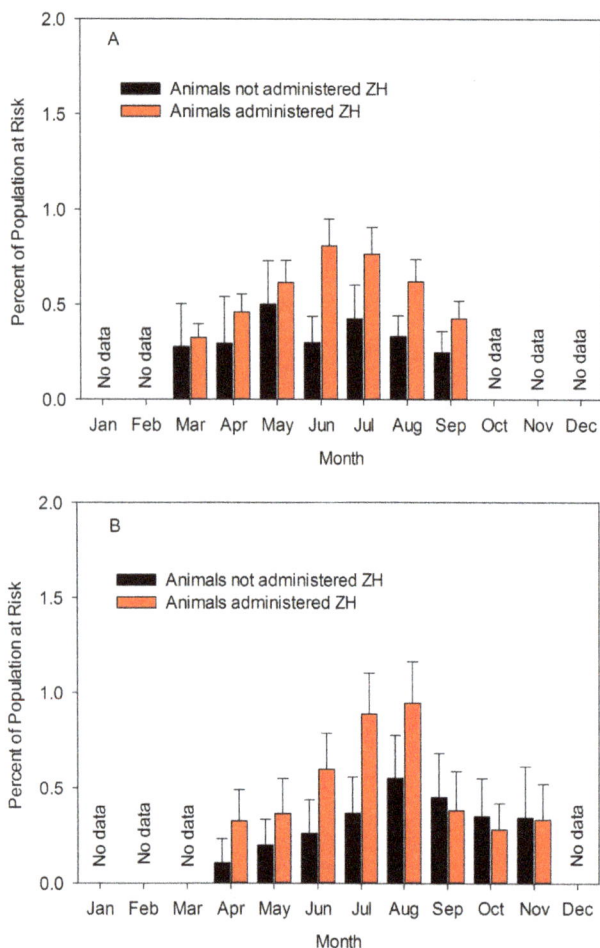

Figure 4. Seasonal modification of the association between β-adrenergic agonist administration and mortality. Model-adjusted estimates of the percentage of cattle that died among groups of animals administered zilpaterol hydrochloride (ZH) compared to a diet without ZH by month in which they were shipped to slaughter. Graph A represents 722,704 animals housed in 9 feedlots and graph B represents 149,636 animals housed in a single feedlot.

Single-feedlot ZH Dataset

Of the 149,636 cattle at risk, 0.38% (n = 571) died during the 24-day exposure period and after accounting for potential over-dispersion in the data, the 95% CL of this estimate were 0.35% and 0.42%, respectively (Table 1). Model-adjusted estimates of the risk of death among those administered ZH and the comparative cohort were 0.48% (95% CL = 0.43, 0.53) and 0.26% (95% CL = 0.22, 0.31), respectively. After adjusting for clustering, administration of ZH was associated with an 85% increase in the risk of death (RR = 1.85 [95% CL = 1.51, 2.27]; $P<0.01$) during the at-risk period. Mortalities were classified as attributable to conditions either of the respiratory system or of the digestive system (this latter category also included all other attributable causes of death). After adjusting for clustering, administration of ZH was associated with an increase in the risk of death attributable to conditions of the respiratory (RR = 2.15 [95% CL = 1.60, 2.91]; $P<0.01$) and digestive (RR = 1.82 [95% CL = 1.31, 2.52]; $P<0.01$) systems.

Overall mortality was associated with sex and month of slaughter; in addition to their interactions with exposure, these

Table 3. Cumulative risk of treatment for disease among the exposed cohort (i.e., groups of cattle administered zilpaterol hydrochloride [ZHl]) and the unexposed cohort.

Dataset	Disease grouping	Cohort	Statistic Cumulative risk (%)	95% confidence limits	Relative risk	95% confidence limits	P value
Multi-feedlot ZH dataset	All diseases	Exposed	1.35	1.13, 1.62	1.33	1.18, 1.50	<0.01
	All diseases	Unexposed	1.01	0.83, 1.24	–	–	–
Single-feedlot ZH dataset	All diseases	Exposed	1.33	1.22, 1.46	1.23	1.07, 1.41	<0.01
	All diseases	Unexposed	1.09	0.98, 1.21	–	–	–
	Respiratory	Exposed	0.86	0.78, 0.95	2.31	0.55, 0.79	<0.01
	Respiratory	Unexposed	0.37	0.31, 0.44	–	–	–
	Digestive and other	Exposed	0.47	0.42, 0.54	0.66	0.55, 0.79	<0.01
	Digestive and other	Unexposed	0.72	0.63, 0.81	–	–	–

main effects were included in a final multivariable model. The final model included sex, month and the interaction between ZH exposure and month. Averaged across other variables, animals exposed to ZH were 56% more likely to die than animals in the comparative cohort (RR = 1.56 [95% CL = 1.25, 1.95]; $P<0.01$). However, this effect was modified by the month in which animals were shipped to the abattoir ($P = 0.01$). Model-adjusted RR estimates were 3.06 ($P = 0.01$; Figure 4); 1.83 ($P = 0.07$); 2.30 ($P<0.01$); 2.42 ($P<0.01$); 1.72 ($P = 0.01$); 0.85 ($P = 0.58$), 0.80 ($P = 0.47$) and 0.97 ($P = 0.94$) for April, May, June, July, August, September, October, and November, respectively.

A number of secondary outcomes were available for analysis in this third dataset (Table 3). Animals administered ZH were 23% more likely to require treatment for any condition during the exposure period (RR = 1.23 [95% CL = 1.07, 1.41]; $P<0.01$). The likelihood of treatment, however, varied by the body system to which the clinical signs were attributed. Animals were 34% less likely to require treatment for conditions attributed to the digestive system (RR = 0.66 [95% CL = 0.55, 0.79]; $P<0.01$) but 2.3 times more likely to require treatment for conditions attributed to the respiratory system (RR = 2.31 [95% CL = 1.89, 2.83]; $P<0.01$). In addition, animals administered ZH were 2.3 times more likely to require more than a single treatment regimen for respiratory disease than contemporaneous controls (RR = 2.34 [95% CL = 1.82, 3.04]; $P<0.01$). As a consequence of the increased burden of treatments in animals administered ZH, there was a 3-fold increase in the percentage of animals subject to a slaughter withholding period at the time the rest of their group was shipped to slaughter (RR = 3.00 [95% CL = 2.31, 3.90]; $P<0.01$). Those animals that could not be shipped to slaughter with their contemporaries were dispersed across many groups rather than clustered within a few; that is, 50.0% of groups administered ZH had one or more animals that could not be shipped with the rest of their group compared to 25.8% of groups not administered ZH.

Once at the abattoir, a greater percentage of carcasses from ZH administered cattle (1.59%) were classified as dark, firm and dry (Table 4), compared to those carcasses from animals not administered ZH (0.53%; RR = 3.02 [95% CL = 2.35, 3.89]; $P<0.01$). As opposed to the 9-feedlot dataset, sex was neither a modifier of this association ($P = 0.21$) nor a significant covariate ($P = 0.34$).

Discussion

Death is a relatively rare event in feedlot cattle [25,26]. Even so, the data presented herein provide compelling evidence that administration of FDA-approved βAA to cattle increased both the cumulative incidence (risk) and incidence rate of death. The various measures of effect used to explore the relationship between βAA and mortality, i.e., RR, IRR and HR where applicable, were similar across the multiple datasets that included both randomized field trials and population-based observational data. The attributable fraction (AF), a measure of the proportion of deaths attributable to βAA administration among those cattle in the exposed cohort, varied little from dataset to dataset, remaining relatively constant at 40–50%.

Of considerable practical interest among those responsible for the care and well-being of cattle intended for slaughter for human consumption is identification of variables that could be exploited to help select or manage groups of cattle for which βAA drugs might be contraindicated. The most consistent modifier of the biological association between βAA administration and mortality was month of year (Figure 4). In the multi-feedlot ZH data set, month was statistically detected as an effect modifier in one model

Table 4. Prevalence of carcasses classified as *dry, dark, and firm* among the exposed cohort (i.e., groups of cattle administered zilpaterol hydrochloride [ZH]) and the unexposed cohort.

Dataset	Cohort	Statistic Prevalence (%)	95% confidence limits	P value associated with main effect comparison	P value associated with interaction with sex	Prevalence among steers (%)	95% confidence limits	Prevalence among heifers (%)	95% confidence limits
Multi-feedlot ZH dataset	Exposed	1.75	1.11, 2.75	<0.01	0.01	1.87	1.19, 2.95	1.30	0.82, 2.05
	Unexposed	0.86	0.53, 1.40	–	–	0.81	0.49, 1.33	1.07	0.60, 1.89
Single-feedlot ZH dataset	Exposed	1.59	1.43, 1.78	<0.01	0.21	1.57	1.39, 1.78	1.70	1.30, 2.22
	Unexposed	0.53	0.42, 0.66	–	–	0.50	0.40, 0.64	0.93	0.44, 1.96

(i.e., population at-risk) but not in the other model (i.e., time at-risk). However, in the latter model, the observed P value (0.14) provided some, albeit weak, evidence of variation in the association across months. In the single-feedlot ZH dataset, month was again detected as a significant modifier of the association between βAA administration and mortality ($P = 0.01$). Furthermore, the consistency of the temporal pattern of this association across the multi- and single-feedlot ZH datasets (Figure 4) provides compelling reasons to explore seasonal factors that might modify the effect of βAA administration on mortality. By this we mean that month is clearly a proxy for other variables with the most probable being thermal heat index. Given the variation in the measure of effect across months, at least for ZH, it seems plausible that greater heat indices may have contributed to a disproportionate increase in the risk of death among animals administered βAA when compared to those not administered this synthetic hormone. It was not possible, however, to test this association in our analysis; clearly this warrants additional prospective exploration. If month is indeed a proxy for a causal biological interaction between some measure of heat index and βAA administration, then mitigation strategies, as yet unknown, need to be developed for a substantial proportion of the year in that a significant relationship was detected in those cattle shipped for slaughter beginning in April (in the single-feedlot ZH dataset) and for those cattle shipped for slaughter through September (in the multi-feedlot ZH dataset).

Force of mortality, which is sometimes referred to as the hazard function, is an instantaneous measure of the risk of death in the next time period, conditioned on having survived to the present. This measure was greater for those animals administered RH than unexposed animals and was relatively constant for both groups across the majority of the exposure period for company C. The apparent late-stage increase (Figure 3) in the hazard function among the RH-treated groups of animals, when compared to the control groups of animals, did not lead to a violation of the proportional hazards assumption of the semi-parametric survival analysis. However, this increase appeared quite marked and bears further examination in any follow-up research. Unfortunately, days of exposure for each animal that died were only available for company C and included 3 large randomized trials of RH of 62,379 animals. Consequently, the force of mortality for those cattle administered ZH could not be evaluated.

A number of broad hypotheses might explain the observed association of βAA drug administration and increased mortality. The first potential hypothesis is that other unmeasured confounding variable(s) gave rise to a spurious relationship. For example, in the ZH datasets, the contemporaneous control cohorts consisted of those animals not administered a βAA. There are various reasons why these animals were not fed a βAA. For example, they may have been destined for a marketing program that precluded the use of a βAA or they were deemed not suitable for βAA administration (e.g., their body weight was sufficient enough that if fed a βAA hormone, their carcass weights would have been excessive). While it is possible that these unmeasured variables confounded the association of βAA use and increased death loss, it seems highly improbable given the strength of association and consistency of effect across feedlots, datasets, and the covariates evaluated in the models. This possibility seems even more implausible in the dataset involving RH. Each of the 12 studies included randomized allocation of animals or groups to the exposed or unexposed cohorts. One of the major benefits of randomization is the unbiased distribution of unmeasured confounders among the treatment groups. Furthermore, apart from company A in which no deaths in either cohort were

reported, statistical variation among the measured associations of RH administration and mortality was not detected among companies B, C, and D. In addition, no statistical variation in the association between βAA and increased death loss was observed across feedlots in the multi-feedlot ZH dataset. This association, therefore, was relatively consistent and predictable from operation to operation despite unmeasured variation in farming practices and other attributes such as feedlot size, geographical location, animal husbandry, and cattle diets.

A second and related hypothesis is that the association was not necessarily due to the drug itself; rather, the association might have been a consequence of those management changes required to administer the βAA in the ration. Such collinearity of effects is virtually impossible to disentangle without purposively designing a study (e.g., a cross-over design) to deal with the phenomenon. For example, although not available in the data described herein, it is possible that the time at which feed was delivered changed for those animals administered a βAA. That is, most modern cattle feedlots have developed strategies to provide a consistent diet in a consistent and timely manner to the cattle. In this scheme, the amount of feed delivered is expected to be consumed within 24 hours. Because a minority of groups of cattle are fed βAA at any one time in an feedlot, one management strategy might be to feed the unexposed cattle first and subsequently feed the ration containing the βAA later in the day. If so, this strategy could have resulted in a relatively sudden change in the time at which the βAA-exposed cattle were fed (possibly up to a 2-hour delay for example). While cattle tend to adapt relatively quickly to changes in routine, such a change might have initially resulted in cattle that were hungry and thus over-consumed readily fermentable carbohydrates. However, the observed force of mortality was relatively constant over the exposure period (i.e., from day 0 up to 42). The feedlots that supplied data for the 2 observational datasets have had a number of years of experience in feeding the FDA-approved βAA and have had the opportunity to develop and adopt management strategies to minimize changes in routine.

A third hypothesis is that the βAA hormones themselves are causally associated with the increased mortality. Clearly, the measure of effects are relatively strong and consistent across the datasets; yet, given that the RH studies were not purposefully designed to investigate an association with mortality and the observational nature of the ZH data, it is difficult to definitively establish a causal relationship nor to identify the mechanistic explanations. However, evidence supporting adverse drug events can be drawn from the aggregated observations of βAA administration in human medicine. For example, authors of various studies that included randomized clinical trials and an FDA-performed meta-analysis of the available data, have concluded that long-acting β2 adrenergic agonists used for asthma contribute to an increased risk of severe asthma events and death [8,9,11,19]. While this association might be somewhat ameliorated by the inclusion of a corticosteroid, the FDA determined this was a class effect and now requires a boxed warning to be included on the labels of all long-acting βAA intended to be administered routinely, e.g., daily for the control of asthma. Furthermore, in the datasets of ZH in which risk of treatment was available, exposed animals were more likely to require treatment during the at-risk period than unexposed animals.

Others have reported an increased risk of myocardial disease in certain patients administered βAA drugs [12]. If a similar association occurs in cattle, one might expect metabolic markers of such an event, elevated creatine phosphokinase (CPK) for example [27]. Indeed, ZH administration is associated with increased serum CPK [2]; unfortunately the isoform(s) were not reported so it is uncertain if the elevated serum CPK resulted from damage to striated muscle, myocardial tissue, or both.

After accounting for the effect of exposure, most of the unexplained variation in mortality occurred at the level of the group rather than at the organizational levels of the study, feedlot, or company depending on the dataset. Moreover, there was almost no (and at times zero) unexplained variation attributed to unmeasured company or feedlot level factors. In other words, the biological association did not vary sufficiently among companies or feedlots to be detected by the statistical methods described herein. Group-level factors, therefore, seem to be important determinants (or modifiers) of mortality and if discovered, may influence the design of management strategies to reduce mortality, particularly in pens administered βAA. Unfortunately, we could not identify any meaningful and consistent effect modifiers, other than month, in the data and further research is needed to identify factors that may modify the observed association between βAA and increased risk of death. Saliently, the statistical variation of groups is a function of both the individuals as well as the interaction among the individuals within the group. In addition to group-level management strategies, therefore, 2 additional lines of investigation ought to be pursued and include animal-level factors, such as genetic variation in response to βAA [28], and how individuals interact to influence the behavior and potentially the response to βAA of other animals.

The data reported have considerable strengths in that the number of observations permitted the detection of a change in a rare event (or events, if one considers the secondary outcomes). When seeking approval for products, it is extremely uncommon to have available such numbers to detect rare adverse drug events. Based on the results observed herein, the number needed to harm, a measure of extent of exposure required for a βAA-related death, was approximately 500 animals or 15,000 animal days. In most reports of well-controlled cattle experiments, the number of animals included is usually insufficient to speak to an association of βAA with mortality, given the rarity of death and estimates of the number needed to harm. As a result, most drug approvals require some post-approval monitoring, often termed the pharmaco-epidemiology or Type IV trials, and the self-reporting by patients of side-effects, either to the company, the FDA, or their doctor, is part and parcel of a holistic drug regulatory framework. Furthermore, our data are from commercial cattle fattening feedlots and as such, provide a degree of validity to the results. However, the number of companies and feedlots is relatively limited and consequently, selection bias is possible in that the decision to provide the data for inclusion in the analyses may have been influenced by a suspicion of increased mortality associated with βAA administration.

Despite the potential limitations of the data, we argue that given the magnitude of the data, and the strength and consistency of the various measures of effect, both RH and ZH are most likely causally associated with increased cumulative incidence, incidence rate, and hazard of death when they are administered in accordance with the FDA-approved label directions. The excess deaths attributed to βAA administration, and potentially the secondary outcomes of illness and occurrence of beef classified as *dark, firm and dry*, represent adverse drug events. If so, we believe a broad and inclusive dialogue that explores the balance between improved production efficiencies achieved through means such as βAA [29] and resultant adverse effects on the welfare of animals we raise for food is needed. This is particularly warranted for those drugs that are approved solely to improve the efficiencies of production yet offer no offsetting health benefits to the animals to which it is administered. For this dialogue to be sufficiently inclusive, it ought to include a broad collection of stakeholders such as animal scientists, cattle and beef producers, animal health specialists, welfarists, ethologists, and consumers.

Author Contributions

Conceived and designed the experiments: GHL. Analyzed the data: GHL HMS. Wrote the paper: GHL DUT HMS.

References

1. Health and Human Services, Food and Drug Administration website. Freedom of information summary. Original new animal drug application. NADA 141–221 ractopamine hydrochloride (OPTAFLEXX 45) type A medicated article for beef cattle. Available: http://www.fda.gov/downloads/AnimalVeterinary/Products/ApprovedAnimalDrugProducts/FOIADrugSummaries/ucm118030.pdf. Accessed 2013 July 10.

2. Health and Human Services, Food and Drug Administration website. Freedom of information summary. Original new animal drug application. NADA 141–258 ZILMAX (zilpaterol hydrochloride) type A medicated article for cattle fed in confinement for slaughter. Available: http://www.fda.gov/downloads/AnimalVeterinary/Products/ApprovedAnimalDrugProducts/FOIADrugSummaries/ucm051412.pdf. Accessed 2013 July 5.

3. Hilton GG, Montgomery JL, Krehbiel CR, Yates DA, Hutcheson JP, et al. (2009) Effects of feeding zilpaterol hydrochloride with and without monensin and tylosin on carcass cutability and meat palatability of beef steers. J Anim Sci 87: 1394–1406. 10.2527/jas.2008-1170.

4. Rathmann RJ, Bernhard BC, Swingle RS, Lawrence TE, Nichols WT, et al. (2012) Effects of zilpaterol hydrochloride and days on the finishing diet on feedlot performance, carcass characteristics, and tenderness in beef heifers. J Anim Sci 90: 3301–3311. 10.2527/jas.2011-4375.

5. Bohrer BM, Kyle JM, Boler DD, Rincker PJ, Ritter MJ, et al. (2013) Meta-analysis of the effects of ractopamine hydrochloride on carcass cutability and primal yields of finishing pigs. J Anim Sci 91: 1015–1023. 10.2527/jas.2012-5647.

6. Scramlin SM, Platter WJ, Gomez RA, Choat WT, McKeith FK, et al. (2010) Comparative effects of ractopamine hydrochloride and zilpaterol hydrochloride on growth performance, carcass traits, and longissimus tenderness of finishing steers. J Anim Sci 88: 1823–1829. 10.2527/jas.2009-2405.

7. Bryant TC, Engle TE, Galyean ML, Wagner JJ, Tatum JD, et al. (2010) Effects of ractopamine and trenbolone acetate implants with or without estradiol on growth performance, carcass characteristics, adipogenic enzyme activity, and blood metabolites in feedlot steers and heifers. J Anim Sci 88: 4102–4119. 10.2527/jas.2010-2901.

8. Nelson HS, Weiss ST, Bleecker ER, Yancey SW, Dorinsky PM, et al. (2006) The Salmeterol Multicenter Asthma Research Trial: a comparison of usual pharmacotherapy for asthma or usual pharmacotherapy plus salmeterol. Chest 129: 15–26. 10.1378/chest.129.1.15.

9. McMahon AW, Levenson MS, McEvoy BW, Mosholder AD, Murphy D (2011) Age and risks of FDA-approved long-acting beta(2)-adrenergic receptor agonists. Pediatrics 128: e1147–1154. 10.1542/peds.2010-1720.

10. Salpeter SR (2010) An update on the safety of long-acting beta-agonists in asthma patients using inhaled corticosteroids. Expert Opin Drug Saf 9: 407–419. 10.1517/14740330903535852.

11. Salpeter SR, Buckley NS, Ormiston TM, Salpeter EE (2006) Meta-analysis: effect of long-acting beta-agonists on severe asthma exacerbations and asthma-related deaths. Ann Intern Med 144: 904–912.

12. Salpeter SR, Ormiston TM, Salpeter EE (2004) Cardiovascular effects of beta-agonists in patients with asthma and COPD: a meta-analysis. Chest 125: 2309–2321.

13. Marchant-Forde JN, Lay DC Jr., Pajor EA, Richert BT, Schinckel AP (2003) The effects of ractopamine on the behavior and physiology of finishing pigs. J Anim Sci 81: 416–422.

14. Poletto R, Rostagno MH, Richert BT, Marchant-Forde JN (2009) Effects of a "step-up" ractopamine feeding program, sex, and social rank on growth performance, hoof lesions, and Enterobacteriaceae shedding in finishing pigs. J Anim Sci 87: 304–313. 10.2527/jas.2008-1188.

15. Poletto R, Meisel RL, Richert BT, Cheng HW, Marchant-Forde JN (2010) Behavior and peripheral amine concentrations in relation to ractopamine feeding, sex, and social rank of finishing pigs. J Anim Sci 88: 1184–1194. 10.2527/jas.2008-1576.

16. Wagner SH, Mostrom MS, Hammer CJ, Thorson JF, Smith DJ (2008) Adverse Effects of Zilpaterol Administration in Horses: Three Cases. J Equine Vet Sci 28: 238–243.

17. Avendano-Reyes L, Macias-Cruz U, Alvarez-Valenzuela FD, Aguila-Tepato E, Torrentera-Olivera NG, et al. (2011) Effects of zilpaterol hydrochloride on growth performance, carcass characteristics, and wholesale cut yield of hair-

breed ewe lambs consuming feedlot diets under moderate environmental conditions. J Anim Sci 89: 4188–4194. 10.2527/jas.2011–3904.

18. Baszczak JA, Grandin T, Gruber SL, Engle TE, Platter WJ, et al. (2006) Effects of ractopamine supplementation on behavior of British, Continental, and Brahman crossbred steers during routine handling. J Anim Sci 84: 3410–3414. 10.2527/jas.2006-167.

19. Beasley R (2006) A historical perspective of the New Zealand asthma mortality epidemics. J Allergy Clin Immunol 117: 225–228.

20. McDermott JJ, Schukken YH, Shoukri MM (1994) Study design and analytical methods for data collected from clusters of animals. Prev Vet Med 18: 175–191.

21. McDermott JJ, Schukken YH (1994) A review of methods used to adjust for cluster effects in explanatory epidemiological studies of animal populations. Prev Vet Med 18: 155–173.

22. Dohoo IR, Martin SW, Stryhn H (2009) Veterinary Epidemiological Research. Charlottetown, Prince Edward Island, Canada: VER Inc.

23. Brown H, Prescott R (2006) Applied mixed models in medicine; Senn S, Barnett V, editors. West Sussex, England: John Wiley & Sons Ltd.

24. University of Bristol, Centre for Multilevel Modeling website. A User's Guide to MLwiN Version 2.26. Available: http://www.bristol.ac.uk/cmm/software/mlwin/download/2-26/manual-web.pdf Available. Accessed 2012 November 2.

25. Loneragan GH, Dargatz DA, Morley PS, Smith MA (2001) Trends in mortality ratios among cattle in US feedlots. J Am Vet Med Assoc 219: 1122–1127.

26. Babcock AH, Cernicchiaro N, White BJ, Dubnicka SR, Thomson DU, et al. (2013) A multivariable assessment quantifying effects of cohort-level factors associated with combined mortality and culling risk in cohorts of U.S. commercial feedlot cattle. Prev Vet Med 108: 38–46. 10.1016/j.prevetmed.2012.07.008.

27. Guzy PM (1977) Creatine phosphokinase-MB (CPK-MB) and the diagnosis of myocardial infarction. West J Med 127: 455–460.

28. Kononoff PJ, Defoor PJ, Engler MJ, Swingle RS, James ST, et al. (2013) Impact of a leptin SNP and zilpaterol hydrochloride (ZH) on growth and carcass characteristics in finishing steers. J Anim Sci. 10.2527/jas.2012–5229.

29. Capper JL, Hayes DJ (2012) The environmental and economic impact of removing growth-enhancing technologies from U.S. beef production. J Anim Sci 90: 3527–3537. 10.2527/jas.2011–4870.

24

Self-Reported Musculoskeletal Disorders of the Distal Upper Extremities and the Neck in German Veterinarians: A Cross-Sectional Study

Agnessa Kozak[1]*, Grita Schedlbauer[2], Claudia Peters[1], Albert Nienhaus[1,2]

1 Institute for Health Services Research in Dermatology and Nursing, University Medical Center Hamburg-Eppendorf, Hamburg, Germany, **2** Department of Occupational Health Research, Institution for Statutory Accident Insurance and Prevention in Healthcare and Welfare, Hamburg, Germany

Abstract

Background: Veterinary work is a physically demanding profession and entails the risk of injuries and diseases of the musculoskeletal system, particularly in the upper body. The prevalence of musculoskeletal disorders (MSD), the consequences and work-related accidents in German veterinarians were investigated. Work-related and individual factors associated with MSD of upper extremities and the neck were analyzed.

Methods: In 2011, a self-reporting Standardized Nordic Questionnaire was mailed to registered veterinarians in seven federal medical associations in Germany. A total of 3174 (38.4%) veterinarians responded. Logistic regression analysis was used to determine the association between risk factors and MSD-related impairment of daily activities.

Results: MSD in the neck (66.6%) and shoulder (60.5%) were more prevalent than in the hand (34.5%) or elbow (24.5%). Normal activities were affected in 28.7% (neck), 29.5% (shoulder), 19.4% (hand) and 14% (elbow) of the respondents. MSD in the upper body occurred significantly more often in large animal practitioners. Accidents that resulted in MSD were most frequently reported in the hand/wrist (14.3%) or in the shoulder (10.8%). The majority of all accidents in the distal upper extremities were caused by animals than by other factors (19% vs. 9.2%). For each area of the body, a specific set of individual and work-related factors contributed significantly to severe MSD: Older age, gender, previous injuries, BMI, practice type, veterinary procedures such as dentistry, rectal procedures and obstetric procedures as well as high demands and personal burnout.

Conclusion: From the perspective of occupational health and safety, it seems to be necessary to improve accident prevention and to optimize the ergonomics of specific tasks. Our data suggest the need for target group-specific preventive measures that also focus on the psychological factors at work.

Editor: Carlos M. Isales, Georgia Regents University, United States of America

Funding: The authors have no support or funding to report.

Competing Interests: The authors have declared that no competing interests exist.

* E-mail: a.kozak@uke.de

Introduction

Recent studies on professional veterinarians have demonstrated that veterinary work is physically demanding and poses an elevated risk of significant injuries [1–4]. A number of physical and psychological risk factors at work, particular in veterinary professions, have been linked to musculoskeletal disorders (MSD): static or awkward postures, repetitive or forceful tasks, animal related injuries, pressure of time, work stress, career structure or after hours duties [5–8]. Equine and bovine practitioners regularly undertake repetitive tasks, such as rectal palpation or obstetric procedures, which require lifting or exerting an upward force and/ or resisting animals' unpredictable movements [4]. Some practitioners work with one or both arms above shoulder level for over one hour daily [7]. These postures and movements may be risk factors for the development of MSD in the upper extremities in veterinarians [6,9]. Ailsby, for instance, assumed that an occupational neck- shoulder- and arm-syndrome is significantly

associated with continuous or repeated strain from repetitive and forceful motions during veterinary work (e.g. procedures such as rectal examinations or calving) [10]. Such microtrauma or minute injuries from repeatedly overusing a specific part of the body result in conditions called "Repetitive Strain Injuries" or "Cumulative Trauma Disorders" (CTD). In the literature, those conditions are summarized under the higher level term of "Work-Related Musculoskeletal Disorders of Upper Extremities" (WRMSDs-UE), which are inflammatory and degenerative disorders responsible for pain and functional impairment in tendons, muscles, joints, nerves or blood vessels [11].

Work-related accidents constitute a further health risk factor. According to the insurance data from the Statutory Accident Insurance in the Health and Welfare Services in Germany (BGW-Berufsgenossenschaft für Gesundheitsdienst und Wohlfahrtspflege) for the 5-year period (1998–2002) of all reported claims, work-related accidents accounted for 87.7% of claims in veterinary practice. Animals (66%) were the main cause of these accidents [12]. Numerous studies have shown that veterinarians are at high risk of significant acute traumatic injury (ATI) from animal contacts - predominantly in the upper extremities [2,13–15]. Large animal practitioners are most likely to suffer severe injuries [8,16]. In particular, palpation is one of the five most common causes of injuries in veterinary practitioners [13]. The risk of job-related injuries in veterinarians is higher than for other professions in the healthcare sector [12].

Therefore, working characteristics may contribute to the prevalence of MSD symptoms in veterinarians. They may suffer from work-related physical impairment or disability in functional tasks and/or the chronic or acute musculoskeletal disease. Veterinarians are more likely to report chronic work-related musculoskeletal problems if they perform clinical work [8]. According to the registration data from the German Federal Veterinary Council, 49% of the veterinarians in Germany work in clinical practice and perform tasks and procedures which can lead to MSD [17]. However, there are no available data on the prevalence of MSD in German veterinarians.

The purpose of the present study was, therefore, to examine the self-reported prevalence for MSD, the resulting physical limitations, and the frequency of injuries in the distal upper extremities and the neck. We also investigated the relationship between demographic, occupation-related risk factors (e.g. practice type, work task or previous injury) and MSD-related impairment of daily activities (severe MSD) in the relevant body regions.

Materials and Methods

Subjects

In 2011 we conducted a survey of registered veterinarians in seven federal states in Germany (medical associations in Baden-Württemberg, Bavaria, Berlin, Brandenburg, Lower Saxony, Schleswig-Holstein, and Westphalia-Lippe). According to the registration data from the German Federal Veterinary Council, there were no statistically significant differences between responders and non-responders with respect to gender and age distribution [17]. None of the seven medical associations of the federal states in the study was overrepresented. Thus, the sample can be considered as representative.

Measurement

We measured the presence and severity of MSD during the preceding 12 months with the Standardized Nordic Questionnaire [18]. This instrument has been applied to various occupational groups to evaluate musculoskeletal problems. An anatomical sketch of labeled body regions allowed the respondents to clearly identify body areas affected by MSD. A dichotomous yes/no answer indicated whether the participants had suffered any symptoms in the queried body area during the preceding 12 months. To assess the severity, the following question was asked: *"What is the total length of time that [neck] trouble has prevented you from doing your normal work (at home or away from home) during the last 12-months?"*. Possible replies to this question were: (1) *"the discomfort was not too severe"*; (2) *"1 to 7 days"*; (3) *"8 to 30 days"* or (4) *"more than 30 days"*. We aimed to distinguish participants who felt a certain discomfort but did not experience longer lasting restrictions in work and daily life from those who were restricted for at least one week in the past 12 months. Participants who replied with *"the discomfort was not too severe"* were allocated to the non-affected group. For each queried body area, we also asked the participants whether these symptoms were caused by a work-related injury during their professional life. Work-related injuries were differen-

tiated into animal-related and other-related injuries during working hours (e.g. falls, motor vehicle accidents). The participants were asked to provide their demographic data (age and gender), anthropometric measures (height and weight), dominant hand, current job status (full-time or part-time), the type of practice (small, mixed or large animal), length of work experience, number of hours worked per week and whether they were involved in sports activities or not. We calculated the body mass index (BMI) and categorized it into normal weight (BMI<25), overweight (25–30), and obese (>30).

The veterinarians were asked to estimate the number (0; <600; 600–2400; 2400–6000; 6000–12,000; >12,000) of examinations and procedures they performed annually. The detailed list of veterinary procedures was adopted from Scuffham et al. and translated into German [4]. The following procedures were queried: (1) obstetric procedures, (2) rectal palpations, (3) inseminations, (4) vaginal examinations, (5) animal handling/lifting, (6) blood sampling, (7) vaccinations, (8) dehorning/velveting, (9) foot trimming, (10) lameness examinations, (11) necropsies, (12) ultrasonography, (13) radiography, (14) endoscopies, (15) dental procedures, (16) surgery lasting <1 hour, and (17) surgery lasting >1 hour. For the analysis, we summarized the number of procedures into three categories (0 or not specified; < 600; ≥600).

Quantitative job demands were measured by a five-point Likert scale from the Copenhagen Psychosocial Questionnaire (COP-SOQ) [19]. This scale measures the amount of work that has to be done in a particular time (e.g. intensive and extensive job demands). The frequency of typical load factors at work were measured with four questions (1. *"Do you have enough time for your work tasks?"*; 2. *"Do you have to do overtime?"*; 3. *"Is your work unevenly distributed so it piles up?"*; 4. *"Do you have to work very fast?"*). The Cronbach's Alpha value was acceptable ($\alpha = .65$). To capture the psychological condition of the veterinarians, the 'personal burnout' subscale from the Copenhagen Burnout Inventory (CBI) was applied. This scale contains six items on general symptoms of exhaustion and is defined as "the degree of physical and psychological fatigue and exhaustion experienced by the person". This five-point Likert scale ($\alpha = .87$) shows good internal consistency [20]. Both scales were transformed into a theoretical range, extending from 0 (never/almost never) to 100 (always) points. This transformation is a standardized procedure and conforms to the German validation study. If at least half of the single items had valid answers, scale scores were computed as the average of the values [21]. For the logistic regression models, we summarized the original scales into tertiles and defined them as low, medium or high. The final questionnaire was pre-tested on ten veterinarians to remove inconsistencies, detect unclear wording and to complement missing aspects.

Ethics Statement

Each questionnaire included an informative letter which clarifies the free participation and anonymity of this study. We did not ask for the written consent of the participants. The voluntary participation was deemed as informed consent. The study protocol was approved by the Hamburg Medical Council Ethics Commission (# PV3839).

Statistical Analysis

Descriptive statistics were used to describe the study sample and to estimate the prevalence of musculoskeletal disorders (MSD), the disorder severity (activities affected) and accident prevalence in the upper extremities and neck. Differences in MSD prevalence were examined using Pearson's chi-square test for categorical variables.

For collinearity analysis, we scanned the Spearman correlation matrix to avoid multicollinearity or redundancy between independent variables (e.g. job tasks). Spearman's correlation coefficients of $\rho \geq 0.6$ were considered as problematic, as they introduce a substantial bias into the estimation of the logistic regression models [22]. Thus, the variable 'job experience' was removed from the analysis, as this strongly correlated with age ($\rho = 0.8$). We found that rectal palpations were frequently mentioned as a risk factor for CTD or ATI in the upper extremities [3,6,13]. As the predictor variables foot trimming, dehorning/velveting, vaginal examinations, and inseminations showed significant moderate correlations with rectal palpations ($\rho \geq 0.6$), we decided to remove these from further analysis. Univariate logistic regressions were calculated to identify associations between severe MSD in the previous 12 months and individual, work-related and psychosocial factors in the respective body parts. As we performed a number of tests, we set the alpha level at $p < 0.01$, in order to lower the probability of type I errors. Predictor variables which significantly affected the rate of MSD severity were selected for multivariate modeling. However, the demographic variables age and gender were included in each tested model, whether or not they had a significant influence in the univariate analysis. Backward stepwise multivariate logistic regression analyses were performed to develop a final explanatory model for each body part. The likelihood ratio statistic was used for variable entry ($p < 0.05$) and removal ($p < 0.1$). Analyses were performed with SPSS Version 17.0.

Results

Study Population

A total of 3174 veterinarians responded to the self-administered questionnaire (response rate 38.4%). Complete information was provided by 3051 subjects (96% of the responses). Table 1 describes the study population. The mean age of the participants was 47.6 (± 10) years, with an average of 18.0 (± 10.2) years of job experience in veterinary practice. Of the 3051 participants in the survey, the majority (97.1%) worked in a clinical practice and 82% were self employed. Most study participants were small animal practitioners (48.6%). The proportion of women working in small animal practices was significantly higher (75.2%) than in mixed (38.9%) and large (31.8%) animal practices ($p < 0.001$) and vice versa (25% of men worked in small, 61% in mixed and 68% in large animal practices). Thus, there was a gender difference in the tasks performed in veterinary practice. Male practitioners significantly more often performed tasks related to a job profile in mixed and large animal practices (e.g. rectal palpations or obstetric procedures). Table 2 shows relevant veterinary tasks which significantly correlated with practice type (Spearman's correlation of at least $\rho = 0.2$). The tasks are ranked according to their relevance (high to low correlation). Large and mixed animal practitioners more often performed foot trimming, rectal palpations, inseminations, dehorning/velveting, vaginal examinations and obstetric procedures. Small animal practitioners, however, more often performed x-rays, handling and lifting, dental procedures and surgeries.

Prevalence of MSD Symptoms

Of those affected, a quarter reported MSD trouble in one body site, 56% reported two to three body sites, and 8% experienced MSD in four queried body sites. The prevalence of MSD by body site is given in Table 3, stratified by gender and practice type. The prevalences of the MSD symptoms in the upper extremities in the preceding 12 months differed considerably; the highest prevalences were observed in the neck (66.6%) and shoulder region (60.5%).

Table 1. Characteristics of the study population.

Variables		N = 3051 (%)
Sex	Female	1657 (54.3)
	Male	1394 (45.7)
Age*	<30	105 (3.4)
	30–39	561 (18.4)
	40–49	1081 (35.4)
	>50	1304 (42.7)
	>50	1304 (42.7)
BMI	<25	1733 (56.8)
	25–30	1050 (34.4)
	>30	268 (8.8)
Job experience**	<10	693 (22.7)
	10–19	1003 (32.9)
	20–29	936 (30.7)
	>30	419 (13.7)
Practice type	Small	1483 (48.6)
	Mixed	614 (20.1)
	Large	954 (31.3)
Working h/week	>35 h	2471 (81.0)
	15–34 h	465 (15.2)
	<15 h	115 (3.8)
Work setting	Practice	2963 (97.1)
	Industry	57 (1.9)
	University/ Administration	24 (0.8)
	Other	7 (0.2)

Note. *Age: mean 47.6 (SD±10) years; **Job experience: mean 18.0 (SD±10.2) years.

MSD in the hand (34.5%) and elbow (24.5%) were less frequently reported. Neck symptoms were more likely to be reported by female veterinarians ($p < 0.001$). Male veterinarians, however, significantly more often reported symptoms in the elbow ($p < 0.001$). A significantly higher proportion of large animal practitioners reported MSD in the distal upper extremities than did practitioners in mixed and small practices ($p < 0.001$).

Severe MSD (Activities Affected)

Correspondingly, the perceived physical disability in functional tasks (severe MSD) during the preceding 12 months was highest in the neck (28.7%) and shoulder (29.5%), and lowest in the hand/wrist (19.4%) and elbow (14%). Women showed higher MSD severity in the neck ($p < 0.001$) and also in hand/wrist ($p < 0.01$), while men reported significantly higher severe MSD in the elbow region ($p < 0.001$). The proportion of severe MSD in the upper distal extremities increased significantly with the size of the treated animals (Table 3).

Reported Accidents

Work-related accidents that resulted in MSD complaints were most frequently reported in the hand/wrist (14.3%) and shoulder (10.8%); the least reported injuries were in the neck (6.6%) and elbow region (5.5%). Except for the neck, more accidents in the upper extremities were caused by animals than by other factors

Table 2. The frequency of veterinary tasks performed annually, stratified by practice type.

Practice type	Small (%)			Mixed (%)			Large (%)		
Veterinary tasks	0	<600	600–2400	0	<600	600–2400	0	<600	600–2400
Foot trimming	77.8	6.4	1.2	12.8	31.9	25.3	9.5	61.7	73.5
Rectal palpation	81.8	60.7	6.3	9.8	19.7	29.6	8.4	19.6	64.1
Insemination	66.7	12.8	1.3	16.0	28.1	31.2	17.3	59.1	67.4
Dehorning/velveting	65.2	3.7	13.5	15.7	32.7	18.9	19.1	63.7	67.6
Vaginal examination	72.6	41.5	8.9	13.0	22.9	27.5	14.3	35.5	63.6
Radiography	22.4	55.2	69.7	20.0	22.3	15.1	57.6	22.5	15.1
Obstetric procedure	74.5	36.1	22.1	10.9	25.4	14.7	14.6	38.6	63.2
Handling/lifting	39.8	30.4	59.2	14.2	21.1	20.1	46.0	48.5	20.7
Dental procedure	22.4	54.7	57.7	11.8	22.9	18.6	65.8	22.4	23.7
Surgery lasting <1	40.7	44.9	67.2	22.7	19.8	20.2	36.6	35.4	12.6
Surgery lasting >1	37.2	50.2	68.4	18.7	20.8	17.2	44.1	29.0	14.4

Note. The differences between practice types were significant (p<0.05) for all procedures.

(19% vs. 9.2%). Male practitioners were more likely to report injuries in the neck (11.4% vs. 6.5%), shoulders (23.4% vs. 10.1%), elbows (20.7% vs. 12.6%), and hand/wrist (36.5% vs. 30.1%) than female practitioners. Except for the elbow, the accident rate increases proportionally (p<0.05) with the age of the practitioners. Large and mixed animal practitioners were more likely to report accidents in the neck (14%,13% and 3.6%, respectively), shoulder (24.2%, 25% and 6.4%, respectively) and elbow (23.2%, 17.8% and 10.4%, respectively, p<0.001) than small animal practitioners. No significant differences were found for accidents in the hand/wrist (35.2%, 36.2% and 29.6%, respectively; no Table).

Risk Factors for Severe MSD

Logistic regression analysis was used to identify factors influencing the risk of MSD causing restricted movements and restricted daily activities during the preceding 12 months. The analysis was performed separately for individual regions of the upper extremities; the results are shown in Tables 4, 5, 6, 7. As

some predictor variables are the same for different body regions, we describe the results together.

Veterinarians of 40 years and older run a higher risk of having physical disability in the neck (OR 2.0, 95% CI 1.2–3.3), shoulder (OR 2.1, 95% CI 1.2–2.0), elbow (>40 years: OR 11.6, 95% CI 2.8–47.9; >50 years: 13.4, 95% CI 3.2–55.9), and hand (OR 2.1 95% CI 1.0–4.1) than their younger colleagues. Severe MSD of the hand was found more often in women (OR 1.6, 95% CI 1.2–2.1), whereas female veterinarians complained of MSD in the elbow less often than their male colleagues (OR 0.7, 95% CI 0.6–0.9). Furthermore, previous accidents increased the risk of physical impairment in neck (OR 2.1, 95% CI 1.6–2.9), shoulder (OR 1.6, 95% CI 1.2–2.0), and hand (OR 1.5, 95% CI 1.2–1.9). Veterinarians with a BMI of 25–30 had 1.3 (95% CI 1.1–1.7) times the odds of MSD severity in the elbow, compared with those who had normal BMI. Veterinarians in mixed (OR 1.5, 95% CI 1.1–2.1) and large (OR 1.9, 95% CI 1.4–2.7) practices showed a higher risk for severe MSD in the elbow than small animal practitioners.

Table 3. Twelve month MSD prevalence and severe MSD (activities affected) of the upper body, stratified by gender and practice type.

Body region		Neck		Shoulder		Elbow		Hand/Wrist	
12-month prevalence		MSD experience	Severe MSD	MSD experience	Severe MSD	MSD experience	Severe MSD	MSD experience	Severe MSD
		n (%)	n (%)	n (%)	n (%)	n (%)	n (%)	n (%)	n (%)
Female n=1657	Total	1240 (74.8)	527 (31.8)	995 (60.0)	466 (28.1)	336 (20.3)	198 (11.9)	592 (35.7)	350 (21.1)
	Small n=1115	839 (75.2)	356 (31.9)	653 (58.6)	293 (26.3)	196 (17.6)	116 (10.4)	360 (32.3)	219 (19.6)
	Mixed n=239	172 (72.0)	78 (32.6)	149 (62.3)	75 (31.4)	54 (22.6)	31 (13.0)	96 (40.2)	55 (23.0)
	Large n=303	229 (75.6)	93 (30.7)	193 (63.7)	98 (32.3)	86 (28.4)	51 (16.8)	136 (44.9)	76 (25.1)
Male n=1394	Total	793 (56.9)	348 (25.0)	851 (61.0)	433 (31.1)	411 (29.5)	230 (16.5)	460 (33.0)	242 (17.4)
	Small n=368	211 (57.3)	82 (22.3)	183 (49.7)	79 (21.5)	77 (20.9)	30 (8.2)	84 (22.8)	37 (10.1)
	Mixed n=375	217 (57.9)	96 (25.6)	236 (62.9)	114 (30.4)	112 (29.9)	67 (17.9)	123 (32.8)	69 (18.4)
	Large n=651	365 (56.1)	170 (26.1)	432 (66.4)	240 (36.9)	222 (34.1)	133 (20.4)	253 (38.9)	136 (20.9)
Total N=3051		2033 (66.6)	875 (28.7)	1846 (60.5)	899 (29.5)	747 (24.5)	428 (14.0)	1052 (34.5)	592 (19.4)

Table 4. Multivariate analysis of severe MSD in the neck.

Variables		%	Crude OR (95%CI)	Adjusted OR[†] (95%CI)
Age (years)	<30	21.9	1	1
	30–39	31.0	1.6 (0.9–2.6)	1.5 (0.9–2.6)
	40–49	29.0	1.5 (0.9–2.4)	1.6 (1.0–2.7)
	>50	27.9	1.4 (0.9–2.2)	2.0 (1.2–3.3)**
Accidents	No	35.3	1	1
	Yes	55.5	2.3 (1.7–3.1)	2.1 (1.6–2.9)**
Dental procedures	0 or n/s	26.8	1	1
	<600	28.2	1.1 (0.9–1.3)	1.0 (0.8–1.3)
	≥600	34.3	1.4 (1.1–1.9)	1.4 (1.0–1.9)*
Quantitative demands	Low	18.4	1	1
	Medium	25.7	1.5 (1.2–2.0)	1.3 (1.0–1.8)
	High	36.7	2.6 (1.9–3.4)	1.7 (1.2–2.4)**
Personal Burnout	Low	13.6	1	1
	Medium	31.6	2.9 (2.4–3.6)	2.1 (1.7–2.7)**
	High	50.8	6.6 (5.1–8.6)	4.3 (3.2–5.8)**

Note. *p<0.05; **p<0.01. [†]Gender had no effect in the final model.

Veterinarians who frequently performed dental procedures (≥ 600 per year) were at higher risk of being affected by MSD in the neck region (OR 1.4, 95% CI 1.0–1.9), compared to those who less often or hardly ever performed such tasks. Work-related risk factors for MSD in the shoulder increased significantly with the number of annual obstetric procedures (≥600 per year: OR 2.1, 95% CI 1.2–3.5). On the contrary, veterinarians who performed up to 600 radiological examinations per year less often reported severe MSD in the shoulder (OR 0.8, 95% CI 0.6–1.0). The risk of severe MSD in the elbows was associated with frequent rectal palpations (≥600 per year: OR 1.4, 95% CI 1.0–2.0). High quantitative demands and elevated levels of personal burnout showed consistent association with perceived severe MSD severity in all queried body regions, compared with those who less often reported pressure of time due to heavy workload and emotional exhaustion (Tables 4, 5, 6, 7).

Table 5. Multivariate analysis of severe MSD in the shoulder.

Variables		%	Crude OR (95%CI)	Adjusted OR[†] (95%CI)
Age (years)	<30	21.0	1	1
	30–39	23.9	1.2 (0.7–2.0)	1.3 (0.8–2.3)
	40–49	29.6	1.6 (1.0–2.6)	2.1 (1.2–3.6)**
	>50	32.4	1.8 (1.1–2.9)	2.1 (1.2–2.0)**
Accidents	No	42.1	1	1
	Yes	55.5	1.7 (1.3–2.2)	1.6 (1.2–2.0)**
Obstetrics	0 or n/s	22.3	1	1
	<600	32.7	1.7 (1.4–2.0)	1.4 (1.2–1.8)**
	≥600	42.1	2.5 (1.6–3.9)	2.1 (1.2–3.5)**
Radiography	0 or n/s	33.1	1	1
	<600	26.1	0.7 (0.6–0.8)	0.8 (0.6–1.0)*
	≥600	32.3	1.0 (0.8–1.2)	1.2 (0.9–1.4)
Quantitative demands	Low	16.8	1	1
	Medium	27.1	1.8 (1.4–2.5)	1.7 (1.2–2.4)**
	High	37.3	3.0 (2.2–4.0)	2.0 (1.4–2.9)**
Personal Burnout	Low	18.5	1	1
	Medium	31.5	2.0 (1.7–2.5)	2.0 (1.6–2.5)**
	High	46.0	3.8 (2.9–4.8)	3.7 (2.7–5.1)**

Note. *p<0.05; **p<0.01. [†]Gender, BMI, practice type, lameness examinations, and rectal palpations had no effect in the final model.

Table 6. Multivariate analysis of severe MSD in the elbow.

Variables		%	Crude OR (95%CI)	Adjusted OR† (95%CI)
Gender	Male	16.5	1	1
	Female	11.9	0.7 (0.6–0.8)	0.7 (0.6–0.9)*
Age (years)	<30	1.9	1	1
	30–39	6.6	3.6 (0.9–15.3)	3.8 (0.9–16.2)
	40–49	15.3	9.3 (2.3–37.9)	11.6 (2.8–47.9)**
	>50	17.2	10.7 (2.6–43.6)	13.4 (3.2–55.9)**
BMI (kg/m²)	<25	11.3	1	1
	25–30	17.6	1.7 (1.3–2.1)	1.3 (1.1–1.7)*
	>30	17.5	1.7 (1.2–2.4)	1.4 (0.9–1.9)
Practice type	Small	9.8	1	1
	Mixed	16.0	1.7 (1.3–2.3)	1.5 (1.1–2.1)*
	Large	19.3	2.2 (1.7–2.8)	1.9 (1.4–2.7)**
Rectal palpations	0 or n/s	10.4	1	1
	<600	11.6	1.2 (0.9–1.5)	1.0 (0.7–1.3)
	≥600	19.9	2.2 (1.7–2.9)	1.4 (1.0–2.0)*
Quantitative demands	Low	7.6	1	1
	Medium	12.5	1.7 (1.2–2.6)	1.5 (0.9–2.2)
	High	18.5	2.8 (1.8–4.2)	2.0 (1.3–3.2)**
Personal Burnout	Low	9.4	1	1
	Medium	15.4	1.8 (1.4–2.3)	1.8 (1.4–2.4)**
	High	19.1	2.3 (1.6–3.1)	2.3 (1.6–3.3)**

Note. *p<0.05; **p<0.01. †obstetric procedures, radiography had no effect in the final model.

Table 7. Multivariate analysis of severe MSD in the hand/wrist.

Variables		%	Crude OR (95%CI)	Adjusted OR† (95%CI)
Gender	Male	17.4	1	1
	Female	21.1	1.3 (1.1–1.5)	1.6 (1.2–2.1)**
Age (years)	<30	14.3	1	1
	30–39	16.9	1.2 (0.7–2.2)	1.1 (0.6–2.3)
	40–49	17.4	1.3 (0.7–2.2)	1.4 (0.7–2.9)
	>50	22.5	1.7 (1.0–3.1)	2.1 (1.0–4.1)*
Accidents	No	41.2	1	1
	Yes	52.0	1.5 (1.2–1.9)	1.5 (1.2–1.9)**
Rectal palpations	0 or n/s	18.0	1	1
	<600	16.6	0.9 (0.7–1.1)	0.8 (0.6–1.1)
	≥600	23.7	1.4 (1.1–1.8)	1.2 (0.9–1.7)
Quantitative demands	Low	17.3	1	1
	Medium	19.2	1.1 (0.9–1.4)	1.4 (0.9–2.1)
	High	27.5	1.8 (1.3–2.5)	1.8 (1.2–2.8)**
Personal Burnout	Low	13.0	1	1
	Medium	20.9	1.8 (1.4–2.2)	1.6 (1.2–2.1)**
	High	27.6	2.5 (1.9–3.4)	1.9 (1.4–2.9)**

Note. *p<0.05; **p<0.01. †practice type and radiography had no effect in the final model.

Discussion

To our knowledge, this is the first large scale self-reported survey of German veterinarians which examines MSD prevalence, its severity as manifested in restricted daily activities, and work-related accidents. In line with international literature, this study showed that MSD in the distal upper extremities and the neck was frequent in this professional group. The type of veterinary practice was related to MSD prevalence and severity. In addition, work-related accidents that resulted in MSD symptoms were most frequently reported in the hand/wrist and shoulder region. The majority of all injuries in the distal upper extremities were caused by animals. Working and individual characteristics were shown to attribute to MSD severity in the upper body.

Two studies from Australia and New Zealand using the same measuring instrument also found the highest 12-month symptoms prevalence in the neck (57%–58%) and shoulder (52%–59%), followed by the hand (32%–52%) and elbow (17%–29%) [4]. However, a Dutch veterinary cohort reported symptoms in the upper extremities significantly less often (37%, 38%, 14% and 11%, respectively) [23]. The 12-month prevalence in our study was much higher than the values found in comparable professions in international studies (e.g. nurses, farmers, physicians or chiropodists) [24–27]. The prevalence values are also much higher than those found in surveys with other employees. According to a survey in Germany, about 46% of subjects complained of pain in the neck and shoulder region. About 20% of employees had pain in the arms and hands [28]. In agreement with the findings of previous studies, multiple anatomical regions were often affected [1,4,7]. In their large-scale survey in France, Roquelaure et al. found that MSD symptoms of the upper limbs often overlapped two anatomical body regions, particularly the neck and shoulder regions [29]. The type of veterinary practice was related to MSD prevalence and severity, which is in line with the results from other studies on hazards and disorders [3,4,6,8,16,30]. Practitioners in mixed and large animal practices much more frequently reported MSD in the upper body. In a study from the Netherlands, problems related to the musculoskeletal system of the upper body were by far the most important disorders in equine practitioners [1]. We found higher MSD prevalences for women in the neck and hand/wrist and for men in the elbow. Studies on general and working populations have reported higher MSD prevalences in woman than in men. Besides, women more often reported pain at more than one body site [31,32].

A small but considerable number of participants had MSD symptoms which were serious enough to affect their daily activities. From the occupational perspective, this is of critical importance, as it probably affects the veterinarians' quality of life and may also lead to changes in professional activities. This in turn may cause a loss in productivity and/or loss of earnings. The participants of the aforementioned studies less frequently reported that MSD prevented them from carrying out their daily activities than those in our study [4,5]. To some extent, this may be attributed to the differences in the definition of items used. In this context, it should be pointed out that studies with additional diagnostic measuring procedures observed significantly lower values of MSD in the neck-shoulder region and lower back [33–35]. In a study on bovine practitioners, the self reported pathological findings of CTD were also lower than the prevalence of any musculoskeletal problem [6]. Thus, it would be desirable to verify the present results through further investigations with objective procedures. However, by choosing severe MSD as an outcome measure, we aimed to identify those cases with MSD complaints which were serious enough to prevent them from performing their daily activities for at least seven days in the previous 12 months.

The present study demonstrates that hand/wrist and shoulder are frequently affected by work-related accidents. A German study which analyzed the occupational records (accidents and diseases) of veterinary staff over a 5-year period found that the hand (48.3%) and arm (17.3%) were the most affected anatomical locations. They also found that veterinarians and their staff had a 2.9-fold higher risk of injuries than general practitioners [12]. In terms of species-specific injury mechanism, our results are in keeping with previous studies, which report that work-related accidents were most frequent in large animal practices and that the upper extremities were most frequently affected [3,8,16,30]. Langley and Hunter analyzed data from the US Department of Labor on human workplace fatalities associated with animals for the years 1992–1997. They found that large animals (cattle and horses) were primarily responsible for the majority of fatal events among workers. Men and elderly workers were at greater risk of mortality [36]. This is similar to our findings; male and elderly veterinarians significantly more often reported work-related injuries. This is probably because male practitioners more frequently worked with large animals, which exposed them to greater risk of major injuries. However, the results with respect to gender were inconsistent. Some studies on injuries reported a greater risk for men [7,8], while others found that women were more often affected [3,30,37]. Some authors have argued that women are at greater risk due to their small size and limited physical strength [3,37]. In contrast to our results, previous findings showed that increasing years of experience were associated with decreasing injury-related events [13,30]. This might be explained by the higher proportion of elderly veterinarians in our study. However our results on accidents were limited, because we did not differentiate the origin and severity of the accidents in detail.

Our findings demonstrate that for each part of the body a specific set of personal and work-related factors contribute significantly to severe MSD. Older age, gender, previous injuries, BMI, practice type, veterinary procedures such as dentistry, rectal palpation, obstetrics as well as quantitatively high demands and personal burnout increased the likelihood of severe MSD in the upper extremities and the neck. Older veterinarians more often reported severe MSD in all queried body parts than their younger colleagues. The age effect described in the present study on MSD is confirmed by other studies with veterinarians [4,38]. For ageing workers, a progressive decline in physical work capacity, characterized by diminished muscular capacity, has been reported – especially for physically demanding occupations [39]. In general, the MSD are likely to become more prevalent in the veterinary profession as the working population ages and a shortage of young professionals is to be expected, especially in the large animal practices [40]. With respect to gender, women showed a higher risk of severe MSD in the hand and men in the elbow. This could be due to different mechanical patterns of procedures undertaken and/or differences in physique. According to Berry et al., women and men reported different procedures which caused them CTD; men more often reported rectal palpation and calving manipulation while women reported holding instruments, computer work and other causes [3]. The activity profile that causes MSD is greatly dependent on the type of practice. Scuffham et al. asked veterinarians about routine activities that triggered MSD in them. Large and mixed animal veterinarians mostly considered that rectal examinations, obstetric treatment, ultrasound examinations and diagnostic testing on the hoof and lameness were stressful activities. On the other hand, small animal veterinarians found that lifting and transporting animals was stressful, together with surgeries [41]. In a subsequent study, it was shown that large animal veterinarians and veterinarians who only worked with horses exhibit the greatest prevalence of MSD periods in comparison to veterinarians in other practices or organizations [4]. Cattell found that 71% of CTD and 31% of ATI to veterinarians in large animal practices were related to rectal examinations [6]. Thus, in view of the activity profile, it is plausible in the present study that mixed and large animal veterinarians, who also performed rectal palpations, significantly more often reported symptoms in the elbows. Symptoms in the shoulders correlate with frequent vaginal investigations, whereby the type of practice played a lesser role in the corresponding analysis model. In addition, dental examinations correlated with symptoms in the neck. It is known that this region is susceptible for MSD - not only for human dentists, but also for veterinarians specializing in dentistry [42,43].

Furthermore, participants in our study who reported previous work-related accidents had a higher chance of developing MSD in the neck, shoulder and hand/wrist. These results were also supported by Randall et al., who examined ergonomic risk factors among veterinary sonographers [38]. Thus, trauma acquired at work may have serious long-term consequences. Precautionary measures, such as training in body posture and handling animals, are of increasing importance in this profession. Ergonomics of the work environment can also be considered to decrease the incidence of injuries to the neck (e.g. for practitioners that have higher incidence of neck pathology).

In the current study, quantitative demands and personal burnout were associated with significant increases in MSD in all queried body regions. The association between psychosocial factors and MSD is well documented [44]. The relationship between MSD period prevalence and quantitative demands caused by time pressure and work overload was consistent with two recent studies from Australia and New Zealand [4,5]. The assumption is that a mismatch of the amount of work and the time available to do it may lead to stress [45]. Thus, MSD is not only triggered by physical factors (e.g. lifting, repetitive tasks), but also by emotional and psychosocial demands. For instance, Loomans et al. found an intermediate correlation in veterinarians between emotional work load and MSD of the lower body [1]. In addition, psychosocial stress in the veterinary setting is also associated with increased consumption of alcohol, tobacco and medication [46]. For these reasons, it is strongly recommended that preventive measures should be implemented to sustain and improve not only the physical but also the psychological well-being of veterinarians. However, we cannot rule out the possibility of reverse causation. Although the cross-sectional design is sufficient for making initial associations, it is ineligible to derive causal relationships.

Strengths and Limitations

Our study includes a large number of participants and is one of the most extensive international studies of veterinarians. The response rate of 38.4% corresponds well with the average response rate of 38.5% in other studies with veterinarians [4]. By using registration data, the sample size can be considered representative with respect to gender and age. The use of a common standardized questionnaire enables us to compare these results with other studies among veterinarians and other occupational groups. However, some limitations should be pointed out. The retrospective data collection of exposure and complaints is susceptible to recall bias, because of the potential for misreporting the number of veterinary procedures and MSD related events in the preceding 12 months. Our study, like others, was limited by

the inability to survey the non-respondents in depth due to methodological and organizational issues. We cannot rule out the possibility that veterinarians who suffered from MSD had greater motivation to participate in the study than those who were not affected, so that we were prone to overestimate the MSD burden in this occupational group. In addition, a healthy worker effect might potentially have resulted in minor underestimation of MSD, as some veterinarians might previously have left their occupation or remained on sick leave due to MSD or other diseases. The results may have been influenced by other potential work-related factors which were not considered when collecting data, in particular, insufficient recreation time, career structure, client interaction, perceived peer support, use of auxiliary devices or specific work activities (e.g. working in cold environments or working postures) [4,5]. This lack of data limits the ability to broadly explore the association between work-related factors and severe MSD in the upper extremities and the neck. A further limitation consists in the redundant predictors. As some veterinary procedures correlated highly with each other, we omitted a few explanatory variables in the multivariate models. The omission of the variables may limit the explanatory power of the model. However, we did not observe significant changes in the R-squared values of the analyzed models when we removed these factors. In general, causal relationships between variables cannot be derived in cross-sectional studies, although these allow us to quantify the magnitude of MSD prevalence and to identify initial associations. In order to establish causal explanations for MSD, a longitudinal study will be required, which has not yet been performed in this occupational group.

Conclusions

Our study contributes to the available evidence on the MSD and shows that these disorders are highly prevalent in the upper body of German veterinarians. The overall prevalence appears to be similar to that found in other international studies. From the perspective of occupational health and safety, it seems to be necessary to improve accident prevention and to optimize the ergonomics of specific tasks. In order to prevent MSD in the upper body, our data suggest the need for target group-specific (e.g. gender and practice type) preventive measures that also focus on the psychological factors at work. As a consequence of demographic changes, employees are remaining in their professions for longer. In particular, this applies to independent veterinarians in Germany, which emphasized the importance of preventive measures. Veterinary associations and organizations should provide their members with adequate training and information, so that they can work safely with animals and equipment. Preventive measures should be incorporated into the curriculum and explain to future veterinarians about the permanent and seasonal challenges in the individual veterinary practices and the related activities. Further research work must concentrate on the long-term consequences of veterinary work for the musculoskeletal system. The resulting knowledge could, for example, provide evidence-based aids for decision when determining and evaluating exposure in occupational diseases.

Acknowledgments

The authors would like to thank the German Federal Chamber of Veterinary Surgeons for their cooperation and support. We specifically acknowledge the Veterinary Medical Associations from Berlin, Brandenburg, Baden-Württemberg Lower Saxony, Bavaria, Westphalia-Lippe, and Schleswig-Holstein for the provision of addresses and/or consignment of the questionnaires. We thank all veterinarians for their substantial participation in the study.

Author Contributions

Conceived and designed the experiments: AK GS AN. Performed the experiments: AK GS CP AN. Analyzed the data: AK GS CP AN. Wrote the paper: AK GS CP AN.

References

1. Loomans JBA, Weeren-Bitterling MS, Weeren PR, Barneveld A (2008) Occupational disability and job satisfaction in the equine veterinary profession: How sustainable is this "tough job" in a changing world? Equine Vet Educ 20: 597–607.
2. Lucas M, Day L, Shirangi A, Fritschi L (2009) Significant injuries in Australian veterinarians and use of safety precautions. Occup Med Oxf Engl 59: 327–333. doi:10.1093/occmed/kqp070.
3. Berry SL, Susitaival P, Ahmadi A, Schenker MB (2012) Cumulative trauma disorders among California veterinarians. Am J Ind Med 55: 855–861. doi:10.1002/ajim.22076.
4. Scuffham AM, Legg SJ, Firth EC, Stevenson MA (2010) Prevalence and risk factors associated with musculoskeletal discomfort in New Zealand veterinarians. Appl Ergon 41: 444–453. doi:10.1016/j.apergo.2009.09.009.
5. Smith D, Leggat P, Speare R (2009) Musculoskeletal disorders and psychosocial risk factors among veterinarians in Queensland, Australia. Aust Vet J 87: 260–265. doi:10.1111/j.1751-0813.2009.00435.x.
6. Cattell MB (2000) Rectal palpation associated cumulative trauma disorders and acute traumatic injury affecting bovine practitioners. Bov Pr 34: 1–5.
7. Reijula K, Räsänen K, Hämäläinen M, Juntunen K, Lindbohm M-L, et al. (2003) Work environment and occupational health of Finnish veterinarians. Am J Ind Med 44: 46–57. doi:10.1002/ajim.10228.
8. Fritschi L, Day L, Shirangi A, Robertson I, Lucas M, et al. (2006) Injury in Australian veterinarians. Occup Med 56: 199–203. doi:10.1093/occmed/kqj037.
9. Singleton G (2005) Shoulder injuries in veterinary surgeons. Vet Rec 157: 491–492.
10. Ailsby RL (1996) Occupational arm, shoulder, and neck syndrome affecting large animal practitioners. Can Vet J 37: 411.
11. Aptel M, Aublet-Cuvelier A, Claude Cnockaert J (2002) Work-related musculoskeletal disorders of the upper limb. Joint Bone Spine 69: 546–555. doi:10.1016/S1297-319X(02)00450-5.
12. Nienhaus A, Skudlik C, Seidler A (2005) Work-related accidents and occupational diseases in veterinarians and their staff. Int Arch Occup Environ Health 78: 230–238. doi:10.1007/s00420-004-0583-5.
13. Poole AG, Shane SM, Kearney MT, McConnell DA (1999) Survey of occupational hazards in large animal practices. J Am Vet Med Assoc 215: 1433–1435.
14. Landercasper J, Cogbill TH, Strutt PJ, Landercasper BO (1988) Trauma and the veterinarian. J Trauma 28: 1255–1259.
15. Jeyaretnam J, Jones H (2000) Physical, chemical and biological hazards in veterinary practice. Aust Vet J 78: 751–758.
16. Norwood S, McAuley C, Vallina VL, Fernandez LG, McLarty JW, et al. (2000) Mechanisms and patterns of injuries related to large animals. J Trauma 48: 740–744.
17. Deutsches Tierärzteblatt (2012) Statistik 2011: Tierärzteschaft in der Bundesrepublik Deutschland. Available: http://www.freie-berufe-berlin.de/vfb.de/Verweisseiten-VFB/Tieraerzte_2011. Accessed 23 June 2013.
18. Kuorinka I, Jonsson B, Kilbom A, Vinterberg H, Biering-Sørensen F, et al. (1987) Standardised Nordic questionnaires for the analysis of musculoskeletal symptoms. Appl Ergon 18: 233–237. doi:10.1016/0003-6870(87)90010-X.
19. Kristensen TS, Hannerz H, Høgh A, Borg V (2005) The Copenhagen Psychosocial Questionnaire–a tool for the assessment and improvement of the psychosocial work environment. Scand J Work Environ Health 31: 438–449.
20. Kristensen TS, Borritz M, Villadsen E, Christensen KB (2005) The Copenhagen Burnout Inventory: A new tool for the assessment of burnout. Work Stress 19: 192–207. doi:10.1080/02678370500297720.
21. Nübling M, Stößel U, Hasselhorn H-M, Michaelis M, Hofmann F (2006) Measuring psychological stress and strain at work - Evaluation of the COPSOQ Questionnaire in Germany. GMS Psycho-Soc Med 3. Available:/pmc/articles/PMC2736502/?report = abstract. Accessed 20 May 2013.
22. Stoltzfus JC (2011) Logistic Regression: A Brief Primer. Acad Emerg Med 18: 1099–1104. doi:10.1111/j.1553-2712.2011.01185.x.
23. Meers C, Dewulf J, De Kruif A (2008) Work-related accidents and occupational diseases in veterinary practice in Flanders (Belgium). Vlaams Diergeneeskd Tijdschr 77: 40.
24. Lipscomb J, Trinkoff A, Brady B, Geiger-Brown J (2004) Health Care System Changes and Reported Musculoskeletal Disorders Among Registered Nurses. Am J Public Health 94: 1431–1435. doi:10.2105/AJPH.94.8.1431.
25. Walker-Bone K, Palmer KT (2002) Musculoskeletal disorders in farmers and farm workers. Occup Med 52: 441–450.
26. Oude Hengel KM, Visser B, Sluiter JK (2011) The prevalence and incidence of musculoskeletal symptoms among hospital physicians: a systematic review. Int Arch Occup Environ Health 84: 115–119. doi:10.1007/s00420-010-0565-8.
27. Losa Iglesias ME, Becerro De Bengoa Vallejo R, Salvadores Fuentes P (2011) Self-reported musculoskeletal disorders in podiatrists at work. Med Lav 102: 502–510.
28. Beermann B, Brenscheidt F, Siefer A (2007) Arbeitsbedingungen in Deutschland - Belastungen, Anforderungen und Gesundheit. Available: http://www.baua.de/cae/servlet/contentblob/672584/publicationFile/48431/GIZ2005-Arbeitsbedingungen.pdf. Accessed 20 May 2013.
29. Roquelaure Y, Ha C, Leclerc A, Touranchet A, Sauteron M, et al. (2006) Epidemiologic surveillance of upper-extremity musculoskeletal disorders in the working population. Arthritis Care Res 55: 765–778.
30. Gabel CL, Gerberich SG (2002) Risk factors for injury among veterinarians. Epidemiol Camb Mass 13: 80–86.
31. Wijnhoven HAH, de Vet HCW, Picavet HSJ (2006) Prevalence of musculoskeletal disorders is systematically higher in women than in men. Clin J Pain 22: 717–724. doi:10.1097/01.ajp.0000210912.95664.53.
32. De Zwart BCH, Frings-Dresen MHW, Kilbom Å (2000) Gender differences in upper extremity musculoskeletal complaints in the working population. Int Arch Occup Environ Health 74: 21–30. doi:10.1007/s004200000188.
33. Toomingas A, Németh G, Alfredsson L (1995) Self-administered examination versus conventional medical examination of the musculoskeletal system in the neck, shoulders, and upper limbs. J Clin Epidemiol 48: 1473–1483.
34. Lee CE, Simmonds MJ, Novy DM, Jones S (2001) Self-reports and clinician-measured physical function among patients with low back pain: a comparison. Arch Phys Med Rehabil 82: 227–231. doi:10.1053/apmr.2001.18214.
35. Michel A, Kohlmann T, Raspe H (1997) The association between clinical findings on physical examination and self-reported severity in back pain. Results of a population-based study. Spine 22: 296–303.
36. Langley RL, Hunter JL (2001) Occupational fatalities due to animal-related events. Wilderness Environ Med 12: 168–174.
37. Epp T, Waldner C (2012) Occupational health hazards in veterinary medicine: physical, psychological, and chemical hazards. Can Vet J Rev Vétérinaire Can 53: 151–157.
38. Randall E, Hansen C, Gilkey D, Patil A, Bachand A, et al. (2012) Evaluation of ergonomic risk factors among veterinary ultrasonographers. Vet Radiol Ultrasound 53: 459–464. doi:10.1111/j.1740-8261.2012.01942.x.
39. De Zwart BC, Frings-Dresen MH, van Dijk FJ (1995) Physical workload and the aging worker: a review of the literature. Int Arch Occup Environ Health 68: 1–12.
40. Kostelnik K, Heuwieser W (2009) Changing faces of veterinary medicine - shortage of food animal veterinarians. Dtsch Tierärztliche Wochenschr 116: 412–420.
41. Scuffham A, Firth E, Stevenson M, Legg S (2010) Tasks considered by veterinarians to cause them musculoskeletal discomfort, and suggested solutions. N Z Vet J 58: 37–44. doi:10.1080/00480169.2010.64872.
42. DeForge DH (2002) Physical ergonomics in veterinary dentistry. J Vet Dent 19: 196–200.
43. Hayes M, Cockrell D, Smith DR (2009) A systematic review of musculoskeletal disorders among dental professionals. Int J Dent Hyg 7: 159–165. doi:10.1111/j.1601-5037.2009.00395.x.
44. Bongers PM, Ijmker S, van den Heuvel S, Blatter BM (2006) Epidemiology of work related neck and upper limb problems: psychosocial and personal risk factors (part I) and effective interventions from a bio behavioural perspective (part II). J Occup Rehabil 16: 279–302. doi:10.1007/s10926-006-9044-1.
45. Kristensen TS, Bjorner JB, Christensen KB, Borg V (2004) The distinction between work pace and working hours in the measurement of quantitative demands at work. Work Stress 18: 305–322. doi:10.1080/02678370412331314005.
46. Harling M, Strehmel P, Schablon A, Nienhaus A (2009) Psychosocial stress, demoralization and the consumption of tobacco, alcohol and medical drugs by veterinarians. J Occup Med Toxicol Lond Engl 4: 4. doi:10.1186/1745-6673-4-4.

PERMISSIONS

LIST OF CONTRIBUTORS

Richard Cuthbert
Royal Society for the Protection of Birds, Sandy, United Kingdom

Rhys E. Green
Royal Society for the Protection of Birds, Sandy, United Kingdom
Conservation Science Group, Department of Zoology, University of Cambridge, Cambridge, United Kingdom

Rafael Mateo
Instituto de Investigación en Recursos Cinege´ticos, IREC (CSIC-UCLM-JCCM), Ciudad Real, Spain

Mark A. Taggart
Instituto de Investigacio´n en Recursos Cinege´ ticos, IREC (CSIC-UCLM-JCCM), Ciudad Real, Spain
Department of Plant and Soil Science, School of Biological Sciences, University of Aberdeen, Aberdeen, United Kingdom

Soumya Sunder Chakraborty, Parag Deori and Vibhu Prakash
Bombay Natural History Society, Mumbai, India

Mohini Saini, Devendra Swarup and Suchitra Upreti
Centre for Wildlife Conservation, Management and Disease Surveillance, Indian Veterinary Research Institute, Izatnagar, Uttar Pradesh, India
Conservation Science Group, Department of Zoology, University of Cambridge, Cambridge, United Kingdom

Florian Roeber, Garry A. Anderson, Robin B. Gasser and Aaron R. Jex
Faculty of Veterinary Science, The University of Melbourne, Parkville, Victoria, Australia

Angus J. D. Campbell
Faculty of Veterinary Science, The University of Melbourne, Parkville, Victoria, Australia
Mackinnon Project, The University of Melbourne, Werribee, Victoria, Australia

John W. A. Larsen and Norman Anderson
Mackinnon Project, The University of Melbourne, Werribee, Victoria, Australia

Kyung-Ha Ahn
Department of Neurology, Seoul National University, Seoul, Republic of Korea

Kyoung-Min Lee
Department of Neurology, Seoul National University, Seoul, Republic of Korea
The Smith-Kettlewell Eye Research Institute, San Francisco, California, United States of America

Edward L. Keller
The Smith-Kettlewell Eye Research Institute, San Francisco, California, United States of America

Colin Robertson
Department of Geography and Environmental Studies, Wilfrid Laurier University, Waterloo, Ontario, Canada
Spatial Pattern Analysis and Research Laboratory, Department of Geography, University of Victoria, Victoria, British Columbia, Canada

Trisalyn A. Nelson
Spatial Pattern Analysis and Research Laboratory, Department of Geography, University of Victoria, Victoria, British Columbia, Canada

Kate Sawford and Craig Stephen
Faculty of Veterinary Medicine, University of Calgary, Calgary, Alberta, Canada

Walimunige S. N. Gunawardana
Faculty of Veterinary Medicine and Animal Science, University of Peradeniya, Peradeniya, Central Province, Sri Lanka

Farouk Nathoo
Department of Mathematics and Statistics, University of Victoria, Victoria, British Columbia, Canada

Gretel Torres de la Riva, Thomas B. Farver and Lynette A. Hart
Department of Population Health and Reproduction, School of Veterinary Medicine, University of California-Davis, Davis, California, United States of America

Benjamin L. Hart
Department of Anatomy, Physiology and Cell Biology, School of Veterinary Medicine, University of California-Davis, Davis, California, United States of America

Anita M. Oberbauer
Department of Animal Science, College of Agriculture and Environmental Sciences, University of California-Davis, Davis, California, United States of America

Locksley L. McV Messam
Department of Public Health Sciences, School of Medicine, University of California-Davis, Davis, California, United States of America

Neil Willits
Statistics Laboratory, Department of Statistics, University of California-Davis, Davis, California, United States of America

Alain Lazartigues and Eric Lemonnier
CHRU de Brest, Hôpital de Bohars, Centre de Ressources Autisme, Bohars, France

Marine Grandgeorge
CHRU de Brest, Hôpital de Bohars, Centre de Ressources Autisme, Bohars, France
UMR-CNRS 6552, Laboratoire Ethologie Animale et Humaine, Rennes, France

Martine Hausberger
UMR-CNRS 6552, Laboratoire Ethologie Animale et Humaine, Rennes, France

Sylvie Tordjman
CHRU Guillaume Régnier, Rennes, France

Michel Deleau
Centre de recherches en psychologie, cognition et communication, Rennes, France

Mark C. Eisler
School of Veterinary Sciences, Faculty of Medicine and Veterinary Medicine, University of Bristol, Bristol, United Kingdom

Joseph W. Magona
Bulindi Zonal Agricultural Research and Development, Hoima, Uganda

Crawford W. Revie
Atlantic Veterinary College, University of PEI, Charlottetown, Canada

Edris Bazrafshan, Ferdos Kord Mostafapour and Kamal Aldin Ownagh
Health Promotion Research Center, Zahedan University of Medical Sciences, Zahedan, Iran,

Mehdi Farzadkia
School of Public Health, Tehran University of Medical Sciences, Tehran, Iran

Amir Hossein Mahvi
School of Public Health, Tehran University of Medical Sciences, Tehran, Iran
Center for Solid Waste Research, Institute for Environmental Research, Tehran University of Medical Sciences, Tehran, Iran
National Institute of Health Research, Tehran University of Medical Sciences, Tehran, Iran

Jonathan Massey, Simon Rothwell, William E. R. Ollier and Lorna J. Kennedy
Centre for Integrated Genomic Medical Research (CIGMR), Institute of Population Health, Faculty of Medical and Human Sciences, The University of Manchester, Manchester, United Kingdom

Robert G. Cooper
Centre for Integrated Genomic Medical Research (CIGMR), Institute of Population Health, Faculty of Medical and Human Sciences, The University of Manchester, Manchester, United Kingdom
Rheumatic Diseases Centre, Manchester Academic Health Science Centre,The 6 University of Manchester, Salford Royal NHS Foundation Trust, Salford, United Kingdom

Clare Rusbridge
Stone Lion Veterinary Hospital, London, United Kingdom

Anna Tauro
Alcombe Veterinary Surgery, London, United Kingdom

Diane Addicott
Hungarian Vizsla Breed Club, Royal Tunbridge Wells, United Kingdom

Hector Chinoy
Rheumatic Diseases Centre, Manchester Academic Health Science Centre,The 6 University of Manchester, Salford Royal NHS Foundation Trust, Salford, United Kingdom

Nicholas H. Bexfield, Penny J. Watson, Jesús Aguirre-Hernandez, David R. Sargan, Laurence Tiley and Jonathan L. Heeney
Department of Veterinary Medicine, University of Cambridge, Cambridge, United Kingdom,

Lorna J. Kennedy
Centre for Integrated Genomic Medical Research, University of Manchester, Manchester, United Kingdom

Christopher Simpson and Henk R. Braig
School of Biological Sciences, Bangor University, Bangor, Wales, United Kingdom

Peter Masan
School of Biological Sciences, Bangor University, Bangor, Wales, United Kingdom
Institute of Zoology, Slovak Academy of Sciences, Bratislava, Slovakia

M. Alejandra Perotti
School of Biological Sciences, University of Reading, Reading, United Kingdom

Mohamed M. H. Abdelbary, Christiane Cuny, Franziska Layer, Kevin Kurt, Ulrich Nübel and Wolfgang Witte
Robert Koch Institute, Wernigerode, Germany

Lothar H. Wieler, Birgit Walther and Anne Wittenberg
Institute of Microbiology and Epizootics, Free University Berlin, Berlin, Germany

Robert Skov and Jesper Larsen
Microbiology and Infection Control, Statens Serum Institut, Copenhagen, Denmark

Henrik Hasman
National Food Institute, Technical University of Denmark, Lyngby, Denmark

J. Ross Fitzgerald
The Roslin Institute, University of Edinburgh, Edinburgh, United Kingdom

Tara C. Smith
Department of Epidemiology, College of Public Health, the University of Iowa, Iowa City, Iowa, United States of America

J. A. Wagenaar
Department of Infectious Diseases and Immunology, Faculty of Veterinary Medicine, Utrecht University, Utrecht, the Netherlands

Annalisa Pantosti
Istituto Superiore di Sanitá, Rome, Italy

Marie Hallin
Centre National de Référence Staphylococcus aureus, Microbiology Department, Erasme University Hospital, Université Libre de Bruxelles, Brussels, Belgium

Marc J. Struelens
European Centre for Disease Prevention and Control, Stockholm, Sweden

Giles Edwards
Department of Microbiology, Scottish MRSA Reference Laboratory (SMRSARL), Glasgow Royal Infirmary, Glasgow, United Kingdom

R. Böse
Labor Dr. Böse GmbH, Harsum, Germany

Maarten O. Blanken, Elisabeth E. Nibbelke and Louis Bont
Department Pediatric Immunology and Infectious Diseases, University Medical Center, Utrecht, Utrecht, The Netherlands

Hendrik Koffijberg
Department Julius Center for Health Sciences and Primary Care, University Medical Center Utrecht, Utrecht, The Netherlands

Maroeska M. Rovers
Departments of Epidemiology, Biostatistics & HTA, and operating rooms, Radboud University Nijmegen Medical Center, Nijmegen, The Netherlands

Fernanda C. Dórea, J.T. McClure, Javier Sanchez and Crawford W. Revie
Department of Health Management, Atlantic Veterinary College, University of Prince Edward Island, Charlottetown, Prince Edward Island, Canada

C. Anne Muckle
Department of Pathology and Microbiology, University of Prince Edward Island, Charlottetown, Prince Edward Island, Canada

David Kelton
Department of Population Medicine, University of Guelph, Guelph, Ontario, Canada

Beverly J. McEwen
Animal Health Laboratory, University of Guelph, Guelph, Ontario, Canada

W. Bruce McNab
Animal Health and Welfare Branch, Ontario Ministry of Agriculture Food and Rural Affairs, Guelph, Ontario, Canada

Burak K. Pekin
Division of Applied Plant Ecology, Institute for Conservation Research, San Diego Zoo Global, Escondido, California, United States of America

Michael J. Wisdom, Bridgett J. Naylor and Catherine G. Parks
Pacific Northwest Research Station, USDA Forest Service, La Grande, Oregon, United States of America

Bryan A. Endress
Division of Applied Plant Ecology, Institute for Conservation Research, San Diego Zoo Global, Escondido, California, United States of America
Department of Forest Ecosystems and Society, Oregon State University, Corvallis, Oregon, United States of America

Peter Muir, Zeev Schwartz, Sarah Malek, Abigail Kreines, Jason A. Bleedorn, Susan L. Schaefer, Gerianne Holzman and Zhengling Hao
Comparative Orthopaedic Research Laboratory, and the Department of Surgical Sciences, School of Veterinary Medicine, University of Wisconsin-Madison, Madison, Wisconsin, United States of America

Sady Y. Cabrera
Department of Surgery, VCA West Los Angeles Animal Hospital, Los Angeles, California, United States of America

Nicole J. Buote
CaliforniaAnimal Hospital, Los Angeles, California, United States of America

Chang Wang, Chichao Huang, Jian Qian, Jian Xiao, Huan Li, Yongli Wen, Wei Ran,
Qirong Shen and Guanghui Yu
National Engineering Research Center for Organic-based Fertilizers, Jiangsu Collaborative Innovation Center for Solid Organic Waste Resource Utilization, Nanjing Agricultural University, Nanjing, PR China

Xinhua He
School of Plant Biology, University of Western Australia, Crawley, Australia

Amber N. Barnes
College of Public Health and Health Professions, University of Florida, Gainesville, Florida, United States of America

Ali M. Messenger and Gregory C. Gray
College of Public Health and Health Professions, University of Florida, Gainesville, Florida, United States of America
Emerging Pathogens Institute, University of Florida, Gainesville, Florida, United States of America

Dan G. O9Neill and Dave C. Brodbelt
Veterinary Epidemiology, Economics and Public Health, Royal Veterinary College, London, United Kingdom

David B. Church
Small Animal Medicine and Surgery Group, Royal Veterinary College, London, United Kingdom
Paul D. McGreevy and Peter C. Thomson
Faculty of Veterinary Science, University of Sydney, Sydney, New South Wales, Australia

Robert D. Campbell
Calgary Animal Referral and Emergency Centre, Calgary, Alberta and the Faculty of Veterinary Medicine, University of Calgary, Calgary, Alberta, Canada

Kent G. Hecker
Veterinary Clinical and Diagnostic Sciences, Faculty of Veterinary Medicine, University of Calgary, Calgary, Alberta, Canada

David J. Biau
Département de Biostatistique et Informatique Médicale, Hôpital Saint-Louis, AP-HP Paris, France

Daniel S. J. Pang
Veterinary Clinical and Diagnostic Sciences, Faculty of Veterinary Medicine, University of Calgary, Calgary, Alberta, Canada

Hotchkiss Brain Institute, University of Calgary, Calgary, Alberta, Canada

Cristina P. Araújo, Ana Luiza A. R. Osório, Kláudia S. G. Jorge and Antonio Francisco S. Filho
Programa de Pós-graduação em Ciência Animal FAMEZ, UFMS, Campo Grande, MS, Brazil

Carlos Alberto N. Ramos
Bolsista DTI, CNPq, Campo Grande, MS, Brazil

Carlos Eugênio S. Vidal
PPGMV, UFSM, Santa Maria, RS, Brazil

Eliana Roxo
Instituto Biológico de São Paulo, São Paulo, SP, Brazil

Christiane Nishibe and Nalvo F. Almeida
Faculdade de Computação, UFMS, Campo Grande, MS, Brazil

Antônio A. F. Júnior
Laboratório Nacional Agropecuário, Pedro Leopoldo, MG, Brazil

Marcio R. Silva
Embrapa Gado de Leite, Juiz de Fora, MG, Brazil

José Diomedes B. Neto and Valíria D. Cerqueira
UFPA, Castanhal, PA, Brazil

Martín J. Zumárraga
Instituto de Biotecnología, Instituto Nacional de Tecnología Agropecuaria, Buenos Aires, Argentina

Flábio R. Araújo
10 Embrapa Gado de Corte, Campo Grande, MS, Brazil

Laser Antônio Machado Oliveira
Laboratório de Pesquisas Clínicas, Ciências Farmacêuticas, Escola de Farmácia, Universidade Federal de Ouro Preto, Morro do Cruzeiro, Ouro Preto, Minas Gerais, Brazil

Henrique Gama Ker, Bruno Mendes Roatt, Rodrigo Dian Oliveira Aguiar-Soares, Gleisiane Gomes de Almeida Leal and Nádia das Dores Moreira
Laboratório de Pesquisas Clínicas, Ciências Farmacêuticas, Escola de Farmácia, Universidade Federal de Ouro Preto, Morro do Cruzeiro, Ouro Preto, Minas Gerais, Brazil

Laboratório de Imunopatologia, Núcleo de Pesquisas em Ciências Biológicas, Instituto de Ciências Exatas e Biológicas, Universidade Federal de Ouro Preto, Morro do Cruzeiro, Ouro Preto, Minas Gerais, Brazil

Evandro Marques de Menezes Machado
Laboratório de Imunopatologia, Núcleo de Pesquisas em Ciências Biológicas, Instituto de Ciências Exatas e Biológicas, Universidade Federal de Ouro Preto, Morro do Cruzeiro, Ouro Preto, Minas Gerais, Brazil

Maria Helena Franco Morais
Secretaria Municipal de Saúde, Prefeitura de Belo Horizonte, Belo Horizonte, Minas Gerais, Brazil

Alexandre Barbosa Reis
Laboratório de Pesquisas Clínicas, Ciências Farmacêuticas, Escola de Farmácia, Universidade Federal de Ouro Preto, Morro do Cruzeiro, Ouro Preto, Minas Gerais, Brazil
Laboratório de Imunopatologia, Núcleo de Pesquisas em Ciências Biológicas, Instituto de Ciências Exatas e Biológicas, Universidade Federal de Ouro Preto, Morro do Cruzeiro, Ouro Preto, Minas Gerais, Brazil
Instituto Nacional de Ciência e Tecnologia em Doenças Tropicais (INCTDT), Salvador, Bahia, Brazil

Rodrigo Corrêa-Oliveira
Laboratório de Imunologia Celular e Molecular, Centro de Pesquisas RenéRachou, Fundação Oswaldo Cruz, Belo Horizonte, Minas Gerais, Brazil
Instituto Nacional de Ciência e Tecnologia em Doenças Tropicais (INCTDT), Salvador, Bahia, Brazil

Mariângela Carneiro
Infectologia e Medicina Tropical, Faculdade de Medicina, Universidade Federal de Minas Gerais, Minas Gerais, Brazil
Laboratório de Epidemiologia de Doenças Infecciosas e Parasitárias, Departamento de Parasitologia, Instituto de Ciências Biológicas, Universidade Federal de Minas Gerais, Belo Horizonte, Minas Gerais, Brazil

Wendel Coura-Vital
Laboratório de Pesquisas Clínicas, Ciências Farmacêuticas, Escola de Farmácia, Universidade Federal de Ouro Preto, Morro do Cruzeiro, Ouro Preto, Minas Gerais, Brazil,

Infectologia e Medicina Tropical, Faculdade de Medicina, Universidade Federal de Minas Gerais, Minas Gerais, Brazil
Instituto Nacional de Ciência e Tecnologia em Doenças Tropicais (INCTDT), Salvador, Bahia, Brazil

Guy H. Loneragan
International Center for Food Industry Excellence, Department of Animal and Food Sciences, College of Agriculture and Natural Resources, Texas Tech University, Lubbock, Texas, United States of America

Daniel U. Thomson
Department of Clinical Sciences, College of Veterinary Medicine, Kansas State University, Manhattan, Kansas, United States of America

H. Morgan Scott
Department of Diagnostic Medicine/Pathobiology, College of Veterinary Medicine, Kansas State University, Manhattan, Kansas, United States of America

Agnessa Kozak and Claudia Peters
Institute for Health Services Research in Dermatology and Nursing, University Medical Center Hamburg-Eppendorf, Hamburg, Germany

Albert Nienhaus
Institute for Health Services Research in Dermatology and Nursing, University Medical Center Hamburg-Eppendorf, Hamburg, Germany
Department of Occupational Health Research, Institution for Statutory Accident Insurance and Prevention in Healthcare and Welfare, Hamburg, Germany

Grita Schedlbauer
Department of Occupational Health Research, Institution for Statutory Accident Insurance and Prevention in Healthcare and Welfare, Hamburg, Germany

Index